Praise for The Building Blocks of Health

"Finally, an up to date, science-based book about your health that is very accessible to the public. Joe Speidel, MD, MPH, is imminently qualified to inform us. He has an impeccable education in medicine and public health and a distinguished and long academic career with over 300 articles published. Equally important, he cares deeply about the public's health and his efforts are reflected in this wonderful and important book."

–John Swartzberg, MD, FACP
Clinical Professor Emeritus, School of Public Health, University of California, Berkeley–University of California, San Francisco, Joint Medical Program
Chair, Editorial Board, University of California, Berkeley, Health & Wellness Publications

"Dr. Speidel has spent his career saving lives. Now, he's empowering you to save your own. In The Building Blocks of Health, Dr. Speidel breaks down the science of disease prevention into accessible advice that will help you live a longer, healthier life."

–Neal D. Barnard, MD
President, Physicians Committee for Responsible Medicine
Adjunct Professor, George Washington University School of Medicine

"Dr. Speidel's treatment of lifestyle as medicine in The Building Blocks of Health is thoughtful, balanced, empowering and remarkably thorough. Anyone looking for reliable ways to optimize years in life, and life in years, should own this book, and refer to it routinely."

–David L. Katz, MD, MPH
Past President, American College of Lifestyle Medicine
President, True Health Initiative

"Professor Joe Speidel's new book is sensible, easy to understand, grounded in science and, most importantly, a useful guide that will help you transform your life so that you become happier and healthier — for longer!"

–Stefano M. Bertozzi, MD, PhD
Dean Emeritus and Professor of Health Policy & Management
University of California, Berkeley, School of Public Health

The Building Blocks of Health

How to Optimize Wellness with a Lifestyle Checklist

1st edition

J. Joseph Speidel, M.D., M.P.H.

The Building Blocks of Health

How to Optimize Wellness with a Lifestyle Checklist

1st edition

J. Joseph Speidel, M.D., M.P.H.

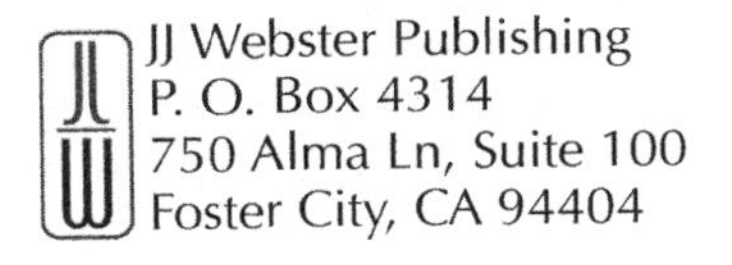

JJ Webster Publishing
P. O. Box 4314
750 Alma Ln, Suite 100
Foster City, CA 94404

This book presents the opinions and ideas of its author. It is intended to provide helpful general information on the subjects that it addresses. Neither the author nor the publisher are engaged in rendering advice or services to the individual reader. The ideas, procedures and suggestions in this book are not in any way a substitute for the advice and care of the reader's own physician or other medical professional based on the reader's own individual conditions, symptoms or concerns. If the reader needs personal medical, health, dietary, exercise or other assistance or advice the reader should consult a physician and/or other qualified health professionals. The author and publisher specifically disclaim all responsibility for any injury, damage or loss that the reader may incur as a direct or indirect consequence of following any directions or suggestions given in the book or participating in any programs described in the book.

Written by J. Joseph Speidel
The Building Blocks of Health: How to Optimize Wellness with a Lifestyle Checklist
1st Edition

Publisher's Cataloging-In-Publication Data
(Prepared by The Donohue Group, Inc.)
Names: Speidel, J. Joseph (John Joseph), 1937- author.
Title: The building blocks of health : how to optimize wellness with a lifestyle checklist / J. Joseph Speidel, M.D., M.P.H.
Description: 1st edition. | Foster City, CA : JJ Webster Publishing, 2020. | Includes index.
Identifiers: ISBN 9781952762000 (paperback) | ISBN 9781952762017 (ePub) | ISBN 9781952762024 (Kindle)
Subjects: LCSH: Self-care, Health. | Medicine, Preventive. | Nutrition. | Exercise. | Weight loss. | BISAC: HEALTH & FITNESS / Healthy Living. | MEDICAL / Preventive Medicine. | HEALTH & FITNESS / Diet & Nutrition / General.
Classification: LCC RA776.95 .S64 2020 (print) | LCC RA776.95 (ebook) | DDC 613--dc23

Paperback ISBN 978-1-952762-00-0
Ebook-EPUB ISBN 798-1-952762-01-7
EBook-Kindle ISBN 978-1-952762-02-4
Library of Congress Control Number: 2020916887

Editor: Ann S. Ferren
Cover and Interior Design: Melissa Webster Speidel

Published 2020 by JJ Webster Publishing
P. O. Box 4314
100 Alma Ln, Suite 100
Foster City, CA 94404

Dedication

To MJ my muse

CONTENTS

CHAPTERS

1
Introduction to a Healthy Lifestyle

The goal of this book is to help you take charge of your health by adopting a healthy lifestyle. Healthy behavior is essential for a long healthy life. The U.S. spends more than $200 billion a year on diabetes and heart disease.[1] Healthy behaviors could eliminate 90% of the diabetes, 80% of the coronary heart disease, and nearly half of the cancers that afflict Americans.[2] With a healthier lifestyle, many of us could live 10 to 15 years longer. The benefits of a healthy lifestyle are amazing. This book presents the science that underlies a health-restoring, health-preserving lifestyle and warns against unproven claims, like those for "superfoods" and harmful supplements that are promoted in advertising, social media or on the internet. Acting on misinformation—false, inaccurate, or incomplete health information can be harmful to your health.[3] [4]

A book can't take the place of a well-trained health care provider, but your doctor or nurse practitioner is usually just not given enough time to convey all of the advice you need to get and stay healthy. In many health care systems, the concept of a 15-minute visit has become the norm. And not everyone has easy access to health information when they need it. As a recent article in the *Journal of the American Medical Association* pointed out, "Even in countries with the best public health infrastructure (such as Switzerland), many people know only a small portion of the most essential facts about health."[5] I hope this book can provide much of the information your doctors would give you if they had enough time.

This book is organized around the multiple lifestyle factors, the Building Blocks of Health, that are essential for good health. Each chapter will help you put in place the Building Blocks of Health—the behaviors and health factors on the Lifestyle Checklist. They include good nutrition, weight control, and getting plenty of physical activity. But, you can't rely on doing just one thing, like getting a lot of exercise, to keep yourself healthy. Even marathon runners get heart attacks if their nutrition and other health behaviors are unhealthy. And you can't rely on avoiding just one risky behavior, like not smoking, to stay healthy. Multiple factors are at work to make us sick or keep us healthy—the Lifestyle Checklist in chapter 2 can help you monitor progress on the road to good health.

When several health risk or health-enhancing factors are present, their effect is usually more than additive; their effect usually changes exponentially. For example, a high cholesterol level by itself or a high blood pressure by itself might double heart disease risk. But if a person had both high cholesterol and high blood pressure, the increased risk for heart disease would likely be increased not by four times, but by six times or more. If that person also smoked, a third risk factor, the risk could increase more than 20-fold.

Optimizing your health is not just about preventing disease; lifestyle changes can also be therapeutic and reverse some disease conditions. Medicine and health are complex subjects. I hope to make them as understandable as possible by distilling a large volume of scientific information into advice that is easy to grasp and act on. This is a book about how to avoid disease and illness. It is not a medical textbook on how to diagnose and treat disease—you need a doctor or other health care professional for that.

What to expect from adopting a healthy lifestyle

Fortunately, the principles of healthy living are not complicated or difficult to learn. In fact, the main principles are so simple they can be summarized in one sentence. What you have to do is maintain a normal weight; adopt a diet low in added sugar and saturated fat, and high in natural unrefined whole plant-based foods, (fruits, vegetables, legumes, soy and whole grains); get enough sleep and physical activity; manage stress; and avoid high risk behaviors like misuse of drugs, alcohol and tobacco.

By adopting a healthy lifestyle, you can substantially increase your chances of:

- Losing weight
- Getting physically active and in shape
- Looking better
- Feeling more energetic
- Sleeping better
- Better sex life
- Avoiding major illness like heart attack, cancer, and stroke
- Avoiding physical pain and disability
- Avoiding mental disability from depression, a stroke or dementia

- Long life
- Contributing to humane farming practices and greener living

There are no guarantees, but the odds of reaching all of these desirable objectives go up when you adopt an optimal healthy lifestyle based on sound science. Getting to a healthy lifestyle depends on learning the principles of healthy living and behavioral change. Most of us will need to adopt a healthier lifestyle. This book or your doctor can't make the needed changes for you—it will be up to you.

Scientific evidence and clinical experience make the case for behavioral change

Perhaps you are already asking, would a major lifestyle change really work to improve my health? Is it worth it? I was already convinced by my medical studies, but I became even more a believer in a healthy lifestyle as the road to wellness after seeing it work for sick patients when I evaluated a healthy living program. Dr. George Melcher, the founder of the Continental Health Enhancement Center (CHEC) in Colorado, based his program on the very low-fat, whole-food, plant-based diet popularized by Nathan Pritikin. In addition to healthier food, patients were encouraged to engage in as much physical activity as they could tolerate and given stress management counseling. So, what happened? The patients' blood pressure, cholesterol, and weight all declined markedly to healthier levels, and diabetics who were on insulin needed much less.[6] But the most striking thing was what happened to patients with the debilitating cardiac symptoms of chest pain (angina) and shortness of breath. Their symptoms disappeared!

A retired dentist who could not walk across the room without severe angina told me he thought he was just waiting to die. But after ten days his angina went away and never came back! Another patient said that after two bypass operations on his coronary arteries, he was told there was nothing more that could be done for him to relieve his cardiac symptoms. He too became symptom free and able to live a normal life.

In their book, *How Not to Die*, Michael Greger and Gene Stone, describe the experience of Greger's grandmother, who at age sixty-five, was sent home with the expectation of imminent death from end-stage heart disease. Although she was confined to a wheelchair with crushing chest pain, she somehow made it to Nathan Pritikin's center. According to Greger, she was described in Pritikin's biography as one of the "death's door people:[7]

> Frances Greger, from North Miami, Florida, arrived in Santa Barbara at one of Pritikin's early sessions in a wheelchair. Mrs. Greger had heart disease, angina, and claudication; her condition was

> so bad she could no longer walk without great pain in her chest and legs. Within three weeks, though, she was not only out of her wheelchair but was walking ten miles a day.[8]

Greger went on to say, "Thanks to a healthy diet and lifestyle, she was able to enjoy another thirty-one years on this earth with her six grandchildren. The woman who was once told by doctors she only had weeks to live didn't die until she was ninety-six years old."[9]

Many studies show what I saw firsthand at CHEC, that the human body has a remarkable ability to heal when an individual stops the chronic damage caused by unhealthy nutrition, lack of exercise, and other injurious health habits. To attain optimal health, most Americans need a new healthier lifestyle.

Before you say, "I could never make all of the needed changes," keep in mind that millions of people have. Yes, behavioral change can be difficult—it takes commitment. But for many people, it does not take a lot of willpower after you get started. Starting is the hard part. You will probably have to give up some favorite dinner table and restaurant dishes and comfortable processed "junk" foods, get your body moving, and if you smoke, you will have to quit. But men and women who have successfully adopted the dietary, exercise, and other changes needed for a healthy lifestyle usually become "converts." They enjoy their new foods and are not very hungry on their new diet. And they are so pleased with their new feelings of energy and wellbeing, and their new slimmer bodies that they never want to go back to their old way of living! When you put in place the Building Blocks of Health and adhere to an optimal lifestyle, you will gain much more than you give up.

My Story

Perhaps you are wondering about me—why follow the advice in this book when there are hundreds of diet, health, and self-help books out there, some with conflicting advice, exaggerated claims and promises of quick results? I hope that my background will convince you that my advice is, as it should be, based on evaluation of scientific evidence. My undergraduate major at Harvard College was in the sciences, chemistry and physics, and my M.D. is from a top medical school—Harvard.

My medical internship year, caring for patients at St. Luke's Hospital in New York City, convinced me that it was much better to prevent rather than to treat and try to cure ill health and disease. Most of medicine is focused on trying to "put together broken pieces" by curing illness and patching up damaged bodies. Caring for men in their forties with heart attacks, and alcoholics with damaged brains and cirrhosis of the liver, made it clear to me that the most logical, efficient and and important thing that we could do for health was to focus on prevention.

After my internship year at St. Luke's Hospital, I went back to school to study public health—again at Harvard. I had excellent training in preventive medicine, especially the science of nutrition, to this day a specialty of the Harvard T. H. Chan School of Public Health, and a subject still largely absent from medical school curricula.[10] After my public health studies, I directed a multimillion-dollar reproductive health research and services program for the U.S. Agency for International Development (USAID) and served as president of Population Action International, an organization that specializes in making the scientific findings of research accessible to policymakers and the public. After Population Action International, I directed the population program at the William and Flora Hewlett Foundation, where I was responsible for making decisions about which program and research projects to fund. For 17 years, I conducted research on reproductive health as a professor at the University of California, San Francisco (UCSF) medical school, and until recently was Co-Director of the UCSF Bixby Center for Global Reproductive Health. I am now a UCSF professor emeritus.

And although my lifestyle is not perfect, thanks to a plant-based diet and statins, my total cholesterol is 124 milligrams per deciliter of blood (mg/dL), (150 mg/dL or lower is optimal) and my low density lipoprotein cholesterol (LDL Cholesterol or LDL-C) is 59 mg/dL (70 mg/dL or lower is optimal). My exercise routine is to alternate daily cycling over a 16-mile route with walking 4 miles. A test found that my estimated fitness age was 18 years younger than my chronological age. With knowledge and discipline, you can have similar results.

Prevention is neglected

Most of medicine is focused on curing, rather than preventing disease. Depending on what is included in the estimate, only from 3% to 9% of health expenditures go to prevention,[11 12] yet 75% of our health care costs are related to treating preventable conditions.[13] Even though studies confirm that health promotion and disease prevention programs are cost-effective, saving more than $3.00 for every $1.00 invested,[14] most U.S. health expenditures are directed toward curing already established disease, not to their prevention. The U.S. spends about $4 trillion a year on health with half of that spending for hospital care, physician and clinical services, and 10% for prescription drugs. About 5% of the population — those most frail or ill — account for nearly half the spending in a given year, whereas half the population has little or no health care costs, accounting for just 3% of spending.[15] We pay for care because individuals need it, and we empathize with their plight. But we fail to invest in preventive measures, for example, diabetes prevention and smoking cessation programs, in part because the people who will benefit are not yet sick, unknown, unseen, and therefore, easier to ignore.[16]

Recommendations for health should be evidence-based – understanding scientific data

As it should be, this book is based on medical science and my review of more than 2,500 scientific articles over the past four years. Readers should be wary of exaggerated claims about a new food, drug or diet and be cautious about interpreting health news stories. The news media is enamored with stories about a new therapeutic breakthrough or a new study that seems to show that everything that we thought we knew about some aspect of health is wrong. But no one study is likely to provide the last word on health. Considering the difficult challenge of keeping up with health research, reporters do a fine job. But at times, they can't put new research findings in their proper context in brief news stories.

Throughout this book, you will find presentations of the results of scientific studies. I have included the references for many of these studies, as would be found in a peer-reviewed scientific publication, but some have been omitted. For the sake of simplicity, I have usually not presented data on the statistical significance of findings (i.e., the likelihood that a result is not caused by random chance); or confidence intervals (that usually show with a 95% probability a result would be in a certain numerical range). Many studies present the percentage of an increase or decrease in an event. This is useful information but the absolute risk of a good or bad event is more valuable. It is good to keep in mind that a very large percentage change in risk of an event with a very low absolute risk, i.e., a very rare event, is not important. Doubling or tripling the risk of a rare event is still a rare event. Please consult Chapter 16, "Understanding Scientific Data," for a more detailed discussion of how to understand the scientific information presented in each of the chapters.

An important word of warning

The main purpose of this book is to help you reduce or eliminate health risks you can control. Your health care provider can and should be a partner in your quest for good health. They should be well-trained, for example, a physician, osteopath, or an advanced practice clinician (a licensed physician's assistant, licensed nurse practitioner, or licensed nurse midwife) that practice scientific, evidence-based medicine. They will provide information, diagnosis of health problems, and treatments you may need to get and stay healthy. I would not seek help from homeopaths or other poorly trained purveyors of so-called alternative medicine.

Expert health care providers are needed to conduct physical examinations, order necessary laboratory tests, and provide some of the other needed preventive measures and therapies. Some significant health-threatening conditions, for example, high blood pressure and high cholesterol, do not cause symptoms. Testing is necessary to detect them. Screening for cancer is also needed. And although conditions that lead to illness are often responsive to lifestyle modification, they may also require and benefit greatly from treatment with drugs or other forms of modern scientific medicine.

Healthy adults can usually follow this book's advice about nutrition and other lifestyle changes without difficulty. But getting the advice and approval of your physician before a lifestyle change is always a good idea. Anyone taking medication or with a health problem must obtain medical advice and supervision when changing their lifestyle. New patterns of diet and exercise may present risks for some people. A lifestyle change may decrease or even eliminate the need for medication for conditions such as high blood pressure or diabetes. Users of anti-hypertensives or insulin could experience problems unless their drug dosages are adjusted under medical supervision, and a person with heart disease may be at risk if they undertake an unsupervised exercise program.

Some of the following chapters of this book will not be highly relevant to each reader. For example, if your weight is normal, you may want to focus on chapters other than the one on obesity. With the coronavirus pandemic raging, you may want to turn to Chapter 11 on preventing infectious diseases. I do suggest, however, that everyone starts by reading Chapter 2 that provides an overview of the Building Blocks of Health and the Lifestyle Checklist before moving on in the book.

2
Lifestyle Checklist

This chapter provides an overview of the behaviors relating to health that contribute to illness and premature death and introduces the behaviors that can keep us healthy—they are the Building Blocks of Health. It describes how a Lifestyle Checklist can help you to get and stay healthy.

The causes of disease and death

Causation of important diseases, including cancer and heart disease, is not fully understood. Despite much progress, we are still working on unraveling the exact biological mechanisms of cause and the best strategies for the prevention and cure of major illnesses. Even with this limitation, we can prevent and even reverse and cure many diseases through our personal behavior—our lifestyle.

My Story

When I attended the Harvard Medical School, they told us, "half of what you learn here will turn out to be wrong. Unfortunately, we don't know which half." That jocular aphorism itself turned out to be wrong. Very little of what was taught was wrong. It was just incomplete and missing much information about the amazing complexity of the biological systems in the human body. Likely, continuing progress in the scientific understanding of disease will further elucidate rather than invalidate what we know now. The recommendations in this book are based on what we know now, but some of the advice in this book will probably turn out to be imperfect in the light of new knowledge. And some of the advice may not be entirely appropriate for everyone. It is not likely, however, that the broad thrust of the principles for enhancing health through a healthy lifestyle is in error.

So, let us now take a more detailed look at what is making us sick, what is killing us, and what we can do about it. It turns out that we in the U.S., and people in many other wealthy countries, have evolved a lifestyle that is toxic to our health. Our health habits can be likened to ingesting a slow-acting poison that over time makes us sick and kills us prematurely. Fortunately, just by adopting a better way of eating, exercising, and living, we can stop and largely reverse much of the ongoing damage to our health.

At the beginning of the 20th-century, pneumonia, tuberculosis, and diarrheal diseases were the three leading causes of death in the U.S.; heart disease was fourth on the list.[1] Over the century, the disease pattern among Americans has shifted markedly—improved sanitation, vaccination, antibiotics, and other health measures have cut infectious (communicable) disease rates, at least in most years. Communicable diseases are still important, with thousands of deaths from influenza each year, and, as of October 2020, hundreds of thousands of deaths and great uncertainty about the ultimate impact of the coronavirus (COVID-19) pandemic.

Chronic diseases, also called noncommunicable diseases (NCDs), are a leading cause of death and disability in the U.S. and an increasing burden in developing countries as they adopt our unhealthy lifestyle. In the U.S., NCDs have been causing 7 out of 10 deaths each year. Heart disease, cancer, and stroke alone have been causing more than 50% of all U.S. deaths,[2] and many NCD deaths occur prematurely—defined as before age 70.[3]

Modifiable behavioral risk factors, including misuse of tobacco and alcohol, physical inactivity, and an unhealthy diet high in sodium (salt), saturated fat, and added sugar, are important causes of NCDs. These lifestyle factors lead to unhealthy changes in the body's metabolism that increase the risk of NCDs, including the health "biomarkers," high blood pressure (hypertension), overweight and obesity, hyperglycemia (high blood sugar) and hyperlipidemia (high cholesterol and triglycerides). These changes in the body's physiology, in turn, lead to the four main types of noncommunicable diseases that account for more than 80% of NCDs worldwide: cardiovascular diseases (e.g., heart attacks and stroke), cancers, chronic respiratory diseases (e.g., chronic obstructed pulmonary disease and asthma) and diabetes.[4]

As can be seen from Table 2.1, in 2017, the leading killers in the U.S. were heart disease, cancer, respiratory diseases, accidents, and cerebrovascular diseases, including stroke, Alzheimer disease and diabetes. Our health habits influence most of these leading causes of disease; they are diseases of our way of life. As noted, the COVID-19 pandemic threatens to rapidly increase infectious disease deaths, and is already the third most frequent cause of death in 2020.

Table 2.1. 2017 U. S. Deaths and Death Rates for the 15 Leading Causes of Death[5]

	Cause of Death	Number of Deaths	Percentage of All Deaths
	All Causes	2,813,503 (100)	100.0
1	Diseases of heart	647,457	23.0
2	Malignant neoplasms (cancer)	599,108	21.3
3	Accidents (unintentional injuries)	169,936	6.0
4	Chronic lower respiratory diseases	160,201	5.7
5	Cerebrovascular diseases (stroke)	146,383	5.2
6	Alzheimer disease (dementia)	121,404	4.3
7	Diabetes mellitus	83,564	3.0
8	Influenza and pneumonia	55,672	2.0
9	Kidney diseases	50,633	1.8
10	Suicide	47,173	1.7
11	Chronic liver disease and cirrhosis	41,743	1.5
12	Septicemia (systemic infection)	40,922	1.5
13	Essential hypertension and hypertensive renal disease	35,316	1.3
14	Parkinson's disease	31,963	1.1
15	Pneumonitis due to solids and liquids	20,108	0.7
	All Other Causes	561,920	20.0

Source: National Vital Statistics Reports, Vol. 68, No. 9, June 24, 2019

Another prominent and rapidly increasing cause of death is poisoning from prescription and illicit drug overdoses, mostly from opioids. In 1990 there were fewer than 10,000 drug-related deaths. By 2015 that figure had increased to more than 52,000 and is estimated to have reached more than 70,000 and to have become one of the top ten causes of death in 2017.[6] The wider use of fentanyl, and its analogs such as carfentanil, a dangerous elephant tranquilizer 5000 times more potent than heroin, are among drivers of the epidemic of deaths.[7]

Unintentional injuries (e.g., motor vehicle crashes, poisoning, and drowning), suicide, and homicide are the three leading causes of death in teenagers and young adults 15 to 34 years old. Among this age group, unintentional deaths from poisoning, including opioid-related deaths, have surpassed deaths related to motor vehicle crashes.[8 9]

Poor health and disability

Many diseases are not ultimately fatal, but as chronic diseases, they can have a severe impact on the quality of life. Other diseases may lead to substantial periods of ill health before ultimately causing death. In 2008, 107 million Americans—almost 1 out of every 2 adults age 18 or older—had at least 1 of 6 reported chronic illnesses: cardiovascular disease (CVD), arthritis, diabetes, asthma, cancer, or chronic obstructive pulmonary disease (COPD).[10] The data in Table 2.2 shows that a higher proportion of Americans will be afflicted by many diseases than will die from them.

Table 2.2. Lifetime Occurrence and Risk of Death from Health Conditions and Injuries

Condition	LifeTime Occurrence		Lifetime Risk of Death
	Male	Female	
Cardiovascular Disease[11 12]	60%	55%	1/4 (23%)
Cancer[13]	42%	35%	1/4 (22%)
Stroke[14]	10%	16%	1/17 (5.2%)
Respiratory Disease (COPD)[15]	30%	26%	1/18 (5.6%)
Diabetes[16]	54%	54%	1/34 (2.9%)
Kidney Disease[17]	54%	54%	1/55 (1.8%)
Auto Crash[18]	18%/yr		1/66 (1.5%)
Suicide			1/61 (1.6%)

Christopher Murray and his Burden of Disease Collaborators assessed the major health problems in the U.S. in the period from 1990 to 2010.[19] The diseases and injuries with the highest number of years of life lost due to premature mortality in 2010 were ischemic heart disease, lung cancer, stroke, chronic obstructive pulmonary disease, and road injury. The study found that morbidity (illness) and chronic disability accounted for nearly half of the U.S. health burden. In 2010 Americans were living about three years longer than in 1990 but not longer without disabilities. Age-standardized years lived with disability rates increased for Alzheimer disease, drug use disorders, chronic kidney disease, kidney cancer, and falls. The study suggests that, on average, Americans will be faced with a decade of living when they are not in good health. They will suffer from conditions in decreasing order of frequency: low back pain, major depressive disorder, other musculoskeletal disorders, neck pain, anxiety disorders, chronic obstructive pulmonary disease, drug use disorders, diabetes, osteoarthritis, asthma, falls, Alzheimer disease, alcohol use disorders, and many other disease related disabilities that impair the quality of their lives.

In spite of much higher per capita spending on health, of the 34 developed countries in the Murray study, between 1990 and 2010, the U.S. lost ground in health status. The U.S. rank for the age-standardized death rate declined from 18th to 27th. For healthy life expectancy, Japan remained in 1st place, but the U.S. fell from 14th to 26th. Although there have been improvements in population health in the United States, other wealthy nations have made greater improvements.

Most people in wealthy countries have an unhealthy lifestyle–occurrence of high-risk conditions and behaviors

Studies reveal that more than 90% of adult Americans have at least some unhealthy behaviors or unhealthy conditions. The U.S. Center for Disease Control and Prevention (CDC) used data from 395,343 U.S. adult respondents to the 2013 Behavioral Risk Factor Surveillance System (BRFSS) to assess adherence to five healthy behaviors: not smoking cigarettes, meeting the aerobic physical activity recommendation (at least 150 minutes per week of moderate or, 75 minutes per week of vigorous-intensity physical activity), consuming no alcohol or only moderate amounts (up to 2 drinks per day for men, up to 1 drink per day for women), maintaining a normal body mass index (BMI 18.5 to 24.9), and sleeping at least 7 hours per 24-hour period.[20] The study found that only 6.3% of study subjects reported all five healthy behaviors; 24.3% had four; 35.4% had three; 24.3% had two; 8.4% had one, and 1.4% of respondents engaged in none of the five healthy behaviors.

Most of us could improve our health by changing how we live. So, what is wrong? We are over-stressed, under-exercised, and overfed on a red meat-based, high-saturated fat, high-sugar, high-salt, processed-food diet. Most of us are not sufficiently aware of what our fast-food burgers and fries are doing to our health. Far too many of us have a lifestyle that leads to unhealthy conditions such as high cholesterol, diabetes, high blood pressure, and obesity that make it much more likely that we will suffer major illnesses including heart disease, cancer, and stroke, face long periods of disability, and die prematurely.

So now, let us now take a look at how often some of the leading causes of illness and death are present in our lives (see Table 2.3) and what their consequences are for health. Later chapters provide more details about the causes and prevention of major illnesses and conditions.

Table 2.3. The occurrence of Common High-Risk Health Conditions and Behavior in the U. S. (BMI=body mass index)

Condition	Prevalence
Overweight or Obese (BMI over 25)[21]	72% (men), 64% (women)
Obese (BMI over 30)[22]	36.6% (men), 41% (women)
Physically Inactive[23]	45% get no health benefits 80% do not meet guidelines
Smoking (2018)[24]	15.6% (men), 12.0% (women)
Diabetes[25] (adults)	13% (men), 12% (women)

Risky behaviors and conditions related to cardiovascular disease

Heart disease and stroke are made more likely by unhealthy nutrition, smoking, high blood pressure, obesity, and sedentary physical activity habits. Only 54% of Americans with high blood pressure have it under control. Suboptimal nutrition resulting in high blood cholesterol is very common. According to the American Heart Association, more than 98 million adult Americans have a total cholesterol level of 200 mg/dL or higher. Although some physicians consider a total cholesterol level of 200. mg/dL to be "normal" and not of concern, it carries a substantial level of risk of heart disease. A cholesterol level of greater than 150 mg/dL entails some degree of risk of cardiovascular disease.

It is likely that fewer than 5% of Americans have a truly heart-healthy diet that emphasizes plant-based unprocessed foods. Only 5% of American adults consider themselves to be vegetarians, and 2% consider themselves to be "vegans." i.e., those who do not consume any animal products such as eggs and dairy products.[26] Altogether, according to one National Health and Nutrition Examination Survey (NHANES) data, 99% of Americans have at least one cardiovascular disease risk factor.[27]

Prevalence of smoking

Although smoking has declined in the U.S., in 2018, 13.7% (34.2 million) of adult Americans still smoked cigarettes.[28] Smoking is considered the cause of one out of every three cancers, 90% of lung cancer deaths in men, and 80% of those in women. Cigarette smoking is also considered to be the cause of about 90% of all deaths from chronic obstructive pulmonary disease (COPD) that includes emphysema and chronic bronchitis. In 2019, an estimated 27.5% of high school students and 10.5% of middle school students vaped, a practice that is unhealthy.[29]

Prevalence of overweight and obesity

Among those surveyed by the CDC, not even 30% of Americans manage to maintain a normal weight, and overweight and obesity are more common:[30 31]

- Percent of adults aged 20 and over with overweight: 31.8% (BMI 25.0-29.9) in 2015–2016
- Percent of adults aged 20 and over with obesity: 39.8% (BMI 30.0-99.8) in 2015–2016
- Percent of adults aged 20 and over with overweight or obesity: 71.6% in 2015–2016

Body mass index (BMI) is a measure of body fat based on height and weight that applies to adult men and women. Being overweight or obese raises the risk for heart disease, stroke, type 2 diabetes, and the risk of several cancers, including colon, breast, endometrial, and gallbladder cancers. Obesity also leads to osteoarthritis, hypertension, high cholesterol, gallstones, and sleep apnea.

Adherence to physical activity guidelines

Exercise helps control weight, reduce the risk of cardiovascular disease, diabetes, dementia, and some cancers. Among those surveyed by the CDC, inadequate physical activity was common: almost half (48%) did not participate in 150 minutes of moderate intensity or 75 minutes of vigorous intensity aerobic physical activity per week, and 79% did not participate in enough both aerobic and muscle strengthening exercises to meet guidelines. In 2014, 28% of adults (31 million persons) aged 50 and older reported no physical activity such as calisthenics or walking for exercise.[32] Not only does exercise improve physical strength, mental health, and prevent illness, it helps you look better, feel better, and have more energy. Staying physically fit increases the chances of a more vigorous and longer life.[33]

Misuse of alcohol and other substances

Among those surveyed by the CDC, misuse of alcohol was common: 18% of Americans are binge drinkers, defined as five or more drinks for men and four for women on one or more occasions in the past month; and 7% of Americans are heavy drinkers, defined as 60 or more drinks per month among men and 30 or more per month among women. Excessive use of alcohol contributes to injuries and potentially fatal alcohol poisoning. Long-term effects of excessive consumption of alcohol include increased risk of dementia, stroke, heart attack, hypertension, gastritis, pancreatitis, liver disease, and a variety of cancers. Alcoholism all too often leads to depression and other psychiatric problems, as well as unemployment and other social problems.

According to the 2018 National Survey on Drug Use and Health, 15.9% of people aged 12 or older reported that they had used marijuana in the past year. Of people aged 12 years and older, an estimated 20.3 million had a substance use disorder, including 14.8 million with an alcohol use disorder; 8.1 million with an illicit drug use disorder, most commonly involving marijuana (4.4 million); and 2 million with an opioid use disorder, mostly involving prescription pain medications.[34]

The health effects of multiple risk factors

Numerous studies have considered the implications of multiple risk factors on mortality and specific diseases and found that their impact on health is greater than just additive.

In 2010, the American Heart Association (AHA) set national goals for cardiovascular (CV) health promotion according to 7 behaviors and metrics that define CV health:[35 36]

1. Never smoked or quit more than one year ago
2. Body mass index no greater than 25 kg/m2
3. Physical activity of at least 150 minutes (moderate intensity) or 75 minutes (vigorous intensity) each week
4. Four to five key components of a healthy diet consistent with current AHA guidelines:
   - fruits and vegetables: at least 4.5 cups per day
   - fish (preferably oily): at least two 3.5-oz servings per week
   - fiber-rich whole grains (1.1 g fiber per 10 g carbohydrate): at least three 1-oz–equivalent servings per day
   - sodium: less than 1500 mg per day
   - sugar-sweetened beverages: no more than 450 kcal (36 oz.) per week
   - saturated fat: less than 7% of total energy intake
   - nuts, legumes, and seeds: at least four servings per week
   - processed meats: no more than two servings per week
5. Total cholesterol: less than 200 mg/dL
6. Blood pressure: less than 120/80 mm Hg
7. Fasting blood glucose: less than 100 mg/dL

Behavior change provides important health benefits.

Many studies show that health can improve, and mortality can fall rapidly after modification of risk factors. Studies have considered how well Americans are meeting the AHA's seven components of good cardiovascular (CV) health. One such study among adults from the 2003 to 2008 National Health and Nutrition Examination Surveys (NHANES), found that fewer than 1% of adults exhibited ideal CV health for all seven metrics.[37] Another similar study among 4754 participants in New Ulm, Minnesota, also found that only 1% of study participants met all seven metrics, whereas 7.1% met only one or none of the metrics.[38] And another study found that only 1.2% of those studied in 2005-2010 met all seven metrics.[39] In this study, among participants who met none or only one of the cardiovascular health metrics, mortality risk was 14.8 deaths per 1000 person-years from all causes—nearly three times higher than the mortality rate of 5.4 per 1000 person-years among those who met six or seven metrics.

Other studies have considered multiple lifestyle behaviors and health. A prospective study considered four health behaviors: smoking, being physically active, moderate alcohol intake, and a blood level of vitamin C that indicated fruit and vegetable intake of at least five servings a day. The all-cause mortality risk for those with four compared to zero healthy behaviors was 4-fold lower and equivalent to being 14 years younger in chronological age.[40]

A study that considered just three lifestyle behaviors related to health (not smoking, healthy diet, and adequate physical activity) also demonstrated the power of healthy habits to influence death rates. Although not many people died during the short study (an average of 5.7 years), study subjects with two out of three healthy behaviors cut their chances of dying by more than half, and those with all three healthy behaviors reduced their chances of dying during the study by 82%.[41]

A meta-analysis is a statistical process that combines data from many different individual research studies (see Chapter 16, "Understanding Scientific Data" for a discussion of the strengths and weaknesses of each type of study). A 2012 meta-analysis evaluated the findings of 15 prospective studies that had at least three of the following five lifestyle factors: obesity, alcohol consumptions, smoking, diet and physical activity. The studies had more than half a million participants from U.S., Europe, and Asia. The meta-analysis found that a combination of at least four healthy lifestyle factors was associated with a 66% reduction in all-cause mortality.[42]

A study in Germany compared participants with and without any of these four healthy lifestyle factors: never smoking, having a body mass index lower than 30, 3.5 hours per week or more of physical activity, and adhering to a healthy diet (high intake of fruits, vegetables, whole-grain bread, and low meat consumption).[43] Only 9% of participants had all four factors. Compared to participants without any healthy factors, participants with all four had a 78% lower risk of developing a chronic disease. The decreased risk for diabetes was by 93%; for heart attack (myocardial infarction) 81%; for stroke 50%; and for cancer 36%.

A Dutch study investigated the association between adherence to the Mediterranean diet and three additional healthy lifestyle factors (weight, smoking, and physical activity) and premature death. Fewer than 15% of women and 12% of men had all four healthy behaviors. When the mortality of those with the least healthy and the healthiest lifestyle scores was compared, it was found that the healthiest women lived 15.1 years longer and the healthiest men 8.4 years longer than the least healthy.[44]

A 2018 study in the journal *Circulation* that followed U.S. study subjects for more than 30 years found that adherence to five low-risk lifestyle-related factors at age 50 could prolong life expectancy. Those who never smoked, had a healthy weight, regular physical activity, a healthy diet, and only moderate alcohol consumption lived 14.0 years longer to age 93 for females and 12.2 years longer to age 87 for males than individuals who had no low-risk lifestyle factors.[45] The study found that each factor contributed to longevity, and compared with those who didn't have any of the healthy lifestyle habits, those who with all five were 74% less likely to die during the 30 years of the study.

Still, more evidence comes from a study of Seventh-Day Adventists who ate a vegetarian diet for at least half of their lives. They lived about 13 years longer than a comparison group of non-smoking Californians consuming a typical American diet.[46 47] The good news from all of these studies is that someone with a healthy lifestyle is likely to live about a decade longer and to be in better health than the average American.

The elements of a healthy lifestyle are synergistic

The studies that considered multiple lifestyle health factors linked to good health provide strong evidence that no one health-enhancing factor is decisive and that the more beneficial factors—the Building Blocks of Health—that are present in a person's life the healthier they will be. Fortunately, the elements of a healthy lifestyle are not in conflict; they are mutually reinforcing or synergistic. Healthy behavior patterns, when practiced together, have a beneficial effect that is greater than the sum of each individual effect.

No diet or lifestyle can guarantee good health, but the drawbacks and sacrifices of lifestyle modification are minimal compared to the potential benefits. Studies reveal how few of us adhere to all of the behaviors associated with longevity and health;

however, a healthy lifestyle is not an all or nothing phenomenon. Some—probably most—people will find it difficult or impossible to adopt an optimal lifestyle, at least not all of the time. Keep in mind that any progress toward an improved lifestyle will make some contribution to enhanced health and wellbeing.

It may take many years for the silent damage from high blood cholesterol or high blood pressure to result in clinical cardiovascular disease and symptoms. Fortunately, as has been noted, lifestyle changes, such as those brought about by adherence to the very low-fat, whole-food, plant-based diet Pritikin program,[48] can rapidly improve health. Restrictions on smoking have been found to affect hospital admissions for acute coronary syndromes and mortality within a few months.[49] A healthy lifestyle can quickly improve health, and it is effective at any age.

Screening for health risk and monitoring our risks

Although much of what you need to do to prevent illness is up to the lifestyle you choose, the help of a health care provider, for example, a physician or licensed nurse practitioner, is also important. A routine physical exam will include a detailed medical history, a check of your blood pressure, weight, and various laboratory tests, including a blood lipid profile. A lipid profile is recommended for adults over age 20 every five years—or more often if indicated. The profile will help you to assess the risk of cardiovascular diseases by including at least a measurement of total cholesterol, low-density lipoprotein cholesterol (LDL-C), high-density lipoprotein cholesterol (HDL-C), and triglycerides. A wide variety of other tests for cardiovascular disease and screening for cancer may be indicated. Depending on age, sex, and individual circumstances, other screening tests and preventive measures are likely to be indicated. These tests will help you use the Lifestyle Checklist to monitor risk and track improvements in your level of risk after lifestyle modification.

In addition to helping identify aspects of your present lifestyle that are harming your health, a medical evaluation may also help guide just how and how much you need to change to minimize these risks. Age and gender-specific recommendations on ways to stay healthy can be found at Healthfinder.gov.[50]

The Lifestyle Checklist

The Lifestyle Checklist includes both behaviors like healthy nutrition and factors, sometimes called biomarkers, that are indicators of good health, such as blood pressure values. For each health behavior or factor, you can keep track of compliance with a simple yes or no. And for each indicator there is a reference to the book chapter that provides the information you need to adhere to the item on the checklist. At times two measures of the same indicator of health are listed. For example, "LDL-Cholesterol is no higher than 100 mg/dL" and "LDL-Cholesterol is no higher than 70 mg/dL" to indicate both a good level of LDL-C and a more optimal level.

It is good to keep in mind that there are no numerical scores attached to the checklist, just a simple yes or no. This is because the importance to health of each factor is not the same, and there is no way to scientifically numerically rank or sum the factors. How frequently you use the checklist is up to you but, perhaps, monthly monitoring will suffice to alert you to progress and show where improvement is needed. Just keep in mind that the more "yes" answers you have, the healthier you will become and stay.

Table 2.4. The Lifestyle Checklist

Healthy Behavior or Indicator	**Yes**	**No**
I don't smoke or use tobacco (see Chapter 7, "Preventing Cancer")		
My diet is healthy (see Chapter 3, "Optimal Nutrition" and Chapter 6, "Preventing Cardiovascular Disease")		
I am not obese–BMI 30 or greater (see Chapter 4, "Weight Control")		
I am not overweight–BMI 25-29.9 or greater (see Chapter 4, "Weight Control")		
I am physically active with aerobic exercise (see Chapter 9, "Benefits of Physical Activity")		
I am physically active with resistance exercise (see Chapter 9, "Benefits of Physical Activity")		
I do not misuse alcohol or other drugs (see Chapter 7, "Preventing Cancer")		
My blood pressure is normal—120/80 or lower (see Chapter 6, "Preventing Cardiovascular Disease")		
My LDL-Cholesterol is no higher than 100 mg/dL (see Chapter 6, "Preventing Cardiovascular Disease)		
My LDL-Cholesterol is no higher than 70 mg/dL (see Chapter 6, "Preventing Cardiovascular Disease")		
My triglyceride is less than 100 mg/dL (see Chapter 6, "Preventing Cardiovascular Disease")		
I protect my brain from dementia (see Chapter 8, "Preventing Dementia")		
I manage stress (see Chapter 10, "Stress and Mental Health")		
I protect the health of my skeleton (see Chapter 12, "Preventing Osteoporosis")		
I get recommended cancer screening (see Chapter 7, "Preventing Cancer")		
I get enough sleep (see Chapter 14, "More Advice about Healthy Living")		

Healthy Behavior or Indicator	Yes	No
I safeguard my reproductive health (see Chapter 13, "Sexual and Reproductive Health")		
I avoid unneeded dietary supplements (see Chapter 5, "Vitamins and Other Supplements")		
I get vaccinated and protect against infectious diseases (see Chapter 11, "Preventing Infectious Disease")		
My fasting blood glucose is 100 mg/dL or lower (see Chapter 3, "Optimal Nutrition")		
I avoid harmful environmental exposures (see Chapter 14, "Environmental Pollutants and Toxins")		
I practice accident prevention (see Chapter 15, "More Advice about Healthy Living")		
I protect my hearing and vision, (see Chapter 15, "More Advice about Healthy Living")		
I protect my oral health (see Chapter 15, "More Advice about Healthy Living")		

Beyond prevention through behavior change

Of course, various illnesses will benefit greatly from treatment with modern scientific medicine that goes beyond lifestyle choices and their modification. Depending on your health condition, you may need the expert care of a health care provider. There are many common, and often very bothersome, health conditions that I don't address in this book because they usually are not as likely to be serious or life-threatening, not easily amenable to prevention by lifestyle modification, or are mainly addressed through the advice and care of a health care provider. They include, for example, back pain, seasonal allergies, irritable bowel syndrome, colds, arthritis, and headaches.

Premature death: the role of behavior, socioeconomic status, heredity, environment, and health care

One estimate is that almost half of lost life expectancy is attributable to behavior, but good health depends on more than just healthy lifestyle behaviors.[51] Studies show that both having a sense of purpose that goes beyond self-interest and positive social relationships are correlated with avoidance of disease and longevity.[52] Studies have attributed 40% of premature deaths—those before age 70—to behavior that you can change, 30% to heredity, 15% to social circumstance, and surprisingly just 10% to the health care we receive. Of modifiable behaviors, smoking, obesity, and physical inactivity are causing the largest number of premature deaths.[53]

Social variables, including income, education, social status, housing, occupation, and access to transportation, have an important influence on health and life expectancy.[54] Perhaps you are wondering how does your social setting make you likely to be less or more healthy—what is the biological mechanism? To some degree, poor social circumstances lead to unhealthy behaviors. In addition, the odds are higher that you will suffer from chronic stress if you are socially isolated, suffering from adverse childhood experiences, poorly educated, experiencing job insecurity, subject to racial bias, crime, and violence, or live in poor housing and "food deserts" without easy access to healthy food. The factors that contribute to the wear and tear of everyday life are called "allostatic load." High levels of stress contribute to allostatic load and increase the risk of physical and mental ill-health and death.[55]

Chronic stress leads to overeating, obesity, high blood pressure, insulin resistance, diabetes, and the chronic inflammation that is associated with cardiovascular and many other diseases. Other environmental factors related to socioeconomic status may also be important if they lead to smoking, drug misuse, undiagnosed high blood pressure, physical inactivity, and a high saturated fat, high salt, junk food diet. People with low socioeconomic status are also more likely to live in communities with environments that have polluted air and water and are exposed to toxins such as lead. They are also less likely to have the knowledge and means to stay healthy and have less access to high-quality health care.

One estimate is that the wide-ranging and unhealthy effects of stress and chronic inflammation caused by poverty and low social status contribute as much as half of the gap in health compared to those who are better off.[56] Although Americans with higher incomes are likely to live longer, the gap is much lower in some places, like New York City, and it is narrowed by healthier lifestyles, including avoiding obesity, not smoking, and getting exercise.[57] Unfortunately, this book cannot improve many of the socioeconomic variables associated with ill health. Still, it can help an individual adopt many preventive health behaviors that avoid or minimize the environmental risks of low socioeconomic status. In the ongoing debate about who should pay for health care, consider that it is estimated that only 10% to 20% of health outcomes are attributed to health care, and most disease is more closely linked to the modifiable lifestyle behaviors described in this book.[58 59]

What about heredity?

What about good or bad heredity and just plain good or bad luck? Certainly, for some people, heredity boosts the risk of several diseases, including heart disease, some forms of cancer, obesity, and Alzheimer dementia. But usually behavioral, social, and environmental factors are much more important than heredity. This effect can be seen by what happens when people move from an environment with a low risk of a disease, and they adopt the less healthy lifestyle of a new environment. Their risk of illness goes up to more closely match that of others living in the new environment. For example, one study found that the incidence of heart attack among Japanese men age 45-49 living in Hawaii was as high as for Japanese men 20 years older living in Japan. And the age-adjusted rate of heart attack for Japanese men living in California was an additional 50% higher than for those living in Hawaii.[60]

Genetics may increase the propensity to get a certain disease, but for most diseases among populations at high risk because of an unhealthy lifestyle, as much as 80% to 90% of the disease risk is from non-genetic factors. We know that a set of factors that are modifiable, including smoking, inactivity, unhealthy nutrition, high blood pressure, and overweight, account for over 70% of stroke and colon cancers, over 80% of coronary heart disease, and over 90% of adult-onset diabetes.[61] It is increasingly clear that although we cannot change our genetic makeup, changing our behaviors can change the ways that genes are expressed and counteract the hereditary propensity for a variety of diseases. Such factors such as exercise, diet, aging, obesity, and stress have epigenetic effects, that is to say, they influence which of an individual's genes may be turned on or turned off.

Can we slow down aging?

Behavior, heredity, access to quality health care, and social circumstances do not account for all health conditions. There is also a general decline in the body's overall functional capability with age. Nearly all of the diseases discussed in this book are more likely as we age. Aging weakens physical work capacity, the ability of the immune system to fight off infectious diseases, and the functional capacity of other bodily systems such as the kidneys and the respiratory system. An article in the *Journal of the American Medical Association* (*JAMA*) noted that "Chronological age is also the main risk factor for the geriatric syndromes, including frailty and immobility as well as decreased physical resilience, which is manifested by delayed or incomplete recovery from stressors, such as surgery, hip fracture, and pneumonia."[62] The article went on to point out that features of the aging process include: chronic, low-grade inflammation; various forms of cell dysfunction; reduced capacity of stem cells to repair or replace tissues; and cellular senescence. Ultimately if we don't die from an accident or disease or some other external cause, we will die from the gradual accumulation over time of unrepaired molecular and cellular damage that causes multiple body systems to fail.[63]

My colleague here at the University of California, San Francisco (UCSF), Elizabeth

Blackburn, was awarded the Nobel Prize in Medicine in 2009 for her discoveries relating to telomeres, a component of chromosomes that changes in length and gets shorter with cellular aging. Research at UCSF and elsewhere indicates that chronic stress and chronic inflammation are associated with the cellular aging that predicts early onset of cardiovascular disease, diabetes, dementia, some cancers and many other diseases associated with aging. Blackburn's work, and that of another UCSF colleague, Dean Ornish, showed that eating a whole-food, plant-based diet, increased exercise, and stress management slows telomere shortening and even reverses it.[64] Other studies also suggest that managing stress, being physically active, and eating a plant-based diet are important lifestyle behaviors that can slow cellular aging.[65]

Currently, many Americans average a decade of ill health and disabilities prior to their death, and in old age, multiple concurrent disease conditions are common. However, based on research in animals, it appears that someday it may be possible to develop new therapeutic interventions that target biological aging processes. If successful, they could prevent, or at least delay, the onset and progression of multiple chronic diseases and infirmities of old age.[66] For now, the best we can do is optimize our lifestyle by putting in place the Building Blocks of Health.

When the risk of death from one disease linked to aging decreases, the risk of death from other diseases increases. For example, finding a cure for cancer may cause an unintended increase in the prevalence of Alzheimer disease. A concept advanced by Olshansky is that because death is inevitable, the goal of public health and medicine should not be to extend the lifespan but to extend the healthspan—the number of years of healthy living.[67] He suggests that "life extension should no longer be the primary goal of medicine when applied to people older than 65 years of age. The principal outcome and most important metric of success should be the extension of healthspan."

A study that found a slowing and a plateauing of the trend toward longer human lifespans estimated that age 115 is the upper limit of longevity.[68][69] Until drugs and other therapies that slow aging are available—and perhaps even after they are—a healthy lifestyle is the best insurance against aging.[70] Your personal habits and behavior—your health lifestyle, including healthy nutrition and regular exercise, can slow, or even stop and sometimes reverse, many of the effects of aging and prevent or delay illness. Your lifestyle can help you flourish and live up to your potential for vitality, health, and long life.

Summing up

For most of us, our health habits are so far removed from what would be optimal that they can justifiably be compared to exposure to a slow-acting poison. We have a lifestyle that is making us ill and killing us prematurely. That is the bad news. The good news is that we know a lot about what to do to get healthy. We can change our health habits, our lifestyle, and quickly get much healthier and live longer. To a large extent, *prevention* of illness is up to our own efforts—we can't rely on anyone else. Although scientific understanding of the causes of many diseases remains incomplete, enough is known that we can adopt the health habits that markedly increase our chances of good health and live 10 or 15 years longer than those without healthy behaviors. A healthy lifestyle can slow or even stop and reverse many of the chronic degenerative processes that cause much sickness and death. The human body has a remarkable recuperative and repair capacity. We just need to stop the insults to our health caused by health-damaging behaviors that are prominent features of the lifestyle of Americans. This same healthy lifestyle will help you feel better, look better, and function better. It can help you attain a level of health that, according to the World Health Organization, is not merely the absence of disease, but "... a state of complete physical, mental, and social wellbeing."

In the following chapters, I will present additional data about how an unhealthy lifestyle is causing the major illnesses that plague us and describe the science behind the optimal lifestyle that makes up the Building Blocks of Health. I will explain how to achieve a healthy lifestyle by eating properly, exercising, and adopting other strategies for healthy living—the behaviors you need to say "yes" to each of the items on the Lifestyle Checklist.

3
Optimal Nutrition

Many of us search for a fountain of youth, a perfect slender figure, and good health—all based on the food we eat. Perhaps we believe philosopher Ludwig Feuerbach (1804–1872), who proclaimed "Der Mensch ist, was er isst" (Man is what he eats). Maintaining a lifetime of healthy nutrition is among the important things we can do to improve and preserve our health. In his book, *How Not to Die*, Michael Greger presents evidence that a whole-food plant-based diet will help prevent, treat, or reverse all but one of his list of the fifteen leading causes of death.[1] An optimized pattern of nutrition can help avoid cardiovascular disease (CVD), prevent obesity, diabetes, and certain cancers. Yet as we have seen from the research reports in the introductory chapters, eating a healthy diet is a health-supporting behavior that is probably the least likely among Americans, and overweight and obesity have reached epidemic proportions.

This chapter considers the drawbacks of a typical American diet; presents basic information about nutrition; explores the health implications of consuming a variety of dietary components such as fat, carbohydrates, and protein; describes the best diets and what research tells us about a variety of popular diets, and finally explore topics like organic foods and gluten-free eating. Chapter 4, considers how to avoid and reverse overweight. Chapter 5, on vitamins and other dietary supplements, presents the evidence that although they can provide benefits, supplements often cause harm.

This chapter presents information about healthy eating that may differ from your usual diet. As was pointed out in the introduction to this book, Anyone taking medication or with a health problem must obtain medical advice and supervision when changing their lifestyle.

The typical American diet

The typical American diet, the TAD, is not healthy. It contains too much saturated fat, red meat, refined grains, sodium (salt), added sugars, processed food, and too many calories. Americans don't eat enough fruit, vegetables, and whole unprocessed or minimally processed plant-based foods. Our unhealthy diet is an important reason that high blood cholesterol, elevated blood pressure, and obesity are common among people in the U.S. These are the unhealthy conditions that contribute to the noncommunicable diseases that are the leading causes of disability and death in the U.S.: heart disease, cancer, stroke and diabetes.[2 3 4]

One widely publicized source of nutritional guidance is found in the U.S. government's *2015-2020 Dietary Guidelines for Americans*. Although the *Guidelines have much useful information and sound advice, the recommendations of the Dietary Guidelines* at times deviate from the best nutritional science. This deviation may reflect scientific controversies, but the recommendations are also subject to the political influence of the food industry and meat and dairy interests.

The *2015-2020 Dietary Guidelines for Americans* is based on the *Scientific Report of the 2015 Dietary Guidelines Advisory Committee*. This latter report is a more objective source of reliable information on nutrition and diets than the *Dietary Guidelines*.[5] David Katz, founding director of Yale University's Prevention Research Center and founder of the True Health Initiative made the following comment about the *Guidelines*: "I want to start out by saying what a fan I am of the 2015 DGAC report...I invite every citizen who wants to eat in accord with expert guidance to refer to the DGAC report, and ignore the Dietary Guidelines!"[6]

In 2015, the Dietary Guidelines Advisory Committee (DGAC) came to conclusions that are consistent with those of most nutrition experts, "On average, current dietary patterns are too low in vegetables, fruit, whole grains, and low-fat dairy, and too high in refined grains, saturated fat, added sugars, and sodium." The 2015 DGAC found that overconsumption by the U.S. population of two nutrients—sodium and saturated fat—poses health risks. High consumption of sugar-sweetened foods and beverages, and refined grains, was also identified by the 2015 DGAC as detrimental to health and concluded that there was moderate to strong evidence that higher intake of red and processed meat was detrimental to health compared to lower intake.[7]

In 2020, the Dietary Guidelines Advisory Committee (2020 DGAC) released an updated report8 to provide the basis for the 2020-2025 Dietary Guidelines for Americans that is scheduled to be released late in 2020. The 2020 committee report confirmed the conclusions of the 2015 report, noting that Americans overconsume calories, saturated fats, sodium, added sugars, and some Americans overconsume alcohol. The 2020 DGAC confirmed that "Common characteristics of dietary patterns associated with positive health outcomes include higher intake of vegetables, fruits, legumes, whole grains, low- or non-fat dairy, lean meat and poultry, seafood, nuts, and unsaturated vegetable oils and low consumption of red and processed meats, sugar-sweetened foods and drinks, and refined grains." The Committee also found that higher intake of red and processed meats, sugar-sweetened foods and beverages, and refined grains had negative consequences for health.

The Committee recommended a shift from saturated to unsaturated fats within the context of a healthy dietary pattern consisting of higher intakes of vegetables, fruits, legumes, whole grains, nuts and seeds, with some vegetable oils, low-fat dairy, lean meat and poultry, and fatty fish and lower intakes of red and processed meats, sugar-sweetened foods and drinks, and refined grains.

The Committee cited increased evidence that among those who drink, consuming higher average amounts of alcohol is associated with increased mortality risk compared to drinking lower average amounts. Accordingly, the Committee tightened the previous recommendation that women should limit alcoholic drinks to one per day and men to two per day by recommending that both men and women who drink alcohol should limit it to one drink a day on days when alcohol is consumed. The Committee concurred with the recommendation of the 2015-2020 Dietary Guidelines for Americans that those who do not drink should not begin to drink because they believe alcohol would make them healthier.

In another change, the Committee suggests that no more than 6% of energy should come from added sugars rather than the previous advice to avoid more than 10% energy from added sugars.

Unhealthy processed foods make up a large proportion of the American diet. In his entertaining book, *Salt, Sugar, Fat—How the Food Giants Hooked Us*, Pulitzer Prize-winning author Michael Moss convincingly documents that manufacturers of processed foods are more concerned with maintaining and growing their $1 trillion in annual sales and substantial profits than they are with optimizing the health of Americans.[9] Extensively advertised processed foods from corporations stock the shelves of grocery stores and convenience outlets. Processed foods are "engineered" to be tasty, convenient, low cost, and have long shelf lives. But these desirable traits come with a cost to health. Typically, processed foods are packed with large amounts of added salt, sugar, and fat, ingredients that make foods less healthy but highly palatable, and some would even say addictive. How many of us can stop after eating just a few crunchy salt and fat-laden potato chips?

Moss explains that food scientists have discovered that the "mouth feel" of a crunchy food, like potato chips, is something we enjoy. Adding salt, sugar, and fat to foods is even more important to enhancing their desirability and enjoyment. Research has shown that there is a "bliss point" for certain optimal levels of added sugar and salt. These are the levels that make food the most pleasurable. For fat, there does not seem to be a bliss point—food preference research suggests that the more fat in or added to a food, the greater our gustatory pleasure.[10]

A French study looking specifically at the health effects of eating processed food found that a 10% increase in the proportion of "ultraprocessed" food consumption was associated with a 14% higher risk of all-cause mortality over the 10-year duration of the study.[11]

An additional problem is that when we eat out at restaurants or buy "fast food," we don't have many healthy options. We usually end up with extra-large portions of unhealthy food.[12] Over the past 30 years, portion sizes and calorie count averages of fast food offerings have increased substantially.[13] Most of our home cooking is guided by cookbooks and cooking shows that present recipes that are optimized for variety, taste, and enjoyment, but not for health.

Surveys over the period 2009-2012 showed that where, on average, Americans are getting their calories is far from ideal.[14] Almost half of total energy calories came from these seven categories of food: burgers and sandwiches (13.8%); desserts and sweet snacks (8.5%); sugar-sweetened beverages (6.5%); rice, pasta, and grain-based mixed dishes (5.5%); chips, crackers, and savory snacks (4.6%); pizza (4.3%); and meat, poultry, and seafood mixed dishes (3.9%).[15]

The average American gets about a third of total daily calories by consumption of fat. Some experts recommend that for optimal nutrition, the total amount of fat consumed should be limited to 10% to 15% of total daily calories.[16] [17] [18] Other experts call for substituting unsaturated fats rather than limiting the amount. There is, however, general agreement on the benefits of limiting trans and saturated fat. Yet a high proportion (71%) of the American population consumes more than the 2015 DGAC recommended maximum of 10% of daily calories from saturated fat. The American Heart Association recommendation is even lower, only 5% to 6% of daily calories should be supplied by saturated fat.

U.S. sugar consumption averages about 66 pounds a year per person or 19.5 teaspoons (32 grams), supplying 328 calories a day.[19] [20] This greatly exceeds the recommended 100 calories per day for women and 150 calories per day for men and the recommendation that, ideally, only 5% of daily calories should come from added sugars.

The typical American's diet far exceeds recommended levels of salt.[21] Americans consume an average of 8,500 milligrams (8.5 gm) of salt (sodium chloride) a day. The American Heart Association recommends 2,400, or even better, a 1,500 mg of sodium per day limit for everyone, including children.[22]

The Centers for Disease Control and Prevention found that most adults in the U.S. consume fewer than the recommended number of servings of fruits (2 cups/day for a 2400 calorie diet) and vegetables (3 cups/day for a 2400 calorie diet). A 2013 survey found that fewer than 15% of U.S. citizens had the recommended fruit intake, and only 8.9% met the recommendations for vegetables.[23 24] Only in a few age ranges do as many as 20% of older Americans meet the recommended goals for either fruit or vegetables.

Good nutrition supports health

Scientists studying the link between nutrition and health agree on many aspects of what comprises healthful nutrition. But diets vary so much over a lifetime that dietary studies are difficult, and areas of uncertainty and disagreement remain. When addressing some topics, rather than providing definitive guidance, this book will describe the data that underlies differences in research findings and recommendations.

Most nutrition experts agree that a healthy diet eliminates all trans-fats, minimizes red meat and saturated fats, is low in sodium, added sugars and products made from refined grains, and avoids excess calories. There is also a consensus that a healthy pattern of nutrition includes high levels of consumption of whole unprocessed or minimally processed plant-based foods: legumes (legumes are beans, peas, lentils and more than 100 other edible plant foods), whole grains, fruits, and vegetables. These whole, mainly plant foods, provide high-quality carbohydrates and fiber.

Many nutrition experts consider that consumption of non-fat dairy, seafood, nuts, healthful oils (monounsaturated and polyunsaturated fats) and limited amounts of unprocessed meat can also be considered to be components of healthy nutrition. Others make the case that an optimal diet is entirely whole-food plant-based and eliminates trans-fats, saturated fats, meat, seafood, most dairy, and added sugars. Other experts advocate a diet that is extremely low in oils and fats with no more than 15% or better yet 10% of total calories coming from fat—a diet shown to reverse the atherosclerosis that leads to, angina, heart attack, stroke and other forms of cardiovascular disease.

Although Americans are exposed to an unhealthy food environment with too much low-cost hyper-palatable food, we can attain good nutrition by making wise and healthy decisions about what to eat. We don't eat individual nutrients, we eat food, so our focus should be on selection and consumption of healthy foods that are plant-based, high in dietary fiber, healthy fatty acids, vitamins, and low in refined carbohydrates, added sugars, salt, saturated fatty acids (SFAs), dietary cholesterol, and trans-fat.[25]

Dariush Mozaffarian, a leading nutritional scientist, has offered the following summary statement about healthful nutrition: "The focus of modern dietary recommendations to prevent chronic diseases should be on healthful foods and dietary patterns, including greater consumption of fruits, vegetables, nuts, fish, moderate dairy, and vegetable oils; consumption of whole-grain foods in place of refined starches and sugars; and avoidance of sugar-sweetened beverages, processed meats, and foods that contain partially hydrogenated vegetable oils. Such diets are naturally higher in beneficial fatty acids, minerals, vitamins and antioxidants, phytochemicals, and dietary fiber, and lower in salt, saturated fat, and trans-fat."[26]

Basic facts about food and nutrition

The two general categories of food are macronutrients and micronutrients. Calories are the usual way that the energy content of a food is measured. Micronutrients are not a source of energy, so while they are essential to health, they do not have a calorie content number. Some other important components of food, such as water and fiber, do not supply energy, so they do not have a calorie content, but they too are essential to or contribute to good health.

Micronutrients: vitamins and minerals

Vitamins are micronutrients that are essential for the proper function of the body's metabolism. Only small amounts are needed to maintain health. Most Americans do not suffer from vitamin deficiencies, and high doses of vitamins may cause harm rather than improve health; see Chapter 5, "Vitamins and Other Supplements," for the details.

Minerals, such as calcium, iodine, sodium, and iron are essential to the structure and proper functioning of the body. For example, iron is an essential component of the hemoglobin that carries oxygen in red blood cells. Calcium is a major component of bones and teeth, and it also has a wide variety of other functions relating to blood clotting, nerve conduction, and muscle contraction. Sodium is essential to metabolism, but as described in Chapter 6, "Preventing Cardiovascular Disease," high amounts of sodium in the diet increase the risk of high blood pressure, and CVDs.

Macronutrients

There are three main types of macronutrients: carbohydrates, proteins, and fats. Some nutrition experts also include alcohol, water, and fiber in the category of macronutrients. Relatively large amounts of macronutrients are needed in the diet to provide the energy necessary for physical activity, to support the body's metabolism, and to build and maintain the structure of the body. As is shown in Table 1, below, carbohydrates and proteins contain about four calories per gram of weight. Fats are calorie-dense, they contain nine calories per gram. Alcohol is also calorie-dense, it contains seven calories per gram.

Table 1. Energy content of macronutrients

Macronutrient	Calories per Gram	Calories per Ounce
Carbohydrate	4	113
Protein	4	113
Fat	9	255
Alcohol	7	198

Carbohydrates

Carbohydrates are starches (complex carbohydrates), sugars (simple carbohydrates), and fibers obtained from plants. Other than fiber, carbohydrates are broken down in the intestine and converted by the liver to glucose, the form of sugar used by the body's cells for energy or other metabolic processes, or converted into glycogen or fat, forms that are stored in the body and serve as reserve sources of energy. Starches are composed of many glucose units linked together and are often metabolized more slowly than simple sugars, but not when they are highly refined. Complex carbohydrates are less apt to over-stimulate a strong insulin response, and so are less likely to lead to obesity and diabetes. Carbohydrates are healthiest when consumed in whole, unprocessed forms, such as those in vegetables, beans, peas, and grains, such as brown rice, oats, wheat, and barley. Less healthy sources are found in processed foods, such as white bread, most pastas, white potatoes, and white rice.

Sugar

Sugars come in many forms. The ingredients listed on food-product labels that end in "-ose," such as glucose, sucrose, galactose, dextrose, lactose, fructose or maltose, are sugars. Sugars are healthful components of food when found naturally in milk, fruit, and vegetables. But sugar becomes unhealthy when added in large amounts to foods, most often in the form of sucrose or high-fructose corn syrup. Common table sugar, or sucrose, is a disaccharide molecule—a combination of the monosaccharides glucose and fructose linked together. High fructose corn syrup has a similar composition to sucrose except that the ratio of fructose to glucose is increased with 55% to 65% fructose. As with other sugars, sucrose is digested into its two components. The next section of this chapter will explain the negative effects of added sugar and why we don't need it in our diets.

Fiber

Fiber is not digestible by humans, and in general, it does not provide nutrients or calories except when it is broken down to some extent by intestinal bacteria. There are two types of fiber: insoluble fiber and, the more beneficial form, water-soluble fiber that absorbs large amounts of water. Both types of fiber provide bulk and other benefits that aid digestive tract function and health. Most plants contain some of each type of fiber. Fiber is present in fruits, vegetables, grains, and legumes, but not in meats. Soluble fiber is the predominant form found in legumes, barley, oats, and fruits. Insoluble fiber (cellulose, hemicellulose, lignin) is the predominant form found in wheat, other whole grains, and some vegetables. The Institute of Medicine recommends an intake of 30-38 grams of fiber per day for men and 21-25 grams per day for women, but the average American consumes about 15 grams of fiber a day.

High fiber consumption is associated with a lower risk of cardiovascular disease. A study of people over age 65 found that the fifth of the study participants with the highest intake of fiber was at a 21% lower risk of a CVD event than the lowest fifth.[27] A meta-analysis of 193 studies involving 135 million person-years of observation published in 2019 in *Lancet* found that a high intake of dietary fiber from whole grains and other sources is associated with a wide array of health benefits. People who consumed the most fiber (25 to 30 grams a day or more) had a 15% to 30% lower death rate, and a lower incidence of heart disease, stroke, diabetes, colorectal and breast cancer than people who ate the least fiber (less than about 15 grams a day). High fiber intake was also linked to healthy biomarkers, including lower blood cholesterol, blood pressure, and body weight. In absolute terms, this translated to about 13 fewer death per 1000 participants over the duration of the studies.[28] There is little doubt that fiber is good for health.

Protein

Proteins are the body's building materials. Skin, muscle, and bones are made of protein in various forms. When food is digested, the proteins in food are broken down into smaller units called amino acids. Amino acids are either derived from food or are synthesized by the body and reassembled into the body's proteins. There are 22 different amino acids. Thirteen of these can be synthesized, but the other nine, called essential amino acids, must come from food.

Because proteins form the body's muscles and other structures, food advertisers often tout their products as being better for health because they are "high protein." The U.S. sales of sports nutrition high protein powders and other products is estimated at $6.6 billion a year. However, very few Americans fail to get enough protein, and some of us may get too much. There is scant evidence that protein bars or powders that provide more than the recommended minimum of about 10% to 15% of total calories are beneficial. This is the equivalent of about 46 grams per day for women and 56 grams for men. The Recommended Dietary Allowance (RDA) for protein is a modest 0.8 grams of protein per kilogram of body weight. The RDA is the amount of a nutrient you need to meet your basic nutritional requirements and stay healthy— not the specific amount you are supposed to eat every day. To determine your RDA for protein, you can multiply your weight in pounds by 0.36.

To avoid loss of muscle, if you are elderly or losing weight by restricting calories, or when weight training to build muscle, it may be advisable to consume about twice the recommended level. But consuming 300 grams a day of protein will not help build muscle faster than 100 grams a day. Although the long-term effects of protein excess are unknown, there is concern that it will increase the risk of kidney disease and cancer.[29] Most Americans consume enough protein for good health. We don't need meat or dairy foods for protein; plant foods are a perfectly good source.

Fats, oils, and cholesterol

Fats and oils are lipids. Their essential role includes being a source of stored energy, a component of cell membranes, serving as the building blocks for hormones, and facilitating the absorption of the fat-soluble vitamins A, D, E, and K. If food calories beyond those needed for energy are consumed most of the extra calories are stored in the liver and muscles as glycogen, a ready energy source, or as fat—the major storehouse of energy. Some fat, and some essential types of fat that the body cannot synthesize, is required for good health, but fat need not make up more than 5% of total calories.[30]

Cholesterol is a fatty substance synthesized in the liver and carried throughout the body in the blood bound to proteins called lipoproteins. Cholesterol is a necessary building block for the production of hormones, cell membranes, and some parts of the body, such as the brain. Cholesterol is also a component of the bile acids that help the body absorb fats from the intestines. Cholesterol is not found in plant foods, only in animal foods, sources that are usually also high in saturated fats, such as meat, poultry, shellfish, egg yolks, butter, cheese, and milk. There is no need to obtain cholesterol through food. The human body can synthesize enough cholesterol for good health. Large amounts of dietary cholesterol, but not usually consumed amounts of cholesterol, raise blood cholesterol levels.[31]

The metabolic processes that involve fat and cholesterol are complicated, but the basic physiology is that lipids are transported in the bloodstream by a type of protein called lipoproteins. Dietary fat is broken down into triglycerides and carried by very-low-density lipoproteins (VLDL) throughout the body where some are converted to cholesterol-laden particles of low-density lipoprotein cholesterol (called LDL-Cholesterol or LDL-C or LDL). The higher the level of LDL-C, the more likely the formation of the cholesterol-laden blood vessel plaques that cause narrowing of coronary and other arteries and make a heart attack or stroke more likely. High intake of saturated fat increases unhealthy LDL-C.

Cholesterol is also transported linked to high-density lipoproteins (called HDL-Cholesterol or HDL-C or HDL). HDL-C is sometimes called "good" cholesterol because a high HDL-C helps prevent the formation of plaques and removes cholesterol from blood vessel plaques. HDL-C seems to work to limit the damage caused by high LDL-C, but if LDL-C is low, a low level of HDL-C does not seem to increase the risk of arterial damage or a heart attack. Clinical trials of drugs that increased HDL-C have not shown benefit, nor do individuals genetically predisposed to produce high levels of HDL-C have a lower risk of heart attacks. However, actions that increase HDL-C naturally, through exercise, weight loss, moderate or no alcohol and, avoidance of trans-fats, refined carbohydrates, and smoking, are associated with heart health.

In summary, high levels of triglycerides and LDL-C and low levels of HDL-C are associated with an increased risk of atherosclerosis and cardiovascular disease. The main concern for cardiovascular health is avoiding high LDL-C and high triglycerides. Attaining a high HDL-C is beneficial but of lesser importance to health and probably of little or no importance when LDL-C is in a healthy low range.

There are different types of dietary fat with differing implications for health based on their varying impact on blood levels of triglycerides, LDL-C, and HDL-C. Fats are classified as saturated or unsaturated. Although in a particular food one form of fat may predominate, foods contain a mixture of the various types of fat.

Saturated fat is sometimes called "bad fat" based on its health effects. Saturated fat molecules have no chemical double bonds between carbon atoms because they are filled or "saturated" with hydrogen. Saturated fats are usually solid at room temperature and tend to raise LDL-C, the unhealthy form of cholesterol in the bloodstream. Saturated fats come mainly from animal sources, including meat (beef, lamb, pork, lard, poultry) and dairy products (butter, cream, cheese, whole and reduced-fat milk). Meats that are highest in fat content include ground beef, bacon, liver, and other organ meats. Tropical oils such as coconut, palm kernel, and palm oil may come from plants, but they have a high content of saturated fatty acids and are solid or semi-solid at room temperature. Saturated fatty acids are also found in some other plants, such as nuts.

Unsaturated fats are sometimes called "good fats" based on their relatively benign health effects. Unsaturated fats are classified as monounsaturated or polyunsaturated depending on if they have a single or multiple unsaturated chemical bonds. Unsaturated fats are usually the predominant form of fat found in vegetable oils that are liquid at room temperature.

Trans-fats, also called partially-hydrogenated oils, are a harmful form of unsaturated fat that is synthesized in a chemical process that adds hydrogen to liquid vegetable oils to make them more solid. Since 1911, when Crisco was introduced by Procter and Gamble, trans-fats have been a prominent feature of the American food supply. Like saturated fats, trans-fats raise markers of inflammation (interleukin-6 and C-reactive protein), increase unhealthy LDL-C levels, and lower healthy HDL-C levels. Studies suggest that a 2% increase in energy intake from trans-fatty acids was associated with a 23% increase in the incidence of coronary heart disease (CHD).[32] Because they improve taste and shelf life, trans-fats have been used to make shortening and many commercially prepared baked goods such as pastries, pizza dough, pie crust, cookies, crackers, snack foods, fried foods, and margarine.

Because they harm health, in 2015, the U.S. Food and Drug Administration (FDA) ruled that partially-hydrogenated oil is no longer "generally recognized as safe" (GRAS) and must be phased out of food by 2018 unless approved as food additives on a case-by-case basis.[33 34 35 36] The FDA labeling rules allow foods that have up to 0.49 grams of trans-fats to list their trans-fat content as zero. As little as 0.5% of the total energy intake 10 calories (1 gram) of trans-fat may incur adverse health effects.[37] The best advice is to completely avoid any food containing trans-fats.

Monounsaturated fatty acids (MUFAs) and polyunsaturated fatty acids (PUFAs) are usually liquid at room temperature. They have more favorable blood lipid and health effects than saturated fats. Plant sources rich in MUFAs include vegetable oils (e.g., canola, peanut, olive, high oleic safflower, and sunflower), avocados, peanut butter, and most nuts. Primary sources of PUFAs are vegetable oils (corn, soybean, cottonseed); some nuts (walnuts, pine nuts); and some seeds (sesame, pumpkin, flax). When substituted for trans and saturated fats, monounsaturated or polyunsaturated fats bring about a reduction in LDL-C. They are sometimes called "good" fats or "healthy" fats.

There are three types of n-3 PUFAs, also called omega-3 fatty acids: alpha-linolenic acid (ALA) is an n-3 fatty acid that the body converts into the other two types, Eicosapentaenoic acid (EPA) and docosahexaenoic acid (DHA). EPA and DHA are found in fish and shellfish. ALA sources include some green vegetables (Brussels sprouts, kale, spinach) soybean oil, canola oil, walnuts, and flaxseed. ALA cannot be synthesized by humans and, therefore, is considered essential in the diet.

Figure 3.1. Fatty Acid Profiles of Common Fats and Oils[38]

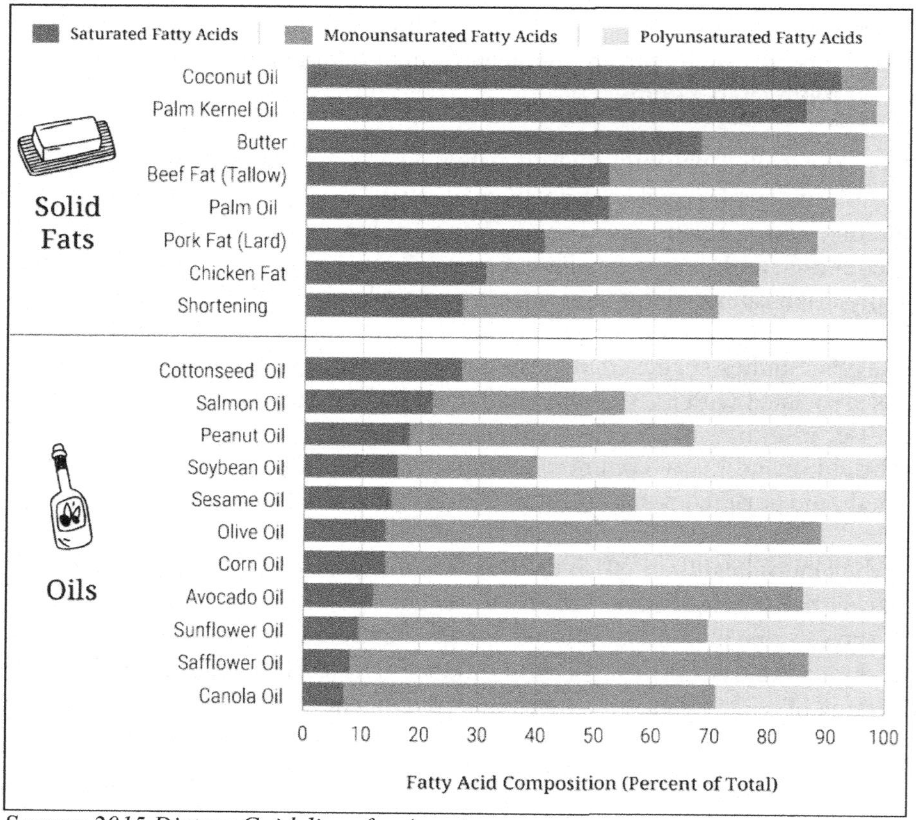

Source: 2015 Dietary Guidelines for Americans

Figure 3.1, from the *2015-2020 Dietary Guidelines for Americans*, shows that foods and oils contain a mixture of the various types of fatty acids.[39] Ingestion of any of the oils listed in the figure above will result in some intake of saturated fatty acids.

Note that the tropical oils, coconut, palm kernel, and palm, are called oils because they come from plants. However, they are solid or semi-solid at room temperature due to their high content of short-chain saturated fatty acids. They are considered solid fats for nutritional purposes. Also, shortening may be made from partially hydrogenated vegetable oil, which contains trans-fatty acids.

Water

Water is essential for life and the stability of the body's physiology. Water is needed to maintain circulation and the functioning of the kidneys and liver, and to remove wastes. Abundant intake of water protects against kidney stones and decreases the risk of bladder cancer. Dehydration can adversely affect mentation, including concentration, reaction time, learning, memory, mood, and reasoning, and can also cause disorientation, headaches, fatigue, and anxiety.[40 41] Adequate hydration is needed during physical exercise, and when exposed to temperature stress.

Water needs vary greatly depending on environmental conditions and physical activity, so there is not a fixed recommended level of healthy intake of water. The Institute of Medicine (IOM) has suggested that an adequate daily intake for total water, including water in food, is about four quarts for men and about three quarts for women. Although thirst is a good guide to water needs, and most people can meet their water needs by drinking at meals, and when they get thirsty, substantially more fluid may be needed in hot environments because body water deficits and dangerous heatstroke can occur rapidly.

It is also possible to consume too much fluid and cause water toxicity by exceeding the kidney's maximal excretion rate of approximately 0.7 to 1.0 quart per hour. Water toxicity is a dangerous condition characterized by low blood sodium resulting in a transfer of water to the body's cells by osmosis. This causes the cells to swell and can cause seizures, brain damage, coma, and even death.[42 43] Some athletes who overheat or develop muscle cramps drink too much and end up overhydrated and ill with water intoxication, and some have died. Dehydration in sports is not a cause of muscle cramps. Overheated athletes need to cool off resting in the shade or, if necessary, submerged in cool water.[44]

The role of nutrients in health

To help us understand the complex links between nutrition and health, this chapter section will consider additional evidence about the health effects of the nutrients sugar, other carbohydrates, proteins and fats. Later in the chapter, the pros and cons of various diets will be presented.

Added sugar harms health

The naturally occurring sugars found in fruits, vegetables, and milk are not added sugars, and there is general agreement that they are beneficial components of a healthy diet. They come with "their own antidote," fiber, that slows absorption and helps avoid a spike of insulin release.[45 46] Large amounts of added sugars, have harmful consequences: increased risk of cardiovascular diseases, obesity, diabetes, some types of cancer, high blood pressure, gout, Alzheimer disease and liver damage.[47 48]

Humans did not evolve with a metabolism suited to eating large amounts of added sugars. It was not until the 19th century that sugar became widely available at low cost and consumed in large amounts throughout the world. Sugar "toxicity" is highly dose-related. When ordinary white sugar (sucrose) is metabolized in the body, it is broken into its two components, glucose and fructose. Glucose is the essential energy source metabolized by every cell in the body. Glucose elicits the secretion of insulin, a hormone that promotes the uptake of sugar by the cells of the body. Fructose, which tastes twice as sweet as glucose, does not directly cause the release of insulin. It must undergo other chemical changes in the liver before it can be used for energy or other metabolic purposes. When too much fructose hits the liver, for example after consumption of a "big gulp" supersized sugar-sweetened soft drink, the harmful consequences can include increased serum triglycerides, liver cell damage, accumulation of fat in the liver, abdomen, muscles and elsewhere in the body, and an addictive-like stimulation of food intake beyond energy needs.

Chronic overeating of added sugars increases the risk of obesity, insulin resistance that leads to type 2 (adult-onset) diabetes, and the metabolic syndrome.[49 50] The metabolic syndrome is characterized by the presence of three or more of the following five health risk factors: a large waist circumference (abdominal obesity), high blood glucose, high triglyceride levels, low HDL-C and high blood pressure. The metabolic syndrome is an unhealthy condition that has been linked to the development of type 2 diabetes and heart disease. It is alarming that more than 40% of Americans over age 40 have the metabolic syndrome.[51]

Sugar-sweetened beverages present a unique risk

Sugar-sweetened beverages (SSBs) provide only "empty" calories without healthful nutrients, and sugar in liquid form is likely to be less satiating. This leads to the consumption of excess calories and obesity. Since 1950 consumption of SSBs has increased by a factor of five and now contributes nearly 50% of added sugars in the American diet. Between 1965 and 2002, the proportion of total dietary calories provided by beverages increased from 11.8% to 21.0%,[52] and the epidemic of overweight and obesity in America became much worse. Studies, including meta-analysis, have concluded that consumption of sugar-sweetened beverages is associated with an increased risk of obesity, diabetes, cardiovascular disease, metabolic syndrome, and nonalcoholic and fatty liver disease.[53 54 55] Men also have an increased risk of gout.[56] According to one estimate, in 2010, sugar-sweetened beverages caused 25,000 excess deaths in the U.S.[57]

Sugar, obesity and diabetes

Globally, the prevalence of diabetes has nearly doubled from 108 million adults in 1980 to 422 million in 2014.[58 59] According to the American Diabetes Association, 1.7 million U.S. adults and more than 5,000 children are newly diagnosed with diabetes each year, adding to the total of 30.3 million Americans, or 9.4% of the U.S. population with diabetes in 2015.[60] An additional 84 million Americans age 18 and older have prediabetes, a condition with blood sugar higher than normal, and a greatly increased risk of developing diabetes.

Diabetes is the 7th leading cause of death in the United States, killing about 79,500 Americans in 2015 and contributing to an additional 253,000 deaths.[61] In 2012, one in five health care dollars was spent to support the care of patients with diabetes at a total estimated cost of $245 billion.[62] Much of this expense is caused by the severe long-term complications of the disease.[63] At current rates of increase, the U.S. Centers for Disease Control and Prevention (CDC) estimates that as many as one in three people in the United States could have diabetes by the year 2050.[64]

Obesity is the strongest risk factor for developing metabolic syndrome and type 2 diabetes; 85% of Americans with type 2 diabetes are overweight or obese.[65] Independent of body weight, sedentary behavior, or alcohol use, high sugar intake is associated with the development of type 2 diabetes in a dose-response manner. A study in 175 countries found that every extra 150 calories per person per day increase in sugar intake (about one can of a sugar-sweetened soda a day) was associated with an increase in diabetes prevalence by 1.1%. Other food types did not increase the risk.[66] However, U.S. observational studies found that those who increased their consumption of red meat by a half serving a day increased their risk of diabetes by 48%, and those who reduced their consumption by a half serving a day reduced their risk by 14%.[67]

Insulin, produced by the pancreas, regulates blood sugar and is required to transport glucose from the bloodstream into the body's cells where it is used for energy, metabolic processes, or stored as an energy reserve in the form of glycogen or fat. When constantly buffeted by overloads of sugar that elicit insulin surges, the body's cells develop insulin resistance, a condition that requires an ever-greater release of insulin. Too much sugar overworks, damages, and eventually wears out the insulin-producing cells in the pancreas. Lack or ineffectiveness of insulin in a person with diabetes means that elevated levels of glucose remain circulating in the blood. When either the pancreas does not produce enough insulin (or none as in juvenile-onset type 1 diabetes) or the body cannot effectively use the insulin the pancreas produces because of insulin resistance, the result is type 2 diabetes (90% to 95% of diabetes cases). Over time, high glucose causes damage to many tissues in the body and leads to heart attack, stroke, kidney failure, vascular insufficiency and amputations, vision loss, hearing loss, nerve damage, and premature death. Diabetes is the leading cause of blindness, kidney failure, and amputations.[68 69]

Data from the Nurses' Health Study suggests that 90% of type 2 diabetes is preventable by adopting a lifestyle that features 30 minutes or more of daily physical activity, avoidance of overweight (body mass index, BMI, less than 25), not smoking, a healthy diet rich in whole grains with minimal added sugars and refined carbohydrates, avoiding red meat and having about three alcoholic drinks per week.[70 71 72 73] However, the value of alcohol in the prevention of diabetes is questionable. A recent advisory on preventing diabetes from the Harvard T. H. Chan School of Public Health noted, "If you already drink alcohol, the key is to keep your consumption in the moderate range, as higher amounts of alcohol could increase diabetes risk. If you don't drink alcohol, there's no need to start—you can get the same benefits by losing weight, exercising more, and changing your eating patterns."[74 75]

For individuals that are prediabetic, with a fasting blood glucose of 100 to 125, weight loss, increased physical activity, and avoidance of added sugars can usually decrease insulin resistance and reverse the prediabetic condition in three to six months. The same lifestyle changes can often decrease and sometimes even eliminate the use of insulin among those who have diabetes.[76 77] Weight loss from bariatric surgery is an even more effective treatment for type 2 diabetes (a "cure" in about one-third of cases) and for reducing its cardiovascular and other complications.[78]

Sugar, cardiovascular disease and arthritis

Cardiovascular disease (CVD) is also linked to the consumption of sugar. A 2009 meta-analysis found a positive association between sugar-sweetened beverage intake and coronary heart disease among women.[79] A 2010 study found that there was a linear trend with increasing added sugar consumption and substantially lower levels of cardio-protective HDL-C, higher triglycerides, but there was little influence on LDL-C.[80] A 2014 meta-analysis of 37 randomized controlled trials considered the effects of the modification of dietary added sugars on lipids.[81] Higher compared with lower sugar intakes significantly raised triglycerides, total cholesterol, LDL-C, and HDL-C slightly.

The Health Professionals' Follow-Up Study of nearly 43,000 men found that participants in the top quartile of sugar-sweetened beverage (SSB) intake (about 6.5 drinks per week) had a 20% higher relative risk of coronary heart disease than those in the bottom quartile. Moreover, those who consumed the greatest amount of sugar-sweetened drinks also had higher triglyceride and C-reactive protein (a marker of inflammation) levels and lower HDL-C levels. No increase in the risk of heart disease was found among men who drank artificially sweetened beverages (ASB).[82]

A 2014 study in the *Journal of the American Medical Association, Internal Medicine*, found that between 2005 and 2010, most adults (71.4%) consumed 10% or more of daily calories from added sugar.[83] Comparing the risk of CVD mortality among those who consumed less than 10% of calories from added sugar to those who consumed 10% to 25%, the study found a 30% increase in the risk of CVD mortality. Among the 10% of adults who consumed more than 25% of calories from added sugar, the CVD risk was 2.75 times greater.

A more recent study, published in 2019, evaluated associations between consumption of SSB with the risk of total and cause-specific mortality among 37,716 men from the Health Professional's Follow-up study (from 1986 to 2014) and 80,647 women from the Nurses' Health study (from 1980 to 2014). The study found that CVD mortality was 31% higher, and the total death rate was 28% higher among those who consumed two or more SSB a day compared to those who rarely drank them.[84]

Sugar-sweetened beverage intake may also increase the risk of some forms of arthritis. According to data from the Nurses' Health Study and the Nurses' Health Study II, women who drank as little as one sugar-containing soft drink a day had a highly significant 71% increased risk of developing seropositive rheumatoid arthritis than those who drank none or less than one such drink a month.[85]

How much sugar is too much?

Currently, added sugar contributes 15% to 25% of total calories consumed in the U.S., an average of 66 pounds annually![86 87] Recommendations for the maximum level of added sugar in the diet differ. The 2020 DGAC *Dietary Guidelines for Americans* suggest consumption of less than 6% of total calories per day from added sugars.[88] The American Heart Association's (AHA) advice is that women should consume no more than 100 calories per day of added sugars and men no more than 150 calories per day of added sugar.[89] The World Health Organization (WHO) strongly recommends reducing the intake of free (added) sugars to less than 10% of total energy intake and suggests that a further reduction to 5% could have additional health benefits.[90]

Table 3.2. Recommended daily maximum of added sugar for a 2000 calorie per day diet

Authority & Percent of Total Energy from Sugars	Teaspoons/day	Calories/day
U.S. average 15-25%	19.5	328
2020 DGAC: 6% of calories	7.2	120
American Heart Association	6 (for women), 9 (for men)	100 (for women), 150 (for men)
WHO 10% & 5% of calories	12 & 6	200 & 100

The health implications of carbohydrates: quantity and quality matters

According to the *Scientific Report of the 2020 Dietary Guidelines Advisory Committee*,[91] diets high in low-quality carbohydrates (added sugar and highly refined carbohydrates) are of concern because they are generally associated with high triglycerides and low HDL-C, biomarkers associated with increased rates of CVDs. As of 2015-2016, 42% of U.S. energy intake was from low-quality carbohydrates.[92] Nutritional science suggests that it is important to reduce consumption of sugar-sweetened beverages, processed foods with added sugars and refined grain products such as chips, crackers, cereals, and bakery desserts, including those that are often considered healthy such as white bread, white rice, and white potatoes.[93 94]

Although the metabolic and health effects of consuming sugar have often been compared unfavorably with consumption of complex carbohydrates, according to Mozaffarian et al., "Among the most important new insights related to diet and cardiometabolic health is the growing evidence characterizing the importance of carbohydrate quality."[95] It seems that many other additional, but not fully understood, characteristics of complex carbohydrates are relevant in determining their health effects. These include fiber content, bran and germ content, glycemic index, glycemic load, the way they are metabolized by the liver and their structure. For example, if carbohydrates are whole and unprocessed, minimally processed, highly refined, or liquid affects how they are metabolized by the body.

Mozaffarian et al. observed that because multiple characteristics appear to be relevant, health effects are unlikely to be replicated by simple extraction of individual factors (e.g., fiber) or nutrients and consumption of these as supplements or food additives. And that "...consuming individual constituents as supplements, is unlikely to produce the same benefits as substituting whole-grain, higher-quality carbohydrates for refined, lower-quality carbohydrates."[96]

Meat, high protein diets and health

Numerous studies have considered the health effects of high meat and high animal protein consumption.[97] Evidence shows that higher red meat consumption, especially processed red meat (e.g., bacon, hot dogs, and sausages), is associated with an increased risk of type 2 diabetes, cardiovascular disease, certain types of cancer, including colorectal cancer, and mortality. Additional health outcomes associated with consumption of processed red meat include chronic obstructive pulmonary disease, heart failure, and hypertension. Consuming processed red meat may entail a greater risk because along with high amounts of saturated fats, there are adverse effects from preservatives (e.g., sodium, nitrites, and phosphates) and preparation methods (e.g., potential cancer-causing polycyclic aromatic hydrocarbons from high-temperature commercial cooking/frying) that could influence health outcomes.[98 99 100]

In one observational analysis, both unprocessed and processed meat consumption was associated with higher heart disease risk when meat replaced foods, such as low-fat dairy, nuts, and fish.[101] A meta-analysis of prospective studies indicates that high consumption of red meat, especially processed meat, may increase all-cause and CVD mortality.[102 103] In one study, the substitution of one serving per day of other foods (e.g., fish, poultry, nuts, legumes, low-fat dairy, and whole grains) for one serving per day of red meat was associated with a 7% to 19% lower mortality risk.[104 105] A related study evaluated 85,168 women and 44,548 men without heart disease, cancer or diabetes from the Nurses' Health Study and the Health Professionals' Follow-Up Study. It concluded, "A low-carbohydrate diet based on animal sources was associated with higher all-cause mortality in both men and women whereas a vegetable-based low-carbohydrate diet was associated with lower all-cause and cardiovascular disease mortality rates."[106]

A 2014 study published in *Cell Metabolism* concluded that "Respondents aged 50–65 reporting high protein intake had a 75% increase in overall mortality and a four-fold increase in cancer and diabetes death risk during the following 18 years. These associations were not found in the older population studied, and they were either abolished or attenuated if the proteins were plant-derived." The study noted that people over 65 might benefit from more protein, perhaps because they tend to be frail and malnourished. The authors also reported that among those of all ages without type 2 diabetes at baseline, those in the high animal protein group had a 5-fold or greater increase risk of diabetes mortality during the 18-year study period.[107]

A 2015 meta-analysis of prospective cohort studies found an association between processed meat consumption and a 15% increased risk of all-cause and cardiovascular mortality in U.S. populations.[108] And a 2017 NIH-AARP study found that high intakes of red and processed meat and elevated all-cause mortality and mortality from nine different causes including cardiovascular disease, diabetes, cancer, and hepatic, renal, and respiratory diseases.[109] The strongest association was death from chronic liver disease, which more than doubled with the highest intake. The fifth of the study participants consuming the most red and processed meat had a 26% greater all-cause mortality than the fifth of the study subjects consuming the least. The study also showed reduced risks were associated with substituting white for red meat, particularly unprocessed white meat.

Similar findings were reported from a long-term Spanish study of older adults with cardiovascular risk factors that assessed protein consumption for roughly five years. The study found that when protein replaced carbohydrates, the eating pattern was linked to a 90% greater risk of gaining more than 10% of body weight and to a 59% higher risk of death from any cause. When protein replaced fat, the risk of death rose by 66%. The study authors concluded that "These results do not support the generalized use of high-protein diets as a good strategy for losing weight," and suggested that "Long-term efficacy and safety of these diets deserve more attention,"[110]

A meta-analysis of randomized clinical trials published in 2019 in the journal *Circulation* found that replacing red meat with nuts, legumes, and other plant-based protein foods (but not with fish or low-quality carbohydrates), reduced levels of CVD risk factors such as total cholesterol and LDL-C.[111] A long-term epidemiologic study published in 2019 in the *British Medical Journal*, found that increases in red meat consumption over eight years were associated with a higher mortality risk in the following eight years. An increase in total red meat consumption of at least half a serving per day was associated with a 10% higher mortality risk. For processed meat, the risk was increased by 13%, and, for unprocessed red meat consumption, there was a 9% higher mortality risk. An increase in consumption of whole grains, vegetables, or other protein sources was associated with a lower risk of death.[112]

Additional information on the CVD effects of processed meat, unprocessed red meat, poultry, or fish intake comes from a 2020 analysis of six prospective cohort studies.[113] Two or more servings of processed meat, unprocessed red meat, or poultry, but not fish, per week was significantly associated with a small (about 4% to 7%) increased risk of CVD, and higher intake of processed meat or unprocessed red meat, but not poultry or fish, was significantly associated with a small increased risk of all-cause mortality.

A controversial report questioning the importance of any risk posed by processed and red meat made headlines in late 2019.[114] A series of articles published in the *Annals of Internal Medicine* showed that people on diets low in red and processed meat had lower CVD, cancer, and all-cause mortality. However, the *Annals* authors claimed that the research showed that consumption of processed and red meat caused only trivial increases in CVD risk, the research methodology of studies was too flawed, and overall, the evidence was too weak to serve as guidance for the public. The study concluded that the health benefits were just not clear enough or great enough to suggest changing diets to reduce or giving eating up red and processed meat.

The push back from leading nutrition scientists was immediate and scathing.[115] Some of them demanded the retraction of the articles. They pointed out that the most scientifically sound research methods, such as randomized controlled trials of people on a fixed diet over many years, are just not feasible for nutritional research.[116] Critics of the *Annals* article noted that the conclusions of the observational research methods that are used in much nutritional research are valid. The vast majority of studies show that red and processed meat consumption increases the risk of all-cause and cardiovascular mortality. Critics of the *Annals* article also pointed out that the lead author had industry funding that constituted an undisclosed conflict of interest. My advice is to stick with the recommendations of the nutrition experts and minimize the consumption of red and processed meat.

Veggie burgers or meatless burgers are a rapidly growing option that in 2019 were available at 20,000 restaurants across the U.S. Some of these products may be highly processed and high in sugar, salt, and fat. For example, Beyond Meat's ingredients for its plant-based patties are high in sodium and saturated fat. They include water, pea protein isolate, expeller-pressed canola oil, refined coconut oil, rice protein, and other natural flavors. Ingredients for Impossible Foods burgers are also high in sodium and saturated fat. They include water, soy protein concentrate, coconut oil, sunflower oil, potato protein, soy leghemoglobin, and natural flavors. Artificial meats may or may not be healthy for the environment but do not always fit the profile of healthy foods for human consumption.[117] It is important to read the labels of meatless burgers because some may be healthy foods, but others are not.

Another important reason to cut back on eating meat, especially from ruminants such as beef cattle and sheep that emit large amounts of methane, is because global livestock production is the source of about 18% of all greenhouse gas emissions.[118] There is little evidence that more than the recommended minimum of about 10% to 15% of total calories from protein a day are beneficial. Avoiding high red and processed meat consumption is advisable to support both human health and the health of the planet.

Fat in the diet—some experts say focus on the type not the amount

Some nutrition experts say only the type of fat matters to health, but others recommend very low-fat diets. According to some popular media, the longstanding concern about large amounts of fat in the diet as a detriment to health is an obsolete concept, an unfortunate error that has harmed public health. For example, Nina Teicholz the author of the book *The Big Fat Surprise: Why Butter, Meat and Cheese Belong in a Healthy Diet*, blamed epidemiologic studies that showed an association between high-fat diets and CVD, (and not irrefutable causation), for subjecting Americans to a "...vast, uncontrolled diet experiment with disastrous consequences."[119 120] A *New York Times* op-ed by Mozaffarian and Ludwig made a reasonable suggestion to "Stop Fearing Fat" and advanced a proposition for which there is much relevant evidence, that is that the type of fats consumed influences cardiometabolic health more than the proportion of calories consumed from total fat.[121 122]

The primary rationale for limiting total fat to 30% in the *1980 U.S. Dietary Guidelines* and a range from 20% to 35% of total calories in the *2005 Guidelines*, was to lower saturated fat and dietary cholesterol, which were associated with increased cardiovascular risk. But as Mozaffarian and Ludwig pointed out in a 2015 editorial in the *Journal of the American Medical Association* (*JAMA*), ".... the campaign against saturated fat quickly generalized to include all dietary fat."[123]

With regard to total fat in the diet, the 2015 DGAC reported that diets with a lower percentage of energy from fat did not improve lipid profiles or reduce the risk of heart disease, diabetes, cancer, or adiposity (overweight or obesity).[124 125] The Food and Agriculture Organization also noted that several randomized control trials had not found evidence for the beneficial effects of low-fat diets. For example, a low-fat (27% to 30% of energy from fat), high-carbohydrate diet did not favorably affect serum lipids, fasting serum glucose, fasting serum insulin, or blood pressure, compared with higher fat diets.[126]

The longstanding advice to eat low-fat foods, and the marketing of a spate of highly processed low-fat foods, undoubtedly has played a part in the decline in consumption of dietary fat in the U.S. from about 40% of calories to near the often-recommended limit of 30% total energy. But there were unintended consequences. As fat has been lowered in the American diet, it has almost always been replaced with processed foods that have large amounts of added sugar and other refined carbohydrates. This is a prominent reason for the current criticism of low-fat diets. Studies suggest that substitution of saturated fat with highly processed carbohydrates (e.g., added sugar and refined grains) does not lower cardiovascular risk, whereas substitution of saturated fat with unprocessed plant-based foods or the "healthful" unsaturated fats found in nuts, vegetable oils, and fish reduces the risk of cardiovascular disease.[127 128]

Because different types of fat have different health effects, the 2015 DGAC report suggests that dietary advice should put the emphasis on optimizing types of dietary fat and not reducing total fat.[129] In keeping with the conclusions of the 2015 DGAC report, the *2015-2020 U.S. Dietary Guidelines* eliminated the advice to limit total dietary cholesterol and to limit total dietary fat that were prominent features of previous reports.

So perhaps the well-intentioned advice to eat low-fat may have backfired and harmed rather than improved health because we substituted sugar and refined carbohydrates for the fat eliminated from our diets. At least over the past few decades, sugar, highly refined carbohydrates, and calorie intake has increased substantially, the prevalence of obesity tripled, and the incidence of type 2 diabetes increased many-fold. Other lifestyle factors such as less physical activity, more eating out, and the consumption of ever-larger food portions probably also influenced these trends. Still, there is evidence that the added sugars and refined grains of processed foods are major contributors to the metabolic dysfunction, obesity, diabetes, and cardiovascular disease epidemics that characterize health in America.[130 131]

So, is the advice to limit total fat in the diet wrong and obsolete? One problem with almost all of the studies cited that show lack of benefit from low-fat eating is that they define low-fat as up to 30% of total calories from fat. The clinicians who have seen remarkable improvements in both cardiovascular health and biomarkers such as LDL-C with very low-fat diets would argue that a diet with 30% of energy from fat is not low enough in fat to bring about substantial improvement in health. I use the term ultra-low-fat (ULF) diets to describe diets with 10%, or at most 15%, of daily calories supplied by fat.

The view of ULF advocates is that a reduction in fat to 10% to 15% of total calories, and importantly, replacement of the missing fat calories with unprocessed or minimally processed plant-based foods, is required to obtain the favorable health changes they have seen but ultra-low-fat diets are unlikely to be healthy if they substitute refined carbohydrates for fat. Mozaffarian et al. have observed that a very low-fat, high-carbohydrate diet does have the potential to be cardio-protective as long as most of the carbohydrates are minimally processed.[132] A later section in this chapter on diets describes the benefits of the ULF eating plans of Pritikin,[133] Ornish,[134] Esselstyn,[135] and others.

In summary, a prominent problem with reducing fat calories in the American diet is that it that the calories have been replaced with unhealthy refined grains and added sugars. But the response to this situation should not be to go back to a high saturated fat burgers and butter diet, rather to focus on plant-based eating that includes healthy (mono and polyunsaturated) fats and the carbohydrates found in whole foods, such as beans, legumes, fruit and vegetables.

Different fats have different health effects

If total fat in the diet is considered to be less of a concern, at least according to many nutrition scientists, does the type of fat matter? We know that trans-fats are harmful, but what are the health implications of monounsaturated fatty acids (MUFAs), polyunsaturated fatty acids (PUFAs), and saturated fatty acids (SFAs)?

Consumption of saturated fat is not needed for good health, and the preponderance of evidence indicates that high consumption of saturated fat (sometimes called a "bad" fat) increases harmful LDL-C and increases the risk of cardiovascular disease and some cancers. The 2015 DGAC recommends that less than 10% of total daily calories should come from saturated fat.[136] The American Heart Association recommends aiming for a dietary pattern with only 5% to 6% of total calories derived from saturated fat.[137] According to this recommendation, of a 2,500 calorie a day diet, fewer than 150 calories or 17 grams a day should be saturated fat. A McDonald's Big Mac has 540 calories and a total of 30 grams of fat, of which 10 grams is saturated fat.

Research based on the Nurses' Health Study cohort found that higher consumption of red meat and high-fat dairy products, together, the main sources of saturated fatty acids in the diet, was also associated with greater risk of coronary heart disease (CHD) events. In contrast to eating red meat, higher consumption of poultry and fish and low-fat dairy products was associated with a lower risk, and that a higher ratio of polyunsaturated to saturated fat was strongly associated with lower CHD risk.[138]

A 2012 Cochrane meta-analysis, a study design generally considered to be of exceptionally high scientific validity, found that reducing saturated fatty acids by reducing or modifying dietary fat reduced the risk of cardiovascular events by 14%.[139] Studies among high-risk individuals have shown that greater consumption of MUFA and PUFA lowered the risk of cardiovascular disease and death, whereas saturated fat and trans-fat were associated with increased risk of cardiovascular disease.[140] [141] [142] [143] The evidence is not as clear for the replacement of SFA by monounsaturated fatty acids or replacement with carbohydrate and likely depends on the type and source.

Prospective cohort studies and randomized controlled trials have found lower rates of CVD when polyunsaturated fatty acids (PUFAs) from soybean, corn, and other vegetable oils replaced saturated fatty acids (SFAs).[144] [145] A 2010 meta-analysis of randomized controlled trials found that increasing PUFA consumption as a replacement for SFA reduced the occurrence of CHD events by 19%.[146]

A 2015 Cochrane meta-analysis of 15 trials of at least 2 years duration found that replacing saturated with polyunsaturated fats led to an estimated 27% reduction in cardiovascular disease, but no benefits were seen for replacement of saturated fat with carbohydrates or proteins. A dose-response analysis showed that this protection was proportional to the reduction of total cholesterol, which in turn depended on the extent of reduction in saturated fat consumption.[147]

A long-term study (24 to 30 years of follow-up), published in 2015, found that higher intakes of polyunsaturated fatty acids and carbohydrates from whole grains were significantly associated with a lower risk of CHD. Replacing 5% of energy intake from saturated fats with equivalent energy intake from polyunsaturated fatty acids was associated with a 25% lower risk of coronary heart disease, replacement with monounsaturated fatty acids decreased risk by 15%, and replacement with carbohydrates from whole grains a 9% lower risk of CHD.[148]

Fish oils

Omega-3 (n -3) polyunsaturated fats are found in seafood, such as salmon, trout, herring, tuna, and mackerel, and in walnuts, soy, canola oils, and flaxseed oils. Some nutrition experts advocate for increased consumption of omega-3 polyunsaturated fats for their benefits on blood lipid biomarkers, including lowering triglyceride levels, reducing the risk of potentially fatal abnormal heart rhythms, and because they may make platelets less likely to form the blood clots that can cause a heart attack or stroke. Increased consumption of omega-3 fatty acids from fish, fish oil supplements, or plant sources has been considered to be a dietary strategy to prevent coronary heart disease. However, randomized placebo-controlled studies have had mixed results, and fish seems to be more likely to improve cardiovascular health than the consumption of fish oil supplements.[149] [150] [151] [152] [153] [154] [155]

According to a 2013 review, with the advent of the wide use of statins and other medical therapies for CVD prevention, the use of fish oil supplements or even eating fish to prevent CVDs is less likely to be an efficacious strategy.[156] A carefully carried out 2018 meta-analysis has found that fish oil supplements provide no benefit with regard to cardiovascular disease or all-cause mortality.[157] This finding confirms the similar conclusion of the U.S. Agency for Healthcare Research and Quality.[158]

A 2018 Cochrane systematic review considered the results of 25 trustworthy randomized trials[159] The Cochrane researchers came to the same conclusion, i.e., that increasing consumption of the omega-3s Eicosapentaenoic acid (EPA) and docosahexaenoic acid (DHA), has little or no effect on all-cause mortality or cardiovascular health (coronary heart deaths, coronary heart disease events, stroke or heart irregularities). The review observed that long-chain omega-3 fats probably did reduce triglycerides and HDL cholesterol.

In 2019, after five years of study, VITAL, a well-designed clinical trial of supplementation with a high dose (1 g per day) of n–3 fatty acids, did not find a lower incidence of major cardiovascular events or cancer than a placebo.[160] However, an analysis that excluded the first two years of follow-up found a lower hazard ratio (0.89) for major cardiovascular events in the n–3 group as compared to the placebo group. Although secondary endpoint conclusions are less reliable, the data also suggested that compared to the placebo group, Blacks and those with low fish intake in the n-3 group had a significantly lower risk of myocardial infarction. Additional analyses from the VITAL study are planned, and confirmation of the secondary findings by future trials is needed.

A 2019 meta-analysis that included the findings from VITAL found that daily marine omega-3 supplementation is moderately effective. After an average of five years of use, omega-3 supplementation provided a modest 3% to 8% reduction in CVD endpoints.[161] The study found lower rates of myocardial infarction, coronary heart disease death, total coronary heart disease, cardiovascular disease death, and total cardiovascular disease, but no benefits were found for stroke. Risk reductions were linearly proportional to the dose of marine omega-3 supplementation, suggesting that greater cardiovascular benefits may be achieved at higher doses of marine omega- 3 supplementation. The study authors concluded that "Despite the modest effect sizes for some of the CVD outcomes, the use of marine omega-3 supplementation may still help prevent large absolute numbers of CVD events, given the high incidence rates of CVD worldwide."

A reasonable conclusion is that additional research on high doses of marine omega-3 supplementation is needed. So far, the research suggests that there are health benefits from eating fish, and, perhaps small benefits from consuming high dose fish oil supplements.

Is butter really back?

The long-standing concern that high consumption of saturated fats increases the risk of cardiovascular disease was weakened by several meta-analyses that, with the exception of trans-fats, found no clear relationship between total fat, and a weak relationship or no relationship between saturated fatty acid intake and cardiovascular events or deaths.[162 163 164] For example, a 2015 systematic review and meta-analysis of evidence from studies the authors considered to be generally well designed observational studies did not support a robust association of saturated fats with all-cause mortality, CHD, CHD mortality, ischemic stroke, or diabetes in healthy individuals.[165]

A 2014 meta-analysis, published in the *Annals of Internal Medicine* by Chowdhury et al., found no association between most dietary and circulating fatty acid types and coronary artery disease events. The study found that saturated fats were not associated with increased CVD risk, and polyunsaturated and monounsaturated fats were not cardio-protective.[166] The Chowdhury study, with findings at odds with years of advice linking dietary fat and health, and published in a leading medical journal, generated a great deal of publicity, controversy, and confusion. The Chowdhury study conclusion that available evidence did not support limiting saturated fat was repeated in a *New York Times* commentary proclaiming, "Butter is Back," and a *Time* magazine cover displaying an artistic butter swirl and the bold headline, "Eat Butter" even though butterfat is very high in saturated fatty acids (70%). The following year, a Gallup poll registered a sharp decline in the number of U.S. adults limiting fat in their diets. The "butter is back" episode seems to be another unfortunate example of the media unduly publicizing a flawed study that purports to demonstrate that "everything we thought was true is wrong." It is also a lesson on the need for caution in interpreting meta-analysis studies.

The University of California, Berkeley Wellness Letter's lead story summarizing the Chowdhury study was titled "The end of the debate? Fat chance."[167] According to the *Wellness Letter*, the studies reviewed usually did not explicitly specify the nutrients that replaced saturated fatty acids when their intake was lowered, and the replacement foods may have been high in the added sugars and refined carbohydrates that are as unhealthy as the fats they replaced. An editorial in *Lancet* made the same point, that to understand the effects of changed levels of saturated fat, requires taking into account the nature of the replacement energy source.[168 169] Another criticism of the Chowdhury study is that the authors did not compare the effects of saturated fat with those of polyunsaturated fat.[170] Other critics also noted the importance of the nature of replacement energy sources was not considered, that a few key papers were omitted from the study, and some included studies were misinterpreted.[171]

Doubt about the validity of the Chowdhury study also comes from a *JAMA* article by Barnard, Willett, and Ding that suggests caution about the use of meta-analysis, especially when studying links between diet and various disease conditions.[172] They point out most people's diets are quite variable, recall is difficult, and that nutrition intervention studies vary in many methodological details, weakening the argument for combining their results. They noted that the Chowdhury meta-analysis gave weight to both a Malmö Diet and Cancer cohort study where barely 1% of participants got less than 10% of energy from saturated fat intake,[173] and to the Oxford Vegetarian Study[174] that included participants with reported saturated fat intake ranging from 6% to 7% of energy among vegans to approximately twice that amount in the other diet groups.

In contrast to the Chowdhury meta-analysis, the Oxford study found that study participants in the group with the highest one-third of saturated fat intake had nearly triple the risk of fatal ischemic heart disease compared with the lowest one-third. Although the Malmö study found no significant association between saturated fat intake levels and risk of cardiovascular events, there were no participants with low saturated fat intake. Consumption ranged from 13% to more than 22% of calories. The Malmö study authors stated that saturated fatty acids-cardiovascular disease hypothesis "is thus not fully testable in this population." Barnard, Willett, and Ding noted that, nevertheless, the Malmö study was given substantial weight in the Chowdhury meta-analysis, which concluded that available evidence did not support limiting saturated fat.

More data on specific dietary fats and mortality comes from a long-term study that used 83,349 women from the Nurses' Health Study and 42,884 men from the Health Professionals Follow-up Study to examine this relationship.[175] The study found that participants with the highest intake of total fat (about 42% of calories) were 16% less likely to have died over the study period than those with the lowest total fat consumption (about 25% of calories). Polyunsaturated omega-6 fatty acids (found in corn, sunflower, and soybean oils) were more strongly associated with lower death rates than were omega-3s. Replacing 5% of energy from saturated fats with equivalent energy from PUFA and MUFA was associated with estimated reductions in total mortality of 27% and 13%, respectively. The study authors concluded that their findings support current dietary recommendations to replace saturated fat and trans-fat with unsaturated fats.

The bottom line on saturated fat consumption

We know that almost all diets that have been shown to be heart-healthy are low in trans and saturated fats and emphasize whole plant-based foods, including vegetables, fruits, beans, whole grains, and nuts that have unsaturated fats. Consumption of trans-fats should be as close to zero as possible. The advice of the American Heart Association is to strive for a diet with only 5% to 6% of total calories derived from saturated fat and replace the calories with high-quality carbohydrates such as whole grains or with polyunsaturated fats. Replacing saturated fats with the refined carbohydrates and added sugars, found in the typical American diet, will not decrease CVD risk.[176 177] So if polyunsaturated fats and monounsaturated fats should replace trans and saturated fats, does total fat matter at all? It may. The case for ultra-low-fat diets is presented in a following section on rating diets.

What is the latest advice about dietary cholesterol?

As we have noted, cholesterol causes atherosclerosis when there is too much LDL-C in the blood. According to the *2015-2020 Dietary Guidelines for Americans*, "Strong evidence from mostly prospective cohort studies but also randomized controlled trials has shown that eating patterns that include lower intake of dietary cholesterol are associated with reduced risk of CVD, and moderate evidence indicates that these eating patterns are associated with reduced risk of obesity."[178] However, both because dietary cholesterol only weakly influences blood cholesterol levels and because very few Americans consume enough cholesterol to increase their blood levels, the *2015-2020 Dietary Guidelines* have dropped the previous advice found in the 2010 edition to limit the consumption of dietary cholesterol to 300 mg per day.[179]

Some nutrition experts recommend continuing attention to dietary cholesterol because it can increase blood cholesterol levels.[180] A review of some 40 studies found that high dietary cholesterol statistically significantly increased both serum total cholesterol and LDL-C.[181] However, dietary cholesterol was not statistically significantly associated with coronary artery disease, ischemic stroke or hemorrhagic stroke.

Eggs are a cholesterol-rich food. One large egg contains approximately 200 mg of dietary cholesterol. However, a review of the health effects of egg consumption that considered 30 individual studies found that many studies showed no association between egg consumption and CVD.[182] The review suggests an adverse effect in sub-groups of the population, notably in those with diabetes. However, the authors concluded that the preponderance of evidence suggests that a diet including eggs may be used safely as part of a healthy diet in both the general population and for those at high risk of cardiovascular disease, those with established coronary heart disease, and those with diabetes.

Other study authors have also concluded that egg consumption, although a major source of dietary cholesterol, is not significantly associated with clinical cardiovascular events in the general population.[183] Three large international prospective studies, including about 177,000 individuals, 12,701 deaths, and 13,658 CVD events from 50 countries, did not find significant associations between egg intake and blood lipids, mortality, or major CVD events.[184] However, some of the studies excluded participants with preexisting CVDs. Recent review articles also suggest abandoning the previous advice to avoid eggs.[185]

Other studies about the health effects of eggs are inconclusive, and others suggested negative health effects. For example, a study from Korea found that those with high consumption of eggs, seven eggs per week compared to zero to one eggs per week, had an 80% increase in the risk of having detectable coronary artery calcification.[186]

A 2019 study among nearly 30,000 U.S. adults from six prospective cohort studies with a median follow-up of 17.5 years, found that each additional 300 mg of dietary cholesterol and each additional half an egg consumed per day were each significantly associated with a 17% increase in risk of incident CVD and an 18% increase in all-cause mortality. The study authors concluded that among U.S. adults, higher consumption of dietary cholesterol or eggs was significantly associated with a higher risk of incident CVD and all-cause mortality in a dose-response manner.[187]

However, a high-quality 2020 multivariable analysis of three studies with up to 32 years of follow-up found that consumption of at least one egg per day was not associated with incident cardiovascular disease risk after adjustment for updated lifestyle and dietary factors associated with egg intake.[188]

Some but not all nutrition experts suggest that if your diet is otherwise healthy and your blood lipids low, eating eggs will not increase CVD risk. The current average intake of dietary cholesterol in the United States is approximately 270 mg per day.[189] It would appear that although consumption of dietary cholesterol is not a major health risk, avoidance of exceeding 300 mg of cholesterol per day remains the optimal strategy for health. With regard to eggs, eating three, four or even seven eggs a week does not appear to have a substantial effect on blood cholesterol or risk of CVD unless a person already has high cholesterol or diabetes.

Is alcohol a benefit to health?

Moderate alcohol intake is often claimed to be beneficial to health, particularly for the prevention of heart disease, but this is mostly wishful thinking. The *2020 Dietary Guidelines Advisory Committee Report* notes that although moderate intake of alcohol (among adults) is associated with positive health outcomes, many of these studies have serious problems. According to the 2020 DGAC, "Although it is possible that alcohol consumption at low levels may have some benefits, the likely direction of confounding and selection bias in observational studies means that associations with better health among low average drinkers compared with never drinkers may be a statistical artifact." Therefore, the 2020 DGAC does not recommend that anyone begin drinking alcohol or drink more frequently on the basis of potential health benefits because moderate alcohol intake also is associated with increased risk of violence, drowning, injuries from falls, motor vehicle crashes, and breast and at least six other types of cancer.

The 2015 DGAC report points out that there are many circumstances in which people should not drink alcohol:

- Individuals who cannot restrict their drinking to moderate levels
- Anyone younger than the legal drinking age
- Women who are pregnant or who may become pregnant
- Individuals taking prescription or over-the-counter medications that can interact with alcohol
- Individuals with certain specific medical conditions (e.g., liver disease, high triglycerides, pancreatitis)
- Individuals who plan to drive, operate machinery, or take part in other activities that require attention, skill, or coordination or in situations where impaired judgment could cause injury or death (e.g., swimming)

Approximately 60% of individuals report alcoholic beverage consumption in the past month, and of those, approximately 40% binge drink—consuming 5 or more drinks for men or 4 or more drinks for women during a drinking occasion—often multiple times per month. The lost productivity, medically-related costs, and costs to the legal and criminal justice systems from excessive alcohol consumption add up to $224 billion annually in the United States. As noted, the 2020 DGAC cited new scientific evidence about the harms of alcohol and strengthened previous recommendations to limit consumption of alcohol. The new recommendation for those who drink, is to limit consumption to just one drink a day for both men and women. In addition to the health risks of consuming alcohol, the 2020 DGAC considers alcohol to be an important risk factor for, or contributor to, a variety of social and mental health problems, including depression, child abuse and neglect, fetal alcohol spectrum disorder, motor vehicle crashes, domestic violence, sexual assault, vandalism and other property crimes, and nuisance violations.

The following chapters discussing cardiovascular disease, cancer and dementia describe why the drawbacks of consuming alcohol nearly always outweigh the benefits.

Rating the diets—can we describe a best dietary pattern?

Of the myriad nutritional patterns and thousands of diets that have been, and are still being promoted, many can best be described as diets with unproven claims and poorly understood effects on health. Often these diets have the singular goal of weight loss and have little regard for their impact on other aspects of health, in particular their long-term implications for cardiovascular health. Unfortunately, because nutrition research is so difficult, we do not have definitive evidence about what constitutes optimal nutrition.

To help the public choose the best diet, with the help of a panel of health experts, in 2020 *U.S. News & World Report* ranked diets in nine categories, such as best plant-based diet, best for weight loss, or just eating for good health.[190] Of the 35 diets evaluated, the Mediterranean diet was number one, and the similar DASH diet and the Flexitarian tied for second in the Best Diet Overall category. Other top-ranked diets were Weight Watchers, the Mayo Clinic diet, and the Volumetrics diet. The top-ranked diets emphasize fruits, vegetables, whole grains, and plant-based protein.

Weight Watchers was tops in the Weight Loss Diet category, Vegan and Volumetrics were tied in second place. Other highly ranked weight-loss diets were the Flexitarian, Jenny Craig, and Ornish diets. The ultra-low-fat vegetarian Ornish diet was ranked the best Heart Healthy Diet followed in second place by the Mediterranean diet, and the DASH diet ranked third. In the best Plant-based Diet category, the Mediterranean diet was ranked first, the Flexitarian second and the Nordic, Ornish, and Vegetarian diets tied for third. Significantly, the popular Paleo diet was ranked near the bottom at number 29 in the Best Diet Overall category. And the Keto diet, a low-carb, high-fat regimen, was ranked number 35, in last place, in the Best Diet for Healthy Eating category.[191]

Studies of indigenous hunter-gatherers from many parts of the world indicate that it is likely that there is no singular diet optimal to provide excellent metabolic health and freedom from chronic diseases such as heart disease, diabetes, and obesity.[192] Populations, such as the Hadza in Tanzania, Shuar, hunter-gatherer/farmers in the rainforest of Ecuador, and the Tsimane in Bolivia eat a variety of diets. They all have a lifestyle characterized by very high levels of physical activity, and all are mostly free from the degenerative diseases that afflict Americans and other people in industrialized countries. They rely on subsistence hunting, gathering, and farming, and a high proportion of the foods that they eat are plant-based. They do not lead sedentary lives or consume processed foods loaded with fat, salt, highly refined carbohydrates, and added sugars. In general, hunter-gatherers do not have convenient access to large amounts of food and, as is described later in this book, any calorie-restricted diet, regardless of the proportion of carbohydrates, fats and protein, improves metabolic biomarkers—but some weight-loss diets are not healthy for long-term consumption.

Most of us will not want or have a lifestyle similar to that of hunter-gatherers, so more attention to diets in the context of modern living is warranted. Our choices have important health implications, and knowledge of the health implications of individual nutrients can help guide food choices. But nutrients are consumed in the form of foods that are made up of a multitude of complex constituents, and their interactions and health effects are not fully understood. Since we eat food, our focus should be on the selection and consumption of healthy foods. There is substantial evidence that the adoption of several overall dietary patterns can improve health, prevent some cancers, improve multiple cardiovascular risk factors, and prevent or even reverse CVD. The *2015 Dietary Guidelines Advisory Committee Report* concluded that healthy eating patterns can be achieved with a variety of eating styles, including the "Healthy U.S.-style Pattern," the "Healthy Mediterranean-style Pattern," and the "Healthy Vegetarian-style Pattern."[193]

The 2015 DGAC found what they called "remarkable consistency" in the findings and implications of their examination of the association between dietary patterns and various health outcomes.[194] The 2015 DGAC report states "Common characteristics of dietary patterns associated with positive health outcomes include higher intake of vegetables, fruits, whole grains, low- or non-fat dairy, seafood, legumes, and nuts; moderate intake of alcohol (among adults); lower consumption of red and processed meat, and low intake of sugar-sweetened foods and drinks, and refined grains."

Katz and Meller have identified seven basic dietary pattern varieties: low-fat (including vegetarian and traditional Asian); vegan; Mediterranean; mixed and balanced; low glycemic; low carbohydrate; and Paleolithic.[195] Among these, epidemiologic and clinical research suggests that those that are plant-based are the most likely to improve and preserve health. Two general diet patterns stand out as having much in common and being much better than the typical American diet—the TAD. 1) whole-food plant-based, including vegetarian, vegan, and traditional Asian diets—they all may be ultra-low-fat, and; 2) Mediterranean, and the nutritionally similar mixed and balanced diets. There are differences between them, and discerning, which is superior is difficult, if not impossible, with the available evidence. In part, this is because different bodies of evidence from research are referred to and underlie our knowledge about the links between these differing dietary patterns and health. For example, some nutrition experts (e.g., Ornish, Esselstyn) advocate for ultra-low-fat diets, with no more than 10% of total calories from fat. Other top nutrition experts (e.g., Willett, Hu, Mozaffarian) recommend more mainstream diets that substitute "healthier" PUFA and MUFA fats for trans and saturated fats. The pros and cons of these different dietary recommendations are discussed in the following sections.

The case for vegetarian and vegan diets

Vegetarian diets are consistent with most recommendations for healthy eating. They emphasize plant-based foods, in particular fruits, vegetables, legumes, nuts, and vegetable oils, no meat, and little processed food. Typically, they are low in total fat, low in saturated fat, high in fiber, and plant protein replaces animal protein.

Assessing the role of diet in the health outcomes for vegetarians is complicated by their often-major differences in other health-conscious lifestyle behaviors such as avoidance of smoking, high levels of physical activity, and low incidence of overweight and obesity. Determining their impact is also complicated by the variety of vegetarian diets that are consumed around the world, including by pesco-vegetarians (who also consume fish); lacto-ovo-vegetarians (who also consume milk and eggs); and strict vegans (who consume no animal products). Not much is known about possible differences in health outcomes between these differing vegetarian diets.

As Katz and Meller[196] and Hu[197] have noted, the scientific literature on plant-based diets supports the conclusion that they have favorable effects on a wide array of health outcomes.[198 199 200] They improve blood lipids (lower LDL-C and non-HDL-C), facilitate weight loss, and help prevent various cardiovascular diseases and cancers and provide the benefits of a high intake of fiber.[201 202] The long-term Nurses' Health Study and the Health Professionals Follow-up Study found that intake of plant protein was associated with lower cardiovascular and all-cause mortality.[203] Diets high in animal protein, especially processed red meat (but not fish and poultry), were associated with higher cardiovascular mortality, but perhaps only in those with one or more lifestyle-related health risk factors.

Populations in low-resource settings with vegetarian or mostly plant-based dietary patterns have been observed to have low cardiovascular and cancer disease risk.[204 205 206] Similar observations have been made about groups with vegetarian diets in the U.S., such as Seventh-Day Adventists.[207 208] A meta-analysis of seven studies relating to CVD mortality and vegetarian diets found that heart disease mortality was 29% lower in vegetarians than in non-vegetarians.[209]

The Oxford Vegetarian Study was a prospective study of 6,000 vegetarians and 5,000 non-vegetarian control subjects in the U. K. between 1980 and 1984.[210] The study found that vegans had the lowest total cholesterol and LDL-C; vegetarians and fish eaters had similar intermediate values and meat-eaters the highest. Meat and cheese consumption was associated with high, and dietary fiber intake was associated with low total cholesterol levels. After 12 years of follow-up (and adjusting for smoking, body mass index, and social class), death rates from all causes were 20% lower and cancer deaths 39% lower in non-meat-eaters than in meat-eaters. Greater intakes of total animal fat, saturated animal fat, and dietary cholesterol were associated with increased mortality from heart disease.

A 2013 Swedish study found that those who never consumed fruit or vegetables had three years shorter lives and a 53% higher mortality rate than did those who consumed five servings of fruit and vegetables per day.[211] Although vegetables and fruit are often considered together as components of a healthy plant-based diet, several studies have found that eating fruit is protective against high blood pressure, stroke, diabetes, weight gain, some cancers, and age-related muscle loss (sarcopenia).[212] A study among Chinese adults found that a higher level of fruit consumption was associated with lower blood pressure and blood glucose levels.[213] The risk of a cardiovascular event was 25% to 40% lower among those with daily consumption of fruit compared to those who ate none.

Another study documented that in just four weeks, a plant-based diet can rapidly reduce heart disease risk factors.[214] Systolic and diastolic blood pressure declined, and LDL-C decreased from 143.0 mg/dl to 118.4 mg/dL. Other CVD risk factors, including weight, waist circumference, heart rate, insulin, glycated hemoglobin, and high–sensitivity C–reactive protein, were also reduced.

A review of the impact of vegetarian dietary patterns on CVD suggested that healthy lifestyle choices may reduce the risk of myocardial infarction by more than 80%, and that vegetarian dietary patterns alone could reduce CVD mortality and the risk of coronary heart disease by 40%.[215] According to the American Dietetic Association, "...appropriately planned vegetarian diets, including total vegetarian or vegan diets, are healthful, nutritionally adequate and may provide health benefits in the prevention and treatment of certain diseases."[216]

Vegetarian and very-low-fat diet advocates also note the evidence that human anatomy and physiology is most suited to a diet of plant-based foods. This evidence is provided by the fact that humans have long intestines, whereas carnivores have short intestines, and that our tooth and jaw structures are similar to those of other primates living on mainly plant-based diets in natural settings. However, it must be acknowledged that after two million years of mainly plant-eating, about two million years ago, our hominid predecessors evolved to homo Erectus, with the anatomical features of a runner's build and a spear-throwing arm suited to hunting and eating meat.[217]

Not all vegetarian diets optimize health

A vegetarian or vegan diet may not embody other important characteristics of a healthy diet. For example, they may not be low sodium, low in added sugars, low in highly processed carbohydrates such as white flour, or high in whole, unprocessed plant-based foods. Evidence that plant-based diets can vary considerably in their implications for health comes from a 2017 study in the *Journal of the American College of Cardiology*.[218] The 20-year study examined the association between diet and coronary heart disease (CHD) among more than 200,000 adults. The researchers compared CHD risk with how closely diets fit into three categories of plant-based diets outlined below.

An overall plant-based diet

The study assessed the level of consumption of all plant foods compared to intake of all animal foods and foods that contain animal products. The study found that the greatest relative increase in consumption of all plant foods was associated with up to an 8% decrease in CHD.

A healthful plant-based diet

The study assessed the level of consumption of healthy plant foods, such as whole grains, fruits, vegetables, nuts, legumes, healthy oils, tea and coffee, while reducing intake of less healthy plant foods as well as animal foods. The study found that the greatest relative increase in consumption of healthy plant foods was associated with up to a 25% decrease in CHD.

An unhealthful plant-based diet

The study assessed the level of consumption of less healthy plant foods, such as fruit juices, refined grains (pasta, white rice, and processed breads, rolls and cereals), potatoes (French fries and potato chips), sweets, desserts, and sugar-sweetened beverages, while reducing the relative intake of healthy plant foods as well as animal foods. The study found that the greatest increase in consumption of unhealthy plant foods was associated with up to a 32% increase in CHD.

An implication of this study is that less healthy plant foods and animal foods are both associated with increased CHD risk, with, at least in this study, a greater risk for less healthy plant foods. The study authors concluded "This highlights the wide variation in nutritional quality of plant foods, making it crucial to consider the quality of plant foods consumed in plant-rich diets."

Although vegetarian, vegan, and traditional Asian diets are often low-fat, they may not be if large amounts of oils and fats are used in food preparation or if they are consumed with condiments and sauces that are high in fat. And most important: only animal foods like meat and dairy provide vitamin B-12, so people on vegan diets need to consume fortified foods or vitamin supplements.

The case for ultra-low-fat plant-based diets

A long-standing common but somewhat arbitrary goal from the American Heart Association, WHO, and other groups has been to define a diet with 30% or fewer total calories from fat to be the definition of a low-fat diet.[219 220] A group of investigators and clinicians, including Pritikin,[221] Ornish,[222] Esselstyn,[223] Connor,[224] McDougall,[225 226] Fuhrman,[227] Barnard[228 229 230] Campbell,[231] Jenkins,[232] Greger[233] and Shintani[234] advocate for a very low-fat, whole-food, or minimally processed plant-based diet with a much more restrictive definition of low-fat than the AHA. They maintain that modest decreases in total fat in the diet will have only a modest effect on biomarkers such as total cholesterol and LDL-C. They consider a diet to be truly low-fat when no more than 15%, or better yet 10%, of daily calories comes from fat.[235 236 237] I call these diets ultra-low-fat (ULF) diets.

The investigators advocating ULF diets are likely to base their conclusions about the health benefits of ULF plant-based diets on the clinical outcomes of small-scale research trials among highly motivated individual patients, usually with established CVD, who adhere closely to their restrictive diet recommendations. Although the impacts of ULF diets on health are impressive, the evidence supporting ULF eating is not as well supported by many large-scale, long-term epidemiologic studies or multiple randomized controlled trials as some other dietary patterns. One reason is that existing large-scale diet studies do not include a group of study subjects consuming an ultra-low-fat diet because there are just not enough people eating in this way to serve as study subjects. For example, in the study of dietary fat and mortality in the Nurses' Health Study the Health Professionals Follow-up Study, the lowest quintile of fat consumption among those studied was 24% to 25% of energy from fat.[238]

Advocates of very-low-fat diets often cite the low cardiovascular and cancer disease risk of traditional populations with vegetarian or mostly plant-based dietary patterns, for example, the groups with low cardiovascular disease incidence in rural China described by T. Colin Campbell in his book *The China Study*.[239] Similar diets and low risk of CVDs and cancer are found among some of the long-lived populations featured in Blue Zone[240] studies and Seventh-Day Adventists.[241 242] Another example is found in Mexico's Tarahumara Indians, a highly physically active group, sometimes known as "super-runners" for their long-distance running feats. They have been found to be essentially free from cardiovascular risk factors and free from CVDs.[243] Their usual diet provided less than 10% of calories from fat and consisted of corn, beans, fruit other vegetables, and small quantities of game, fish, and eggs.

A traditional high carbohydrate low-fat Japanese dietary pattern is associated with longevity.[244] These diets emphasize soy products, fish, seaweeds, vegetables, fruits, and green tea and are low in meats. An unfavorable characteristic of Japanese diets is often high sodium from soy sauce and salt added to other foods such as fish, likely contributing to a relatively high incidence of high blood pressure, stroke, and some cancers.[245 246] Japanese living in Okinawa have a long life expectancy and are reputed to have the world's longest disability-free lifespan. Their traditional daily diet is low in calorie density, low in fat, and rich in plant-based foods. It features about seven daily servings of green leafy and orange-yellow root vegetables, an equal number of servings of grain-based foods, many of which are whole grain, as well as soy, fruit, and seaweed. By weight, fish make up 11% of their diet and meat, poultry, and eggs, just 3%. In addition to a healthy diet, many Okinawans are reported to be physically active and lean even at age 100.[247 248]

Pritikin, Ornish and Esselstyn—ultra-low-fat whole-food plant-based diets

In the 1970s, Nathan Pritikin created the ultra-low-fat Pritikin diet based on unprocessed or minimally processed straight-from-nature foods like fruits, vegetables, and legumes. Dean Ornish and Caldwell Esselstyn, Jr. are among the physicians who have conducted pioneering and careful clinical trials of similar diets that demonstrated that a lifestyle intervention based on diet could usually halt the progression of coronary heart disease and even reverse it.

The Ornish program lifestyle modifications include:[249]

- Whole-foods, plant-based diet (naturally low in fat and sugar)
- Stress management techniques (including yoga and meditation)
- Moderate exercise (such as walking)
- Social support and community (love and intimacy)

The ULF diet that Ornish and Esselstyn and others advocate features "beans and greens." It limits fat intake to 10% to 15% of total calories, avoids saturated and trans-fats, meat, oils, refined grains and refined grain products, minimizes non-fat dairy or eliminates dairy, eliminates added sugars, seafood (in some versions), and most processed foods—typically they are high in added fat, sugar and salt.[250] Esselstyn's advice is to not eat "anything with a face or a mother." The diet consists mainly of natural unrefined plant-based foods, including fruits, vegetables, legumes, whole grains, soy, and cereals. Their whole-food plant-based diet is high in fiber and low in rapidly absorbed added sugars, so it has a low glycemic index.[251 252 253 254 255]

Ornish emphasizes that a very-low-fat diet that is high in refined carbohydrates like sugar, white flour, white rice, and pasta, increases harmful LDL-C and triglycerides and that replacing fat in the diet with "low-fat" foods that are high in sugar and other refined carbohydrates will not decrease and may increase cardiovascular risk.[256 257]

Beginning in 1977, Ornish studied patients with heart disease and symptoms like angina and coronary artery disease that was documented by angiograms. As described in his book *The Spectrum*, the participants who adopted his program had more than a 90% reduction in the frequency of angina after a few weeks, on average a 40% reduction in LDL-C, and improved blood flow to the heart as shown by quantitative coronary arteriography and heart muscle perfusion studies with positron emission tomography (PET scans).[258 259] A follow-up study of Ornish's Lifestyle Heart Trial published in the *JAMA* showed that after five years, there was more regression of coronary atherosclerosis in the experimental treatment group but a continuing progression of coronary disease in the control group.[260 261 262]

A study among coronary heart disease patients who were eligible for revascularization found that nearly 80% of the patients who chose the Ornish program were able to avoid surgery.[263] A similar larger study found that after 12 weeks on the Ornish program, average LDL-C decreased by 17.6%, total cholesterol by 14.9%, triglycerides by 10.6%, BMI by 6.6%, and functional exercise capacity as measured by METs (metabolic equivalents) improved by 22.2%.[264] According to Ornish, "Over and over, I've seen patients with coronary heart disease so severe that they can't walk across the street or work or play with their kids or make love or do much of anything without getting severe chest pain become pain-free after only a few weeks of making these diet and lifestyle changes."[265 266 267 268]

Some observers of the Ornish program are somewhat skeptical of the impact of the stringent diet requirements because exercise and stress management are also a feature of the program. Ornish has evaluated the relative impact of each of the features of his program, diet, stress management, and exercise.[269 270] His study found that reduced dietary fat intake was the only predictor related to lower LDL-C, and that management of stress was related to a decrease in triglycerides and total cholesterol. Ornish stated that "I'm not aware of any studies showing that walking and stress management techniques alone can reverse heart disease."

Studies similar to those of Ornish have been carried out by Caldwell Esselstyn Jr. of the Cleveland Clinic Foundation with equally impressive results. In his book *Prevent and Reverse Heart Disease*,[271] Esselstyn described patients who, although they were receiving aggressive treatment with surgery and drugs, remained ill with advanced coronary artery disease and were experiencing increasing symptoms such as angina. His goal was to reduce his patient's total cholesterol levels to those seen in populations where heart disease is essentially nonexistent.

Stress management and moderate exercise were not emphasized by Esselstyn's program, but his patients had essentially the same beneficial improvements in cardiovascular health as those in the Ornish program. Within a few months of initiating a very low-fat plant-based diet, the study subjects experienced a rapid decline in their cholesterol levels and relief of their angina symptoms. All patients who maintained the Esselstyn diet achieved a total cholesterol goal of less than 150 mg/dL and had no recurrent cardiac events during a 12-year follow up. Patients who adhered to the program are still free from heart-related symptoms after 20 years. Esselstyn's study also showed that a nutrition-based intervention could stop and reverse the progression of very severe coronary artery disease.[272 273]

Terry Shintani has also carried out studies of the power of proper nutrition to rapidly improve the risk factors for cardiovascular disease. Participants in his study consumed a high carbohydrate, low-fat traditional Hawaiian diet without calorie or portion size restriction for 21 days.[274] The Hawaii diet is high in complex carbohydrates (77% of calories), very low in fat (12% of calories), and moderate in protein (11% of calories). Even though encouraged to eat to satiety, study participants had a significant weight loss, averaging 10.8 lbs. The participants also had improved biomarkers: lower blood pressure, lower total cholesterol, lower LDL-C, lower triglycerides, and lower glucose.

These studies provide an important argument for the adoption of whole-food plant-based ULF diets. They are the only ones demonstrated to bring about regression of coronary atherosclerosis, as shown by objective measurement techniques, including arteriograms.

My Story

As I mentioned in the introductory chapter, when I was at Continental Health Enhancement Center (CHEC), I witnessed the same remarkable clinical results among cardiac cripples who adopted an ULF diet, participated in stress management exercises and undertook physical activity to the extent possible allowed by their physical condition. Patients with the debilitating cardiac symptoms of chest pain (angina) and shortness of breath became free from pain, and improved their exercise tolerance after just a few weeks on an ultra-low-fat whole-food plant-based diet![275]

So, what could be wrong with the argument for ULF diets? The limitations on the type of foods required for an ULF diet are likely to make adherence challenging. There are not enough well-designed large-scale epidemiological studies of ULF diet risks and benefits. Perhaps most of the benefit of ULF eating is because the diet is whole-food plant-based rather than very low in fats. It is unclear if it is really necessary to eliminate those plant-based foods that are associated with health but are high in fat, such as nuts and avocados. Although high in monounsaturated fat, avocados have been shown to be beneficial for cardiovascular health.[276]

There is even stronger evidence that nuts are a healthful food. Total nut intake has been found to be associated with lower overall and cause-specific mortality.[277 278 279] A meta-analysis found that higher nut intake was associated with reduced risk of cardiovascular disease, cancer and all-cause mortality, and mortality from respiratory disease, diabetes, and infections, with most of these diseases showing a 20% to 35% reduction in mortality.[280] However, a Swedish study found that other healthy behaviors accounted for most of the health benefits attributed to nuts.[281]

The case for Mediterranean diets

Mediterranean diets encompass a diverse range of eating patterns based on the traditional diets of the Mediterranean region. They are often found in places that are associated with healthier lifestyles, reduced risk of cardiovascular disease and increased longevity, such as in the Blue Zones, e.g., Ikaria, Greece; and Ogliastra Region, Sardinia.[282] They include both plant and animal foods. Foods that are emphasized include olive oil, vegetables, fruits, whole-grain breads, and cereal foods, nuts and seeds, beans and legumes, selective dairy intake; often fish and other seafood; and quite limited consumption of meat. In some countries, consumption of moderate amounts of alcohol in the form of wine is a feature of Mediterranean diets.[283] The New Nordic diet is predominantly plant-based and very similar to the Mediterranean diet except for the regional choices of a differing spectrum of healthy fruits, vegetables, whole grains, and lean meats.[284]

The Mediterranean diet has been found to have favorable effects on a wide variety of the biomarkers associated with cardiovascular health, including blood cholesterol levels, insulin resistance, and the metabolic syndrome. Reduced progression of cardiovascular disease, preserved cognition, and possibly reduced risk of cancer (See Chapter 7, "Preventing Cancer") have been attributed to a Mediterranean diet.[285 286 287 288]

The Lyon Diet Heart Study found a 50% to 70% reduction in the risk of recurrence of CVD events or deaths from all causes.[289 290] In an 11-year study among elderly men and women, higher levels of compliance with both the DASH (a mixed and balanced diet) and Mediterranean dietary patterns were associated with better cognitive function. Whole grains and nuts and legumes appear to be among the plant-based foods positively associated with brain health.[291]

A study among nurses over about 15 years found that an Alternate Mediterranean diet was associated with "healthy" aging defined as no major chronic diseases or major impairments in cognitive or physical function or mental health.[292] An even longer 26 year follow up of the Nurses' Health Study found that the risk of sudden cardiac death (deaths that make up about half of all heart attack deaths) was about half among those with the highest scores on the Alternate Mediterranean diet which emphasizes high intake of vegetables, fruits, nuts, legumes, whole grains, and fish and moderate intake of alcohol.[293]

The National Institutes of Health (NIH)-AARP study found that a Mediterranean diet was associated with a reduction in all-cause mortality.[294] A study in the Netherlands found that 10 years of adherence to the Mediterranean diet was significantly related to lower mortality.[295] The study scored adherence to four healthy lifestyle factors: Mediterranean diet, not smoking, normal weight (BMI 18.5 to 25), and regular physical activity. The highest-scoring women could be expected to live 15.1 years longer than the least healthy with low scores. The corresponding longer life expectancy for men was 8.4 years. This study suggests that adherence to four modifiable healthy lifestyle factors can substantially reduce premature mortality.

Substantial media attention was given to the PREDIMED (Prevencion con Dieta Mediterreanea) trial when the results were published in the *New England Journal of Medicine* in 2013. The study of subjects with established cardiovascular disease compared the cardiovascular events of a "low-fat" control group with study subjects on a modified Mediterranean diet supplemented with extra-virgin olive oil or nuts. Over the nearly five-year study, the dietary intervention was claimed to have major cardiovascular benefits.[296]

Critics of the original PREDIMED trial noted that the reduction in CVD events was attributable only to a lower death rate from stroke. And although the trends for other cardiovascular events appeared favorable, there was no statistically significant reduction in the rates of heart attack, death from cardiovascular causes, or death from any cause compared to the control group. Furthermore, the study was not a true comparison of low-fat eating compared to the Mediterranean diet because among the low-fat control group, total fat consumption was high and decreased insignificantly, from 39% to 37%.[297] A separate analysis of the PREDIMED trial found a benefit, a decrease in peripheral artery disease among those on the modified Mediterranean diet supplemented with extra-virgin olive oil or nuts.[298]

A 2015 study also indicates that foods prominent in the Mediterranean dietary pattern are beneficial.[299] It found that when unsaturated fats, especially polyunsaturated fats, and/or unrefined whole-grain carbohydrates replace saturated fats, cardiovascular disease risk is reduced. A 2016 meta-analysis of evidence from several randomized controlled trials (RCTs) suggests that a Mediterranean diet with no restriction on fat intake may be associated with reduced incidence of cardiovascular events, breast cancer, and type 2 diabetes, but does not affect all-cause mortality.[300]

Although there is evidence for the CVD and other health benefits of the classic Mediterranean diet, today's inhabitants of Mediterranean countries now eat more meat and other processed foods. It is worth noting that CVD is the leading cause of death in several countries that could be considered to be Mediterranean: Spain, France, Italy, and Greece. Another concern about Mediterranean diets is that among some patients, the high levels of olive oil that are advocated result in a failure to achieve a low level of blood cholesterol.[301] And Mediterranean diets seem somewhat less effective at preventing subsequent CVD events among those at high risk than the ULF diets advocated by Ornish and Esselstyn.

Mixed and balanced diets

Mixed and balanced diets are healthier variations of the typical American or Western diets consumed in the U.S. and other developed countries. They include both plant and animal food but are modified with the goal of improving health, especially by the prevention of CVDs. They generally conform to the healthier diets recommended by nutrition experts. They are promoted in the *2015-2020 Dietary Guidelines for Americans* and the *Dietary Recommendations of the World Health Organization.*[302]

They have been studied in federally funded intervention trials supported by the U.S. National Institutes of Health. Among these interventions are the Dietary Approaches to Stop Hypertension (DASH) diet, the MIND diet, the Diabetes Prevention Program (DPP), the Optimal Macronutrient Intake Trial for Heart Health (OmniHeart) diet, and the low saturated fat Therapeutic Lifestyle Changes Diet (TLC) created by the National Institutes of Health's National Cholesterol Education Program.

The DASH (Dietary Approaches to Stop Hypertension) Eating Plan was designed 20 years ago to be low in sodium and to increase the intake of healthy foods with the main goal of lowering blood pressure. In addition to lowering blood pressure, the DASH diet also lowers LDL-C and reduces cardiovascular disease. The DASH Eating Plan is mostly plant-based, with small amounts of both animal and dairy products. The DASH diet emphasizes fruits, vegetables, and non-fat and low-fat dairy products; it includes whole grains, poultry, fish, and nuts; and it is low in red meat, sweets, and sugar-sweetened beverages. The DASH diet is much lower in sodium than the typical American diet and includes menus with two levels of sodium, 2,300, and 1,500 mg per day.[303 304 305]

The original DASH diet was relatively low in total fat (27% of calories) and higher (55% of calories) in carbohydrate. The OmniHeart study compared the effects of three modified DASH diets, each of which lowered blood pressure and improved blood lipids. One of the three OmniHeart diets emphasized carbohydrates (increased from 48% to 58% of total calories), another diet emphasized protein (increased from 15% to 25% of total calories), and the third emphasized unsaturated fat; with monounsaturated fat increased from 13% to 21%, and total fat increased from 27% to 35% of total calories. The study findings showed that the protein-rich and the unsaturated fat-rich diets provided additional benefits on blood pressure and blood lipids and further reduced the estimated ten-year risk of heart disease more than did the carbohydrate-rich diet. So in controlled feeding trials, each of the several modified DASH diets was found to significantly lower blood pressure and improve blood lipids compared with usual Western diets.[306 307 308 309 310] The DASH diet also reduces the risk of gout and chronic kidney disease.[311]

The Diabetes Prevention Program (DPP) is a fairly similar diet, again emphasizing a mix of foods—especially plant foods and select, mostly lean animal foods—and restrictions on refined starch and added sugar. In combination with routine, moderate physical activity, and associated weight loss, the DPP diet was associated with a 58% reduction in incident diabetes in adults at high risk.[312]

Low-glycemic diets

So how important to healthy nutrition is attention to the glycemic index of food? High glycemic index meals stimulate high insulin levels. They are followed in some individuals by an overshoot of the uptake of glucose, low blood sugar (reactive hypoglycemia), and elevated serum triglycerides. The result may include hunger from the hypoglycemia, excessive food intake, insulin resistance, the pancreatic beta cell dysfunction and damage that leads to diabetes, and, over an extended time, an unhealthy pattern of blood lipids and an increase in the risk for obesity, type 2 diabetes, and heart disease.[313]

The glycemic index (GI) is a measure of the blood glucose-raising potential of the carbohydrate content of a standard amount of a food compared to a reference food (generally pure glucose). The glycemic index indicates how rapidly a carbohydrate is digested and released as glucose (sugar) into the bloodstream. Consumption of high-GI foods causes a sharp increase in blood glucose concentration (and insulin release) after a meal that declines rapidly. In contrast, the consumption of low-GI foods results in a lower blood glucose concentration that decreases more gradually. Carbohydrate-containing foods can be classified as high- (≥70), moderate- (56-69), or low-GI (≤55) relative to pure glucose (GI=100). Sugars and most highly refined starchy foods (e.g., white bread, white potatoes) have a high glycemic index whereas non-starchy vegetables and legumes tend to have a low glycemic index.

The glycemic load (GL) index takes into account the total amount of the carbohydrate actually consumed. It multiplies the glycemic index of the food eaten by the carbohydrate content of the actual serving. The GL of food estimates how much the food will raise a person's blood glucose level after eating it. One unit of GL approximates the effect of consuming one gram of glucose. So, GL may be a better overall indicator of how a carbohydrate food will affect blood sugar. GL's of 10 or below are considered low, and 20 or above are considered high.[314]

Low-glycemic load diets have been shown to provide benefits, including weight loss, improved insulin metabolism, and better diabetes control. Some meta-analyses have concluded that meals with high glycemic load and index are associated with increased risk of cardiovascular disease, especially for women.[315] A meta-analysis of 28 trials has found that lowering the glycemic index of diets consistently reduced LDL-C but did not affect HDL-C or triglycerides.[316]

Table 3.3 Glycemic Indexes (GI) and Glycemic Loads (GL) for Common Foods

Food	GI	Serving Size	Net Carbs	GL
Peanuts	14	4 oz (113g)	15	2
Bean sprouts	25	1 cup (104g)	4	1
Grapefruit	25	½ large (166g)	11	3
Pizza	30	2 slices (260g)	42	13
Low-fat yogurt	33	1 cup (245g)	47	16
Apples	38	1 medium (138g)	16	6
Spaghetti	42	1 cup (140g)	38	16
Carrots	47	1 large (72g)	5	2
Oranges	48	1 medium (131g)	12	6
Bananas	52	1 large (136g)	27	14
Potato chips	54	4 oz (114g)	55	30
Snickers Bar	55	1 bar (113g)	64	35
Brown rice	55	1 cup (195g)	42	23
Honey	55	1 tbsp (21g)	17	9
Oatmeal	58	1 cup (234g)	21	12
Ice cream	61	1 cup (72g)	16	10
Macaroni & cheese	64	1 serving (166g)	47	30
Raisins	64	1 small box (43g)	32	20
White rice	64	1 cup (186g)	52	33
Sugar (sucrose)	68	1 tbsp (12g)	12	8
White bread	70	1 slice (30g)	14	10
Watermelon	72	1 cup (154g)	11	8
Popcorn	72	2 cups (16g)	10	7
Baked potato	85	1 medium (173g)	33	28
Glucose	100	(50g)	50	50

A listing of the GI and GL of 100 foods can be found at: http://www.health.harvard.edu/diseases-and-conditions/glycemic_index_and_glycemic_load_for_100_foods

Low-glycemic diets exclude intake of foods with a high glycemic index and/or glycemic load. These foods include processed foods containing refined starches and/

or added sugars, and usually all fruits and certain high-glycemic index vegetables. However, as Katz and Meller have noted, "Evidence that health benefits ensue from jettisoning fruits, or relatively high-glycemic-index vegetables, from the diet does not exist." Ludwig has noted, "…whereas the concept of glycemic index may be complex from a food science perspective, its public health application can be simple: increase consumption of fruits, vegetables, and legumes, choose grain products processed according to traditional rather than modern methods (e.g., stone-ground breads, old-fashioned oatmeal), and limit intake of potatoes and concentrated sugar. Indeed, these recommendations would tend to promote diets high in fiber, micronutrients, and antioxidants and low in energy density."[317]

In their assessment of the seven dietary patterns that they have identified, Katz and Meller reinforce this idea. They suggest that low-glycemic eating "…tends to occur as a by-product of favoring minimally processed, direct-from-nature foods and avoiding refined starch and added sugars. This basic approach to achieving reduced glycemic-load is compatible with all or nearly all of the other dietary approaches…"[318]

Low-carbohydrate diets

Low-carb eating has been popularized by many diet books. Katz and Meller note that, as is the situation with many diet categories, there is no agreed-on or fixed definition of a low-carbohydrate diet. They suggest that a diet with a carbohydrate intake below 45% of total calories would qualify as low-carbohydrate.[319] The original Atkins diet called for replacing carbohydrates with an unrestricted intake of meat and dairy.

A 2016 meta-analysis of randomized controlled trials assessed the effects of low-fat vs. low-carbohydrate diets on weight loss and risk factors of CVD. The low-carbohydrate diet was defined in accordance with the Atkins diet, or carbohydrate intake of <20% of total energy intake. The dietary goal for the low-fat diets was typical, with <30% of total energy as fat; however, a few studies had as low as 10% of total energy as fat. Compared with participants on low-fat diets, participants on low-carbohydrate diets experienced a greater reduction in body weight but a greater increase in HDL-C and unhealthy LDL-C. The study authors suggest that the beneficial changes of low-carbohydrate diets must be weighed against the possible detrimental effects of increased LDL-C.[320] Although good evidence from long-term studies is not available, an Atkins style high-protein, high fat, low-carbohydrate diets without calorie restriction can be expected to cause the adverse long-term health effects of the excessive saturated fat and protein found in typical American diets.[321]

In 2018, Professor Maciej Banach presented a study at the European Society of

Cardiology, stating: "We found that people who consumed a low carbohydrate diet were at greater risk of premature death. Risks were also increased for individual causes of death, including coronary heart disease, stroke, and cancer. These diets should be avoided."[322] The study found that compared to those in the highest carbohydrate group, those who ate the lowest carbohydrates had a 32% higher risk of all-cause death over six years, and risks of death from heart disease and cancer were increased by 51% and 35%, respectively. Banach said: "Low carbohydrate diets might be useful in the short term to lose weight, lower blood pressure, and improve blood glucose control, but our study suggests that in the long-term they are linked with an increased risk of death from any cause, and deaths due to cardiovascular disease, cerebrovascular disease, and cancer." In considering the reason for the difference in risk, he stated that: "The reduced intake of fiber and fruits and increased intake of animal protein, cholesterol, and saturated fat with these diets may play a role."

Newer, presumably healthier, versions of low carb eating, such as the Eco-Atkins diet studied by Jenkins and colleagues, emphasized consumption of high-protein plant rather than animal foods. A study of the Eco-Atkins diet that featured calorie restriction and plant-based low carbohydrate foods that included soy protein and nuts found that bodyweight declined and total cholesterol, LDL-C, triglycerides, and other cardiovascular biomarkers improved.[323]

The Portfolio Diet is a similar diet developed by the same team of researchers. It is based on the theory that putting together four dietary components, each shown to lower cholesterol by 5% to 10%, will be additive and maximize their effect. Based on a 2,000-calorie daily diet, the daily servings are:

- Plant protein: 50 grams a day, from soy foods such as tofu, soy milk, and soy meat analogs, plus legumes like beans, peas, and lentils
- Nuts: 45 grams a day of tree nuts of all kinds, including peanuts, as well as nut butters
- Viscous soluble fiber: 20 grams a day, from oats, barley, eggplant, okra, apples, berries, oranges, and psyllium
- Plant sterols: 2 grams a day, from fortified foods such as margarine spreads, juices, and yogurt, or from supplements with and without monounsaturated fats providing 26% of energy

A meta-analysis of seven clinical trials of the Portfolio Diet found that after four to 24 weeks, LDL-C declined by 27%.[324] The trials used a National Cholesterol Education Program (NCEP) diet with moderately low total fat (30% of calories) and low-saturated-fat (7% of calories) as a baseline comparison. Those on the NCEP diet reduced LDL-C by just 10%. The study authors concluded that the plant-based

Portfolio Diet reduced the estimated 10-year risk of heart disease by 13% and that the 33% reduction in LDL-C from the Portfolio Diet was a result comparable to that from statin therapy.

Paleolithic diets

The theory of Paleolithic diets is that by adhering to a diet prevalent in the Stone Age, when humans evolved, we will be consuming a diet to which our bodies are best adapted and, therefore, consuming the healthiest diet. Paleolithic diet versions vary considerably, but most feature avoidance of dairy, grains, and processed foods, and they emphasize consumption of vegetables, fruits, nuts and seeds, eggs, and lean meats. The Paleo diet also recommends avoiding some healthy foods, such as whole grains, dairy products, and beans.[325 326]

The theoretical basis for Paleo diets is shaky because of considerable uncertainty about the nature of a Stone Age dietary pattern. The Paleolithic period lasted 2.5 million years (2.6 million to 10,000 years ago), and many of the plant and animal foods consumed during the Stone Age are now extinct. The proportion of meat from hunting that was consumed compared to consumption of gathered plant foods is unknown, but plant microfossils have been found on the teeth of Neanderthals, and starches from grains and tubers have been found on Paleolithic grinding stones that predate agriculture by more than 10,000 years. Furthermore, most meat available today is from relatively sedentary animals bred for human consumption, raised on farms and ranches, and often fattened in feedlots. Therefore, currently available meat has different fat and other nutrient content compared to meat from wild animals, and it is highly likely to be even more different from the meat consumed in the Stone Age.

The nutritional health experts who participated in the 2019 *U.S. News & World Report* ranking of diets were not impressed with the Paleo diet.[327] In eight of nine categories, it ranked near the bottom at between 30 and 37 out of the 41 diets evaluated. The highest-ranking was 26 for Best Fast Weight-Loss Diet.

There is little long-term evidence of the health effects of currently advocated Paleo dietary patterns, but one study suggests that the Paleo diet would not be heart healthy over the long-term. A study of 44 subjects on the Paleo diet for just 10 weeks found that there was a significant increase in LDL-C by 12.5 mg/dL and total cholesterol by10.1 mg/dL.[328] Additional evidence comes from the work of professor Banach, whose previously described study suggests that low carbohydrate diets are unsafe because they increase LDL-C and should not be recommended.[329]

However, other short-term studies have found improvements in the metabolic syndrome biomarkers associated with poor health.[330 331] Evidence that the Paleo diet is healthy also comes from a study that found that diets that are the most Paleolithic- or Mediterranean-like may be associated with about a 25% lower risk of all-cause, cardiovascular-specific, cancer-specific, and other noninjury or accident-specific mortality.[332] The study found that the observed associations were slightly stronger for the Mediterranean diet pattern. The study also found that, especially the Paleolithic diet, higher consumption of nuts, and lower consumption of red and processed meats more strongly contributed to lower mortality than did other individual components of the diets.

Katz and Meller's summary comment on Paleolithic diets suggests commonality with other healthy diets. "Although superficially a departure from the other contending diets, a reasonable approximation of a true Paleolithic diet would, in fact, be relatively low in fat; low in the objectionable carbohydrate sources—namely, starches and added sugars; high in vegetables, fruits, nuts and seeds, and fiber; and low glycemic. An emphasis on lean meat remains distinctive, however, and may provide an advantage related particularly to satiety."[333]

In part, because most of the calories in a usual American diet come from carbohydrates, low-carb diets are almost invariably calorie-restricted. High-protein intake contributes to the preservation of muscle mass during weight loss, and adherence to the diet is facilitated by the high consumption of protein that provides a relatively high level of satiety. The beneficial metabolic effects of low carb and all other low-calorie diets are probably in part the result of calorie restriction and weight loss. For many people, low carb diets are effective at least for short duration weight loss. But longer-term, if low-carb eating includes large amounts of meat, it presents the CVD risk of increased LDL-C from the saturated fat in meat, also a feature of the TAD.

Ketogenic diets

Some high-meat, high-protein, low-carbohydrate diets, like the Atkins, South Beach, and Zone diets, are mistakenly referred to as ketogenic or "keto" diets. A true ketogenic diet must be very low-carb, with no more than 20 to 50 grams of carbohydrates a day, and up to 90% of daily food calories provided by fat. With usual nutrition, the body converts consumed or stored carbohydrates into glucose, the body's main source of energy. In the absence of carbohydrates (because they are restricted in the diet or during starvation), the liver makes ketone bodies from fat. They become the primary source of energy, and fat loss leads to weight loss. The body also converts some of the amino acids in protein into glucose—first from recently consumed food but when needed from the protein in muscles.

Problems with keto eating include the potential loss of muscle mass, increased LDL-C because they are likely to be high in saturated fat, nutrient deficiencies, and liver and kidney problems. Keto diets are deficient in important healthy foods, including fruits, legumes, and whole grains. Ketosis typically takes a few days to occur. It is usually unpleasant, with fatigue, confusion, irritability, sleep disturbances, muscle cramps, nausea, constipation, and other symptoms that are sometimes called "keto flu."

The keto diets advocated by their adherents are somewhat higher in carbs than true ketogenic diets. Typically, they derive 5% to 10% of calories from carbohydrates, 70% to 75% of calories from fat, and 20% from protein. Keto diets are likely to be low in calories, may suppress appetite, and undoubtedly help some people lose weight but cannot be considered a healthy long-term diet. They should not be undertaken except under medical supervision by individuals who are diabetic or so obese that they need to lose more than 50 pounds.[334] The expert panel advising U.S. News & World Report ranked the Keto diet in the last place in the Best Diet for Health category.[335]

Choosing a healthy diet

We have considered the typical American diet and reviewed the science about how nutrition affects health. Following is additional detail about food choices for my candidates for the two top diets: the ultra-low-fat, and the Mediterranean or mixed/balanced diets are similar to the Mediterranean diet).

The ultra-low-fat (ULF) plant-based diet

Ornish,[336] Esselstyn,[337] Connor,[338] McDougall,[339] Fuhrman,[340] and other clinicians and researchers who work directly with patients advocate the whole-food plant-based ultra-low-fat (ULF) diet. They have the experience of evaluating and helping many patients who have adopted the whole-food, plant-based, ULF diet they recommend. Their patients have lost weight, found relief from cardiac symptoms such as angina, and have improved their biomarkers, such as blood pressure, LDL-C, and other indicators of cardiovascular health. Uniquely ULF plant-based diets have been documented to bring about improved coronary artery blood flow.[341] The ULF plant-food advocates also cite the epidemiologic finding of a very low risk of cardiovascular diseases among indigenous populations that subsist on whole-food plant-based very-low-fat diets.

It should be acknowledged that the most extreme versions of ULF eating require more drastic changes from the typical American diet than other healthful diets. This raises the issue of adherence to the diet with dropouts at one year of about 50% found in two studies.[342 343] Dean Ornish recognizes that sticking to his diet recommendations at all times is not likely to be possible for many people.[344]

Diets shown to reverse atherosclerotic heart disease will almost certainly prevent it. And since, as we age, almost everyone develops some degree of atherosclerosis with the attendant cardiovascular impairments to health, it can be argued that everyone would be better off consuming the diet advocated by Ornish and Esselstyn. A summary of what to eat and what to avoid on the Ornish/Esselstyn ultra-low-fat (ULF) plant-based diet follows, for more details, see their publications and websites.[345 346]

An Ornish/Esselstyn diet consists of whole, unrefined, unprocessed plant-based foods, i.e., fruits, vegetables, whole grains, beans, soy, and legumes. The simplest description of a healthful ULF diet is "Beans and greens." Esselstyn's advice is to not eat "anything with a face or a mother."[347]

An Ornish/Esselstyn diet recommends:

- No oils, saturated or trans-fats, limit fat intake to 10-15% of total calories
- No refined grains or refined grain products (e.g., white bread, white rice)
- Minimal non-fat dairy or no dairy
- No nuts (although there is substantial evidence that nut consumption supports CV health)
- Minimal added sugars; especially avoid added sugars in the form of sodas and juices[348]
- Limiting sodium to 1,500 mg per day
- No processed foods—typically, they are high in added fat, sugar, and salt[349]
- No meat and (for some diets) no seafood
- No or limited alcohol

The Physician's Committee for Responsible Medicine advocates a very-low-fat vegetarian diet based on fruits, grains, legumes, and vegetables. The food guidance below is reproduced from their publication *Healthy Eating for Life: Food Choices for Cancer Prevention and Survival*.[350]

- Vegetables (4 or more servings a day), Serving size: 1 cup raw vegetables; 1/2 cup cooked vegetables
- Whole Grains (5 or more servings a day), Serving size: 1/2 cup hot cereal; 1 ounce dry cereal; 1 slice bread
- Fruit (3 or more servings a day), Serving size: 1 medium piece of fruit; 1/2 cup cooked fruit; 4 ounces juice
- Legumes (2 or more servings a day), including beans, peas, and lentils. This group also includes chickpeas, baked and refried beans, soymilk, tempeh,

and texturized vegetable protein. Serving size: 1/2 cup cooked beans; 4 ounces tofu or tempeh 8 ounces soymilk
- A good source of vitamin B-12, such as fortified foods or vitamin supplements

Mediterranean diets

A well-respected group of top nutrition experts, including a group in the Department of Nutrition at my old school, the Harvard T.H. Chan School of Public Health, including Stampfer, Willett, Hu, and Mozaffarian (now at Tufts), as well as authoritative studies by the FAO and 2020 Dietary Guidelines Advisory Committee (DGAC) advocate for the Mediterranean diet and healthful modifications of typical American diets.[351 352 353 354]

While there is general agreement that trans and saturated fats are harmful, and monounsaturated and polyunsaturated fats are relatively healthful, the Mediterranean diet advocates consider these "healthy fats" appropriate sources of a substantial amount of calories. In contrast, the ULF advocates would minimize the intake of all fats. They point out that merely restricting total fat calories has little impact on blood lipid biomarkers. Their overall conclusion is that the type of fats consumed appears to be far more relevant for cardiac and metabolic health than the proportion of calories consumed from total fat.[355 356] Their dietary advice concerning fat is to focus on the type of fat rather than the total amount, and they emphasize the risks of replacing fat with sugar and refined carbohydrates.[357] If your CVD biomarkers are not in a healthy range, the Mediterranean diet may be all that is needed to bring them to an ideal range.

What to eat when on a Mediterranean diet:

- Whole, unrefined, unprocessed plant-based foods, i.e., fruits, vegetables, whole grains, beans, and legumes.
- Healthier oils, polyunsaturates and, mainly, monounsaturates (e.g., olive oil)
- Limited dairy (mostly yogurt and cheese)
- Nuts and seeds
- Moderate seafood and poultry
- Moderate wine

What to avoid when on a Mediterranean diet:

- Processed foods
- Limit red meat
- Added sugars
- Trans and saturated fats

The Harvard Health Letter suggests measuring daily food totals in cups, ounces, and tablespoons rather than servings.[358] Depending on needed calorie intake, the Letter recommends the consumption of 2.5 to 3 cups of vegetables, including legumes, 1.5 to 2 cups of fruit, half a cup of whole grains, 5 to 6 ounces of poultry, or fish, and 1 to 2 tablespoons of healthy oils.

EAT-Lancet Commission Recommendations

Twenty experts prepared the EAT-Lancet Commission report, *Our Food in the Anthropocene: Healthy Diets from Sustainable Food Systems*.[359] The Commission developed global targets for healthy diets and sustainable food production. The science-based target for healthy diets is those composed largely of vegetables and fruits, whole grains, legumes, nuts, and unsaturated oils; low to moderate consumption of seafood and poultry; and zero to low consumption of red meat, processed meat, added sugar, refined grains, and starchy vegetables. The Commission noted that currently, the average intake of healthy foods is far below recommended levels, overconsumption of unhealthy foods is increasing, and that healthier diets would reduce the environmental degradation and contribution to climate change arising from food production.

The Commission concluded that dietary patterns with the following characteristics reduce risk of major chronic disease and promote overall wellbeing:

- Protein sources primarily from plants, including soy foods, other legumes, and nuts; fish or alternative sources of omega-3 fatty acids several times per week, with optional modest consumption of poultry and eggs; low intakes of red meat, if any, especially processed meat
- Fat, 15% (7% to 29%) of energy, largely from unsaturated plant sources, with low intakes of saturated fats; no partially hydrogenated oils
- Carbohydrates primarily from whole grains up to 60% of energy with limited intake refined grains and sugar less 5% of energy
- At least five servings of fruits and vegetables per day, not including potatoes
- Moderate dairy consumption as an option

The Commission report noted that there is strong scientific evidence that food production is the single largest cause of global environmental damage. Agriculture occupies nearly 40% of global land, is responsible for up to 30% of global greenhouse gas (GHG) emissions, especially those caused by ruminant farm animals, 70% of freshwater use and extensive degradation of land. The conversion of natural ecosystems to croplands and pastures is the single largest cause of biodiversity loss and species to be threatened with extinction.

Diets that are both unhealthy and environmentally unsustainable are high in calories, added sugars, saturated fats, highly processed foods and red meats. A new global food system that provides healthier diets for a growing world population and preserves essential natural systems is needed and possible. It requires improving crop yields, zero-expansion of agriculture into natural ecosystems and species-rich forests, better management of the world's oceans and fisheries, and cutting food losses and wastage.

The Nutrition Facts Label can help to make the best food choices

Because most processed foods are loaded with sugar, salt, and fat, the best food to buy is whole unprocessed and plant-based produce that does not need a Nutrition Facts Label (NFL). Consumers can make better choices when they consider the NFL label and understand the meaning of the NFL food label terms.

Daily Value (DV): This is the percentage that a serving of the labeled food contributes to a healthy diet. For example, it is recommended that in a 2000 calorie diet, saturated fat should be limited to 20 grams, so if a portion of food had 5 grams of saturated fat, the DV would be listed as 25%. You might want to consume less than the DV of some nutrients. The 2015 DGAC recommended consuming a maximum of 10% of daily calories from saturated fat. This would be 22 grams of saturated fat. However, the American Heart Association's recommendation is that only 5% to 6% of daily calories should be supplied by saturated fat.

Sugar: The NFL provides a listing of total sugar and separately list the amount of the healthy sugars found in fruits and vegetables and the amount of unhealthy added sugars.

Calories per serving: The NFL lists the calories in a serving to reflect the amounts of food people actually eat. "Low calorie" on the label means 40 or fewer calories per serving, "reduced calorie" means 25% fewer calories than in a same-size serving of the original food, and "light or lite" means 33% fewer calories than in a same-size serving of the original food.

Fat: "Reduced fat" on the label means at least 25% less fat per serving compared to the original food; "low-fat" signifies 3 grams of fat or less per serving; "fat-free" is 0.5 grams or less fat per serving; and "trans-fat free" signifies 0.5 grams of trans-fat or less per serving.

Sodium: "Reduced sodium" means 25% less sodium than in a same-size serving of the original food; "light in sodium or lightly salted" signifies 50% less sodium than in a same-size serving of the original food. "Low sodium" means 140 mg or less per serving; "very low sodium" means 35 mg or less per serving, and "salt/sodium free" means less than 5 mg sodium per serving. "No salt added or unsalted" means no salt was added in processing, but it does not mean that the product is sodium-free.

Vitamins and minerals: "Excellent source of" means the food has at least 20% of the daily value of that vitamin or mineral per serving: "good source of" means the food has 10-19% of the daily value; "enriched with" lists added vitamins and/or minerals; and "fortified with" signifies adding vitamins and/or minerals that are not in the product naturally. Consumers should be aware that while it is not likely, it is possible to get too much of a specific dietary supplement from fortified foods.

A side-by-side comparison with the old label and key changes of the new NFL is shown in Figure 3.2.

Figure 3.2. The Nutrition Facts Label

The New and Improved Nutrition Facts Label – Key Changes

The U.S. Food and Drug Administration has finalized a new Nutrition Facts label for packaged foods that will make it easier for you to make informed food choices that support a healthy diet. The updated label has a fresh new design and reflects current scientific information, including the link between diet and chronic diseases.

1. Servings

The number of "servings per container" and the "Serving Size" declaration have increased and are now in larger and/or bolder type. Serving sizes have been updated to reflect what people actually eat and drink today. For example, the serving size for ice cream was previously ½ cup and now is ¾ cup.

There are also new requirements for certain size packages, such as those that are between one and two servings or are larger than a single serving but could be consumed in one or multiple sittings.

2. Calories

"Calories" is now larger and bolder.

3. Fats

"Calories from Fat" has been removed because research shows the type of fat consumed is more important than the amount.

4. Added Sugars

"Added Sugars" in grams and as a percent Daily Value (%DV) is now required on the label. "Added Sugars" include sugars that have been added during the processing or packaging of a food. Scientific data shows that it is difficult to meet nutrient needs while staying within calorie limits if you consume more than 10 percent of your total daily calories from added sugar.

5. Nutrients

The lists of nutrients that are required or permitted on the label have been updated. Vitamin D and potassium are now required on the label because Americans do not always get the recommended amounts. Vitamins A and C are no longer required since deficiencies of these vitamins are rare today. The actual amount in grams in addition to the %DV must be listed for vitamin D, calcium, iron, and potassium.

The daily values for nutrients have also been updated based on newer scientific evidence. The daily values are reference amounts of nutrients to consume or not to exceed and are used to calculate the %DV.

6. Footnote

The footnote at the bottom of the label has changed to better explain the meaning of %DV. The %DV helps you understand the nutrition information in the context of a total daily diet.

Current Label

Nutrition Facts

Serving Size 2/3 cup (55g)
Servings Per Container About 8

Amount Per Serving	
Calories 230	Calories from Fat 72
	% Daily Value*
Total Fat 8g	**12%**
Saturated Fat 1g	**5%**
Trans Fat 0g	
Cholesterol 0mg	**0%**
Sodium 160mg	**7%**
Total Carbohydrate 37g	**12%**
Dietary Fiber 4g	**16%**
Sugars 1g	
Protein 3g	
Vitamin A	10%
Vitamin C	8%
Calcium	20%
Iron	45%

* Percent Daily Values are based on a 2,000 calorie diet. Your daily value may be higher or lower depending on your calorie needs.

	Calories:	2,000	2,500
Total Fat	Less than	65g	80g
Sat Fat	Less than	20g	25g
Cholesterol	Less than	300mg	300mg
Sodium	Less than	2,400mg	2,400mg
Total Carbohydrate		300g	375g
Dietary Fiber		25g	30g

New Label

Nutrition Facts

1 8 servings per container
Serving size 2/3 cup (55g)

2 **Amount per serving**
Calories 230

	% Daily Value*
3 **Total Fat** 8g	**10%**
Saturated Fat 1g	**5%**
Trans Fat 0g	
Cholesterol 0mg	**0%**
Sodium 160mg	**7%**
Total Carbohydrate 37g	**13%**
Dietary Fiber 4g	**14%**
Total Sugars 12g	
4 Includes 10g Added Sugars	**20%**
Protein 3g	
5 Vitamin D 2mcg	10%
Calcium 260mg	20%
Iron 8mg	45%
Potassium 235mg	6%

6 * The % Daily Value (DV) tells you how much a nutrient in a serving of food contributes to a daily diet. 2,000 calories a day is used for general nutrition advice.

Manufacturers will need to use the new label by July 26, 2018, and small businesses will have an additional year to comply. During this transition time, you will see the current Nutrition Facts label or the new label on products.

July 2016

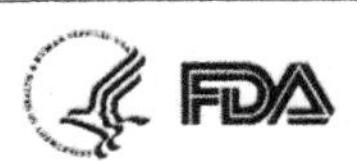

For more information about the new Nutrition Facts label, visit:
www.fda.gov/Food/GuidanceRegulation/GuidanceDocumentsRegulatoryInformation/LabelingNutrition/ucm385663.htm

Are there categories of foods that we should emphasize or eliminate?

What about dairy, fish, organic foods, artificial sweeteners, gluten, genetically modified organisms (GMOs), coffee, tea, and the microbiome? Many Americans have strong feelings about these foods. What does science say? Are they good for us, or harmful, or neither?

Dairy foods

Dairy foods contain a variety of nutrients, including vitamins, fatty acids, protein, calcium, potassium, and in the U.S. they are often fortified with vitamin D. Low-fat dairy foods have been associated with lowered blood pressure, improved blood lipid profiles, improved insulin resistance and lower incidence of diabetes. Milk consumption is associated with an increased risk of prostate cancer,[360] probably no increased risk of endometrial (uterine) cancer,[361] a reduced risk of colorectal cancer,[362] and has been inconsistently associated with cardiovascular disease,[363 364 365] and type 2 diabetes.[366 367] Milk consumption does not appear to reduce the risk of hip fractures.[368]

A 2013 meta-analysis of 20 randomized trials showed a non-significant increase in LDL-C with either higher intake of whole-fat dairy or low-fat dairy.[369] A 2015 meta-analysis considering links between milk consumption and mortality found no consistent association between milk consumption and all-cause or cause-specific mortality.[370] A 2016 meta-analysis found that total dairy products intakes have no significant impact on increased all cancer mortality risk, but whole milk intake in men contributed to significantly elevated prostate cancer mortality risk.[371] The naturally occurring hormones in milk may be the link between high consumption of milk and any increased risk of cancer. A 2017 meta-analysis combining data from 29 prospective cohort studies demonstrated no association between dairy products and cardiovascular and all-cause mortality.[372]

A Swedish study found that mortality rates were up to nearly three times higher among women with high consumption of milk who also had low consumption of fruits and vegetables. A less pronounced increase in risk was found among men. The authors consider that D-galactose is the component of milk that harms health because it causes oxidative stress damage and chronic inflammation; and that the antioxidants in fruits and vegetables mitigate that risk.[373] One study found that the replacement of 5% of energy intake from dairy fat with equivalent energy intake from polyunsaturated fatty acid (PUFA) or vegetable fat was associated with a lower risk of CVD, whereas a 5% energy intake substitution of other animal fat with dairy fat was associated with a 6% increased CVD risk.[374] In addition, the replacement of dairy fat with high-quality carbohydrates from whole grains is associated with a lower risk of CVD.

A 2018 meta-analysis study (PURE) questions the long-standing dietary advice to avoid full-fat dairy products in favor of non-fat or low-fat products.[375] The PURE study was conducted in 21, mostly low or middle-income countries. The study found that over a nine-year follow-up, compared to no intake, two or more daily servings of full-fat dairy foods were associated with a 22% lower risk of heart disease, a 34% lower risk of stroke, and a 23% lower risk of death from cardiovascular disease. In the PURE study, cheese or butter intake was not significantly associated with decreased or increased risk. The relevance of the PURE study for North America and Europe is questionable because dairy consumption and saturated fatty acids intake in these regions is high compared to most of the regions of the world in the study. In addition, the study did not adjust for socioeconomic variables, and in many of the 21 countries, wealthier residents may have both higher consumption of dairy and other foods and other factors that lead to better nutritional and health status and lower death rates.

Neal Barnard has evaluated the health impacts of cheese, and warns against the overconsumption of cheese, a high saturated fat, high sodium, high cholesterol, calorie-dense food that he considers can be addictive.[376] However, some research suggests cheese has less impact on raising LDL-C than butter.[377] Cheese is a fermented dairy product, and, in a cohort study, total fermented food intake was not found to be associated with mortality due to all causes.[378] Some studies have found a lower risk of CVD among high consumers of cheese, and a meta-analysis found no significant association between cheese consumption and all-cause mortality.[379]

The possible varying health effects of specific dairy foods such as milk, yogurt, cheese, and butter have not been well established. The most that can be said is that research on the links between dairy foods and health are inconclusive and are still being investigated. Because low-fat and non-fat dairy has a lower content of calories, SFA, and cholesterol than whole-fat dairy, they are recommended by most dietary guidelines and scientific organizations.[380] Chapter 12, "Preventing Osteoporosis," discusses the role of dairy foods on osteoporosis.

Fish

Fish is rich in the long-chain polyunsaturated omega-3 fatty acids, eicosapentanoic acid (EPA) and docosahexonoic acid (DHA) and low in saturated fatty acids. The American Heart Association recommends eating one serving (3.5 oz. cooked, or about ¾ cup of flaked fish) of a variety of fish at least twice a week. Omega-3 fatty acids from fish are associated with decreased risk of abnormal heartbeats (arrhythmias), which can cause sudden death, decreased triglyceride levels, and decreased risk of diabetic retinopathy and atherosclerotic plaque.[381] [382] [383] [384] [385] [386] [387] A meta-analysis of 19 different studies found that consumption of fish was associated with about a 20% decrease in unstable angina and heart attack among those who ate the most fish, four times per week.[388] The discussion of omega-3 fatty acids earlier in this chapter presented evidence that fish oil supplements do not seem to provide that same benefits that fish do.[389]

The omega-3 content of fish varies according to their species and whether they are farmed or not. Fatty fish like salmon, mackerel, herring, lake trout, sardines, and albacore tuna are high in omega-3 fatty acids. Other fish are lower in omega-3 content. For example, tilapia has about 0.2 grams of omega-3s per serving compared to wild or farmed salmon with more than 1.5 grams.

Fish is not risk-free. Some types of fish may contain high levels of mercury, mostly in the form of methylmercury, PCBs (polychlorinated biphenyls), dioxins and other environmental contaminants. Levels of these substances are generally highest in animals at the top of the food chain that are older, larger, and in predatory fish. Mercury is of concern, especially for children and pregnant women, because of the potential for adverse effects on fetal and child neurodevelopment and adult cardiovascular disease.[390] Children and pregnant women are advised by the FDA to avoid eating fish with the potential for the highest level of mercury contamination (e.g., shark, swordfish, king mackerel or tilefish); and to only eat up to 12 ounces (two average meals) per week of a variety of fish and shellfish that are lower in mercury. Low mercury seafood includes shrimp, scallops, sardines, salmon, oysters, tilapia canned light tuna, pollock, and catfish. [391] [392] [393]

An increasing share of fish sold in the U.S. is farmed and imported. These sources also entail risks to health. Aquaculture feeds fish with an unnatural diet that may include high levels of pesticides, antibiotics, and other toxins. China supplies almost 60% of the $90 billion global aquaculture trade, and contamination of Chinese seafood with antibiotics is not uncommon. Foreign countries provide 90% of the shrimp consumed in the U.S., and that too is sometimes rejected by the FDA because of antibiotic contamination. Fish farmed in Canada and European countries have a better safety record than those from Asian and Latin American countries that have less rigorous standards for the avoidance of contamination and for minimizing the environmental impact of their farming methods.[394] [395] [396] [397]

There are a variety of guides to assist consumers in buying seafood that is both healthy and responsibly farmed or wild-caught. The Environmental Defense Fund (EDF) has a Seafood Selector that is available at http://seafood.edf.org/guide/best The Monterey Bay Seafood Watch website at https://www.seafoodwatch.org provides U.S. state-specific guides to sustainable seafood.

Eating fish and other kinds of seafood can be healthy, but making choices that are safe and ecologically responsible requires careful selection. It may be just as beneficial to health to substitute plant-based foods, vegetables, fruit, beans, and nuts for red meat and processed meats as it is to substitute seafood. There is just not enough wild or farmed seafood for all 7.8 billion of us on the planet to eat seafood twice a week.[398]

Organic foods

Organic food is produced according to standards and practices that strive to recycle resources and to be ecologically sound. In 2015, $43.3 billion, or nearly 5% of U.S. food sold was organic. Typically, organic food is produced without the use of most pesticides, harmful fertilizers, food additives, or genetically modified ingredients. Livestock must be fed certified organic food that contains no animal by-products, have liberal access to pasture, and the use of antibiotics (except for illnesses) or growth hormones is not allowed.

The U.S. Department of Agriculture's National Organic Program is responsible for the legal definition of organic and organic certification. If food products claim to be "natural" or "all natural" on their label, it does not mean that they were produced and processed organically.[399] The term natural on a label is mainly an advertising stratagem, and it does not mean very much.

Because organic food production restricts the use of certain chemical fertilizers, herbicides, and pesticides, there is the perception that it may be safer, healthier, and better for the environment. It is generally not recognized by the public that edible plants have evolved natural pesticides as a defense against insects and other hazards, and exposure to natural pesticides is usually much greater than the total daily exposure to synthetic pesticide residues. Because the human body detoxifies these natural and synthetic chemicals similarly, the scientific case for an advantage for the health and safety of organic foods over those produced with conventional farming methods is far from conclusive.[400]

A 2012 meta-analysis noted that "there have been no long-term studies of health outcomes of populations consuming predominantly organic versus conventionally produced food controlling for socioeconomic factors; such studies would be expensive to conduct."[401] A large Million Women Study in the U.K. linked self-reported organic food intake to a 21% lower risk of non-Hodgkin lymphoma.[402] However, the study also found that organic food consumption was linked to a slightly increased breast cancer risk, which raises questions about the meaning of the findings. A French study reported that those eating high amounts of organic foods had a decreased risk of cancer of six cases per 1000 over a 4.5-year period.[403] The association was restricted to the risk of postmenopausal breast cancer and lymphomas among those reporting the highest intake of organic foods. The implications of this study are also uncertain, in part, but those consuming the most organic foods also were likely to have other healthier habits.

Organic foods also appear to provide little advantage with regard to taste, or nutritive value, or freedom from harmful bacteria.[404 405 406] Other reviews have been more positive about possible benefits of organic foods noting that some studies have found that there is neurotoxicity associated with pesticides in farmworker communities, including subtle but important effects on neurological development, including reduced IQs.[407 408 409 410 411 412 413 414]

The American Cancer Society has stated that there is no evidence that eating organic food reduces cancer risk or that the small amount of pesticide residue found on conventional foods will increase the risk of cancer. However, it does recommend thoroughly washing fruits and vegetables. Elena Hemler suggests that "Concerns over pesticide risks should not discourage intake of conventional fruits and vegetables, especially because organic produce is often expensive and inaccessible to many populations."[415]

Although more costly than conventionally produced foodstuffs, organically produced foods may offer some advantages if they are fresh or minimally processed. Organic produce contains fewer pesticide residues than does conventional produce. In keeping with the precautionary principle, that is desirable. But the value of such a reduction in exposure to human health remains uncertain. Organically produced foods may also be better for the environment than those produced by conventional farming practices, and undoubtedly they contribute to animal welfare.[416]

Artificial sweeteners

Because they are widely used and consumed by many people, artificial sweeteners have been extensively studied and require approval by the FDA. The eight FDA approved artificial sweeteners are:[417 418]

- Aspartame (Equal® or NutraSweet®)
- Acesulfame potassium (ACK, Sunett® and Sweet One®)
- Neotame (Newtame®)
- Saccharin (Sweet 'N Low®, Sweet Twin® and Sugar Twin®)
- Sucralose (Splenda® and Equal Sucralose); can be used as a replacement for sugar in cooking and baking
- Stevia (Truvia®, Stevia in the Raw®, SweetLeaf® Sweet Drops™, Sun

Crystals® and PureVia®); extracted from the leaves of the stevia plant
- Luo han guo (Monk fruit extract) (Monk Fruit in the Raw ®); natural sweetener made from crushed monk fruit
- Advantame; not commonly used at this time

The FDA has not permitted the use of whole-leaf Stevia or crude Stevia extracts because these substances have not been proven to be safe but has allowed the use of certain highly refined Stevia preparations in food products.[419] Sugar alcohols, another class of sweeteners, can also be used as sugar substitutes. Examples include sorbitol, xylitol, lactitol, mannitol, erythritol, and maltitol. They are mainly used to sweeten sugar-free candies, cookies, and chewing gums.[420]

The FDA has reviewed hundreds of safety studies, including animal studies with much higher doses than people would possibly consume, and concluded that available evidence shows that they do not cause cancer or pose any other threat to human health.[421 422 423] A National Cancer Institute study found no increase in the risk of lymphoma, leukemia, or brain cancer in the highest categories of consumption of aspartame-sweetened beverages (equivalent to 7 to 11 cans of soft drinks daily) compared with the lowest categories of consumption.[424] Individuals who have phenylketonuria (PKU), an inherited error of metabolism, have a decreased ability to metabolize the amino acid phenylalanine. They should avoid aspartame because it breaks down to form phenylalanine.

Although there is a popular belief that sugar and artificial sweeteners are associated with hyperactive behavior and cognition problems among children, studies have found no evidence that high consumption of sucrose or aspartame affects children's or adult's behavior or cognitive function.[424 425 426 427 428 429 430 431 432 433]

At one time, it was thought and reported in the medical literature that low-calorie sweeteners stimulate appetite or adversely affect mechanisms that regulate hunger and satiety. According to a Canadian Diabetes Association National Nutrition Committee Technical Review, current evidence does not support this belief.[434] Although studies suggest that artificial sweeteners are generally safe, there is little consistent evidence that they assist weight loss or cause weight gain and some evidence that they disrupt gut bacteria and normal bodily metabolism in ways that favor deposition of fat.[435]

The Nurses' Health Study and Health Professionals Follow-up Study found that over 28 years of follow-up for women and 22 years of follow-up for men, a greater consumption of both sugar and artificially sweetened soft drinks was each independently associated with a higher risk of stroke.[436] A 2017 study in the journal *Stroke* reported that consuming a can a day of a low- or no-sugar soft drink, but not sugar-sweetened beverages, is associated with a higher risk of having a stroke or developing dementia.[437] The associations with dementia were not statistically significant after additional adjustment for vascular risk factors and diabetes. A 2019 meta-analysis of 56 studies found that some studies linked non-sugar sweeteners to a reduced risk of diabetes and overweight, but other research suggests that they increase the risk of these conditions and cancer.[438] The study found no evidence of substantial harm, but negative health effects from long-term high dose use could not be ruled out.

The 2015 DGAC report states that aspartame in amounts commonly consumed is safe and poses a minimal health risk for healthy individuals, but that additional study of safety is advisable because limited and inconsistent evidence suggests a possible association between aspartame and risk of some blood cancers (non-Hodgkin lymphoma and multiple myeloma) in men (but not women).[439] In addition, limited and inconsistent evidence indicates a potential for risk of preterm delivery for pregnant women.[440] The 2015 DGAC recommends that individuals should stay below the aspartame Acceptable Daily Intake (ADI) of no more than 50 mg/kg/day or 3500 mg/day for a 70 kg person. Since a 12-ounce diet beverage contains approximately 180 mg of aspartame, this would imply a limit of nineteen 12-ounce servings per day for a 154-pound person.[441]

The bottom line is that for most of us, usual levels of consumption of aspartame, the most commonly used artificial sweetener, probably present a low risk to health. This risk can be eliminated by drinking water, a less expensive drink.

Gluten free eating

Gluten is the major protein found in wheat, barley, and rye. Movie stars and leading sports figures have lauded the health benefits of gluten-free eating, but there is no scientific evidence of a benefit for most people. Even so, the Consumer Reports National Research Center found that 63% of Americans surveyed thought that going gluten-free would help with weight loss or improve their physical or mental health.[442]

Gluten phobia and avoiding gluten makes sense for the fewer than 1% of Americans with a genetic predisposition to celiac disease and perhaps for the 6% of Americans who have a gluten sensitivity that causes celiac disease symptoms without intestinal damage. Celiac disease is an autoimmune condition in which gluten causes intestinal damage that interferes with the intestinal absorption of nutrients.[443]

For others, rather than being a benefit to health, gluten-free foods are likely to be less nutritious than similar conventional foods because many gluten-free foods are not fortified with vitamins and ingredients such as iron. To restore their taste, gluten-free foods are likely to be made with the high levels of unhealthy ingredients, salt, fat, and sugar, often found in processed foods. Consumer Reports also found that half of the gluten-free foods they tested contained rice flour or rice in another form that contained measurable levels of the toxic inorganic chemical arsenic, a carcinogen. Unless rice-free foods are selected, eating a gluten-free diet might lead to the consumption of a significant amount of arsenic.[444 445]

Going gluten-free should be considered an unproven food enthusiasm that is not a good idea for most people because eating whole grains is associated with good health. A slice of 100% whole grain bread weighing one ounce contains about 16 grams of whole grains. A meta-analysis of 45 studies found that a 90 gm/day increase in whole grain intake resulted in a 17% decrease in risk of mortality from all causes.[446] A similar meta-analysis found that compared to those in the lowest category of whole grain consumption, those in the highest category of consumption had a 16% lower risk of all-cause mortality and an 18% lower risk of CVD mortality.[447]

Gluten-free foods cost about twice as much as their conventional counterparts, and they were a $23.3 billion market in the U.S. in 2014. Most of us would be well advised to skip the gluten-free fad and save our money. We should stick to the current Dietary Guidelines for Americans that call for at least three servings per day of whole-grain intake.

Genetically modified organisms (GMOs)—the pros and cons

It appears that a substantial share of the public is disturbed by the prospect of genetic modification of living things and distrustful of the scientific consensus that foods from plants containing genetically modified ingredients are safe to eat and safe for the environment. Even before the U.S. Congress passed a law in 2016, requiring the nationwide labeling of genetically modified food ingredients, consumers saw more and more products labeled "GMO-free." In her *New York Times* article "Fear Not Fact, Behind GMO Labeling," Jane Brody noted that, "As happened with the explosion of gluten-free products, food companies are quick to cash in on what they believe consumers want, regardless of whether it is scientifically justified."[448]

The National Academies of Sciences, Engineering and Medicine (NASEM) found that GMO crops had "no differences that would implicate a higher risk to human health." The World Health Organization also concluded that GMOs are safe to eat. And the FDA has banned claims that GMO free food is "safer, more nutritious or otherwise has different attributes." The marketing of many products as "Non-GMO" may be misleading because genetically modified versions of the same product do not exist.[449] And labeling some other foods non-GMO means little, for example, DNA from genetically engineered feed is not passed on to meat or milk.

Some bioengineered characteristics seem to have little downside. For example, tolerance to drought or irrigation with saltier water or resistance to insect pests that would eliminate the need to spray with insecticides would seem to be mostly advantageous. Since introduction in the U.S. in 1996, by now, more than 90% of the acreage of planted soybeans, cotton, corn, and sugar beets is bioengineered.[450] Most U.S. corn and almost all U.S. soybeans are bioengineered so farmers can spray them with glyphosate (the main ingredient in Roundup) to kill weeds without harming the crop. There is a legitimate concern about the environmental impact of the widespread use of glyphosate, a possible human carcinogen, that reached 113 million kg annually by 2014. Public health experts urge more scrutiny of the practice and careful testing of the use of newer herbicides, including agent orange, that are designed to work with glyphosate to combat herbicide resistance.[451]

An analysis by the using United Nations data showed that in the United States and Canada, bioengineered seeds have yielded no discernible advantage in crop yields—food per acre—when measured against Western Europe, a region with comparably modernized agricultural producers like France and Germany.[452]

Many people are afraid of GMOs, but there is scant evidence that they cause harm to health. Of course, society must continue to ensure that the benefits of GMOs outweigh any risks. The NASEM recommends that new crop varieties—whether genetically engineered or conventionally bred—be subjected to safety testing.[453] Remember that conventionally bred crops undergo no government testing. Just as there is no reason to pay extra for gluten-free foods, so far, there seems to be no reason to select or pay more for GMO-free foods.

The microbiome

The human microbiota consists of the 10 to 100 trillion symbiotic microbial cells in or on each person. They are mostly bacteria and other microorganisms found in the intestinal tract. Our gut microbiota help synthesize essential vitamins, steroid hormones, and protect the intestinal tract from colonization with harmful germs. They also allow us to digest compounds via non-human metabolic pathways, greatly increasing our ability to extract energy from our diverse diets. Certain mixes of gut microbiota may help prevent or predispose a person to obesity, and they may play a role in type 2 diabetes, insulin resistance, and chronic low-grade inflammation.

Although there is increasing evidence that a person's microbiota can affect digestion, and other aspects of metabolism, the influence of gut microbiota on health is not well understood. The modulation of a patient's microbiota to a healthy state with probiotics (live bacteria), prebiotics (that stimulate the growth and activity of beneficial microorganisms), and antibiotics is being explored for weight control and health. However, in spite of extensive health claims, only a few probiotic foods have been shown by sound research to provide any benefits. For example, their utility to treat diarrheal disease in children has been disappointing.[454 455 456 457 458 459 460]

Coffee and tea

Coffee is a giant ($48 billion per year) retail business in the U.S., where about 75% of adults drink coffee from time to time. At an average of about three cups a day, coffee is a pervasive daily ritual for 54% of Americans age 18 and older. Coffee contains more than 1000 chemicals, and the health effects of coffee are still being explored. There may be some modest benefits from drinking coffee, perhaps related mainly to its content of antioxidants, and little evidence of harm beyond the side effects of caffeine habituation.

Coffee has about 100 mg. of the stimulant caffeine in a 6 oz. cup. There is considerable variation in susceptibility to the side effects of caffeine; for example, some people metabolize it up to four times faster than others. Too much caffeine—more than 300 mg per day—may cause insomnia and nervousness, and slow metabolizers may be at increased risk of heart attack and hypertension.[461] Among coffee drinkers, liver disease, type 2 diabetes, colon cancer, prostate cancer, and some other cancers appear to be a little less likely.[462 463] Altogether, the evidence suggests that there is no health-related reason not to drink coffee but no strong reason to start drinking coffee based on health benefits.[464 465 466]

Tea is the most widely consumed beverage in the world after water. Many of the same potential benefits of coffee are similar for tea. Studies have shown inconsistent but mostly beneficial effects of tea on diabetes, heart disease, stroke, neurodegenerative diseases, and obesity. Tea has not conclusively been shown to decrease the risk of cancer.[467 468] Unless it is decaffeinated, tea has, on average, 40 mg of caffeine per 6 oz. cup, less than coffee at 100 mg. per cup, but still a factor for those who are sensitive to caffeine. It is best to avoid green tea supplements. Like many dietary supplements, they are unproven to have benefits and are not proven to be safe. Studies suggest that "Tea's effects in the body are still not fully understood, but don't expect it to prevent heart disease, cancer or any other condition on its own."[469 470]

Summary of the essential facts

- Anyone taking medication or with a health problem should obtain medical advice and supervision when changing their diet.

- Nutrition is an important Building Block of Health, especially cardiovascular health.
- The typical American diet is not healthy. It contains too much saturated fat, meat (especially red and processed meat), refined grains (white bread, white rice), sodium (salt), added sugars, highly processed food, and too many calories.
- The typical American diet contributes to high total cholesterol and high LDL cholesterol, elevated blood pressure, and obesity—unhealthy conditions that increase the risk of leading causes of illness and death: heart disease, cancer, stroke, and diabetes.
- Nutrition experts generally agree that a healthy diet eliminates all trans-fats, minimizes saturated fats and is low in sodium, added sugars and products made from refined grains; and it includes high levels of whole, unprocessed plant-based foods: legumes, whole grains, fruits, beans, and vegetables, all foods that are high in unrefined carbohydrates and fiber.
- Many nutrition experts consider that consumption of non-fat dairy, seafood, nuts, healthy oils (polyunsaturated and monounsaturated oils), and, possibly, limited amounts of lean meat and alcohol can also be considered to be components of healthy nutrition.
- Other nutrition experts make the case that an optimal diet is whole-food, plant-based and eliminates trans-fats, saturated fats, almost all oils, all meat, all seafood, most dairy, and added sugars, and is extremely low in fat with no more than 15% or better yet 10% of total calories coming from fats.
- All weight-loss diets work by limiting calories, and all diets that limit calories improve health biomarkers, but only healthy diets should be considered for long-term nutrition.
- Sustained maintenance of normal weight is much more likely among people who both have healthy diets and are physically active—more on this in Chapter 4, "Weight Control."

Additional reading

Here are some books and references relating to the links between nutrition and health:

Ornish D, *The Spectrum*. New York: Ballantine Books, 2007.

Esselstyn CB. *Prevent and Reverse Heart Disease*. New York: Penguin Group, 2007.

Willett W, Skerrett PJ. *Eat, Drink, and Be Healthy*. New York: Free Press/ Simon

& Schuster, 2017.

Dietary Guidelines Advisory Committee. *Scientific Report of the 2015 Dietary Guidelines Advisory Committee. Advisory Report to the Secretary of Agriculture and the Secretary of Health and Human Services.* U.S. Department of Agriculture, Agricultural Research Service, Washington, DC., 2015.

Dietary Guidelines Advisory Committee. Scientific Report of the *2020 Dietary Guidelines Advisory Committee: Advisory Report to the Secretary of Agriculture and the Secretary of Health and Human Services*. U.S. Department of Agriculture, Agricultural Research Service, Washington, DC., 2020.

2015-2020 Dietary Guidelines for Americans. https://health.gov/dietaryguidelines/2015/guidelines/

The *2015-2020 Dietary Guidelines for Americans* is a nearly 200-page U.S. government report with much good advice about nutrition, but as in the case of previous *Guidelines*, in the opinion of many nutrition experts, in some ways it is a useful advance, but it also falls short of reflecting the best science-based advice about nutrition.

4
Weight Control

You may have skipped forward to read this chapter first because among healthy lifestyle behaviors, attaining and maintaining a normal weight is the Building Block of good health that is the most difficult for many people. Over the past 40 years, an alarming 70% of U.S. adults have become overweight or obese. Because living with a high amount of body fat has serious consequences for health, and because of the frequency of relapses after weight loss, obesity can be classified as a chronic disease.[1]

Most of the obesity epidemic is a result of our behavior and environment: a sedentary TV watching lifestyle and exposure to and availability of calorie-dense hyper-palatable high-fat, high-sugar, high-salt processed food.[2] Among these factors, what we eat, the food environment is probably the most important. As Michael Greger says in his book, *How Not to Diet*, "It's the food."[3] Food scientists have developed ever more palatable processed foods, marketers have become more sophisticated at getting us to buy them, and mass production costs have gone down, so that portion sizes have ballooned.[4]

Coping with too much hyper-palatable food and therefore too much body fat is difficult because evolution has programmed us to eat copiously when food is available to tide us over during food scarcity—but scarcity now never occurs. Science is still unraveling the complex details of our metabolic systems and how our modern lifestyle has conspired to leave many of us overfed and overweight. But even though our environment is conducive to overeating, we know much about how to fight back and craft our own successful strategy to gain the benefits of normal healthy weight.

Unlike exercise, where gradual increases are essential to avoid soreness and injury, for a healthy person, a diet change can be either gradual or all at once. However, before a dramatic change in diet, to avoid health-related problems, it is essential that you consult with your health care provider if you are on medication or are being treated for a health condition, such as high blood pressure or diabetes.

How common and costly is overweight and obesity?

Of a world population of 7.8 billion people in 2020, about 800 million of us are undernourished.[5] But worldwide, even more of us are overweight or obese. That is to say, we are overfat—we have excessive adiposity. Over the past 40 years, the proportion of both children and adults who are overweight or obese has increased rapidly. By 2014, about 72% of men and 64% of women in the U.S. had become either overweight or obese and these conditions have become a costly and pervasive epidemic.[6] American adults average about 25 lbs. heavier than they were in the 1960s.[7] In a nationally representative survey of U.S. adults, the age-adjusted prevalence of obesity, defined as a body mass index (BMI) of 30 or greater, in 2017–2018 was 42.4% among men and women.[8][9]

The values for severe obesity with a BMI of 40 or greater were 6.9% for men and 11.5% for women. A 5-foot 4-inch tall woman weighing 174 pounds is obese and weighing 232 pounds would be severely obese with a BMI of 40. A 5-foot 9-inch man weighing 203 pounds is obese and weighing 270 pounds would be severely obese. The proportion of the U.S. adult population in an obese weight range has more than doubled since 1980 when only 15% of the U.S. adult population was obese.[10][11]

The predicted trend of obesity in the U.S. is a worsening of the epidemic, with nearly one in two adults (48.9%) becoming obese (BMI 30 or greater) by 2030.[12] Nearly one in four (24.2%) of adults are predicted to have "severe" obesity with a BMI of 35 or greater by 2030. One estimate is that the annual global cost of obesity is $2 trillion, and estimates from the U.S. Centers for Disease Control and Prevention (CDC), placed the 2008 annual U.S. medical costs of obesity at $147 billion, 10% of all medical spending.[13][14][15] These medical costs were estimated to have risen to $200 billion in 2010,[16] and could reach $400 billion by the year 2020.[17] Obesity and diabetes cost the U.S. healthcare system $1 billion a day.

The Accurate Measurement of Adiposity

When considering your weight, perhaps the first thing to do is to determine if you have excess fat, or more accurately, excess adiposity. Polling suggests that more than half of people who are overweight or obese are not aware that they are. Not only a high proportion of total body weight that is fat, but also and even more important, an abdominal distribution of fat elevates health risk. There are several ways to determine adiposity. The most accurate would be to measure the weight of body fat as a proportion of total body weight. Since this is not easy, surrogate measures, such as body mass index (BMI) and waist circumference are used. The BMI approximates the percent of a person's body weight that is made up of fat based on their height and weight.

A convenient way to calculate BMI is to go online to the website of the CDC: www.cdc.gov/healthyweight/assessing/bmi/, or consult the table[18] below.

Table 4.1. Body Mass Index (BMI)

Body Mass Index Table

	Normal						Overweight					Obese										Extreme Obesity														
BMI	19	20	21	22	23	24	25	26	27	28	29	30	31	32	33	34	35	36	37	38	39	40	41	42	43	44	45	46	47	48	49	50	51	52	53	54
Height (inches)	Body Weight (pounds)																																			
58	91	96	100	105	110	115	119	124	129	134	138	143	148	153	158	162	167	172	177	181	186	191	196	201	205	210	215	220	224	229	234	239	244	248	253	258
59	94	99	104	109	114	119	124	128	133	138	143	148	153	158	163	168	173	178	183	188	193	198	203	208	212	217	222	227	232	237	242	247	252	257	262	267
60	97	102	107	112	118	123	128	133	138	143	148	153	158	163	168	174	179	184	189	194	199	204	209	215	220	225	230	235	240	245	250	255	261	266	271	276
61	100	106	111	116	122	127	132	137	143	148	153	158	164	169	174	180	185	190	195	201	206	211	217	222	227	232	238	243	248	254	259	264	269	275	280	285
62	104	109	115	120	126	131	136	142	147	153	158	164	169	175	180	186	191	196	202	207	213	218	224	229	235	240	246	251	256	262	267	273	278	284	289	295
63	107	113	118	124	130	135	141	146	152	158	163	169	175	180	186	191	197	203	208	214	220	225	231	237	242	248	254	259	265	270	278	282	287	293	299	304
64	110	116	122	128	134	140	145	151	157	163	169	174	180	186	192	197	204	209	215	221	227	232	238	244	250	256	262	267	273	279	285	291	296	302	308	314
65	114	120	126	132	138	144	150	156	162	168	174	180	186	192	198	204	210	216	222	228	234	240	246	252	258	264	270	276	282	288	294	300	306	312	318	324
66	118	124	130	136	142	148	155	161	167	173	179	186	192	198	204	210	216	223	229	235	241	247	253	260	266	272	278	284	291	297	303	309	315	322	328	334
67	121	127	134	140	146	153	159	166	172	178	185	191	198	204	211	217	223	230	236	242	249	255	261	268	274	280	287	293	299	306	312	319	325	331	338	344
68	125	131	138	144	151	158	164	171	177	184	190	197	203	210	216	223	230	236	243	249	256	262	269	276	282	289	295	302	308	315	322	328	335	341	348	354
69	128	135	142	149	155	162	169	176	182	189	196	203	209	216	223	230	236	243	250	257	263	270	277	284	291	297	304	311	318	324	331	338	345	351	358	365
70	132	139	146	153	160	167	174	181	188	195	202	209	216	222	229	236	243	250	257	264	271	278	285	292	299	306	313	320	327	334	341	348	355	362	369	376
71	136	143	150	157	165	172	179	186	193	200	208	215	222	229	236	243	250	257	265	272	279	286	293	301	308	315	322	329	338	343	351	358	365	372	379	386
72	140	147	154	162	169	177	184	191	199	206	213	221	228	235	242	250	258	265	272	279	287	294	302	309	316	324	331	338	346	353	361	368	375	383	390	397
73	144	151	159	166	174	182	189	197	204	212	219	227	235	242	250	257	265	272	280	288	295	302	310	318	325	333	340	348	355	363	371	378	386	393	401	408
74	148	155	163	171	179	186	194	202	210	218	225	233	241	249	256	264	272	280	287	295	303	311	319	326	334	342	350	358	365	373	381	389	396	404	412	420
75	152	160	168	176	184	192	200	208	216	224	232	240	248	256	264	272	279	287	295	303	311	319	327	335	343	351	359	367	375	383	391	399	407	415	423	431
76	156	164	172	180	189	197	205	213	221	230	238	246	254	263	271	279	287	295	304	312	320	328	336	344	353	361	369	377	385	394	402	410	418	426	435	443

Source: Adapted from *Clinical Guidelines on the Identification, Evaluation, and Treatment of Overweight and Obesity in Adults: The Evidence Report.*

You can also use the following formulae:

English Units BMI Formula:

BMI=Weight in pounds x 703 / height in inches x height in inches
Example for a 130 pound, 5ft 6 in. person
130 x 703 / 66 x 66
91390 / 4356 = 20.98
BMI = 20.98

Metric Units BMI Formula:

BMI = Weight in Kilograms / height in meters x height in meters
Example for an 81 kilogram, 1.8 meter person
81 / 1.8 x 1.8
81 / 3.24 = 25
BMI = 25

A BMI of 18.5–24.9 is considered to be normal. Overweight is commonly defined as a BMI of between 25 and 29.9. Obesity is commonly defined as a BMI of 30 or more. Although BMI is a commonly used way to approximate adiposity, it does have some important limits. For example, it may overestimate body fat in athletes and others who have a muscular build. And, it often underestimates body fat in people who are older, sedentary, or are frail and have lost muscle mass.

Several anthropometric methods that measure adiposity use body measurements to estimate body fat percentages. These methods have the advantage of simplicity. For example, waist circumference has been shown to correlate well with health risks. Even so, the accuracy of determining body fat percentage is limited because body fat is not directly measured. Many of us use what could be considered an anthropometric method when we look in the mirror to evaluate our fatness and when we recognize that our clothes fit too tightly or are getting loose.

A simple way to measure the extra-important visceral fat is by measuring waist and hip size. A good proxy for too much abdominal fat in adults is a waist size of 35 inches or greater for women and 40 inches or greater for men. Another good measure is the waist-to-hip ratio. It should be 0.8 or less. A ratio of 0.85 or greater in women and 1.0 or greater in men is a warning sign of too much visceral adipose tissue (VAT), and potential insulin resistance and metabolic disease.

There are several other ways to estimate adiposity, but they require specialized equipment. Bioelectric Impedance Analysis, or BIA, is based on the fact that muscle is more conductive than fat. Some weight scales you can buy are BIA capable, but the test has considerable variability based on a person's state of hydration.

Hydrostatic Weighing is considered to be an accurate method of body fat measurement. It requires comparing a person's weight on a scale in the air with their weight when underwater. The estimation works because body fat increases buoyancy—a person with a larger percentage of fat-free mass will weigh more in the water than to a person with a larger amount of fat. Air-displacement plethysmography also works on the same principle as underwater weighing. The subject sits in a small machine that measures how much air is displaced by the individual, and this allows a similar calculation of body density.

The gold standard of body fat measurement is Dual Energy X-ray Absorptiometry, known as DEXA Scanning. In addition to measuring fat-free soft tissue mass and fat tissue mass, it can also be used to measure bone mineral mass and can detect osteopenia (mild bone loss) and osteoporosis (severe bone loss). DEXA also makes it possible to see where fat is distributed in the body.

Recent research compared accurate whole-body and abdominal fat data from DEXA with other predictors of whole-body fat and visceral adipose tissue.[19] The study found that the waist-to-height ratio (WHtR) is the best anthropomorphic predictor of both visceral adipose tissue and whole-body fat mass percentage in both men and women. A waistline slightly greater than half of a person's height (0.53 in men and 0.54 in women) was found to indicate whole body obesity. The ratio indicating abdominal obesity was 0.59 in both sexes. In the small sample of the study, a higher proportion of subjects were found to have obesity than was indicated by BMI calculations. The study showed that not only is WHtR more accurate than BMI; it is also easy to use.

One study using the standard of waist measurement greater than half of height found that an alarming 90% of men, 80% of women, and half of children in the U.S. are overfat, a category broader than overweight or obesity because it includes people who seem to be of normal weight but have excessive unhealthy abdominal fat.[20]

Am I Underweight, Normal, Overweight or Obese?

There are several standards for categorizing the percentage of body weight that is made up of fat with regard to healthy weights. The National Heart, Lung, and Blood Institute's weight categories are underweight (BMI of <18.5), normal weight (BMI of 18.5–24.9), overweight (BMI of 25–29.9), obesity (BMI of ≥30) and extreme morbid obesity a BMI of 40 or greater. The World Health Organization uses a different standard, with an obesity cut-off of equal or greater than BMI ≥25 for men and BMI ≥35 for women.

Although widely used in research and for patient counseling, the BMI is not a direct measure of fat and is subject to under-diagnosis of obesity. For example, Shah and Braverman compared BMIs to body fat percentage determined by dual-energy x-ray absorptiometry (DEXA).[21] They found that 39% (22% of men and 48% of women) were not classified as obese according to their BMI, but their fat percentage showed that they were, (the study defined obesity as a BMI of greater than 25 for men and greater than 30 for women).

The loss of muscle mass in older women caused the greatest disparity in classification. In contrast, 25% of muscular men were misclassified as being obese when they were not. The investigators suggest that the diagnosis of obesity based on BMI could be made more accurate by lowering the cut-off threshold for obesity from a BMI of 30 to 28 for men and from a BMI of 30 to 24 for women. According to the revised standard, 64% of American women are obese.

Weight categories based on body mass index (BMI) established by the National Heart, Lung, and Blood Institute, the World Health Organization,[22] the American Society of Bariatric Physicians (ASBP), and suggested by the investigators Shah and Braverman[23] are shown on the Table 4.2 below.

Table 4.2. Fat Percentage Weight Categories for Adults as measured by Body Mass Index (BMI)

	NIH	ASBP Men	ASBP Women	WHO Men	WHO Women	Shah & Braverman Men	Shah & Braverman Women
Underweight	<18.5			<18.5	<18.5		
Normal	18.5–24.9			18.5–24.9	18.5–24.9		
Overweight	25–29.9			25-29.9	25–29.9		
Obese	≥30	≥25	≥30	≥25	≥25	≥28	≥24
Obesity I				30–34.9	30–34.9		
Obesity II				35–39.9	35–39.9		
Morbid Obesity III	≥40			≥40	≥40		

As is shown in Table 4.3, the American Council on Exercise (ACE) has estimated the percentage of body fat that would be present in men and women at various levels of fitness.[24]

Table 4.3. American Council on Exercise (ACE) Body Fat Percent

Description	Women	Men
Essential fat	10–13%	2–5%
Athletes	14–20%	6–13%
Fitness	21–24%	14–17%
Average	25–31%	18–24%
Obese	32%+	25%+

The health risks of overweight and obesity

Being overweight or obese increases the risk of many life-threatening conditions, including type 2 diabetes, hypertension, heart disease, stroke, high blood pressure, nonalcoholic fatty liver disease and breast, colon, endometrial, and kidney cancer.[25] An international study of disease related to BMI in 195 countries found an increased risk of 20 different health outcomes, but more than two-thirds of deaths related to high BMI were due to cardiovascular disease, followed in frequency by diabetes.[26] Excess adiposity also increases the risk of gout, gallbladder disease, and places greater stress on the back, hips, and knees, which may cause or aggravate osteoarthritis of the knees and hips. Obesity is also associated with heartburn, shortness of breath, sleep apnea, sexual dysfunction, and depression. A Johns Hopkins report on nutrition and weight control pointed out that overweight and obesity can, and I would say frequently, leads to mental anguish as a result of poor body image, social isolation, or being the victim of prejudicial social discrimination.[27]

The U.S. has a higher proportion of obese people than Canada, any country in Europe, or in East Asia and a relatively low life expectancy compared to other countries in these regions. In addition to an early death, being severely obese is associated with about 19 years of living with poor health. Studies estimate that severe obesity shortens life by five to 20 years, with the greatest number of years of life lost when obesity occurs at a young age.[28] A longer duration of overall and abdominal obesity is associated with the progression of subclinical coronary heart disease and is a predictor of increased all-cause mortality in men and women.[29 30 31] One study found that compared to normal-weight adults, obese adults had at least a 20% higher risk of dying from all causes or from cardiovascular diseases.[32]

Among Americans, a gradual weight gain of one to two pounds a year during early adulthood is typical. This may be considered benign with regard to health, but research shows that it is not. A study evaluated the health implications of weight gain from early adulthood (age 18 for women, 21 for men) to middle adulthood (age 55) among health professionals.[33] Women gained an average of 22 pounds over early to middle adulthood, and men gained about 19 pounds. Compared to those who had maintained a stable weight across early and middle life, the study found that each 11 lb. (5 kg) weight gain was associated with a 30% increased risk of type 2 diabetes, 14% increased risk of hypertension, 8% increased risk of cardiovascular disease, 6% increased risk of obesity-related cancer (but such associations were not significant for overall cancer), 5% increased risk of dying prematurely (among never smokers), and a 17% decreased odds of achieving healthy aging. Weight gain also increased the risk of cataracts, cholelithiasis (gallstones), and severe osteoarthritis. The study authors concluded that "Among women and men, moderate weight gain from early to middle adulthood was associated with significantly increased risk of major chronic diseases and mortality."[34]

Waist circumference provides a more accurate indication of a health risk than BMI because it better measures the most metabolically active and harmful fat, the visceral fat stored in the abdomen—especially fat in the liver. A study of 350,000 Europeans found that over the average of a 9.7-year follow-up, having a large waistline (greater than 47 inches in men, 39 inches in women) nearly doubled the risk of premature death.[35]

Waist circumference is a better predictor of the risks of insulin resistance, diabetes, high blood pressure, heart disease, and the metabolic syndrome—defined as the presence of three or more of the following five risk factors: a large waist circumference (abdominal obesity), high blood glucose, high triglyceride, a low high-density lipoprotein cholesterol (HDL-C) level and high blood pressure. The metabolic syndrome affects more than 75 million or 40% of Americans over age 40 and it greatly increases the risk of developing type 2 diabetes and heart disease.[36]

After adjustment for BMI, the INTERHEART study attributed 33.7% of heart attacks to an increased waist-to-hip ratio (abdominal obesity) compared with 10.8% of infarctions attributed to overweight and obesity as measured by a BMI over 25.[37] These findings, together with a study of a genetic propensity for a higher waist-to-hip ratio, provide evidence that abdominal adiposity, independent of elevated BMI, is a major driver of diabetes and coronary heart disease.[38]

Can you be normal-weight and metabolically unhealthy?

According to a study, 23.5% of U.S. adults who were normal weight according to their BMIs had the same metabolic abnormalities that are common among the overweight and obese.[39 40] These abnormalities include reduced HDL cholesterol, and increased triglycerides, fasting glucose, C-reactive protein, insulin resistance, and blood pressure. Many, often older, individuals with metabolic abnormalities have lost muscle mass. They have excessive body fat and visceral obesity as measured by waistline girth, despite a normal BMI. A study of the results of weight loss among normal-weight individuals found that even small losses of weight were highly beneficial to multiple measures of their metabolic status.[41]

Can you be obese and metabolically healthy?

Some obesity experts have considered that about 20% of obese people are metabolically healthy (i.e., normal glucose, blood lipids, blood pressure) and may not have increased health risks related to adiposity.[42] Research has shown that their cardiovascular disease risk is considerably lower than those individuals who are obese and have unhealthy metabolic biomarkers. For example, the metabolically healthy but obese participants in one study had a 38% lower risk of death from any cause than those who were metabolically unhealthy and obese.[43]

But some studies question the concept of healthy obesity. One such study found that, compared to normal-weight individuals with no metabolic abnormalities, individuals with metabolically healthy obesity had a 50% increased risk of coronary heart disease; a 7% increased risk of cerebrovascular disease, a doubled risk of heart failure, and excluding cigarette smokers, an 11% increased risk of developing peripheral vascular disease.[44] Dr. Caleyachetty, the study's lead author, noted that "Metabolically healthy obese individuals are at higher risk of coronary heart disease, cerebrovascular disease and heart failure than normal-weight metabolically healthy individuals. The priority of health professionals should be to promote and facilitate weight loss among obese persons, regardless of the presence or absence of metabolic abnormalities."[45]

Is low body weight actually unhealthy?

Many studies show that leanness is associated with better health, a lower risk of developing serious diseases and that death rates are lower. However, a number of epidemiologic studies have found that this link is not true for the lowest weight categories—a situation sometimes called the "obesity paradox."[46]

The finding of lowest mortality in those with a BMI somewhat above the normal range of 18.5-24.9 has been found by a number of studies,[47] including a widely-publicized meta-analysis of 97 studies published in the *Journal of the American Medical Association* (*JAMA*) in 2012.[48] The study found that individuals who were overweight (BMI, between 25 and 29.9) were actually 6% less likely to die from any cause than people whose weight was considered to be normal weight according to their BMI. And even people who were "mildly" obese (BMI 30 to 34.9) were no more likely to die than their normal-weight counterparts. However, for people who were moderately or severely obese (BMI over 35 or 40, respectively), the risk of dying was increased by 29%.

An editorial commenting on the *JAMA* study noted that the body mass index is an imperfect measure of adiposity. It accounts for only about two-thirds of the between-individual variation in total adiposity. Nor does BMI account for the fact that people with the same BMI can have different health risk factors present.[49] For example, one person with a BMI of 28 may be in perfect health while another with the same BMI might be a smoker, have type 2 diabetes and hypertension. So perhaps the higher risk of death among the normal-weight individuals in the *JAMA* study may have been due in part to the inclusion of sick or frail underweight people in the "normal" weight category.[50]

Walter Willett and his colleagues have pointed out that basing guidelines for an optimal healthy weight on mortality rates is misleading.[51] Reverse causation, that is to say illness is the cause of low BMI rather than low BMI causing illness and higher mortality, is the most serious problem. People frequently lose weight as a result of an illness that is ultimately fatal, a situation that creates the appearance of higher mortality among those with lower weights. Confounding factors such as smoking, alcoholism, and physical activity may distort the association between body weight and mortality. Smokers tend to weigh less, so smoking will make leaner persons appear to be at elevated risk. Willett and his colleagues note that "...in analyses adjusted only for age, the relation between body weight and mortality is typically U-shaped, with increased death rates among both the leanest and the heaviest persons. However, because of the potential for bias, these results should not be accepted as evidence that low weight is harmful."

In many studies when reverse causation is accounted for, and the analysis is limited to persons who have never smoked, mortality increased linearly with increasing body-mass index from very lean to clearly obese.[52 53] For example, the long-term Nurses' Health Study and Health Professionals Follow-up Study found that a combination of at least three low-risk lifestyle factors and a BMI that is considered normal weight, 18.5–22.4, was associated with the lowest risk of all-cause mortality.[54]

Evaluating the importance of obesity on overall health is also complicated by the role of cardiorespiratory fitness in attenuating the health risks of overweight or obesity.[55] Studies have found that fit individuals with metabolically healthy obesity are not at significantly higher risk of CVDs than metabolically healthy normal-weight individuals.[56] Maintaining cardiorespiratory fitness appears to be protective against the risks of overweight and obesity.

Although being mildly over-fat may represent a small increment of increased health risk, and if you are physically fit very little or no increase, the last word on this might be found in a large meta-analysis of 230 cohort studies that tracked 3.74 million deaths among 30.3 million participants. It found that the lowest mortality was among never smokers with a normal BMI of 20-22.[57 58 59]

Obesity and liver disease

The U.S. obesity epidemic has brought increased attention to nonalcoholic fatty liver disease (NAFLD), a major health problem that is caused by excessive calorie intake, especially in the form of the fructose in added sugars.[60] The 2004 American documentary film, *Super Size Me*, followed Morgan Spurlock for a 30-day period during which he ate only fast food and consumed an average of 5,000 calories per day. Spurlock gained 24 pounds, his cholesterol increased to 230 mg/dL, he experienced mood swings, and he developed a fatty liver.[61] In a similar small study, healthy volunteers also developed signs of fatty liver after doubling their caloric intake to gain weight by eating at least two fast-food-based meals per day for four weeks. At the end of the four weeks, the researchers reported:

- The fast-food consumers had gained an average of 6.5 kg (14.3 lbs.).
- Their liver enzymes rose to levels indicating liver damage in 11 of the 18 participants.[62]

According to a Swedish study, being overweight as a teenager may increase the risk of liver disease later in life.[63] At an average follow-up time of 29 years, compared with men with a normal BMI (18.5 to 22.5), those with a slightly elevated BMI (22.5 to 25) had a 17% greater risk of severe liver disease, those who were overweight (BMI 25 to 30) had a 49% increased risk, and those who were obese with a BMI of 30 or greater had a 2.17 times increase in risk. Men with obesity who developed diabetes had a 3.28 times higher risk of severe liver disease. The investigators concluded that a high BMI in late adolescent men was associated with an increased risk of future severe liver disease, including liver cancer, and that diabetes further increased the risk.

In the past two decades, the prevalence of nonalcoholic fatty liver disease (NAFLD) has doubled and is now found to occur among 10% of U.S. children and 20% of adults. In about 10% to 20% of cases, the fat accumulation leads to inflammation, sometimes to scarring similar to the cirrhosis caused by chronic alcoholism, and at times, to liver failure. About 2% to 3% of U.S. adults, at least five million Americans, have a more serious form of fatty liver disease, nonalcoholic steatohepatitis (NASH), that in 15% to 20% of cases leads to cirrhosis. NASH is the fastest growing health condition necessitating liver transplants. If caught early, fatty liver is reversible by weight loss, increased exercise, elimination of alcohol, and minimizing added sources of fructose in the diet such as sucrose (table sugar) and high-fructose corn syrup.[64 65 66]

The physiology of obesity: how and why fat is gained and lost

Although we speak in terms of weight gain and loss, we should keep in mind that our concern is fatness or adiposity, especially avoiding visceral fat—the fat that accumulates in our liver, muscles, and around our internal organs. Biologically, the abdominal fat around our waist, where about 20% of fat is found, is more dangerous to health than the 80% of fat that is subcutaneous in other locations.[67 68 69]

There are some infrequent medical causes for obesity such as an underactive thyroid (hypothyroidism), polycystic ovary disease, tumors of the pituitary or adrenal glands, insufficient production of sex hormones, insulin-producing tumors of the pancreas, some drugs (anti-psychotics, anti-epileptics, steroids and some diabetes medications), and some genetic conditions. They should be addressed by a health care provider.

Appetite and the physiology of how we metabolize food relate to our hormones, our nervous system, especially our brains, our level of physical activity, and the hyper-appetizing external food environment we are exposed to. We gain fat when more calories are consumed than the body needs to expend for energy in physical activity and for resting (basal) metabolism. The energy used for basal metabolism maintains body warmth and supports digestion, circulation, breathing, and other requirements for bodily functions. Basal metabolism typically accounts for 60% to 75% of a body's use of energy.

It may be surprising, but the energy requirements of the brain and internal organs such as the heart and kidneys have the greatest energy requirements—not the muscles. About 10% of the body's use of energy is for dietary-induced thermogenesis—the heat generated and work required to process and digest the food you eat. For a typical American, non-exercise physical activity, that is to say, just moving about throughout the day causes the expenditure of about 25% of calories, whereas organized physical activity or exercise consumes about 5% of calories.[70] Of course, the proportion of total calories expended by exercise can be much greater, and people of similar height, weight, age, gender, and muscle mass may have resting metabolic rates that vary by 20% or more. This can add up to a 500 calorie or more a day difference in energy expenditure.

Energy balance, the difference between the food calories consumed and absorbed versus those expended, is the principal determinant of weight gain and adiposity. An intake surplus of 3500 calories over energy expenditure is needed to store a pound of fat, and an energy deficit of 3500 calories is needed to lose a pound of fat. Eating fewer calories than the body needs results in the use of stored energy sources, first glycogen, and then fat to provide the energy for warmth, physical activity, and the body's metabolism, and the result is weight loss. A small but long-term energy imbalance of 50 to 100 extra calories a day may be enough to produce weight gain. It also means that small improvements in energy balance, if sustained over the long term, can prevent or reverse adiposity.[71 72 73 74 75]

Insulin is an important regulator of the metabolism of fat. Digestion breaks down starches (a form of carbohydrate that is made up of long chains of glucose), proteins, fats, and other carbohydrates in food into amino acids, fatty acids and simple sugars (mostly glucose and variable amounts of fructose), all of which are first processed by the liver. Glucose supplies energy to the body's cells, some is converted to glycogen, a ready source of energy, by the liver, and some is converted to triglycerides that may end up stored as fat. When glucose and the other nutrients are not metabolized in the liver and enter the general circulation, the pancreas is signaled to release insulin. Insulin drives energy storage by promoting synthesis of glycogen and its storage in the liver and muscles, and insulin also promotes the clearing of blood lipids into fat cells for storage in the form of triglycerides.

When the body's immediate needs for glucose, the main energy source for all cells, and the capacity to store glycogen are exceeded, the excess calories are stored as fat. When stored energy is needed, the fat cells release triglycerides into the bloodstream. They are then transported to the liver, where they are broken down into ketones that serve as an energy source. My UCSF colleague Robert Lustig has described the process as follows: "Insulin makes fat—the more insulin, the more fat. And there it sits…and sits…as long as there is insulin around. When the insulin levels drop, the process goes into reverse: the triglycerides get broken down, causing the fat cells to shrink—when that happens, that's weight loss!"[76]

Sugars are healthful components of food when found naturally in milk, fruit, and vegetables. But sugar has the potential to harm health when added in large amounts to processed foods in the form of sucrose (table sugar), high-fructose corn syrup, or dozens of other sugar forms that contain the molecule sucrose that is digested into glucose and fructose.

Consumption of fructose increased fivefold in the last century and doubled over the past thirty years, concomitant with the burgeoning obesity pandemic.[77] Lustig notes that in the story of obesity, "Fructose is very sweet and is inevitably metabolized to fat. It is the primary (but not the sole) villain…"[78] He notes that if you are starving or energy depleted after running a marathon, fructose can quickly and healthfully help restore the liver's stores of glycogen. But for most of us, all the extra sugar in the American diet from processed foods, soft drinks, juices, bakery goods, and desserts has major negative implications for health.

Calorie for calorie, the ethanol in alcoholic drinks and fructose are more toxic than other energy sources, especially to your liver. Ethanol is a cellular poison. Most of it is metabolized by the liver. Any amount that is not metabolized for energy gets turned into fat in the liver or muscles and causes liver damage and insulin resistance. Ethanol stimulates the brain's reward system and decreases the brain's executive functioning. This is a recipe for addiction.

Fructose metabolism is similar to that of ethanol. Unlike glucose that can be metabolized throughout the body, almost all fructose is metabolized by the liver into glycogen or triglycerides. Fructose induces liver insulin resistance that in turn leads to high levels of insulin, disruption of leptin signaling by high insulin, (so you want to eat more), failure to decrease ghrelin, (so the "I'm full" signal is not sent), excess fat storage, and over-time, development of the unhealthy metabolic syndrome. Lustig points out that the toxic effects of both ethanol and fructose are dose-dependent, with each having a threshold for damage. "Fructose toxicity" occurs when ingestion of about 50 grams per day is exceeded. Perhaps half of Americans consume more than 50 grams of fructose per day. As is described in Chapter 3, "Optimal Nutrition," epidemiology reveals another important downside of high consumption of sugar—a strong correlation between the amount of sugar consumed and the likelihood of diabetes.

David Ludwig, a Harvard T. H. Chan School of Public Health professor, suggests that the overweight and obesity epidemic is mainly because of our food environment and increased consumption of highly processed foods such as white bread, white rice, cookies, crackers and sugar-sweetened beverages.[79] He suggests that the way that these overly processed high glycemic index foods produce obesity is through causing a surge in levels of blood sugar, the release of insulin, greater incorporation of glucose into fat, and hunger.

Focus on diet composition rather than calories

We have created a food system that makes available large amounts of low-fiber energy-dense foods that have been engineered with added sugar, fat, caffeine, and sodium to be hyper-palatable.[80] Especially important, the large amounts of added sugar lead to chronically high insulin and insulin resistance. Understanding this physiology gives us key information about what we need to change to get to and maintain a normal weight. We need to avoid calorie-dense foods that are high in fats, added sugar, and highly refined carbohydrates.

To facilitate weight loss, focus on diet composition rather than calories. Consumption of whole foods, including high-protein plant foods, leads to a gentle rise in blood sugar and insulin, and the calories are used for energy metabolism rather than being stored as fat, whereas a large dose of added sugars requires the pancreas to produce high levels of insulin. This, in turn, boosts the storage of fat, and over time, it also decreases the responsiveness of the body's cells to insulin, causing insulin resistance. When the body is resistant to insulin, it forces the pancreas to make even more insulin and that leads to even more fat storage and obesity. When it becomes chronic, this unhealthy feedback loop perpetuates insulin resistance, exhausts the cells of the pancreas that synthesize insulin, and results in diabetes.

One reason that losing weight and then keeping it off is difficult is that as calories are restricted, and weight is lost, the body's metabolism slows down by as much as 20%. Of course, this is a valuable characteristic of metabolism that aided human survival in times of food shortage, but it helps to sabotage the weight loss efforts of dieters. This was illustrated vividly in studies of the extreme weight loss experience of "The Biggest Losers." An NIH study found that after losing large amounts of weight, 13 of 14 contestants had very low levels of leptin (the hormone released by fat that decreases appetite), they struggled with food cravings and, over time, regained significant amounts of weight. When evaluated six years after the contest, the "Losers" had a slowed metabolism that averaged expending nearly 500 calories less a day, and four contestants were even heavier than when they started the contest. Our bodies are programmed to hold on to the fat we have gained.[81 82] This suggests that preventing the childhood obesity that ends up in adult obesity is a crucial step in stopping the obesity epidemic.

Additional bad news about obesity is that some people are more genetically predisposed to be fat than others. Heredity seems to influence the number of fat cells in the body, how much and where fat is stored, and how much energy the body uses at rest. According to a Johns Hopkins report, studies show that only 9% of children born to normal-weight parents will become obese. This can be compared to the 60% to 80% rate of obesity among children born to two obese parents. Studies of identical twins confirm that although inheritance increases the risk of becoming obese, the environment of children born to obese parents is more important than heredity. Comparison of the weights of individuals who were adopted with the weights of their biological and adopted parents indicates that the environment accounts for two-thirds and genetic factors are responsible for only about a third of the difference in weight. Our genes have not changed significantly over the last 40 years, during which time obesity rates have skyrocketed. Clearly, for most people, various aspects of our lifestyle and food environment are more important than a genetic tendency to put on weight.[83]

The influence of hormones on appetite

Although science is still unraveling the complex influences of hormones, nerve signals, and other factors that regulate appetite, food consumption, metabolism, storage of energy in the form of fat and body weight, what follows is a simplified description of what is known.

The hypothalamus of the brain receives minute-to-minute information about hunger and satiety, but it also receives longer-term information about the body's fat stores. The hypothalamus monitors and regulates the body's fat stores by responding to levels of various hormones, including insulin and leptin—they are the main messengers.

In addition to leptin, another hormone, ghrelin, regulates appetite. Ghrelin is produced by the stomach when empty, during fasting, or when dieting and often peaks just before meal-times. Ghrelin stimulates appetite and promotes fat storage. A satisfying meal, and also being overweight, decreases the production of ghrelin and reduces appetite. Other hormones are produced by the intestines after a meal. They include cholecystokinin (CCK) and peptide YY (PYY). They have the opposite effect of ghrelin; they suppress appetite. These gut hormones, with their opposing effects, are considered to be the influences mainly responsible for the short-term, hour-to-hour, and minute-to-minute regulation of appetite. Ghrelin influences the hypothalamus and also has been shown to act on the reward centers of the brain.

Leptin is among about a dozen hormones that are synthesized by adipose tissue. Leptin is produced in amounts proportional to the fat that adipose tissue contains, so when the body's level of fat increases, more leptin is synthesized. The hypothalamus responds to leptin messages with one of two signals. High levels of leptin lead the hypothalamus to turn off the vagus nerve, stimulate the sympathetic nervous system to increase physical activity and metabolism to expend more energy, suppress appetite, make us feel good, and lose fat. Low levels of leptin have the opposite effect. They stimulate the parasympathetic system through the vagus nerve that tells our digestive organs to store energy—including stimulating the pancreas to release more of the insulin that promotes energy storage—and make us feel hungry and unwell.

When leptin signaling is normal, you maintain energy balance at what Lustig calls a "personal leptin threshold" that is also sometimes called a set point. The theory is that the brain uses its regulatory mechanisms to maintain a genetically predetermined weight and level of body fat—a set point. When this regulatory system works well, leptin signals the body that you have enough energy on board, to expend any excess energy, and to keep food intake low. But what if leptin signaling doesn't work or your set point is too high? If your hypothalamus does not respond appropriately to leptin, your brain interprets this as too little fat on board—that you need food. This inappropriately turns on the cycle of vagus nerve stimulation and insulin release, more fat storage (to boost leptin), and obesity results. According to Lustig, both obese and starving people have many of the same symptoms—fatigue, malaise, and depression.[84]

Normally leptin suppresses the release of dopamine and reduces the reward of food. But if you are leptin resistant, dopamine is not cleared away, and you will want to keep on eating because food will continue to be rewarding. Insulin also clears away dopamine, so in a normal person, food would induce the release of insulin and attenuate the reward of more food. But if you are insulin resistant, this does not happen, and more food than you need for energy balance will continue to be pleasurable and likely to be eaten. As Lustig has described it, "Starvation and reward conspire to thwart every obese person."[85]

The failure of the hypothalamus to respond appropriately to leptin is one key to the obesity epidemic.[86] The bodies of most overweight people are resistant to the effects of leptin, and leptin has not been an effective drug to help control weight.[87] So then the question is, what causes leptin resistance? It turns out that when insulin levels are chronically high, leptin cannot signal the hypothalamus because high insulin acts as a leptin antagonist. So, then the next question is: Why are insulin levels chronically high? The answer is mainly that the foods we consume are full of added sugars and highly refined carbohydrates.

The role of stress and food addiction

In a famous poem, W. H. Auden called modern times the "age of anxiety." Obesity has increased at the same time that probably many people have experienced increased psychological stress. The normal stresses of everyday life and physical activity cause the release of the beneficial levels of cortisol from the adrenal glands that help your body cope with stress. Small amounts of cortisol over a short period of time are essential to health, but long-term high levels of cortisol are detrimental. Lustig describes two mechanisms by which stress leads to obesity—stress-induced eating and stress-induced fat deposition.[88] "Stress eaters" generate high levels of cortisol in response to stress and eat more high-fat high-sugar "comfort foods." Chronic stress increases the urge to consume comfort foods and the accumulation of high-risk visceral fat.

Richard Friedman, a psychiatrist, writing in the *New York Times,* considered "What Cookies and Meth Have in Common."[89] He notes that evidence from neuroscience confirms the link between stress and addiction. Pleasurable feelings from sex, food, money, drugs, or other positive events come from the release of dopamine in the brain. But adversity and stress reduce the number of D2s, the dopamine receptors in the brain's reward circuits. This makes people less responsive to dopamine and more likely to seek out the greater stimulation of recreational drugs or comfort food to make themselves feel better. To make things worse, people with fewer D2 receptors also show decreased activity in their prefrontal cortex, making it harder for them to exert self-control. Friedman says that "Chronic exposure to high-fat and sugary foods is similarly linked with lower D2 levels, and people with lower D2 levels are also more likely to crave such foods." For them, normal food consumption is insufficiently rewarding.

So, stressors such as low social status, perceived lack of social support, and financial insecurity are half of the addiction equation. The other half is easy access to cheap addicting food and drugs. In recent decades, we have engineered ever more palatable high calorie processed foods and synthesized ever more potent brain-stimulating drugs for recreational use. The consumption of extra-palatable foods, high in fat, sugar, caffeine, and sodium, increase the level of dopamine in the brain and cause feelings of pleasure and reward. The body's response to highly processed fast foods fits many of the criteria for addiction.

A review of the health effects of fructose and fructose-containing caloric sweeteners found that consumption of sugar-sweetened beverages (SSBs) is associated with weight gain.[90] The review noted similarities between the effects of sugar and other addictive substances (including other foods) on the brain's reward systems—perhaps sugar is addictive. Research with functional MRI brain scans has shown that the brain activity patterns of people with addictive-like eating behaviors are similar to those of substance abusers.

So, what can be done? Certainly, the creation of a less stressful social environment would help, and, as Friedman says, "Fortunately, our brains are remarkably plastic and sensitive to experience. Although it's far easier said than done, just limiting exposure to high-calorie foods and recreational drugs would naturally reset our brains to find pleasure in healthier foods and life without drugs."

Fiber—beneficial and no calories

One might ask, what about avoiding the fructose in fruit? Fruit is a healthy food because, in nature, fructose is packaged with fiber—a component of food that Lustig calls half the antidote to the fructose effect and the obesity pandemic. The other half of the antidote is physical activity.

Chapter 3, "Optimal Nutrition," described that fiber is not digested, and except for the extent it is broken down by gut bacteria, it is not used for energy by humans (it is food for herbivores). Fiber makes an important contribution to our health. One type, soluble fiber, is found in oatmeal, lentils, carrots, and many fruits. With the addition of water, it becomes a viscous mass in the digestive tract that slows the digestion and absorption of food. It also binds to bile acids and helps lower blood cholesterol. Insoluble fiber is found in whole grains, seeds, nuts, brown rice, and many vegetables.

In contrast to soluble fiber, it speeds the passage of foods through the small and large intestines. This means that food moves through the small intestine with alacrity and more quickly generates the PYY signal that tells the brain, "I'm full." Waiting for the PYY signal to kick in is why it is advisable to wait 20 minutes before going for seconds. Insoluble fiber can shorten this wait, and if you wait, you may more easily be able to go without second helpings or a dessert.

There is evidence that humans evolved eating, and hunter-gathers still eat, hundreds of grams of fiber a day.[91 92] It can be argued that human physiology is adapted to eating large amounts of plants that are abundant in fiber. The recommended standard of 14 grams of fiber per thousand calories, or about 25 grams per day for women and 38 grams per day for men, is not set very high, but it is not met by 97% of Americans.[93] One reason is that prominent components of the typical American diet, such as meat and cheese, do not contain fiber.[94]

Plant-based high fiber foods are less energy-dense, so you get fewer calories for the same quantity of food. Fiber-rich foods require more chewing, slow down eating, and when your stomach is full, it contains fewer calories when the "I'm full" signals are sent to your brain.[95] Slowing digestion activates what is called the ileal brake—the feeling of fullness that is sent to your brain when undigested food makes is down to the last part of the small intestine, the ileum. Fiber cuts appetite another way. The bacteria in our guts turn fiber into short-chain fatty acids that reduce inflammation and stimulate the production of the leptin that signals the brain to reduce our appetite.[96]

Another benefit of fiber is that when the two kinds of fiber work together to slow digestion, this limits the rapid rise of glucose and attenuates the magnitude of the insulin response. Milling grain to make white flour, white rice, pasta, and breakfast cereal strips out about three-quarters of the fiber and makes these foods more rapidly digestible. These refined foods cause a more rapid increase and higher peak concentration of glucose that the liver has to cope with. In contrast, the consumption of high levels of insoluble fiber decreases insulin resistance. Fruit is a healthy food because it comes with fiber. Destroying insoluble fiber by juicing fruit, or even worse, just drinking plain juice or a sugar-sweetened soft drink, slugs the liver even harder with high concentrations of the fructose and glucose that stimulates the high levels of insulin that lead to obesity.[97] To get the benefits of fiber is one important reason to avoid most processed foods. Skip the juice and eat whole or minimally refined foods.

Fiber helps prevent the calories you eat from expanding your waistline because the body does not use all food sources with equal efficiency.[98 99] The physical properties of a food influence how completely the body can digest and absorb calories, so all calories do not contribute equally to weight gain. For example, the body can extract only about two-thirds of the calories in raw almonds but nearly 100% of the calories in almond butter. The calories in whole grains, oats, and high-fiber cereals are digested inefficiently, and they also bump up metabolism. Fiber also traps calorie-dense fats and oils, so they go through you rather than being digested and ending up stored as fat in your body. [100,101]

Food choices can also influence hunger. Feeding tests show that meals higher in protein and fiber are more satisfying and better at suppressing hunger than meals high in refined carbohydrates that cause a rapid spike in blood glucose. Selecting meals with a low glycemic index is likely to lead to greater weight loss than the typical American diet.[102] A 2017 study in the *American Journal of Clinical Nutrition* compared the metabolic effects of a diet high in whole-grain and fiber content to a refined grain-based diet.[103] The study found that substituting whole grains for refined grains led to a stool energy loss of nearly 100 calories a day—by speeding up metabolism, cutting the number of calories that the body retained, and by changing the digestibility of other foods.

Sleep and adiposity

Lack of sleep spells trouble for avoiding obesity in several ways. It increases ghrelin (that makes you hungry), increases cortisol, reduces leptin, and activates the reward system that, in turn, increases the desire for comfort foods. A study of the role of sleep in obesity published in the *European Journal of Clinical Nutrition* that analyzed 11 intervention trials found that lack of sleep led to overeating the next day by an average of 385 calories.[104] The study was short term, so the implications for long-term weight gain are uncertain. However, other studies suggest that lack of sleep disrupts the reward center of the brain.

My Story

I know that when I was a somewhat groggy medical intern working in a hospital with very little sleep, I ate more than usual in an attempt to feel better. In Chapter 15, "More Advice about Healthy Living," I discuss the many reasons to get enough sleep—to help avoid overweight and obesity is on the list.

The microbiome—an obesity research frontier

An additional complication concerning the metabolism of food and absorption of food calories is evidence that the genes in the bacteria in your body, the microbiome, may play an important role in the genesis of obesity and type 2 diabetes.[105] That gut bacteria synthesize essential vitamins and amino acids and help degrade toxins is well known. Research has shown that the many genes in a human's microbiome (250 to 800 times the number of human genes) allow bacteria to synthesize proteins, including hormones, neurotransmitters, and molecules causing inflammation, that can enter the circulation and affect health.

Human gut enzymes are unable to digest many of the dietary polysaccharides in fiber, but microbial enzymes can make them into digestible monosaccharides and short-chain fatty acids. The microbiota influences the calories the body absorbs, but more research is needed to understand this phenomenon. Farmers give livestock and poultry antibiotics because it makes them grow fatter. And various animal experiments suggest that microbiota may affect obesity in mammals. The type of bacteria that is predominant in the gut is affected to some extent on the nature of your diet, depending on if your diet is based on animal fat and protein or plant foods.[106] It is possible that manipulation of the microbiome with antibiotics, probiotics (live microorganisms), or other means could affect the risk of obesity, but biomedical science is still learning how to do this.

The role of physical activity for weight loss, health, and maintaining weight loss

So, what about exercise, the activity that Lustig calls the second half of the antidote to fructose toxicity? According to him, a fat but physically fit person is healthier than a normal-weight person with insulin resistance and the metabolic syndrome. Exercise has a variety of beneficial health effects: 1) it activates the sympathetic nervous system, increases muscle mass and insulin sensitivity so you burn more calories at rest and 24/7; 2) it improves liver metabolism, so it decreases the amount and negative effects of visceral fat—it improves insulin sensitivity, lowers insulin levels, and improves leptin signaling; 3) it improves many of the metabolic biomarkers associated with the metabolic syndrome and other chronic diseases and improves health (See Chapter 9, "Benefits of Physical Activity" for details); and 4) it heightens endorphins and reduces stress, so you feel better and have less cortisol that makes you hungry and drives obesity.

At a high level of physical activity, we expend more calories than our appetite tells us to eat, and we lose weight. At a lower level of physical activity, one that is typical for Americans, we lose the ability to sufficiently down-regulate our appetites, and we gain weight. One estimate is that when we walk about 7100 steps a day (about 3.5 miles), our calorie expenditure and appetite are in balance.[107] With less exercise, our appetites do not down-regulate enough, so we are likely to gain weight.

Non-exercise activity thermogenesis (NEAT) is an important component of daily energy expenditure. It represents the energy expenditure of common daily activities, such as fidgeting, walking, and standing.[108] The benefits of NEAT include not only the extra calories expended, but also the reduced occurrence of the metabolic syndrome, cardiovascular events, and all-cause mortality. As explained in more detail in Chapter 9, "Benefits of Physical Activity," all physical activity contributes to health, even if it is gentle or of short duration.

Exercise is an inefficient way to lose weight because most energy is consumed by resting (basal) metabolism, and it is a rare person who boosts their calorie expenditure with physical activity by more than an extra 500 calories per day.

My Story

I alternate a daily 16-mile ride on a bike that barely uses an extra 400 calories with a four-mile walk that burns only 200 extra calories. Although cutting intake of calories is more efficient, by expending additional calories through increased exercise, you can reduce the calorie restriction needed to lose weight. For example, to reduce caloric intake by 500 calories a day, enough to lose a pound a week, an addition of enough moderate to vigorous exercise each day to burn an extra 250 calories would reduce the needed restriction of food to only 250 calories a day.

In addition to helping with energy balance, physical activity helps convert fat to muscle, strengthen bone, and avoid or reverse the frailty that accompanies obesity in older adults. So even if your weight does not change much, exercise will help you to lose fat and lose inches, and exercise is crucial to the maintenance of normal weight for many people.[109] For people who are obese, it is very important to start an exercise program gradually to avoid injury. It is also a good idea to vary exercise activities and to include weight-bearing and weight-training activities.

People who are of normal weight tend to get more exercise than those who are obese. Since 1994, the U.S. National Weight Control Registry (NWCR) has studied and is tracking over 10,000 individuals who have lost significant amounts of weight and kept it off for long periods of time. Although there is substantial variation in how NWCR members keep the weight off, most report being attentive to their weight, continuing to maintain a low calorie, low-fat diet, and undertaking high levels of physical activity.[110]

- 98% of Registry participants report that they modified their food intake in some way to lose weight.
- 94% increased their physical activity, with the most frequently reported form of activity being walking.
- 90% exercise, on average, about one hour per day.

A combination of exercise and calorie restriction is employed by the overwhelming majority of individuals in the Registry who have been successful at weight loss and maintenance of the loss.

Covert Bailey asserted in his book *Fit or Fat?* that "The ultimate cure for obesity is exercise."[111] Not only is exercise a valuable contributor to weight loss, it is also essential to succeed at losing weight and keeping it off. Although dietary calorie reduction alone will lead to weight loss, the addition of exercise to a reduced-calorie diet preserves or builds up muscle and results in somewhat greater losses of body weight and, especially, to the more important goal of losing fat. For example, a study of female adolescents and young adults found that participants who just used limitation of portion size were less successful in avoiding weight gain than those who combined portion limitation with frequent exercise.[112]

There is also some evidence that exercise makes brown fat more active. Brown fat has the ability to turn fat calories into heat efficiently. Brown fat helps babies maintain body warmth but is usually mostly lost during childhood. Exposure to cold activates brown fat in adults, but it remains to be seen if turning down the thermostat will both save on the heating bill and help prevent obesity.[113]

A clinical trial tested the efficacy of several exercise modes in reversing frailty and preventing the reduction in muscle and bone mass that is induced by weight loss.[114] Participants in a weight loss program undertook one of three exercise programs — aerobic training, resistance training, or combined aerobic and resistance training — or they were in a control group with no weight-management or exercise program. After 6 months, the study found that body weight decreased by 9% in all exercise groups but did not change significantly in the control group. Lean mass and bone mineral density decreased less in the combination and resistance groups than in the aerobic group.

The investigators were surprised to find that combined aerobic and resistance training improved cardiovascular fitness to the same extent as aerobic training alone and increased strength to the same extent as resistance training alone. Of the three exercise regimens tested, weight loss plus combined aerobic and resistance exercise was the most effective in improving the physical functional status of obese older adults.

A study among 1.7 million survey participants confirms these findings.[115][116] It found that participation in either strength training or aerobic training is associated with a lower prevalence of obesity and that the combination of these activities is associated with an even lower prevalence of obesity. These results are in keeping with the recommendation that both aerobic and resistance physical activity are synergistic in benefiting health (see Chapter 9, "Benefits of Physical Activity").

In theory, to lose fat, it does not matter if the necessary calorie deficit is brought about by dietary calorie restriction or increased energy expenditure through physical activity. But for the average person, the difference in calorie expenditures between a sedentary and an active person may not be very great. Undoubtedly hours of exercise helped "The Biggest Losers," but many studies have shown that exercise alone is not an efficient "real world" way to lose weight compared to the adoption of a diet that causes restriction of calories.[117 118 119]

A review of more than 500 studies, including randomized, controlled trials (RCTs) shows only modest weight loss with exercise programs alone and only modest increases in weight loss when an exercise intervention is added to dietary restriction.[120 121] In most RCTs, the energy deficit from the prescribed exercise was modest, and the calories expended were far smaller than those resulting from dietary restriction. However, in studies that featured high levels of exercise, of sufficient magnitude to produce an energy deficit of 500 to 1,000 calories per day, participants substantially augmented weight loss.

A 2018 study suggests the importance of physical activity of long duration to weight loss.[122] The study was conducted to determine the amount of compensation for exercise energy expenditure either by eating more or moving less at two levels of exercise—the expenditure of either 1,500 or 3,000 calories a week. Overweight-to-obese sedentary men and women exercised expending either 300 calories (taking about 30 minutes) or 600 calories (requiring about 60 minutes) five days a week for four months. The 3,000 calorie/week group decreased both percentage and weight of body fat, while the 1,500 calorie/week group did not. Both groups compensated for the extra expenditure of calories in their workouts by extra eating. The 30 minutes a day group replaced nearly two-thirds of the calories they burned, but the 60 minutes a day group replaced only one-third of the calories they burned, so they lost more fat. The investigators pointed out that even with high levels of exercise, limiting calories is still needed for weight loss.[123]

Studies show a clear dose-response relationship between physical activity and weight maintenance. Similar to the experience of those participating in the NWCR, two rigorous studies found that about 80 minutes per day of moderate intensity activity added to a sedentary lifestyle was needed to prevent weight regain in the year after weight loss.[124 125] Time constraints and physical limitations that may be significant for overweight or obese adults make high levels of physical activity difficult to achieve and sustain. The loss of adipose tissue that occurs when an individual's exercise level increases may not lead to weight loss because of a desirable increase in lean muscle mass. Exercise can reduce body fat, increase lean body mass, and improve cardiovascular biomarkers even if it does not change body weight.

What is a healthy weight-loss diet?

For weight loss, lifestyle and behavioral factors are also important.[126 127] According to a recent review, "…individual, social, and environmental factors are also linked to energy imbalance. These include television watching and lower average sleep duration, especially among children/adolescents; socioeconomic status and race/ethnicity; local environments, such as the presence of fast-food restaurants, grocery stores, crime safety, parks or open spaces, and walking or biking paths; and influences of advertising, social norms, and work and home dynamics. Ultimately, these influences act through changes in diet or activity to influence weight change."[128]

These factors and differences in heredity and in resting metabolic rate may make weight loss and maintenance of a normal weight more difficult for some people than others. And if losing weight were easy, more than two-thirds of Americans would not be overweight or obese. But the factors that affect weight and equally important, maintaining a healthy weight that are under an individual's control are the most important determinates of adiposity. Selection of a healthy balance of nutrients in the diet, especially low levels of added sugar and high levels of fiber, limiting dietary intake of calories, and increasing expenditure of calories by increasing physical activity are actions under our control that are critical to weight loss and maintenance.

Food selection, or a "diet," and a lifestyle that includes a considerable amount of physical activity are the keys to weight loss and maintenance success. All diets that bring about weight loss do so by restricting calorie consumption. Some diets make it easier to limit calories. Among the characteristics of the ideal weight loss and maintenance diet are:

- It must be safe, nutritionally complete, healthy, and sustainable.
- It should be low in calorie density, avoid refined grains, added sugar, and highly processed foods that are loaded with sugars, fats, and salt.
- It should be high in plant-based high fiber foods—fruits, vegetables, legumes, and whole grains.

The composition of the diet is important but equally important is sticking to it.[129][130] That is why long-term control of weight requires the choice of a healthy diet that you can eat over a lifetime. Weight loss and maintenance of normal weight are facilitated by choice of a high proportion of fruits, vegetables, and whole grains in the diet; whereas selection of larger portion sizes and greater intakes of sugar-sweetened beverages, processed snacks, fast food meals, and possibly trans-fat, appear to increase the likelihood of gaining bodyweight. So, various features of dietary type and quality impact the number of calories a person is likely to eat.[131][132][133] To put it succinctly, you can lose weight the hard way, by focusing on limiting the portion sizes of a typical American diet, or the easy way, by changing your food choices.

The average human stomach can hold about a quart of food, roughly four cups. And when your stomach is full, the feeling of satiety kicks in, and you don't want to eat anymore. Filling up with apple slices would supply only a little over 200 calories, a stomach full of oatmeal would provide around 700 calories, but a stomach full of cheese about 4000 calories—more than a day's food needs. Another way of looking at calorie density is to consider how many calories three pounds of differing foods would contribute to your diet over a day—that is, about the average daily weight of food eaten by Americans. As shown in Table 4.4 below, high fat or pure fat foods are calorie-dense, and vegetables, fruits, and legumes are not.

Table 4.4. Number of Calories in One Pound of Various Foods

Foods	Calories/Pound
Vegetables	60–195
Fruit	140–120
Potatoes, Pasta, Rice, Barley, Yams, Corn, Hot Cereals	320–630
Beans, Peas, Lentils, Legumes	310–780
Breads, Bagels, Dried Fruit	920–1360
Meats	600–1500
Sugars, Syrups, Honey	1200–1800
Cheese, Dry Cereals, Pretzels	1480–1760
Nuts, Seeds, Butters	2400–3200
Oils	4000

In Chapter 3, "Optimal Nutrition," I describe the healthful Okinawa diet that is low-calorie-dense and associated with low levels of obesity and long life. I also describe a study of the traditional Hawaii diet that found that with a low-fat, low-calorie density diet, the study participants could eat as much food as they wanted, and they lost an average of 17 pounds over three weeks.[134] According to Michael Greger, "Low-calorie-density diets offer the best of both worlds: higher dietary quality and better weight loss."[135]

An energy deficit of 3500 calories is needed to lose a pound of fat. Although this simple formulation of weight gain and loss is generally valid, some research shows that it matters where you get the extra calories. Although the human body can convert surplus calories into fat from of each of the macronutrient categories (carbohydrates, proteins, fats, and alcohol), the biochemical pathways for metabolizing dietary fat, alcohol, and fructose, make it more likely that extra calories from these sources will end up stored as fat.[136]

There are hundreds of "weight loss" diets. Many of them work in the short term, and when they work, it is by limiting the consumption of calories. For many of these diets, elimination of certain types of foods, such as "carbs" or eating only a limited array of foods, is the way they work to reduce the intake of calories. These diets often give the appearance of very rapid weight loss. When the intake of calories is lower than a person's energy needs, the body first turns to glycogen stores for energy. Stored glycogen accounts for 5% of the liver's weight and makes up 1% of muscle weight. So, the initial loss of weight is not from losing much fat; it is mostly due to the mobilization and loss of glycogen to provide the body with energy that is accompanied by loss of body water—a phenomenon that happens initially on all calorie-restricted diets. After seven to 14 days, weight loss slows because the loss of body fluids ends, and the body's metabolism slows.[137]

The effectiveness and health effects of high-fat (low carb) compared to low-fat diets for long-term weight loss has long been debated. Many randomized controlled trials (RCTs) and reviews have given inconclusive results. Among the popular "named" diets are those that are low carbohydrate (e.g., Atkins, South Beach, Zone), those that are moderate in the proportion of macronutrients (e.g., Biggest Loser, Jenny Craig, Nutrisystem, Volumetrics, and WeightWatchers) and those that are low-fat (e.g., Ornish, Rosemary Conley). A meta-analysis of 48 randomized trials of popular diets showed that both low-carbohydrate and low-fat diets were associated with an estimated 8-kg (17.6 lb.) weight loss at 6-month follow-up compared with no diet. Their research suggests the choice of almost any diet that cuts calories and that you can adhere to will cause you to lose weight.[138 139 140]

As described in Chapter 3, "Optimal Nutrition," high-fat, high-protein, low-carb diets may have risks associated with their long-term use. Editorial comment on the meta-analysis study of the 48 trials noted that "Protein intakes of 30% of kilocalories, or double what the other diets provide, raise questions about possible long-term influences on kidney function, calcium losses, and other questions that should be explored."[141 142]

The Preventing Overweight Using Novel Dietary Strategies (POUNDS LOST) trial compared weight loss from diets made up of healthier food with differing proportions of macronutrients. The trial tested four diets with a 750 calorie per day deficit from estimated requirements: (1) a low-fat, average protein diet (20% fat, 15% protein, and 65% carbohydrate), (2) a low-fat, high protein diet (20% fat, 25% protein, and 55% carbohydrate), (3) a high-fat, average protein diet (40% fat, 15% protein, and 45% carbohydrate), and (4) a high-fat, high protein diet (40% fat, 25% protein, and 35% carbohydrate). The study found that at two years, weight losses were similar across all four diets and that body fat, abdominal fat, and hepatic fat were also similar, and there were no differences in loss of lean body mass. A commentary on the study noted that "...regardless of their macronutrient composition, weight loss was associated with significant reductions in cravings for fats, sweets, and starches while cravings for fruits and vegetables increased" and that, "... over time people not only adapted but actually preferred the taste of the nutrient-dense foods, such as fruits and vegetables, reflecting enhanced adherence to recommended intake of foods."[143 144 145 146]

The finding that either low-fat or low-carb eating can have comparable effects on weight was also found in a 2018 Stanford study published in the *JAMA*.[147] It compared the effect of counseling and a healthy low-fat diet (29% fat) to a healthy low-carbohydrate diet (45% fat) on weight change. The study found that a weight loss averaging 12 to 13 pounds over 12 months was not significantly different for each of the diets. It was also found that neither genotype pattern nor baseline insulin secretion was associated with the dietary effects on weight loss. All study subjects were encouraged to select a healthy diet featuring vegetables, minimally processed foods, and to eliminate or minimize added sugars and refined grain products. The low carb group, who consumed more saturated fats, had an increase in unhealthy LDL-cholesterol, whereas the LDL-cholesterol declined in the low-fat group. Triglycerides declined in both groups but more in the low carb group.

A similar study, published in *Circulation*, compared a lacto-ovo vegetarian (no fish or meat) diet and a Mediterranean Diet that included fish, dairy, poultry, and some red meat.[148] The two diets were equally effective in reducing body weight, BMI, and fat mass. The vegetarian diet was more effective in reducing LDL-cholesterol levels, while the Mediterranean Diet, as in the Stanford study, significantly reduced triglyceride levels.

Low carb (high fat/protein) and ketogenic diets: balancing effectiveness with risk

Currently fashionable low-carbohydrate and paleo diets typically are low in refined grains and added sugars but feature relatively high quantities of red and processed meat and saturated fat. A meta-analysis of randomized controlled trials (RCTs) found that in weight-loss trials, unlike metabolic studies where all eaten food is carefully controlled, low-carbohydrate interventions led to significantly greater weight loss than did low-fat dietary interventions.[149]

Recent formulations of ketogenic diets limit protein to amounts needed to maintain muscle mass, eliminate sugars and refined carbohydrates, and restrict total carbohydrates to 80 to 200 calories a day.[150] A meta-analysis found that individuals consuming very-low-carbohydrate ketogenic diets (less than 200 calories of carbohydrates/day) achieved better long-term body weight loss than individuals assigned to a conventional low-fat diet with less than 30% of calories from fat.[151]

Because low-carb diets are low in calories, they are effective for short-term use and improve some metabolic biomarkers, but with long-term use, they may increase health risk. For example, a meta-analysis that found a greater weight loss in subjects on low carbohydrate diets than those on low-fat diets found that although the low carb dieters had favorable changes in HDL-cholesterol and triglyceride levels, they had unfavorable increases in the LDL-cholesterol levels that are more significant for cardiovascular health.[152] The study authors concluded the beneficial changes of low-carbohydrate diets must be weighed against the possible detrimental effects of increased LDL-cholesterol.

A systematic review of 17 studies found that the risk of all-cause mortality among those with a high low-carbohydrate score was elevated by 30%.[153] A meta-analysis published in *Lancet Public Health* found that low carbohydrate diets with less than 50% to 55% energy from carbohydrate were associated with increased all-cause mortality unless their protein and fat was plant-based.[154] The excessive protein in low-carb diets has the potential to contribute to kidney and liver damage. They cannot be considered heart-healthy for long-term use.

Keto diets have additional important drawbacks. High protein diets have been shown to have detrimental effects on heart disease risk factors, including coronary artery blood flow.[155] [156] They are also not heart-healthy because, like similar low-carb diets, ketogenic diets likely to be deficient in fiber and micronutrients and are also likely to have the detrimental effect of increased LDL-cholesterol.[157] The lack of carbohydrates forces the body to mobilize some fat, but even more water and protein is lost.[158] This results in rapid weight loss, but much of it will be lean-body protein and water, not fat.

Ketosis can make a person feel unwell with "keto flu" (tired, dizzy, nauseated, weak, and poor sleep). Keto diets may be dangerous for people with heart disease, diabetes, or kidney problems. Especially people on medications for diabetes or high blood pressure should not embark on a ketogenic diet without close medical supervision because they may suffer dangerously low blood sugar or blood pressure.

Of the 35 diets evaluated by nutrition experts in the 2020 U.S. News & World Report, the ultra-low-fat vegetarian Ornish diet described below was ranked the best Heart Healthy Diet the Mediterranean Diet was ranked second and the DASH diet ranked third.[159] The Keto Diet — a low-carb, high-fat regimen — was ranked number 35, in last place, in the Best Diet for Healthy Eating category.

Evidence supporting low-fat and vegetarian diets for weight loss

There is evidence that ultra-low-fat diets are the most effective for weight loss. A National Institutes of Health study put people in a metabolic ward where they controlled the composition and calorie content of meals. The short-term study compared an ultra-low-fat diet (8% of calories from fat) and a low carbohydrate diet. Each diet contained an equal number of calories. According to the lead author, "Calorie for calorie, reducing dietary fat results in more body fat loss than reducing dietary carbohydrate when men and women with obesity have their food intake strictly controlled." The reduced-fat diet led to a roughly 67% greater body fat loss. The authors of the study did caution that "We did not address whether it would be easier to adhere to a reduced-fat or a reduced-carbohydrate diet under free-living conditions."[160]

Evidence supporting the effectiveness of low-fat diets for weight loss comes from a meta-analysis of 32 feeding studies with substitution of the same number of carbohydrate calories for fat calories. It found that fat loss was greater with lower fat diets.[161] A similar meta-analysis by Hooper and colleagues concluded that lower total fat intake does lead to small (3.5 lb.), but statistically significant and clinically meaningful sustained greater weight loss than other diet interventions.[162] Ornish notes that the patients in his randomized controlled trial achieved an average weight loss of 24 pounds in the first year.[163] In a larger study of almost 3,000 patients on the Ornish lifestyle program in 24 hospitals and clinics, BMI decreased by 6.6%.[164] Ornish notes that President Bill Clinton lost and kept off more than 20 pounds since following his whole foods, plant-based diet.

Many additional studies support the effectiveness of low-fat diets for weight loss. The BROAD study featured semi-weekly classes that encouraged participants to eat unrestricted amounts of whole, low-fat plant-based foods, fruits, vegetables, whole grains, and legumes. The overweight study subjects lost an average of 19 pounds at the end of the three-month study and were down by 27 pounds six months later.[165] The ultra-low-fat Hawaii traditional food diet featured low-calorie density eating of whole grains, fruits, vegetables, and beans.[166] The study participants could eat as much food as they wanted. They actually ate more, but different, food that cut calories by 40% and lost an average of 17 pounds over three weeks. Other studies have concluded that a plant-based dietary pattern is the most effective approach for weight loss. A review of 12 randomized controlled trials (RCTs) found that compared to non-vegetarian weight-loss diets, those on the vegetarian diets lost the most weight.[167]

Another study of five different diets, vegan, vegetarian, pesco-vegetarian, semi-vegetarian, and omnivorous, found that those following the vegan and vegetarian diet plans lost the most weight over the course of the 6-month study.[168] The authors concluded that vegan diets may result in greater weight loss than other diets.

The Mediterranean dietary pattern also offers advantages for weight control compared to a typical American diet. In a study where mostly olive oil was substituted for saturated fat, the study subjects lost five pounds of fat over a month.[169] Switching from a diet high in saturated fats to one with polyunsaturated and monounsaturated fats contributes to decreased body fat. When consumed, saturated fats may be more likely to end up stored as body fat rather than being metabolized for energy.[170] However, oils such as olive oil that are predominantly made up of unsaturated fats are still calorie-dense and should not be used excessively.

Anderson, Konz, and Jenkins evaluated the advantages and disadvantages of various weight-reducing diets.[171] Writing in the *Journal of the American College of Nutrition*, they noted that long-term consumption of diets high in saturated fats and cholesterol would increase serum cholesterol levels and risk for coronary heart disease (CHD). Diets restricted in added sugar intake would lower serum cholesterol levels and long-term risk for CHD; however, higher carbohydrate, higher fiber, lower fat diets would have the greatest effect in decreasing serum cholesterol concentrations and risk of CHD. They concluded that "While high-fat diets may promote short-term weight loss, the potential hazards for worsening risk for progression of atherosclerosis override the short-term benefits. Individuals derive the greatest health benefits from diets low in saturated fat and high in carbohydrate and fiber: these increase sensitivity to insulin and lower risk for CHD."

Not only are whole-food plant-based diets the most likely to normalize weight, but they are also the most likely to maximize health and longevity.[172]

Saving muscle while losing fat.

If weight loss is rapid, up to one-third of the loss can come from lean body mass (mostly muscle) rather than fat. So it is important to eat adequate amounts of protein and undertake both aerobic and muscle-strengthening physical activity while dieting. Studies have shown that it is possible to retain and build muscle mass during both dieting and when engaged in weight-training. High protein intake has a modest beneficial effect on preserving lean body and muscle mass during weight loss, and both endurance- and resistance-type exercise help preserve muscle mass, and resistance-type exercise also improves muscle strength.[173]

Although some studies have found no benefit to muscle preservation from increased protein,[174] other studies, including an analysis of 17 clinical trials of people over age 60 (average age 73), found that consuming 10 to 35 grams of extra protein per day significantly increased lean muscle mass and leg strength in men but not much in women.[175][176] Six studies found that on average more than 90% of lean body mass losses during calorie-restricted eating could be avoided by resistance training three times a week.[177]

A review of 49 studies found that weight-trainers consuming 1.6 grams of protein per kilogram of body weight a day, about twice the recommended 0.8 gm/kg, had modestly larger increases in muscle size and strength than those consuming lesser amounts.[178] Higher amounts of than 1.6 gm/kg of protein were not beneficial. Consumption of 0.73 grams of protein per pound of body weight (1.6 gm/kg) a day would be 112 grams of protein a day for a (70 kg.) 154-pound man. This is double the USDA nutrition goal recommended 56 grams a day for men and 46 grams a day for women. Consuming 4 grams of protein for every 10 pounds of your weight is another way of estimating recommended daily protein consumption. This is not a difficult goal to reach from plant and animal sources. A cup of beans contains 15 to 18 grams of protein, a chicken breast 43 grams, yogurt 10 to 20 grams per cup, and an 8-ounce glass of fat-free milk contains approximately 8.5 grams of protein—nearly 40% of the total calories of skim milk.

So, what can we conclude from the data on weight-loss diets?

Many studies have found little difference in weight loss among different diets but did find differences in long-term health effects. For example, a meta-analysis of 19 trials found little or no difference in weight loss and changes in cardiovascular risk factors after up to two years of follow-up when overweight and obese adults, with or without type 2 diabetes, consumed low carbohydrate diets and balanced weight-loss diets with the same calorie content.[179] Differences in the effectiveness of various types of diet for just weight loss relate mainly to the degree of adherence to the diet and the extent of calorie restriction rather than their macronutrient composition.[180] [181] [182]

But sticking to a diet that leads to a sustained normal weight is much easier if it is low in calorie density, avoids refined grains, added sugar and highly processed foods that are loaded with sugars, fats, and salt, and is high in plant-based high fiber foods—fruits, vegetables, legumes, and whole grains.

The long-term health effects of some low-carbohydrate diets have the potential to increase cardiovascular disease risk by increasing unhealthy LDL cholesterol, and high-quality diets can reduce CVD risk. Low fat and low carb (and many other diets) work for short term weight loss, but only healthy diets should be considered for long-term nutrition.

We can see and measure the fat in our bodies, but we also need to adopt diets that prevent cancer, high blood pressure and the silent and unseen build-up of arteriosclerosis in our blood vessels that ultimately leads to heart disease or a fatal heart attack—still the leading cause of death in the U.S. Avoiding most processed food and eating a whole food plant-based diet will give you the benefits of being high in fiber, low in added sugars, low in saturated fats and it will not be calorie-dense. Add in substantial exercise, and you have a good recipe for staying healthy, gaining muscle and losing fat, inches, and weight.

For most people, successful weight loss requires a change in lifestyle—a change in behavior. In general, to lose weight requires dietary changes and, if you are sedentary or not very active, increased physical activity. It may take some experimentation to figure out what combination of behavior changes relating to diet and exercise works best for each individual. Your number one goal should be to avoid accumulating or to lose any excess visceral fat—the fat in and around your liver and other abdominal organs that shows up as increased girth. To become metabolically healthy should be your first objective.

Determining appropriate dietary intake of calories for weight loss

Since eating more calories than you expend is the cause of obesity, it is useful to determine how many calories you should eat each day to maintain your current weight and then to decide on a weight loss goal and the average daily calorie intake needed to lose the amount of weight you want. To maintain their current weight, a person who gets at least an average of 30 minutes of physical activity every day requires about 15 calories per pound of body weight. For a completely sedentary person, this figure would drop to about 12 calories per pound to maintain their weight.

The following table from the USDA provides a rough guide of estimated daily calorie needs according to physical activity status. The active category includes physical activity equivalent to walking three or more miles per day at 3–4 miles per hour.[183]

Table 4.5. Calories Needed to Maintain Weight According to Physical Activity

Females Age	Sedentary	Active
14–18	1,800	2,400
19–30	2,000	2,400
31–50	1,800	2,200
51+	1,600	2,200
Males Age		
14–18	2,200	3,200
19–30	2,400	3,000
31–50	2,400	3,000
51+	2,200	2,800

When you cut 3500 calories out of your regular diet, as the weeks go by, the time to lose a pound of weight will increase. This is because the initial weight loss will include body water, and as your weight declines, your metabolism slows as your body tries to preserve energy stores, and it takes less energy to move a lighter body around for daily activities.

Although it is tempting to plan to lose as much weight as possible as quickly as possible, a better strategy is to adopt a lifetime diet plan and limit weight loss to a safe rate of about 0.5 to 1 pound a week, with an upper limit of two pounds per week for the very obese. Since one pound of body fat contains 3,500 calories, to lose 0.5 pounds a week requires a deficit over the week of 1,750 calories or an average of 250 calories a day less than your maintenance intake. To lose one pound a week would require cutting 500 calories a day from your maintenance intake. To maintain adequate nutrition and to avoid loss of lean body mass (muscle), nutrition experts recommend that a person's calorie intake should not be less than 1,200 calories a day for women and 1,500 calories a day for men. Losing gradually is a realistic long-term goal and is also a goal most likely to be met.

Monitoring caloric intake and weight can help you determine the calorie level needed to maintain or lose weight. Computer and phone apps can help with this. A useful website is the NIH Body Weight Planner at https://www.niddk.nih.gov/bwp. It takes into account the slowing of metabolism that occurs as you lose weight. The planner will take into account your body size and physical activity, your weight goal, and when you want to reach it. It will calculate the calories you should eat in order to maintain your current weight, how much you should eat to reach your goal, and how many calories to eat every day to maintain your new weight.

A similar Louisiana State University, Pennington Biomedical Research Center planner, can be found at https://www.pbrc.edu/research-and-faculty/calculators/weight-loss-predictor/. It shows the trajectory of weight loss according to the daily calorie deficit compared to your maintenance diet.

Studies have shown that estimating the calorie content of food is not easy or exact, and most people tend to considerably underestimate the number of calories that they have eaten. Some people find that simply counting calories and stopping at their predetermined limit each day is all they need to do to lose and maintain weight. Some people find that counting calories does not work for them, but eliminating foods with added sugar or eliminating processed foods (or both) and limiting their diet to high-quality plant-based foods is an effective strategy.[184] [185] For still others, additional measures, such as upping physical activity, will be needed, especially to keep weight off.

Make the best food choices

Too much of the American diet is made up of high fat, high sugar junk food that with 50% to 60% of total calories from sugar and other refined carbohydrates, desserts, fast food, and snacks. Minimizing the intake of added sugar is a particularly important strategy for weight loss. High intake of added sugar has been shown to be associated with high body weight and type 2 diabetes. Several randomized controlled trials have demonstrated that reducing consumption of sugar-sweetened beverages intake improves metabolism and weight control in both children and adults.[186 187] One lifestyle intervention found that each serving per day reduction in sugar-sweetened beverages was associated with a 1.4 pound greater weight loss.[188] In a meta-analysis that looked at 30 studies, the authors singled out the consumption of sugar-sweetened beverages as particularly likely to be associated with high body weight, in part because beverages such as juices and soft drinks are less filling (i.e., they cause less satiety) than other forms of food. They also noted that it may not be sugar alone that is associated with high body weight because added sugar is a component of processed foods such as cookies, cakes, and ice cream that are also high in fat.[189]

Although it is best to avoid most processed foods, because they are often loaded with sugar, consumers can make better choices after referring to the Nutrition Facts Label (NFL) on processed foods. The new NFL provides a listing of total sugar, and that separately lists the amount of the healthy sugars found in fruits and vegetables and added sugars. Better yet, buy mainly the whole, unprocessed fruit and vegetables that don't need a label.

In addition to minimizing added sugar, substituting complex carbohydrates for fats in the form of fruits, vegetables, and whole grains for dietary fat will increase bulk and possibly satiety for the same number of calories consumed. Plant-based whole foods contain more water and more fiber, and each gram of protein or carbohydrate will provide four calories compared to nine calories per gram for fat. So, a diet rich in these foods is low in calorie density with fewer calories per gram. More bulk with the same number of calories is more filling and more effective at suppressing appetite. A whole food plant-based diet that avoids refined carbohydrates like sugar will make you less hungry, and adherence to a calorie-restricted diet easier.

Avoiding temptation and other psychological issues

Many people have trouble controlling the consumption of sweets and other favorite foods. For many of us, it is best not to buy them when shopping, not to keep them in the house, and not to order them when eating out. If you can't reach it, you can't eat it. Keep in mind that as was described in detail in Chapter 3, "Optimal Nutrition," the food industry has processed foods to make them as tempting and palatable as possible by loading them with sugar, salt, and fat and engineering their mouth feel. [190] A Johns Hopkins guide to healthy nutrition pointed out that food manufacturers have devised foods that "...override the body's natural satiety-regulating system in a way that eating handfuls of unprocessed foods—like apple slices, baby carrots or celery stalks—simply wouldn't."[191]

As already described, some people, perhaps most people, overeat in certain situations because they use food as a way to cope with boredom, sadness, anxiety, loneliness and various causes of stress, including studying for an exam, work deadlines, watching their favorite team, and lack of sleep. Too often, we use food for comfort, to release tension or as a reward for accomplishing a task such as completing a final exam or work project. Food does not solve problems, and overeating causes them.

Obesity experts note that behavioral therapy for weight loss should include daily monitoring of food intake and physical activity and at least weekly monitoring of weight. The U.S. Preventive Services Task Force concluded, "...with moderate certainty that offering or referring adults with obesity to intensive, multicomponent behavioral interventions (i.e., behavior-based weight loss and weight loss maintenance interventions) has a moderate net benefit."[192] Ideally, behavioral therapy should include the support of a trained interventionist who provides a structured curriculum of behavioral change, including goal setting, problem-solving, stimulus control, regular feedback, and support.[193,194] However, it is unlikely that access to a trained behavioral interventionist will be practical for the more than 155 million Americans who are overweight or obese. With good diet choices and physical activity, you can lose weight and keep it off on your own.

Intermittent fasting

Evidence is emerging that when eating is confined to a 6-hour period, as in an 18-hour fast, metabolism switches from glucose supplied by the liver to adipose cell-derived ketones for energy. Intermittent fasting is associated with health benefits, including weight loss and decreased obesity.[195] Studies in animals have found a decreased incidence of obesity, cardiovascular disease, cancers, and brain diseases. Studies in humans suggest that diets with a variety of fasting intervals can improve the biomarkers that indicate good health and help weight loss.[196,197]

Among weight loss eating strategies are those that incorporate "mini-fasts," such as alternate day caloric restriction or eating just one meal every 24 hours.[198,199,200] Intermittent fasting at 18 hours a day or with food restricted to 500 to 700 calories every other day or two days a week (5:2 fasting) improves cholesterol and triglyceride levels and decreases obesity, insulin resistance, high blood pressure, and inflammation.[201 202] Unfortunately, these fasting patterns bring about loss of lean body (muscle) mass. Avoiding a total fast and taking in 500 to 700 calories a day of foods that include carbohydrates can help preserve lean body mass.[203]

The evidence for the positive human health benefits of intermittent fasting has come mainly from short-term studies, but 5:2 fasting (with some food intake on the two fast days), every other day fasting and eating only in a 6-hour period appears to confer benefits to health including weight loss. Proponents of intermittent fasting claim that the initial side effects of hunger and irritability during fast periods usually disappear after a month.

It should be noted that there is evidence that a total fast of more than one day is unhealthy and intermittent fasting according to any schedule should only be done under the supervision of a physician—especially if you are diabetic or on any medications.[204 205 206] My advice is to avoid long-term total fasting, but some people may be helped by the 5:2 partial fast or the 18-hour fast regimen. I think it is better to adopt a healthy diet that leads to a stable, healthy weight without excess adiposity—one that you can eat every day long-term.

We know from animal experiments that altering metabolism through restriction of food slows aging in many animals. However, the role of chronic calorie restriction on human longevity is not clear. Life extension was not found in experiments at the National Institute of Aging when rhesus monkeys on calorie restricted diets were compared to those on a healthy diet with calories restricted enough to avoid obesity. In similar monkey experiments at the Wisconsin National Primate Research Center, when a control group was allowed to eat a typical U.S. style high sugar diet (sucrose was 28.5% of carbohydrates) without restriction, the calorie restricted monkeys lived longer.[207] These experiments suggest that the nature of the diet and overfeeding were more important than severe calorie restriction. It is not known how relevant these effects are for humans or their potential for extending human life. The monkey experiments suggest that for age extension, eating a healthy diet and avoiding overweight is as healthful as and certainly a lot more pleasant than chronic severe calorie restriction.

Michael Greger's weight loss boosters

In writing his nearly 600-page book, *How Not to Diet*, Dr. Michael Greger reviewed nearly 5000 scientific studies.[208] He identified several additional strategies that can contribute to attaining and maintaining a normal weight that he calls weight-loss boosters. The boosters are additional factors that, for example, may slightly or moderately boost fat metabolism, suppress appetite, or decrease the absorption of calories. They don't take the place of diet and exercise, and some of these suggestions are not well-proven, but they may help some people decrease excess adiposity. For example:

- Get social support for weight loss through coaching, group therapy, and self-monitoring.
- Preload meals by drinking plenty of water and stay hydrated during the day
- Eat more at breakfast—like a king, lunch—like a prince, and less dinner—like a pauper. And don't eat too late in the day, after 7 pm.
- Chew thoroughly, eat slowly, and leave 20 minutes for the "I'm full" signal to kick in before a second helping.
- Avoid liquid calories, but there are some exceptions, such as pureed blended vegetable-based soups.
- Exercise on an empty stomach—that will burn more fat calories than after a meal.
- Boost non-exercise physical activity by more standing and moving about throughout the day.
- Activate brown fat by turning down the thermostat or eating cayenne pepper (1/2 tsp) and/or ground ginger (1 tsp).
- Combat inflammation with nutritional yeast (2 tsp)
- Activate AMPK, the enzyme that boosts the conversion of fat to energy storage in cells. Exercise and more than 100 plant products will do this as will the acetic acid found in vinegar. Greger recommends 2 tablespoons of vinegar with each meal—don't take it straight.
- Eat an ounce of ground flaxseeds daily. To avoid too much cyanide, avoid more than 9 tablespoons of raw flaxseeds a day.
- The spices, cumin (½ tsp), black cumin (1/4 tsp), and garlic powder (1/4 tsp) may help suppress appetite.

Key suggestions for successful weight loss

The following key suggestions for successful weight loss are adapted from the *Johns Hopkins White Paper, Nutrition and Weight Control*,[209] and the *University of California, Berkeley Wellness Letter*.[210]

- Monitor and keep a record of caloric intake, calories expended in physical activity, and weight.[211] Applications on a computer, smartphone, or fitness tracker can help you keep track of calories expended, calories consumed, and weight.
- Occasionally overeating need not derail your overall weight-loss plan. As Alexander Pope (b. 1688) noted, "to err is human." All we can do is just get back on a healthy diet and exercise plan after a lapse at a party or during a holiday.
- When preparing foods, manage portion sizes (keep them small). Measure and

weigh your food—at least until you know the number of calories in a serving of the food you eat. Minimize the consumption of processed food.

- Control your food environment—don't buy tempting foods you should not be eating.
- Eat at home and avoid "bargain" mega-meals and super-sized drinks offered at fast-food restaurants. [212,213]
- When serving food, use small plates, bowls, and glasses.
- Eat high-volume low-calorie density foods. In general, whole or minimally processed plant-based foods have a low caloric density.
- Be wary about drinking high-calorie beverages, including beer, wine, mixed drinks, sugar-sweetened beverages (SSBs), juices, and coffee or tea if they are loaded with sugar and cream. Remember that alcohol is calorie-dense at seven calories per gram or 198 calories per ounce, and after a few drinks, your will power to hold back on consumption of too much food and drink is likely to be impaired.
- Beverages with artificial sweeteners are preferable to SSBs but water is superior to diet drinks for weight control and health.[214,215]
- Involve family, friends, colleagues, and your health care provider in your quest for a healthier lifestyle.[216] Social support, even a friendly competition, may help you to start and stick to a diet and exercise plan and increase the odds that you will be successful.
- Remember that it takes about 20 minutes for the brain to register that you have a full stomach. Okinawans stop eating when 80% full: They call this hara hachi bu.[217]
- Minimize sedentary activities such as television watching, gaming, and the use of other electronic devices.[218,219]
- Avoid processed foods; most have too much added unhealthy fat, sugar, and salt. Sugar is your main enemy. Excess glucose stimulates insulin that increases fat storage, and excess fructose (or ethanol) goes directly to fat.
- Avoid foods that lend to unthinking robotic consumption of food when you are distracted. A good example of this would be munching chips while watching TV.
- Don't use fats or oils for cooking or on your salads. Water on non-stick pans is usually all that is needed for cooking. Remember that fat is calorie-dense at nine calories per gram or 255 calories per ounce.
- Consider whether to make changes gradually or all at once. To avoid any health-related problems, it is important that you consult with your health care provider if you are on medication and are being treated for a health condition such as high blood pressure or diabetes before a dramatic change in diet or other lifestyle changes.
- When it comes to exercise, gradual increases are essential to avoid soreness and injury, but for a healthy person, a diet change can be either gradual or all

at once. Even for healthy individuals, some experts advise to change diets gradually, but I don't think this is necessary. My advice is to find a diet plan that is healthy for the long term and then just start it and maintain it—recognizing that temporary setbacks will occur. Just be careful at parties and holiday eating!

Medications, Surgery and Other Treatments for Obesity

Eating an extremely low-calorie diet, long total fasting, taking medication to lose weight, or having surgery to lose weight are options that carry a significant risk of long-term serious side effects.[220] They should be considered only for people who are seriously obese, when recommended by a physician and only undertaken under medical supervision. Although bariatric surgery is an effective intervention to bring about weight loss, improve metabolism and reduce the risk of diabetes and CVD, so can a healthier lifestyle without the cost, health risks, and the lifetime of unpleasant side effects.[221 222 223 224 225]

Summary of the essential facts

- To identify excess adiposity, use your waist-to-height ratio. Your waist should measure less than half your height.
- The typical American lifestyle and diet is not healthy and leads to overweight and obesity. We are too sedentary, and our food choices contain too much saturated fat, meat, refined grains, sodium, added sugars, highly processed foods, and too many calories. Among these nutrients, high consumption of sugar and other refined carbohydrates make the greatest contribution to overweight and obesity.
- Some nutrition experts assert that an optimal diet for attaining and maintaining normal weight is whole-food plant-based because it is high in fiber, not calorie-dense and reduces hunger by the elimination of refined carbohydrates, e.g., white bread, white rice, cookies, crackers, and sugar-sweetened beverages, and the fats in highly processed foods. The Ornish diet comes the closest to this, and the Mediterranean diet is a close second.
- Successful weight loss requires behavior changes, especially the adoption of a reduced-calorie diet for losing no more than one pound a week and provide at least 1,500 calories a day for men and 1,200 calories a day for women.
- To avoid lean body (muscle) loss when losing weight, consume adequate protein and engage in aerobic (e.g., biking, jogging) and resistance (e.g., weight-lifting) physical activities.
- Maintaining weight loss usually requires a high level of physical activity. Many people who successfully keep weight off exercise an hour a day.

- Many successful dieters have found that consistent monitoring of weight, food intake, and physical activity is an essential strategy.
- Adherence to a calorie restricted diet, regardless of its macronutrient composition, is an important determinant of successful loss of weight.
- All weight-loss diets work by limiting calories, regardless of their composition, and most will provide a short-term improvement in metabolic biomarkers, but only healthy diets should be considered for long-term nutrition.

Additional reading

If after reading this chapter, you are confused about how to lose weight or want additional details about how and why so many of us get fat, I recommend two books:

Dr. Robert H. Lustig, *Fat Chance, Beating the Odds Against Sugar, Processed Food, Obesity and Disease*. New York: Plume, 2012.

Dr. Michael Greger, *How Not to Diet*. New York: Flatiron Books, gv 2019.

5
Vitamins and Other Supplements

Dietary supplements are vitamins, minerals, amino acids, enzymes, herbs and other botanicals, and various other substances that are added to a diet because they are considered to be useful for maintaining or improving health. A botanical is a plant or part of a plant that is supposed to have medicinal or therapeutic properties. Supplements include a variety of vitamins, minerals like calcium and iron, herbs such as echinacea and garlic, and specialty products like glucosamine, probiotics, sports drinks, and fish oils. They come in many forms, including pills, capsules, powders, drinks, and energy bars.[1 2 3 4]

Although many supplements are expensive, and other than vitamins they are seldom needed, the use of supplements by Americans is extensive. A 2016 survey conducted for the dietary supplement industry trade association, Council for Responsible Nutrition (CRN), found that supplements are taken by 71% of U.S. adults—more than 170 million of us. The survey found that 75% of supplement users take a multivitamin and that the next most popular supplements are vitamin D, vitamin C, calcium, and vitamin B/B complex.[5]

With a healthy diet, most people don't need dietary supplements–and they may be harmful

Widespread use does not mean that supplements are needed. Unlike prescription drugs, other than vitamins, very few supplements are scientifically proven to be beneficial to health. An editorial published in the *Journal of the American Medical Association* (*JAMA*) titled "The Supplement Paradox: Negligible Benefits, Robust Consumption," noted that "During the past two decades, a steady stream of high-quality studies evaluating dietary supplements has yielded predominantly disappointing results about potential health benefits, whereas evidence of harm has continued to accumulate."[6] Available scientific evidence indicates that for most people eating a varied healthy diet, supplements are not needed, and they can be dangerous.

Most supplements are not approved by the Food and Drug Administration (FDA) to be safe, pure, and effective. Some supplements, especially vitamins, are useful in certain situations to correct deficiencies and improve health in other ways, but many are known to be harmful. For example, a dietary supplement sold nationwide as a weight loss and body-building aid caused cases of liver damage resulting in hospitalizations, liver failure, liver transplants, and at least one death.[7] A review of 977 events reported to the FDA between 2004 and 2015 found that after taking a single supplement, most often those related to body-building, there were 166 hospitalizations, 39 reports of life-threatening events, and 22 deaths.[8] According to a study in the *New England Journal of Medicine*, 23,000 people per year end up in a hospital emergency room after taking a supplement.[9] [10]

Many supplements can be considered a type of "complementary" or "alternative medicine." Despite the popularity of alternative medicine, and annual expenditures of nearly $15 billion a year on homeopaths and various other healers, alternative medicine is not proven to have a benefit to health beyond a placebo effect.[11] [12] The placebo effect is the relief of symptoms attributable to patients' "participation in the therapeutic encounter, with its rituals, symbols, and interactions."[13] Many symptoms are responsive to placebos that cause the release of substances such as endogenous (intrinsic) opioids and dopamine, but the basic biology of a disease condition is rarely altered by a placebo.[14] The psychological factors that promote beneficial placebo effects also have the potential to cause an increase of symptoms. For example, if a person is warned about possible side effects of a medication, heightened attentiveness to normal background discomforts may be perceived to be side effects of the medication. When this happens, it is called a nocebo effect.[15]

Vitamins are essential to human health, but when added in large quantities as supplements to the diet, they do not enhance health, and they may cause toxicity from an overdose. With some exceptions, such as some elderly, vegans, pregnant women, and infants, it is possible to get the needed vitamins and minerals from healthy nutrition. For those with specific dietary limitations, needs, or deficiencies, as determined by a competent health care professional, and perhaps for those who want insurance against possible deficiencies, a standard-dose multivitamin/multi-mineral or vitamin D supplement that does not exceed recommended levels, is a reasonable and inexpensive choice.

Do supplements work as claimed?

Prescription drugs have labels, package inserts, advertising, and health claims that must be approved by the FDA as scientifically sound, accurate, and balanced, with risks as well as benefits described. But the advertising and information provided to consumers about dietary supplements do not require premarket review or approval by the FDA, and the result has been the frequent development and introduction of unsafe products.[16 17 18] "There's a false perception that supplements fall under the same regulatory umbrella as prescription drugs," said Orly Avitzur, medical adviser for *Consumer Reports.* Although the dietary supplement manufacturer is responsible for ensuring that a dietary supplement is safe before it is marketed, there are many examples of unsafe products being sold. The FDA is responsible for taking action against any dietary supplement that turns out to be an unsafe product after it reaches the market.

Supplements can be advertised and sold without scientific proof of their value to health because, in 1994, the U.S. Congress responded to lobbying by the so-called "health food" industry and passed the Dietary Supplement Health and Education Act. It curtailed the mandate of the FDA to regulate dietary supplements. The result was an explosion of supplement options hitting the market. Their number increased from about 4,000 in 1994 to 90,000 in 2018, with annual sales of $46 billion.[19 20 21 22 23 24] An article in *JAMA* noted that nearly two-thirds of adults over age 70 use supplements and that spending on supplements approaches 10% of all outlays for pharmaceuticals.[25] The author suggested that given their potential for harm, it is time to focus on the safety of supplements.

Dietary supplement labels may and often do carry unproven health-related claims, for example, that a dietary supplement addresses a nutrient deficiency, supports or improves health, is good for body-building, causes weight loss, or is linked to a particular body function, like strengthening the immune system or benefiting sexual, brain or heart health. Although supplement makers can claim their products help maintain the structure or function or health of the body, they cannot claim to cure disease. Labels with these types of claims must include the words, "This statement has not been evaluated by the Food and Drug Administration. This product is not intended to diagnose, treat, cure, or prevent any disease." On a typical supplement label, this language is likely to be written in small print and difficult to find at an obscure part of the label or referred to by an asterisk at the health-related claim.[26 27 28]

An estimated 5 million U.S. adults and 1 million children use a homeopathic product each year. Homeopathy is an alternative medicine practice based on the unproven and biologically implausible theory that "like cures like" and the "law of infinitesimals," wherein extraordinarily diluted substances that supposedly cause the symptoms of a disease in healthy people will cure similar symptoms in sick people. Because they are so dilute, most, but not all, homeopathic products are likely to be safe but have no therapeutic value beyond a placebo effect. As dietary supplements, homeopathic products are also largely unregulated for safety and efficacy by the FDA. However, their unproven claims could be curbed by the Federal Trade Commission (FTC) on the basis of being false advertising.

Some of the poorly regulated homeopathic formulations have resulted in serious harms. The *JAMA* reported that over 6 years, the FDA received more than 400 reports of adverse events—even seizures and deaths— in infants and children associated with homeopathic teething products. Following a warning from the FDA, product manufacturers and some pharmacies voluntarily removed all brands of homeopathic teething products from their online and retail stores. In January 2017, the FDA announced that its laboratory analysis had found elevated belladonna levels in some of the teething tablets that "far exceeded" the amount stated on the label.[29] Beyond being a waste of money, the use of some homeopathic products could harm health and result in avoiding or delaying the diagnosis and treatment of an illness with scientifically proven medical remedies and thus could result in significant harm.[30 31]

Supplement quality control

The FDA does have powers that can be useful in regulating supplements. The FDA requires that manufacturers must follow good manufacturing practices (GMP) to ensure the identity, purity, strength, and composition of their products. They can monitor information on the product's label and package insert and, at least in theory, make sure that information about the supplement's content is accurate and that any claims made for the product are truthful and not misleading. The FDA can require a recall of unsafe products.[32 33 34] Between 2007 and 2016, the FDA ordered recalls of 776 supplements because they contained unapproved, unlabeled drug ingredients that are potentially dangerous.[35] Although the FDA has the mandate to oversee the labeling and manufacture of supplements, it just does not have the funds or workforce to keep up with and appropriately monitor all 90,000 supplements on the market.[36 37]

Independent testing has found that the strength of supplements may vary markedly and that the contents may not even be what is described on the label. The contents may be different, diluted, or even be missing entirely.[38 39] Four out of 5 herbal supplements tested by the New York State Attorney General's office in 2015 did not contain the herbs listed on the labels.[40] A commentary on a 2018 survey of unapproved drugs in supplements noted, "...between 2007 and 2016 the FDA identified 746 brands of supplements adulterated with pharmaceutical agents. The adulterants included prescription medications such as sildenafil and fluoxetine, withdrawn medications including sibutramine and phenolphthalein, and unapproved drugs, including dapoxetine and designer steroids. Twenty percent of the adulterated supplements contained two or more undeclared drugs...Most supplements adulterated with drugs were marketed as weight loss, sexual enhancement, or sports supplements..."[41 42]

A few supplements have obtained an independent evaluation and come with a written guarantee that the product is made under the FDA's good manufacturing practices (GMP) conditions, as well as a Certificate of Analysis (COA) that assures that the label accurately describes what the customer is buying. Consumers can also gain assurance from labeling that shows that the product has been "U.S.P. Verified." This proves the supplement has been inspected and approved under the United States Pharmacopeial Convention. Unfortunately, fewer than 1% of supplements on the market have been U.S.P. Verified.[43]

Paul A. Offit, and Sarah Erush of the Children's Hospital of Philadelphia, reached out to supplement manufacturers for verification of GMP. They found that about 90% of the companies never responded, and of the remainder, many manufacturers refused to provide either a statement of GMP or a COA; "in other words, they refused to guarantee that their products were what they said they were. Others lied; they said they met GMP standards, but a call to the FDA revealed they had been fined for violations multiple times." The FDA estimates that approximately 50,000 adverse reactions to dietary supplements occur every year, but few dietary supplement consumers are aware of this risk.

Offit and Erush concluded, "...until the day comes when medical studies prove that these supplements have legitimate benefits, and until the FDA has the political backing and resources to regulate them like drugs, individuals should simply steer clear. For too long, too many people have believed that dietary supplements can only help and never hurt. Increasingly, it's clear that this belief is a false one."[44]

Understanding nutritional recommendations and the amount of nutrients in food or supplements[45]

Potentially confusing different terms are used when referring to the amount of a particular nutrient (such as calcium or vitamin D) your body needs for good health and when measuring the amount of a particular nutrient in a serving of food or in a dietary supplement. The amount of a vitamin is often listed in International Units (IU) that relate to the biological effects of the vitamin. For example, one IU is equal to 0.3 micrograms (μg) of vitamin A (retinol), but for vitamin D, one IU is equal to 25 nanograms.

Dietary Reference Intakes (DRIs) are a family of nutrient reference values, including the Estimated Average Requirement (EAR)s that are intended to serve as a guide for good nutrition and to provide the basis for the development of nutrient guidelines. The EAR is used for planning and assessing diets of populations; it also serves as the basis for calculating the Recommended Dietary Allowances (RDA). RDAs are the recommended daily intakes of a nutrient for healthy people and a value intended to meet or exceed the requirement for 97.5% of the population. They tell you, on average, how much of that nutrient you should be getting each day. RDAs are developed by the Food and Nutrition Board of the Institute of Medicine of the National Academies. Because RDAs vary by age, gender, and whether a woman is pregnant or breastfeeding, there are many different RDAs for each nutrient.[46]

Tolerable Upper Intake Level (UL) is the highest average daily intake that is likely to pose no risk of adverse effects to almost all individuals in the general population. As intake increases above the UL, the potential risk of adverse effects may increase.

Daily Values (DVs) describe how much (in percentage) of a nutrient a serving of the food or supplement provides in the context of a total daily diet. DVs are established by the FDA and are used on food and dietary supplement labels. For each nutrient, unlike the RDAs, there is one DV for all people ages four years and older. Therefore, DVs aren't recommended intakes, but DVs often match or exceed the RDAs for most people. DVs are presented on food and supplement labels as a percentage. For example, the DV for calcium on a food label might say 20%. This means it has 200 mg (milligrams) of calcium in one serving because the DV for calcium is 1,000 mg/day. The FDA has a web page that lists the DVs for all nutrients.[47]

The Recommended Dietary Allowances (RDA) is the best guide to how much of a nutrient to consume for good health. Still, most people eating a varied plant-based healthy diet do not need to be concerned about the precise content of vitamins and other nutrients in the food they eat.

Sometimes vitamins and other supplements help maintain or improve health

It seems sensible that any drug or dietary supplement should have a scientifically proven therapeutic benefit, and its benefits should outweigh any risks to health. Vitamins are essential to health, but most studies have shown limited or no health benefits from taking extra vitamins.[48] Although most individuals can obtain all the vitamins and minerals they need by eating a variety of healthy foods, some individuals may not, such as vegans, others who choose restricted diets, or individuals in a particular life stage such as being pregnant, breastfeeding, or elderly. Others may have health conditions that affect digestion, appetite, and limit nutrient absorption and use. Individuals with food allergies, gluten or lactose intolerance, malabsorption from celiac disease, and alcoholics may not get adequate nutrients from diet alone. People in some of these circumstances may benefit from taking a specific multivitamin and/or multimineral supplements. It is a good idea to consult a medical professional and follow their advice before taking a dietary supplement.

Some vitamins appear to be harmless, even in high doses, but high potency vitamin-mineral combinations may be harmful with potentially serious results. Some supplements contain "megavitamins" and "meganutrients" that are 10 to more than 100 times the recommended Dietary Reference Intake (DRI) for a vitamin or mineral and cause kidney stones, liver damage, nerve damage, congenital disabilities, and even death.

The fat-soluble vitamins A, D, E, and K are especially harmful in high doses is because excess amounts are not as readily excreted as are overdoses of water-soluble vitamins.[49] Another reason that overdosing may occur is that many of the ingredients found in dietary supplements are added to foods, including milk, breakfast cereals, and beverages. In addition to the dose of a supplement, other factors such as body size, and how long the supplement is taken can influence toxicity. The evidence is clear: vitamins derived from natural food sources are essential to health, but extra high doses of vitamins and most other dietary supplements are either of no value or can be harmful to health.

What are water-soluble vitamins?[50]

Water-soluble vitamins are not stored by the body. Since they are eliminated in urine, the body requires a fairly continuous daily supply of the B-complex group and vitamin C in the diet. Even so, deficiency of the B vitamins and vitamin C is rare in the United States. Water-soluble vitamins are easily destroyed during food storage or washed out during food preparation. To reduce vitamin loss, fresh produce should be refrigerated, and milk and grains kept away from strong light. Your doctor can tell you if supplemental vitamins are needed, but usually, your diet will provide all that you need.

Water-soluble vitamins are commonly thought of as harmless. Vitamins C and B6 can cause serious health problems if taken regularly in large doses. Vitamin B6 can cause nerve damage at the high doses sometimes prescribed for pre-menstrual syndrome (PMS). A 20-year study of women in the Nurses' Health Study taking 15 times the recommended dietary allowances (RDAs) of vitamin B6 had a 40% increased risk of hip fracture; those taking ten times the recommended dose of vitamin B12 had a 26% increased risk and those taking high doses of both vitamins (more than 35 micrograms of B6 and 20 micrograms of B12) had a 47% increased risk of hip fracture.[51] High intakes of folic acid can mask or worsen the symptoms associated with a vitamin B12 deficiency. Consuming large doses of niacin supplements may cause flushed skin, rashes, and liver damage. [52]

B-complex vitamins

Eight of the water-soluble vitamins are known as the vitamin B-complex group. They are thiamin (vitamin B1), riboflavin (vitamin B2), niacin (nicotinamide, nicotinic acid, vitamin B3), vitamin B6 (pyridoxine, pyridoxal, pyridoxamine), folate (folic acid, folacin), vitamin B12 (cobalamin), biotin (B7) and pantothenic acid. The B vitamins are found in many foods. They facilitate many of the body's metabolic processes, including those relating to obtaining energy from food, and supporting normal appetite, vision, skin health, the nervous system, and red blood cell formation. However, consumption of more than recommended amounts of B-complex vitamins has no known benefit.

Good food sources of the B complex vitamins include peas, green vegetables, legumes, whole grains, and enriched grain products. Vitamins B1, B3, and B6 are also found in poultry and meat, foods with the drawback of a high saturated fat content. Pantothenic acid is made by intestinal bacteria. Thiamin is found in whole grains but lost when grains are processed. Many processed grain products such as cereal, bread, pasta, and rice, are fortified or enriched. Thiamin (B1), niacin (B3), riboflavin (B2), folate, and iron are commonly added to these products.

Adequate folate consumption is important for women planning to become pregnant and pregnant women because folate deficiency may increase the risk of congenital fetal malformations of the brain and spine such as spina bifida. Pregnant women are commonly prescribed supplements containing folic acid (folate), iron, or a prenatal vitamin that contains these nutrients. Folic acid can be obtained through fortified foods such as enriched breads and cereals, vitamin supplements, or a combination of both. Excess of some nutrients, such as vitamin A, may be harmful and can cause congenital disabilities. If recommended by a health professional, a prenatal supplement ensures that both mother and fetus are receiving adequate but not toxic doses of nutrients.

Vitamin B12: cobalamin

Vitamin B12 (cobalamin) supports the integrity of the nervous system and is necessary for the formation of red blood cells. B12 is only found naturally in foods of animal origin such as meats, fish, eggs, milk and milk products, and shellfish.[53] [54] [55] Vitamin B12 deficiency is possible among strict vegetarians (vegans)—those who eat no animal products, infants of vegan mothers, and more common among the elderly. B12 deficiency can be avoided by consuming non-fat dairy products or fortified foods such as commercial breakfast cereals or supplements that contain vitamin B12. Inadequate consumption of vitamin D, calcium, iron, and zinc among vegetarians and vegans is also possible but not likely.

Because the body can store a substantial amount of vitamin B12, deficiency can take years to develop. Overt deficiency occurs in about 3% and borderline deficiency in up to 20% of persons over age 50.[56 57] B12 deficiency can cause anemia, cognitive deficits, and peripheral nerve problems. Some people, especially the elderly, develop a B12 deficiency because the stomach does not make enough acid, or enough of a protein, intrinsic factor (IF), that is necessary for the intestines to absorb vitamin B12 properly. Intestinal diseases like celiac and Crohn's disease can interfere with the absorption of vitamin B12 in the small intestine.[58] Vitamin B12 deficiency can be treated with oral vitamin B12, or in the presence of intestinal disease or absence of intrinsic factor, with injected vitamin B12. It is recommended to use the natural form of B12 (methylcobalamin) rather than the synthetic form (cyanobalamin) because cyanobalamin may impair kidney function in those with borderline kidney disease.[59]

Vitamin C: ascorbic acid, ascorbate

Your body needs vitamin C (ascorbic acid) to form blood vessels, cartilage, muscle, and collagen in bones. Vitamin C is vital to support and help heal your body's tissues. Although rare in the U.S., vitamin C deficiency (the cause of scurvy) may occur in alcoholics, the elderly, and in smokers. Good food sources for Vitamin C include citrus fruits and many common plant foods. One orange, or 6 oz. of grapefruit juice provides enough vitamin C for a day. Some conditions may warrant an increase in vitamin C intake, such as exposure to cigarette smoke, environmental stress, periods of rapid growth, and sickness.

Propelled by the advocacy of two-time Nobel Prize winner Linus Pauling, mega doses of vitamin C have been recommended to prevent cancer and to prevent or cure the common cold. But there is no evidence that this therapy is effective in preventing colds or cancer. Studies suggest that mega doses of more than 500 mg of vitamin C per day do not increase a body's overall level of vitamin C. Megadoses of vitamin C should be avoided because they can cause nausea, kidney stones, gout, diarrhea, and rebound scurvy.[60]

What are fat-soluble vitamins?[61]

Unlike water-soluble vitamins that need regular replacement, the fat-soluble vitamins, vitamins A, D, E, and K, are stored and persist for long periods of time in the body's liver and fat and are only slowly eliminated from the body. Diseases caused by a lack of fat-soluble vitamins are unusual in the U.S., and very few people need to supplement their diet with these vitamins.

Because they are not readily excreted in urine, excessive consumption of fat-soluble vitamins generally poses a greater risk for toxicity than water-soluble vitamins. Fat-soluble vitamins are not destroyed by cooking and eating a normal, well-balanced diet will not lead to toxicity. However, supplements that contain mega doses of vitamins A, D, E, and K may lead to toxicity and should be avoided. Rarely, health problems decrease the absorption of fat, and in turn, decrease the absorption of vitamins A, D, E, and K.

Vitamin A

Vitamin A (retinol, retinoic acid) is a vitamin with antioxidant properties that is important to support vision, growth, cell division, reproduction, and immunity. The healthiest source of vitamin A is from plant-based foods that contain beta-carotene, which the body converts to vitamin A. Beta-carotene is found in fruits and vegetables, especially those that are orange or dark green in color. The retinol, retinal, and retinoic acid forms of vitamin A are supplied primarily by foods of animal origin such as dairy products, fish, and liver.

Vitamin A toxicity is unlikely when it is obtained from food. But excess vitamin A from high potency multivitamin supplements can be toxic when consumed at a level over the Tolerable Upper Intake Level (UL) for adults of 3,000 μg/day of preformed vitamin A (also known as retinol). The Recommended Dietary Allowance (RDA) for men and women is 900 and 700 μg retinol activity equivalents (RAE)/day, respectively.[62] Symptoms of vitamin A toxicity include dry, itchy skin, headache, nausea, and loss of appetite. Signs of severe overuse over a short period of time include dizziness and blurred vision. Vitamin A toxicity also can cause liver disease, slowed growth, severe congenital disabilities, reduced bone strength, and may increase the risk for hip fractures.[63] Beta-carotene is a carotenoid and called a provitamin A because the body converts it into vitamin A. Unlike preformed vitamin A (retinol), carotenoids in food are safe. When taking a vitamin A supplement, look for those containing provitamin A and avoid those with more than 2000 IU of preformed vitamin A (retinol).

Vitamin E: tocopherol[64]

Vitamin E benefits the body by acting as an antioxidant, and it was theorized that antioxidants, and vitamin E supplements, in particular, might help prevent heart disease and cancer. Substantial research now indicates that people who take vitamin E and other antioxidant supplements are not protected against heart disease and cancer and may be harmed by large doses of vitamin E. Many studies do show that regularly eating an antioxidant-rich diet full of fruits and vegetables may lower the risk for heart disease, cancer, and other diseases. The evidence indicates that antioxidants and phytonutrients should be obtained from plant-based foods, fruits and vegetables, grains, nuts, seeds, and fortified cereals, not as supplements.

Vitamin E obtained from food is unlikely to pose a risk for toxicity. Clinical trials suggest that supplemental vitamin E may protect against amyotrophic lateral sclerosis,[65] but that high doses are associated with increased risk of death.[66] Megadoses may also pose a hazard to people taking anticoagulants by interfering with the action of medications such as warfarin (Coumadin) and statins.[67]

Vitamin K[68]

Vitamin K is necessary for the production of the proteins needed for blood clotting, and it works with vitamin D to support bone health and possibly cardiovascular health. Vitamin K is naturally produced by the bacteria in the intestines and comes from plant food sources. Animal foods contain limited amounts of vitamin K. Newborn babies lack the intestinal bacteria to produce vitamin K and may need a supplement for the first week of life. Vitamin K deficiency may also occur in people who take anticoagulants, such as warfarin, who are on antibiotic drugs that alter intestinal bacteria, and who have chronic diarrhea. In all of these circumstances, only take vitamin K on the advice of a physician. Although no Tolerable Upper Intake Level (UL) for vitamin K has been established, excessive amounts can cause the breakdown of red blood cells and liver damage. People on anticoagulants should be aware that excess vitamin K can alter blood clotting times.

Vitamin D

Vitamin D increases the amount of calcium absorbed from the small intestine and plays a role in the body's metabolism of calcium and phosphorous in the immune system, and the regulation of cellular growth. Especially for children, adequate amounts are essential to the healthy formation and maintenance of teeth and bone. Vitamin D and calcium are among the few supplements that may be helpful for some Americans. For most people, only 10 to 15 minutes of sunshine 2-3 times weekly on hands, face, and arms (without sunscreen) is needed for the skin to respond to the ultraviolet B in sunlight and synthesize enough vitamin D to meet the body's requirements. Many foods, including milk, milk alternatives such as soy or almond milk, orange juice, and breakfast cereal, are fortified with vitamin D. Other sources are of animal origin, especially oily fish, for example, herring, salmon, sardines, and cod liver oil. People who do not consume these fortified food items, have no animal products in the diet, and do not receive enough exposure to sunlight may need a vitamin D supplement.

Vitamin D toxicity can occur when consumed at more than the Tolerable Upper Intake Level (UL) of 100 mcg (4000 IU) for people 9 years of age and older. Because many foods are fortified with vitamin D, high doses of vitamin D supplements should be avoided. Vitamin D is essential to the normal skeletal growth of children, but excess consumption is particularly risky for them.[69] Excess vitamin D is stored in the liver and can cause liver portal vein hypertension and toxicity with increased intestinal absorption of calcium that leads to high levels of calcium in the blood.[70 71]

High blood calcium can cause:[72 73]

- Calcium deposits in soft tissues such as the heart and lungs
- Slowed mental and physical growth
- Confusion and disorientation
- Damage to the kidneys
- Kidney stones
- Nausea, vomiting, constipation, poor appetite, weakness, and weight loss

Do Americans need more vitamin D and calcium?

An epidemic of vitamin D prescription began in 2007 after a paper by Michael Holick appeared in the *New England Journal of Medicine*. He asserted that vitamin D blood levels of 21 to 29 nanograms per milliliter were in a range insufficient to promote good health.[74] Holick claimed that vitamin D deficiency was linked to a wide variety of illnesses, including an increased risk of cancer, autoimmune disease, diabetes, schizophrenia, depression, low lung capacity, and wheezing. Notably, Holick has received hundreds of thousands of dollars from industries that profit from vitamin D sales.[75] His report and a number of other studies started a flurry of what has turned out to be a mostly unnecessary billion-dollar vitamin D testing and treatment juggernaut that persists.[76 77 78]

Because of the presumed widespread deficiency, the U.S. Institute of Medicine (IOM) was asked to evaluate the evidence linking vitamin D and health. The IOM released their review in 2010 and noted: "... physicians have been ordering blood tests that seem to suggest, based on the use of criteria that have yet to be validated, that many in our North American population are vitamin D deficient."[79 80] If less than 30 nanograms per milliliter of vitamin D is the standard for deficiency, then 80% of Americans would be diagnosed as vitamin D deficient. However, according to the IOM, a vitamin D level of 20 nanograms per milliliter of blood is adequate.[81] The IOM reported, "...surveys show that average blood levels of vitamin D are above the 20 nanograms per milliliter that the IOM committee found to be the level that is needed for good bone health for practically all individuals. ... a majority of the population is meeting its needs for vitamin D." The Committee concluded that the prevalence of vitamin D inadequacy in North America had been overestimated. The IOM report went on to say, "... some subgroups—particularly those who are older and living in institutions or who have dark skin pigmentation—may be at increased risk for getting too little vitamin D and may need 800 IU per day."[82]

The IOM also considered calcium because "...there is concern that some may not be obtaining sufficient amounts given the foods they eat. Calcium has been increasingly added to foods, and calcium supplement use, particularly among older persons, is widespread." According to the IOM, "Adolescents need higher levels to support bone growth: 1,300 milligrams per day meets the needs of nearly all adolescents. For practically all adults ages 19 through 50 and for men until age 71, 1,000 milligrams daily meets calcium needs. Women over 50 and both men and women 71 and older need no more than 1,200 milligrams per day. National surveys in both the United States and Canada indicate that calcium may remain a nutrient of concern, especially for girls ages 9–18."

The IOM concluded that calcium intakes over 2,000 milligrams per day increase the risk for harm and that some postmenopausal women taking supplements may be getting too much calcium, thereby increasing their risk for kidney stones. The IOM report warned: "As North Americans take more supplements and eat more of foods that have been fortified with vitamin D and calcium, it becomes more likely that people consume high amounts of these nutrients."

The IOM looked at a variety of other health conditions, possibly linked to a lack of vitamin D and calcium. They concluded that "Outcomes related to cancer/neoplasms, cardiovascular disease and hypertension, diabetes and metabolic syndrome, falls and physical performance, immune functioning and autoimmune disorders, infections, neuropsychological functioning, and preeclampsia could not be linked reliably with calcium or vitamin D intake."[83]

Since the IOM report was released, a substantial body of research has provided additional information about the links between vitamin D and health. A regimen of high doses of vitamin D given to postmenopausal women found that increased calcium absorption was very small and did not translate into beneficial effects on bone mineral density, muscle function, muscle mass, or falls.[84] The study authors concluded that "We found no data to support experts' recommendations to maintain serum 25(OH)D levels of 30 ng/mL or higher in postmenopausal women."

An analysis of research on vitamin D published in the *British Medical Journal* in 2014 included 107 systemic reviews, 74 meta-analyses, and looked at 137 conditions or other outcomes.[85] The study concluded that nearly all of the proposed benefits of vitamin D supplementation remain uncertain, primarily because of a lack of large, well-designed clinical trials. A 2016 review article considered, "Should adults take vitamin D supplements to prevent disease?"[86] It concluded that based on randomized controlled trials, there is no consistent evidence that vitamin D supplementation improves bone density, nor any consistent effects on falls, total fracture, or hip fracture risk other than in severely vitamin D deficient frail, elderly women in residential care, but not in seven trials of community-dwelling older people. The article's summary statement is that low dose vitamin D supplements (400-800 IU/day) can be considered on an individual basis. Otherwise, current evidence does not support the use of vitamin D supplementation to prevent disease.

Excellent data is coming from VITAL, a long-awaited well-designed NIH sponsored placebo-controlled clinical trial that is testing supplemental vitamin D and omega-3 for their effects on a wide array of diseases.[87] Its first results were published in the *New England Journal of Medicine* in November 2018. After an average of 5.3 years, study subjects taking a high dose of vitamin D (2,000 IU) were compared to those taking a placebo. Vitamin D did not bring about a reduced overall incidence of major cardiovascular events (a composite of heart attacks, strokes, and cardiovascular deaths) or invasive cancer. VITAL included baseline blood levels of vitamin D and found that most participants (12 out of 13) enrolled in the study started with adequate D levels—20 ng/mL or higher. And people with initially low levels did not benefit from supplementation with regard to CVDs or cancer.

In a secondary analysis of subgroups, (considered less reliable and harder to interpret), normal-weight and Black subjects, (but not overweight and obese study subjects) given extra vitamin D had about a 25% lower rate of total cancer deaths compared to the placebo—but only starting after the first two years among those of normal weight. The VITAL researchers noted that the subgroup findings could be due to just to chance, considering that the findings of the primary outcome measures showed no benefit.

Overall, nearly one in five U.S. adults are now taking vitamin D.[88] There is evidence that a substantial proportion of U.S. adults are taking too much. If supplemental vitamin D is needed, the Recommended Dietary Allowance (RDA) for vitamin D appears as micrograms (mcg) of cholecalciferol (vitamin D3). From age 9 to age 70, the RDA is set at 600 IU (15 mcg/day), and for adults, over age 70 years, the RDA is 800 IU (20 mcg/day). Multivitamins typically contain about 400 IU/day. The tolerable upper limit is 4000 IU/day; beyond this level risk of toxic effects increases. National Health and Nutrition Examination Surveys (NHANES) indicate that in 2013-2014 an estimated 6.6% of people age 60 and older were taking at least 4,000 IU of vitamin D daily, as were 4.2% of all women. High doses of vitamin D are associated with an increased risk of side effects, particularly when taken with calcium supplements. Some epidemiologic studies suggest high doses of vitamin D may be associated with increased risk of prostate and pancreatic cancers, and deaths from all causes. [89]

So, what can we conclude about vitamin D? According to a 2019 editorial in the *JAMA*, "Multiple trials have failed to demonstrate significant benefits of vitamin D supplementation....High-dose monthly oral vitamin D3, compared with placebo, did not reduce risk of incident cardiovascular disease or death. In the Vitamin D and Type 2 Diabetes (D2d) trial, vitamin D supplementation, compared with placebo, failed to lower risk of incident type 2 diabetes in patients with prediabetes."[90] Research is underway that may reveal benefits from supplementation, but so far, studies have found that most people do not need extra vitamin D.

Who does need extra Vitamin D?[91] [92] [93]

The Institute of Medicine (IOM) review panel noted that although most people do not need extra vitamin D, several populations are potentially at risk of vitamin D deficiency and may require extra vitamin D in the form of supplements or fortified foods. They include:

- Exclusively breastfed infants: Human milk only provides 25 IU of vitamin D per liter. On the advice of a medical professional, nearly all breastfed and partially breastfed infants will be recommended to be given a vitamin D supplement of 400 IU/day.
- Dark skin: Those with dark pigmented skin synthesize less vitamin D upon exposure to sunlight compared to those with light pigmented skin.
- Elderly: This population has a reduced ability to synthesize vitamin D upon exposure to sunlight, and is also more likely to stay indoors and wear sunscreen that blocks vitamin D synthesis.
- Covered and protected skin: Those who cover all of their skin with clothing while outside, and those who wear sunscreen with an SPF factor of 8 or higher, block most of the synthesis of vitamin D from sunlight.
- Disease: Fat malabsorption syndromes, inflammatory bowel disease (IBD), and obesity are all known to result in a decreased ability to absorb and/or use vitamin D in fat stores.

In all of these circumstances, it is a good idea to get a blood test to see if the serum 25-hydroxyvitamin D (25(OH)D) level is substantially less than the IOM recommended average of 20 ng/ml (50 nmol/liter). In an article titled Vitamin D Deficiency—Is There Really a Pandemic? In the *New England Journal of Medicine*, Manson and her colleagues caution that many people will have a requirement of only16 ng or even less, and that ensuring that 97.5% of the population attain or exceed 25(OH) D levels of 20 ng per milliliter would requiring shifting the entire population to a higher intake and harm people whose intake is pushed above the Tolerable Upper Intake Level of 4000 IU per day. The authors suggest that almost all of those who are potentially at risk (as described above) will have adequate vitamin D with supplementation of the Recommended Daily Allowance (RDA) of 600 to 800 IU per day, as is recommended by the Institute of Medicine.[94 95]

Supplementary vitamins can cause harm

Many studies suggest that supplementary vitamins provide no benefits, and use increases the risk of cancer, cardiovascular disease, and "all-cause" death rates. In his book, *Do You Believe in Magic? The Sense and Nonsense of Alternative Medicine*, Paul Offit, describes a series of major studies that evaluated the health effects of a variety of vitamins and other supplements.[96] He describes research that tested the theory that antioxidants would be beneficial to health. The unexpected finding was that antioxidants were often harmful. One study found that those taking vitamin E, beta-carotene, or both, were more likely to die from lung cancer or heart disease than those who didn't take them. Another found that study subjects taking vitamin A, beta-carotene, or both, were dying from cancer at a rate 28% higher and heart disease at a rate 17% higher than those who didn't take the vitamins.[97] A large study of people who took vitamins A, C, E, and beta-carotene found no evidence that antioxidants could prevent intestinal cancers, rather they found that death rates were 6% higher in those taking vitamins.[98] Offit cites other studies that have found an increased risk of death and heart failure associated with supplemental vitamin E.[99] He notes that "In 2007, researchers from the National Cancer Institute examined 11,000 men who did or didn't take multivitamins. Those who took multivitamins were twice as likely to die from advanced prostate cancer."[100]

A 2007 study published in the *Journal of the American Medical Association* assessed mortality rates in randomized trials of antioxidant supplements. In 47 trials involving 181,000 participants. Mortality was 5% higher among those using the antioxidants vitamin A, beta-carotene, and vitamin E. The studies did not detect a mortality effect of vitamin C or selenium.[101] Offit's summary of the evidence stated that "In 2008, a review of all existing studies involving more than 230,000 people who did or did not receive supplemental antioxidants found that vitamins increased the risk of cancer and heart disease."[102 103]

A January 2009 editorial in the *Journal of the National Cancer Institute* noted that most studies of vitamins had shown no cancer benefits, but some had shown unexpected harms. Two studies of beta-carotene found higher lung cancer rates, and another study suggested a higher risk of precancerous polyps among users of folic acid compared with those in a placebo group.[104] And another study of 36,000 men who took vitamin E, selenium, both, or neither found that those receiving vitamin E had a 17% greater risk of prostate cancer."[105 106 107]

A study published in 2011 in the *Archives of Internal Medicine* assessed the use of vitamin and mineral supplements in relation to total mortality in 38,772 older women in the Iowa Women's Health Study. Sixty-six percent of women participating in the Iowa Women's Health Study used at least one dietary supplement daily in 1986. By 2004, the proportion had increased to 85%, with 27% of women using four or more supplements.[108] The Iowa study found that the use of multivitamins, vitamin B6, folic acid, iron, magnesium, zinc, and copper were all associated with a 2% to 4% increased risk of death. The study authors concluded that "In older women, several commonly used dietary vitamin and mineral supplements may be associated with increased total mortality risk;...".[109]

A U.S. Preventive Services Task Force (USPSTF), examined the evidence about the effectiveness of vitamin, mineral, and multivitamin supplements for the prevention of cardiovascular disease and cancer.[110 111] The Task Force reviewed three trials of multivitamin supplements and 24 single or paired trials of vitamins. The Task Force concluded that there was no clear evidence of a beneficial effect of supplements, including vitamins A, C, or D, folic acid, calcium (with or without vitamin D), or selenium on all-cause mortality, cardiovascular disease, or cancer. The recommendation statement concluded that antioxidants, folic acid, and B vitamins are harmful or ineffective for chronic disease prevention.

The Task Force did find that there was sufficient evidence to recommend against using either beta-carotene or vitamin E for the prevention of cardiovascular disease or cancer. The evidence showed that there is no benefit to taking vitamin E and that beta-carotene can be harmful because it increases the risk of lung cancer in people who are already at increased risk. The Task Force concluded that for most people the best way to get the important nutrients essential for health is through a balanced diet rich in fruits, vegetables, whole grains, fat-free and low-fat dairy products, and seafood, a diet that has been associated with a reduced risk of cardiovascular disease and cancer.

Multiple studies have found that taking beta-carotene for cognition, and vitamins C and E for cardiovascular disease and for cancer, has shown no meaningful benefits.[112 113 114 115 116] An editorial titled "Enough Is Enough: Stop Wasting Money on Vitamin and Mineral Supplements" in the *Annals of Internal Medicine* opined: "The message is simple: Most supplements do not prevent chronic disease or death, their use is not justified, and they should be avoided. This message is especially true for the general population with no clear evidence of micronutrient deficiencies, who represent most supplement users in the United States and in other countries."[117] The editorial concluded: "...beta-carotene, vitamin E, and possibly high doses of vitamin A supplements are harmful. Other antioxidants, folic acid and B vitamins, and multivitamin and mineral supplements are ineffective for preventing mortality or morbidity due to major chronic diseases—supplementing the diet of well-nourished adults with (most) mineral or vitamin supplements has no clear benefit and might even be harmful. These vitamins should not be used for chronic disease prevention. Enough is enough."[118]

Is there still a case for taking a multivitamin for insurance?

One good study, the Physicians' Health Study II (PHS II), compared taking a multivitamin to a placebo. After 12 years of follow up, those taking the multivitamin had a modest 8% decreased risk of cancer incidence, mostly a decline in colorectal cancer, but no effect on cancer mortality and no effect on the risk of prostate cancer, heart attacks, strokes or cardiovascular deaths among male physicians, aged 65 or older.[119] The study suggests that there is little benefit to be gained from routine use of multivitamins, but it is possible that a similar study among men who were less healthy and well-nourished would have shown more benefit.

Editorial comment on the Physicians' Health Study II noted that this single study among physicians does not provide enough evidence to suggest taking multivitamins for cancer prevention for various reasons, including that the majority of similar studies suggest no effect of vitamin supplementation on cancer risk and some, notably, show evidence of harm.[120 121 122]

Some nutrition experts are more enthusiastic about multivitamins. Harvard professor Walter Willett considers that there is evidence about the importance of vitamins to the prevention of chronic diseases and that probably many people do not get enough vitamins.[123] He suggests that by increasing the amount of vitamins we get, mostly from food, but maybe from supplements, we can improve our long-term health. Some support for this position comes from the 2018 VITAL study that found that supplementation with omega-3s and vitamin D did not significantly reduce major cardiovascular events or total invasive cancer but that some subgroups may have benefitted—more research is needed to determine the importance of these findings.[124]

Willett suggests taking a daily standard multivitamin-multimineral as "insurance" against low levels of intake of eight vitamins that some people do not get enough of in their diets. The recommended vitamins and minerals are beta-carotene, folic acid, iron, zinc and vitamins B6, B12, D, and E. Because of poor absorption; vitamin B12 deficiency occurs in about 3% and borderline deficiency in up to 20% of persons over age 50. Vegans who eat no animal-derived foods are also at risk of vitamin B12 deficiency.

What about supplements other than vitamins?

Dietary supplements other than vitamins include minerals like calcium and iron, herbs and botanicals; probiotics; sports drinks; fish oils; and hormones such as estrogen and testosterone (see Chapter 13, "Sexual and Reproductive Health," for a discussion of taking hormones). Although they are claimed to be useful for maintaining or improving health, other than vitamins, almost all supplements have either been proven to be of no value, proven to be harmful or need more study to determine if they are of any value. Most dietary supplements have not been well tested for safety, especially for use by pregnant women, nursing mothers, infants, or children. [125]

Many supplements contain active ingredients that can have powerful effects on the human body. For example, excess iron causes nausea and vomiting and may damage the liver and other organs. Some dietary supplements interact with certain prescription and over-the-counter drugs in ways that might cause harm. For example, St. John's Wort can speed the breakdown of many drugs (including antidepressants and birth control pills) and, thereby, reduce these drugs' effectiveness; ginkgo taken with ibuprofen may lead to spontaneous and/or excessive bleeding, and high doses of garlic may enhance the effects and adverse effects of anticoagulant and antiplatelet drugs including aspirin, and clopidogrel (Plavix). Herbal supplements are especially not recommended for those who may be immuno-compromised (such as the elderly or those with HIV), those with kidney damage or liver disease, anyone who may be undergoing surgery or other invasive procedures, pregnant or lactating women, or children.[126]

Fish oils, rich in omega-3 fats, are among the most widely taken supplements—consumed by about 8% of U.S. adults in 2012. Recent high-quality studies suggest modest benefits for preventing CVDs, but many previous studies did not find protection.[127] [128] [129] Since their presumed utility is to prevent cardiovascular disease, they are discussed in more detail in Chapter 3, "Optimal Nutrition," and Chapter 6, "Preventing Cardiovascular Disease."

Recently, another supplement, cannabidiol or CBD, is being promoted as a miracle cure for depression, anxiety, insomnia, inflammation, chronic pain, and a variety of other ailments. In 2018 it became the top-selling herbal dietary supplement in health food stores and is found in a wide variety of products. The hype about benefits is great, but there is little evidence that CBD is safe and effective. Many of the unregulated products sold as CBD do not contain CBD. Others vary greatly in their content and often contain other compounds, including THC, the active ingredient of marijuana. Because it is a seemingly non-psychotropic component of cannabis but does have neurological effects, CBD is discussed in greater detail in Chapter 10, "Stress and Mental Health."

Some Americans, both meat-eaters and vegetarians, do not consume enough iron. This is most common among women with heavy menstrual bleeding. Vegetarians and vegans who get their iron from plant foods need about twice as much dietary iron each day as do meat-eaters because the heme iron (iron in blood) in animal foods is more easily absorbed than the nonheme iron that comes from plant foods. Vegetarians may be at a higher risk for developing iron deficiency for an additional reason, the fiber in plant foods may bind to iron and make it less easily absorbed. Among plant foods, dark green leafy vegetables have the highest iron content. Dried fruits are also high in iron. Vitamin C and foods high in vitamin C increase the availability and intestinal absorption of iron. Zinc deficiencies are seldom a problem for vegetarians and can be avoided by including a wide variety of foods in their diet, such as soy products, legumes, grains, cheese, and nuts. Iodine deficiency can be a problem for vegans, but vegans can get iodine from iodized salt, seaweeds, soybeans, sweet potatoes and cruciferous vegetables such as broccoli and cabbage.[130]

Resveratrol is the component of red wine thought to be an anti-aging compound. A study of the supplement resveratrol found that after two months of exercise, men in a control group taking a placebo showed significant and favorable changes in their blood pressure, cholesterol profiles, and a 45% greater exercise capacity, as shown by maximal oxygen uptake. But resveratrol prevented the positive effects of exercise.[131] According to *New York Times* writer Gretchen Reynolds, one theory for these counterintuitive findings is that free radicals "... serve as messengers, nudging genes and other bodily systems into starting the various biochemical reactions that end in stronger muscles and better metabolic health." When antioxidant supplements absorb most of the free radicals produced by exercise, those reactions don't begin.[132]

You should be especially cautious about taking plant-based supplements. According to Bellows, Moore, and Gross of Colorado State University: "Current research shows limited health benefits from taking herbal and botanical supplements, and no conclusive evidence that herbals should be used to treat or prevent any type of medical condition. There is no data to suggest that herbs are more beneficial than conventional drugs for treating illnesses." They note that "The body of well-controlled research is growing, but the short-term and long-term benefits and risks, as well as active or beneficial ingredients, are still largely unknown."[133]

Although 71% of surveyed Americans say supplements are "safe," the FDA has issued a warning for the following herbs that are considered toxic and should be avoided by everyone:[134 135]

- Aristolochic Acid: kidney damage and a carcinogen. It may be found in products with guan mu tong, ma dou ling, birthwort, Indian ginger, wild ginger, colic root, and snakeroot.
- Chapparal: irreversible liver damage
- Comfrey: liver toxicity, carcinogenic effects, and damage to a fetus if used during pregnancy
- Ephedra/ma huang (ephedra sinca): hypertension, myocardial infarction, seizure, stroke, psychosis
- Germander: liver damage and death
- Kava: liver damage, especially risky for those with liver problems
- Lobelia (Indian tobacco): breathing problems, rapid heartbeat, low blood pressure, coma, death
- Magnolia-stephania preparation: kidney disease and permanent kidney failure
- Willow bark: Reye's syndrome in children and allergic reaction in adults
- Wormwood: seizures, numbness of legs and arms, delirium, and kidney failure
- Yohimbe: hypotension (low blood pressure), heart conduction disorders, kidney disorders, nervous system disorders, death

The independent product-testing organization, Consumer Reports (CR), worked with experts from the Natural Medicines Comprehensive Database, also an independent research group, to identify a dozen supplement ingredients (out of nearly 1,100 in the database) linked to the most serious adverse events as determined by clinical research or case reports. The dozen are aconite, bitter orange, chaparral, colloidal silver, coltsfoot, comfrey, country mallow, germanium, greater celandine, kava, lobelia, and Yohimbe. The CR study noted that the FDA had warned about at least eight of them, some as long ago as 1993. CR easily found all of these dangerous supplements for sale in June 2010 when they shopped for them online and in stores near their Yonkers, N.Y. headquarters.[136]

When CR asked why these products were still for sale, they found: "Two national retailers we contacted about specific supplements said they carried them because the FDA has not banned them." CR also noted that "Most of the products we bought had warning labels, but not all did. A bottle of silver we purchased was labeled 'perfectly safe,' with an asterisked note that said the FDA had not evaluated the claim. In fact, the FDA issued a consumer advisory about silver (including colloidal silver) in 2009. Although silver is sold for its supposed immune system 'support,' it can permanently turn skin bluish-gray."[137]

A recent target of FDA scrutiny and ban from use and sale is kratom, a botanical that has been promoted as a treatment for pain, mood disorders and as a way for opioid users to avoid withdrawal symptoms. According to the CDC, between July 2016 and December 2017, kratom alone or more frequently was one of multiple drugs, including fentanyl and heroin, that caused 152 overdose deaths in the U.S.

Sports and Energy Drinks

Beverages called energy drinks are a multibillion-dollar industry based on aggressive marketing strategies that mainly target teens and young adults. In 2010, 34% to 51% of those aged 18 to 24 in the U.S. reported regular consumption of energy drinks, a total of 6 billion drinks.[138][139] A typical 16 oz. energy drink contains 150-200 mg. of caffeine, about equal to the same amount of brewed coffee. In contrast, a 20-oz. bottle of Coke would contain only 58 mg. of caffeine. Energy drinks also contain a variety of herbs, vitamins, and usually large amounts of sugar. Like other dietary supplements, energy drinks are not regulated by the FDA. They are associated with a substantial array of health risks, including increased heart rate, palpitations, high blood pressure, insomnia, and high blood sugar levels.[140][141]

Children should not consume energy drinks. Adolescents should be advised to limit caffeine intake to 100 mg. per day and adults to 500 mg. a day.[142] Because the millions of persons consuming energy drinks are likely to be unaware of the amount of caffeine or risks of the caffeine they are ingesting, caffeine overdoses have caused serious illness and rare deaths—probably from heart irregularities. Assuming that ingestion over a brief time of 3 to 10 gm of caffeine might be lethal, then it would probably take 12 or more energy drinks to reach a lethal dose in a healthy adult. But in the presence of liver disease or other drugs, a fatal dose could be lower.[143]

Mixing energy drinks and alcohol is especially dangerous because caffeine offsets the sedating effects of alcohol, and drinkers may not realize that they are intoxicated, keep on drinking, and drink too much. A group of students who consumed both energy drinks and alcohol approximately doubled their risk of experiencing or committing sexual assault, riding with an intoxicated driver, having an alcohol-related motor vehicle crash, or requiring medical treatment.[144][145]

The International Olympic Committee published a statement in 2015 that it is "inappropriate and unacceptable to encourage dietary supplements for performance enhancement with youth athletes." However, studies have found use by between 22% and 71% of child and adolescent athletes. Although there is little evidence that sports-nutrition supplements are effective, they are marketed with promises of improved athletic performance. They are a growing market, estimated at $6.7 billion of annual sales in the U.S. in 2016.[146]

What about dietary supplements for infants and children?

This book is focused on teens and adults, but parents are so apt to believe that it is important to give their children vitamins or other dietary supplements to protect or enhance their health, that a brief discussion of the need for vitamin supplements for infants and children may be helpful.

The first rule is not to play doctor and give an infant or child supplements that are not recommended by a pediatrician or other competent health care professional who understands the dietary needs of infants and children and if supplements are indicated. Other than recommended doses of vitamins, very few supplements have been tested in infants and children, and there is reason to think that infants and children may be more susceptible than adults to the harms caused by high doses of vitamins and other dietary supplements.[147] Decisions about vitamins for breast and bottle-fed babies should be guided by the advice of a pediatrician or other professional health care provider.[148 149 150 151 152 153] ,

Human milk provides enough of most vitamins, especially vitamin C, E, and the B vitamins. Although human milk contains small amounts of vitamin D, the American Academy of Pediatrics (AAP) recommends that breastfed babies receive oral vitamin D drops which provide 400 IU (International Units) of vitamin D a day in infants less than one year of age and 600 units/day for children over one year of age until they are drinking vitamin D-fortified formula or milk.

Most babies are born with sufficient reserves of iron, and breastfeeding supplies enough easily-absorbed iron, but it is recommended that bottle-fed babies get iron-fortified formula through the first year of life. Children between 6 months and two years and teenage girls, especially athletes, tend to be more susceptible to iron deficiency, so ensuring an appropriate diet is important.

The AAP considers that after infancy, healthy children receiving a normal, well-balanced diet do not need vitamin supplementation over and above the recommended dietary allowances. Megadoses of vitamins—for example, large amounts of vitamins A, C, or D—are of no benefit and can produce toxic symptoms, including nausea, rashes, headaches, and sometimes other even more severe adverse health effects.[154 155 156]

Adequate calcium intake during childhood and adolescence is important for the attainment of peak bone mass and the avoidance of osteoporosis later in life. Nonfat milk and vegetables, such as broccoli and spinach, are good sources of calcium. Some fruit juices are now fortified with calcium, but most have the drawback of high sugar content.

The AAP has warned adults not to give children or adolescents sport drinks or nutrition bars. Because they are highly fortified, a child who eats even "kid-friendly" nutrition bars regularly can get too much vitamin A or too much vitamin B6. The nutrition that is vital to a child's health and development should come from food that includes fruit, vegetables, and whole grains. This diet will almost certainly deliver sufficient amounts of all of the essential vitamins and minerals. Unless blood tests and a pediatrician's evaluation reveal a specific deficiency, it's preferable for children to obtain nutrients from food instead of from dietary supplements. One reason for this is because, unlike supplements, vegetables, fruits, and grains contain phytochemicals and many other beneficial nutrients.

Summary of the Essential Facts[157]

- Most people can obtain the recommended dietary intakes of the vitamins and minerals needed for good health by eating a variety of foods.
- Vitamin deficiency may occur in the elderly; when nutrients are limited in one's diet, for example, B12 deficiency among vegetarians; as a result of a health problem; or caused by tobacco or alcohol use.
- Dietary supplements, including multivitamins, multiminerals, herbs, and sports drinks, usually do not preserve or enhance health, boost athletic performance, or protect against disease.
- Large doses of either single nutrient supplements or high potency vitamin and mineral combinations may be harmful.
- Be especially wary of the risk of supplements other than vitamins, especially herbal and botanical supplements—most are unproven to be beneficial, and many are harmful.
- Do not self-prescribe, consult a medical professional before taking any type of supplement other than a standard low-dose multivitamin/multimineral.

6
Preventing Cardiovascular Disease

Cardiovascular diseases (CVDs), such as heart attack and stroke, involve the heart and blood vessels. Worldwide, cardiovascular disease is a leading cause of death,[1] and in the U.S., heart disease is the most frequent and stroke the fifth most frequent cause of death. CVD kills more than 800,000 Americans every year, and these deaths take an average of 15 years off of the normal lifespan.[2] Even among young people in their twenties, heart attacks are one of the top ten causes of death.[3] Together, heart disease and stroke accounted for more than $500 billion in health care expenditures and related expenses in 2010.[4] Fortunately, the commonest types of cardiovascular disease, those caused by atherosclerosis, are among the most preventable. This chapter will help you prevent CVD with the Building Blocks of Health.

What causes cardiovascular diseases?

Most cardiovascular disease results from the complications of atherosclerosis, (commonly called arteriosclerosis), and high blood pressure. Atherosclerosis results from the slow, progressive, and usually silent accumulation of cholesterol and calcium in the walls of arteries that forms a plaque that thickens arterial walls. The resultant loss of flexibility, scarring, and narrowing of the artery cuts down on or even blocks the ability of the vessel to carry blood. Atherosclerosis can disrupt and limit the flow of blood to any part of the body. When the coronary arteries that supply blood to the heart's muscle are narrowed, one result can be chest pain, or angina, caused when the blood supply to the heart cannot keep up with the extra oxygen demand of exertion. According to the American Heart Association (AHA), an estimated 10 million people in the U.S. suffer from angina. Atherosclerosis can also cause limited exercise tolerance or heart failure because the heart muscle's ability to pump blood is weakened by an inadequate supply of blood or previous damage to the heart's muscle.

When an unstable plaque in a narrowed coronary artery ruptures into the lumen of the artery, the body may attempt to "heal" the break by forming a blood clot, and the clot may partially or completely block the artery. The sudden loss of blood flow to the heart causes a "heart attack" that is usually painful, often weakens the pumping ability of the heart and may cause a myocardial infarct—the death of some of the heart's muscle. If a heart attack affects a large area of the heart, the ability of the heart to pump blood may be so compromised that heart failure or death results.

Death can also occur if a heart attack causes a disruption of the electrical signals that coordinate the heart's pumping action. The result may be irregular uncoordinated heartbeats, called ventricular fibrillation. This prevents the heart from pumping enough blood to sustain life. Unfortunately, often the first sign of heart disease is a heart attack, and about half of first-time heart attacks result in sudden death within the first hour after the attack.[5]

There is also another form of heart disease, more common in women, that is caused by microvascular dysfunction and poor blood flow through the small blood vessels of the heart. The condition is called ischemia and no obstructive coronary artery disease (INOCA). It may cause cardiac dysfunction, decreased exercise tolerance, and angina. INOCA does not show up on arteriograms but carries a high risk for heart attack, heart failure, and death.[6]

High blood pressure and atherosclerosis increase the risk of a disruption of blood circulation to the brain, either because an artery is blocked or because of a weak or damaged artery ruptures and causes bleeding in the brain. The result is a stroke. Other sites where narrowed or blocked arteries commonly cause serious problems are the blood vessels supplying the kidneys, the carotid arteries in the neck that carry blood to the brain, and the arteries that supply the muscles in the arms or legs. Peripheral artery disease that limits the blood supply to the legs can cause claudication—leg pain on walking or more strenuous exercise. This is a problem for an estimated 8.5 million Americans with annual hospital costs estimated to be more than $21 billion.[7,8]

Other forms of cardiovascular disease include the impaired ability of the heart to pump blood due to congenital defects, damage to the valves of the heart, or disruption of the regularity of the heart's beat as occurs with atrial fibrillation. CVD also includes blood clots. Those that form in a leg vein can travel to the lungs and cause a potentially fatal pulmonary embolism. Atrial fibrillation makes it more likely that a blood clot will form in the heart, and if it breaks loose, it can go to the brain and cause a stroke.

The progression of atherosclerosis

Atherosclerosis often starts in childhood and frequently continues to increase in severity throughout life. The 1992 Bogalusa Heart Study examined the blood vessels of children who died in accidents. It found that the children, who ate a typical American diet, already had fatty streaks and plaques on their arteries—the signs of early atherosclerosis.[9] A 1998 autopsy study found that the prevalence of fatty streaks in the coronary arteries increased with age, from approximately 50% at age 2 to 15, to 85% at age 21 to 39; and the prevalence of coronary raised fibrous-plaque lesions increased from 8% at ages 2 to 15 years to 69% at ages 26 to 39.[10]

In a 1953 study, pathologists examining the coronary arteries of young men (average age 22) who were killed in the Korean War were surprised to find that 77.3% of American soldiers had easily visible evidence of atherosclerosis—and sometimes it was severe. In contrast, the dead Korean and Chinese soldiers who lived on a plant-based diet were virtually free from atherosclerosis.[11] In 1971, similar studies among Vietnam War combat dead found that 45% of those examined had evidence of coronary atherosclerosis, and among 5%, the disease was severe.[12]

A more recent study among U.S. servicemen who died from accidental injuries found lower levels of coronary atherosclerosis.[13] While not entirely comparable to the earlier studies, autopsies carried out between 2001 and 2011 found coronary atherosclerosis of any severity among 8.5% of those studied. It was minimal in 1.5%, moderate in 4.7%, and severe in 2.3%. The low levels of atherosclerosis may be accounted for by the low levels of risk factors present in this young (average age 27) population compared to the general public. Only 4% were obese, 3% smoked, 1% had high blood pressure, 0.7% had cholesterol levels higher than 240 mg/dl, and 0.2% had high fasting blood glucose levels.

The 2001 to 2011 studies of U.S. servicemen should not be considered a reason for complacency about cardiovascular disease. Those aged 40 or older were seven times more likely to have coronary atherosclerosis than those age 24 and younger. Among those ages 30 to 39, the prevalence of aortic and/or coronary atherosclerosis was 22.1%, and among those aged 40 or older, it was 45.9%.

As shown in the chart below, the progression of cardiovascular disease with advancing age was documented in the National Health and Nutrition Examination Survey that found that the percentage of Americans with cardiovascular disease progressed with age.[14]

Fig. 6.1 Prevalence of Cardiovascular Disease

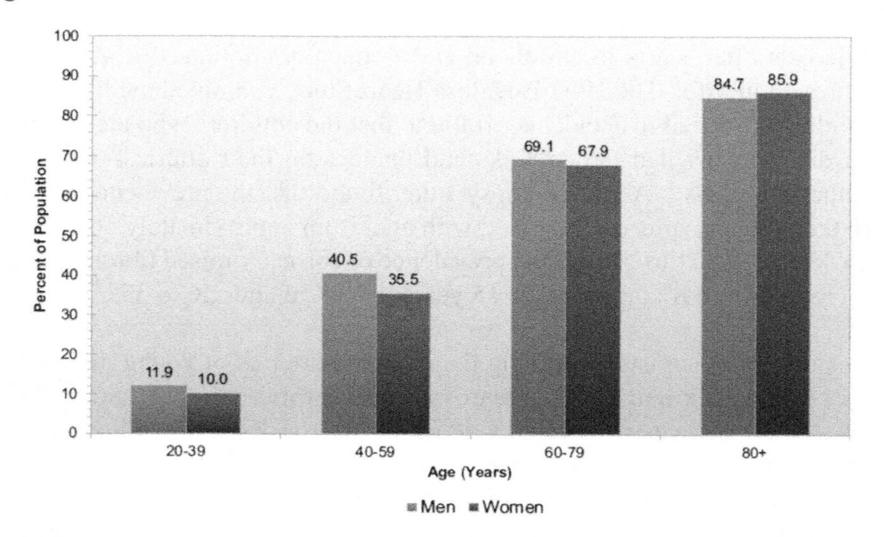

Prevalence of cardiovascular disease in adults ≥ 20 years of age by age and sex (National Health and Nutrition Examination Survey: 2009-2012). These data include coronary heart disease, heart failure, stroke, and hypertension. Source: National Center for Health Statistics and National Heart, Lung and Blood Institute.

How to prevent cardiovascular disease

It was once thought that the development and progression of atherosclerosis was a "normal" or unavoidable part of aging. But, we now know that its occurrence and progression with age can mostly be avoided by putting in place the Building Blocks of Health.

Multiple health factors increase the risk of cardiovascular disease. Research begun in the 1940s by Ancel Keys demonstrated a link between cardiovascular disease, diet, and lifestyle. He documented that elevated blood pressure, elevated blood cholesterol levels, and cigarette smoking increase the risk of heart attack and stroke. Subsequent studies showed that a low LDL cholesterol (LDL-C), not being overweight or obese, and physical activity helps prevent CVDs.[15]

The Framingham Heart Study, begun in 1948 with 5,209 adult subjects, confirmed that high blood pressure, elevated serum cholesterol, and cigarette smoking were major contributors to the development of heart disease. Patients with total cholesterol levels of less than 150 milligrams per deciliter (mg/dl) had the lowest coronary artery disease risk. In the first 50 years of the Framingham study, only five subjects with total cholesterol levels of less than 150 mg/dl developed coronary artery disease. The study also suggested that up to 90% of coronary heart disease deaths could be prevented if total cholesterol remained below 182 mg/dl, systolic blood pressure was under 120 mmHg, and no smoking or diabetes was present.[16 17]

CVD risk factors you can't change

The risk factors predisposing a person to cardiovascular diseases include some that cannot be altered.[18] These risk factors include:

- Family history of early heart disease
- Age
- Sex (males are at greater risk at ages below 65)
- Race (South Asians and Black Americans are often at greater risk)
- Having already had a heart attack
- Chronic kidney disease
- Presence of some blood clotting factors relating to fibrinogen and factor VII, and certain rare variant forms of genes

Age is among the strongest predictors of cardiovascular risk because of the longer duration of exposure to risk factors such as high LDL-C and high blood pressure. Another age-related risk is the genetic mutation disorder called clonal hematopoiesis of indeterminate potential or CHIP. CHIP is rare in persons younger than 40 but may exist in up to 10% of persons age 70 or older. For reasons that are not clear, CHIP carriers have about double the risk of coronary heart disease, and carriers younger than age 50 have been found to have four times the risk of heart attack as noncarriers.[19 20]

CVD risk factors you can change

Many of the most important risk factors for cardiovascular diseases can be modified so as to decrease risk. These risk factors include:

- High blood cholesterol, (primarily low-density lipoprotein cholesterol, LDL-C)
- Unhealthy diet, (a diet high in saturated and trans-fat, sugar, salt, red meat, highly refined carbohydrates, and processed foods)
- High blood pressure
- Smoking and air pollution
- Lack of physical activity
- Diabetes
- Obesity
- Heavy alcohol consumption

- Stress, anger, and depression
- Inflammation and elevated C-reactive protein (CRP)—a marker of inflammation

Smoking is a major cause of increased risk of CVD, and smokers have about triple the risk of a heart attack compared to nonsmokers. Smoking is considered to be the cause of about 20% of CVD deaths.[21] New research shows that e-cigarettes are also dangerous in that daily users nearly double their risk. Among those who both smoke cigarettes and vape, the risk of a heart attack is almost five times that of a nonsmoker.[22 23] When heavy smokers quit, it reduces their risk of a CVD event by about 40% by five years after quitting, but their CVD risk remains higher than never smokers for 10 to 15 years.[24]

Both emotional and physical stress cause many of the same bodily responses: the release of adrenalin and other physiological changes that prepare the body for vigorous physical activity in response to stressful or dangerous situations. This is called the "fight or flight" response. The changes include increased heart rate, increased blood pressure, and arterial contraction from blood platelet clumping. Rarely, stress can cause coronary artery spasm and a fatal heart attack. Coronary spasm is most likely when coronary arteries are already damaged and narrowed from atherosclerosis. In addition to emotional stress, cigarette smoking and the use of cocaine are associated with coronary spasm.[25]

Air pollution, such as high levels of particulates, increases the risk for heart attack or stroke in several ways: impaired blood vessel function, increased blood clotting, disrupted heart rhythms, and increased blood pressure. People at high risk of heart attack should avoid exposure to air pollution when the Air Quality Index is in the unhealthy range (151 to 200).[26 27]

There are other conditions associated with increased risk of cardiovascular disease. They include elevated blood levels of the amino acid homocysteine. Through a poorly understood mechanism, elevated levels of homocysteine may promote atherosclerosis and blood clotting. Blood tests that are not routine may reveal high levels of lipoproteins and enzymes that are linked to an increased risk of coronary heart disease. They include studies of lipoprotein(a) (Lp[a]), apoB, and lipoprotein-associated phospholipase A2 (Lp-PLA2).[28]

High Lp(a) increases the lifetime risk of CVD by about 50%.[29] It is inherited and, unfortunately, cannot easily be decreased by exercise, diet, or statin therapy. The proportion of people with Lp(a) at high levels (>30 mg/dl) is estimated to be between 7% and 26%.[30] The best way to treat elevated Lp(a) is not well established but presumably by aggressively addressing other CVD risk factors, including avoiding smoking, optimizing diet, normalizing blood pressure, and physical activity.[31][32] New drug treatments for Lp(a) are being developed but are not available yet.[33] Among other conditions associated with increased heart attack risk are sleep apnea, influenza, rheumatoid arthritis, and lupus. In men, the presence of erectile dysfunction (ED) may also indicate risk, presumably because ED is caused by plaque in arteries throughout the body, including in the penis.[34]

Multiple risk factors cause an exponential increase in CVD risk

A single risk factor may predispose to cardiovascular disease. For example, inadequate physical activity may contribute to obesity, elevated blood pressure, and an unhealthy pattern of blood cholesterol—all of which are associated with a higher risk of atherosclerotic heart disease. When several cardiovascular risk factors are present, their effect often increases exponentially. The metabolic syndrome is a somewhat ill-defined cluster of CVD risk factors. It is usually diagnosed when an adult has any three or more of the following five cardiovascular disease risk factors:

- Central or abdominal obesity (measured by waist circumference) of greater than 40 inches in men or greater than 35 inches in women
- Triglyceride level of 150 mg/dL or greater
- HDL cholesterol of less than 40 mg/dL in men or less than 50 mg/dL in women
- Systolic blood pressure of 130 millimeters of mercury (mm Hg) or greater, or diastolic blood pressure of 85 mm Hg or greater
- Fasting glucose of 100 mg/dL or greater

When a person has three or more of these risk factors, the chances for heart attack, stroke, and other cardiovascular diseases, type 2 diabetes, and other health problems are much greater than if any one factor alone were present. Individuals with metabolic syndrome have a two-fold increase in risk for heart attack or stroke and a five-fold increased risk for developing diabetes. Although more than one in three U.S. adults has metabolic syndrome,[35] it can be treated and usually reversed by addressing the factors on the Lifestyle Checklist, especially maintaining a healthy weight, eating a heart-healthy diet, getting adequate exercise, and controlling blood pressure through exercise, nutrition, and drugs.

Can a healthy lifestyle prevent heart attacks?

The American Heart Association (AHA) considers lifestyle modification to be the foundation for CVD risk reduction.[36][37] The AHA defines ideal cardiovascular health by the presence of a healthy diet, not smoking, body mass index 25 kg/m2 or lower, physical activity at U.S. recommended levels, and biomarkers of untreated total cholesterol of 200 mg/dl or lower, untreated blood pressure of 120/80 mm Hg or lower, and fasting blood of glucose no higher than 100 mg/dl.[38 39] These seven Building Blocks of good cardiovascular health are sometimes called Life's Simple 7.

A study of the heart health of Americans found that diet and physical activity were the metrics least likely to be ideal.[40] The prevalence of six or seven of the ideal cardiovascular health metrics was as low as 0.5% in a population of Black Americans, and in only one of 14 U.S. study sites did more than 10% of those studied have ideal metrics. Compared with persons with zero to one cardiovascular health metrics, persons with five to seven cardiovascular health metrics had a 23% to 79% reduction in the risk of all-cause mortality and a 42% to 90% reduction in the risk of CVD mortality. In addition, persons with six to seven ideal cardiovascular health metrics had a 51% reduction in cancer risk, and persons achieving five to seven ideal metrics had a 36% reduction in the odds of depressive symptoms.

The INTERHEART study,[41] a major Canadian-led global study of heart disease in 52 countries, identified nine easily measured diet and lifestyle-related risk factors that account for over 90% of the risk of an acute heart attack:

- Smoking
- Blood cholesterol
- Hypertension
- Diabetes
- Obesity
- Diet
- Physical activity
- Alcohol consumption
- Psychosocial factors

The INTERHEART investigators, led by Salim Yusuf, found that these risk factors are the same in almost every geographic region and every racial/ethnic group worldwide and are consistent in men and women. Referring to the INTERHEART study in his book *The Spectrum*, Dean Ornish notes that cardiovascular heart disease "…is almost completely preventable by changing diet and lifestyle…"[42]

More evidence that heart attacks are largely preventable comes from an 11-year Swedish study.[43] It found that adherence to a combination of healthy dietary and lifestyle practices could prevent nearly four of five heart attacks in men. Low-risk behavior included five factors: a healthy diet (top quintile of a Recommended Food Score), moderate alcohol consumption (10 to 30 g/day), no smoking, being physically active (walking/bicycling 40 or more minutes/day and exercising one or more hours/week), and having no abdominal adiposity (waist circumference <95 cm., 37.4 inches). Compared with men having none of five low-risk factors, men having all five low-risk lifestyle factors had a 79% lower heart attack risk. But even in this Nordic country with excellent health information and services, only 1% of the men studied had all five low-risk factors present.

A healthy lifestyle is of particular importance for those with inherited risk for coronary artery disease. Risk can be up to 91% greater compared to those with low genetic risk. A study to determine if a healthy lifestyle could offset high genetic risk considered four healthy lifestyle factors: no current smoking, no obesity (BMI <30), physical activity at least once weekly, and a healthy diet pattern.[44] The study found that among those at high genetic risk, a healthy lifestyle lowered the risk of coronary artery events by 46%.

The importance of lifestyle is shown by the very low risk of CVD among indigenous populations living without the conveniences and stresses of modern society. In Chapter 3, "Optimal Nutrition," I described several traditional populations with low cardiovascular disease risk. Fortunately, most heart attacks are largely preventable when a person adheres to the Building Blocks of Health.[45] And starting a healthy lifestyle in childhood maximizes the odds that it will be effective in preventing cardiovascular disease. We also know that by modifying the risk factors for cardiovascular disease and lowering cholesterol, atherosclerosis can even be reversed.

The role of blood lipids—cholesterol and triglycerides

People and populations with favorable blood lipid patterns have low rates of cardiovascular disease. Like Mexico's Tarahumara and Bolivia's Tismane, people living on whole-food plant-based diets in the poor developing countries in Asia and Africa typically have total-cholesterol levels in the range of 100-140 mg/dl, and they almost never develop clinically significant coronary artery disease.[46 47 48]

About 38% of adult Americans have total cholesterol levels of 200 mg/dl or higher. About 12% of the adult U.S. population 20 years of age or older have total cholesterol levels of 240 mg/dl or higher and more than twice the heart attack risk of someone whose cholesterol is 200 mg/dl.[49] For years it was thought, and the public was led to believe that a blood cholesterol level of 200 mg/dl was normal, of no particular concern to health, or even a desirable level. In fact, this level is just an average among Americans with our usual high-risk, unhealthy diet and lifestyle.

Fully 35% of heart attacks occur among people with total cholesterol between 150 mg/dl and 200 mg/dl. Evidence from the Framingham Heart Study and many subsequent investigations strongly suggest that atherosclerotic heart disease is extremely rare among individuals with a total cholesterol of 150 mg/dl or lower.[50] There is good evidence that lowering LDL-C, whether it is by drugs such as statins or diet and weight loss, is associated with lower CVD risk. The Coordinating Committee of the National Cholesterol Education Program recommends attaining an LDL-C level of 70 mg/dl or lower for those at high risk of cardiovascular heart disease—and that includes almost all of us.[51] In short, a lower level of total cholesterol and LDL-C is healthier.[52 53]

High HDL-C is associated with protection against heart attack. Smoking, obesity, and being sedentary, lowers HDL-C levels, exercise raises HDL-C levels. According to one guideline, an HDL-C level of 60 or above is protective, and levels of HDL-C less than 40 mg/dl for men and less than 50 mg/dl for women are correlated with an increase in the risk of heart disease. At one time, it was a common practice to assess CVD risk by measuring total cholesterol and HDL-C levels and then dividing the total level by the HDL-C level. The Framingham study and other studies suggest that ideally, the ratio of total cholesterol to HDL-C should be less than four to one or even better, less than three to one, the average ratio for American men is higher than that, vegetarians, on the other hand, average only about 2.8 to 1.3.[54 55 56]

As noted in the Chapter 3, "Optimal Nutrition," if LDL-C is in a healthy low range, a high HDL-C does not seem to provide additional benefits for CVD prevention. High levels of HDL may just be a sign that the body is better at disposing of excess cholesterol and preventing the build-up of plaque in the presence of unhealthy high levels of LDL-C. Additional evidence that high HDL-C is not cardioprotective comes from studies of individuals with a genetic predisposition to high HDL-C. Their high HDL-C does not seem to lower the risk of CVD, and some research has found that very high HDL-C, 80 mg/dl or higher, increases CVD risk.[57] Trials of drugs that more than doubled levels of HDL-C failed to reduce the rate of cardiovascular events.[58]

Many people who have heart disease or diabetes have high blood triglyceride levels and other biomarkers associated with high cardiovascular disease risk, including a high total cholesterol level, a high LDL-C level, a low HDL-C level. A triglyceride level of 150 mg/dl or higher is one of the risk factors of the metabolic syndrome that is associated with an increased risk for heart disease and diabetes.

High triglycerides are mainly a lifestyle-related risk factor, but some people have a genetic predisposition to high triglycerides. Being overweight or obese, low levels of physical activity, cigarette smoking, and excess alcohol consumption all contribute to elevated triglyceride levels. Lowering triglycerides is possible by adherence to the factors on the Lifestyle Checklist, especially controlling weight, eating a heart-healthy low saturated fat, plant-based diet, getting regular exercise, avoiding tobacco, eliminating alcohol or at least limiting it to one drink per day and limiting beverages and foods with added sugars.[59]

There is good evidence that lowering triglyceride levels reduces the risk of coronary heart disease events. Still, the link between triglycerides and CVD is variable in part because triglycerides vary considerably in composition and particle numbers.[60] Not all genetic variants that lead to high triglycerides are associated with an increased risk of CVD.

What are the appropriate goals for a blood lipid profile?

Expert review committees have not conclusively recommended a specific target level for total cholesterol, LDL-C or HDL-C to prevent cardiovascular diseases.[61 62] However, the epidemiology of cardiovascular disease and many clinical studies, strongly suggests that the lower the level of LDL-C, the lower the risk, regardless of the therapy used to reduce levels of LDL-C.[63 64 65 66]

Total cholesterol targets

The American Heart Association 2013 categories for total cholesterol and heart disease risk are shown in Table 6.1.[67 68] In my opinion, up to 200 mg/dl should not be considered "desirable" and could lead to complacency because any level above 150 mg/dl entails an increased risk for coronary heart disease. Table 6.1. shows my suggested ranking of risk categories for total cholesterol under "Best Lifestyle."

Table 6.1. Total Cholesterol Level Recommendations

Total Cholesterol Level	American Heart Association Category	"Best Lifestyle" Category
150 mg/dL or Less		Desirable, Low Risk
Less than 200 mg/dL	Desirable	Moderate Risk
200 to 239 mg/dL	Borderline high	High risk
240 mg/dL and above	High blood cholesterol	Very High Risk

LDL cholesterol targets

LDL cholesterol is a better indicator of cardiovascular risk than total cholesterol. The American Heart Association also made lenient definitions of the risk of various levels of LDL-C. As is shown in Table 6.2, the AHA considered an LDL-C level of 100 to 129 mg/dl to be "near or above optimal." If the mean level of LDL cholesterol for American adults age 20 and older is 112.1 mg/dl, then a high proportion of the American public is, according to the AHA, "near or above optimal" and not at the "borderline high" level.[69]

Is there is a level of LDL-C at which there are essentially no adverse cardiovascular events related to atherosclerosis? One estimate is that the threshold for progression of atherosclerosis is approximately 70 mg/dl.[70] Another estimate is that the LDL-C level at which cardiovascular event rates may approach zero is about 60 mg/dl for primary prevention (no previous clinical coronary disease), and 30 mg/dl for secondary prevention (previous clinical coronary disease).

The average level of LDL-C for American adults age 20 and older is 112.1 mg/dl. In populations of hunter-gatherers, LDL-C is estimated to be 50-75 mg/dl, and that of newborn babies is 30-70 mg/dl. Atherosclerotic vascular disease almost never occurs in people with the inherited disorder (familial hypobetalipoproteinemia) that causes very low LDL-C levels, 30-40 mg/dl. They can expect a lifespan that is 15 years longer than average.[71]

A large 2009 study of 136,905 hospital patients with heart attacks found that 72.1% of those admitted had LDL-C levels lower than 130 mg/dl, a level that the AHA would call "near or above optimal." And the same study found that half of the patients with a history of heart disease had LDL-C levels lower than 100 mg/dl, a level the AHA would consider "optimal." Even an LDL-C below 70mg/dl was not fully protective against heart attack, 17.6% of patients had LDL-C below this level.[72] My suggested ranking of risk categories is shown under "Best Lifestyle" in Table 6.2. For optimal heart health, the goal for LDL-C should be 70 mg/dl or lower.

Table 6.2. LDL Cholesterol Level Recommendations

LDL Cholesterol Level	American Heart Association Category	"Best Lifestyle" Category
70 mg/dL or Less		Desirable, likely to halt progression or reverse Cardiovascular Disease (CVD)
Less than 100 mg/dL	Optimal	Low, but not no risk
100 to 129 mg/dL	Near or above optimal	Significant risk
130 to 159 mg/dL	Borderline high	High risk
160 to 189 mg/dL	High	Very high risk
190 mg/dL and above	Very high	Extremely high risk

HDL cholesterol targets

The American Heart Association guidelines for HDL-C "good" cholesterol indicate that higher levels are healthier and that a low HDL-C, less than 40 mg/dl for men, and less than 50 mg/dl for women, increases the risk for heart disease.[73] But as already noted, low HDL-C is probably not an indicator of increased CVD risk if LDL-C is very low.

Triglycerides

The 2013 recommendations of the American Heart Association about triglyceride levels are shown in Table 6.3 below.[74]

Table 6.3.

Triglyceride Level	Category
Less than 100 mg/dl	Optimal
Less than 150 mg/dl	Normal
150–199 mg/dl	Borderline high
200–499 mg/dl	High
500 mg/dl and above	Very high

The average 2013-2016 level of triglycerides for American adults age 20 and older is 95.6 mg/dl, and 22 % of adults have high triglycerides of 150 mg/dl or higher.[75]

Preventing and reversing cardiovascular disease with a healthy diet

As is described in Chapter 3, "Optimal Nutrition," a healthy diet is among the most important lifestyle behaviors that can be adopted to reduce the risk of CVD. A cardioprotective diet is based on the unrefined plant-based foods that are high in fiber. They are either very low in fat or substitute healthier monounsaturated and polyunsaturated fats for saturated and trans-fat, and they are low in refined carbohydrates, added sugars, and sodium. In contrast, long-term low-carbohydrate eating, based on meat, increases cardiovascular risk because it boosts LDL-C.

Omega-3 fatty acid supplements have been recommended as a way to prevent CVD. Most research has shown that eating fish may benefit CVD health. The benefits, if any, of marine omega-3 supplementation (fish oil) supplementation are less clear. A meta-analysis of 10 randomized trials involving 78,000 patients found that that n–3 fatty acids did not lower the risk of major adverse cardiovascular events.[76] A similar study among people with diabetes, ASCEND (A Study of Cardiovascular Events in Diabetes), also found little effect from daily marine omega-3 administration.[77]

The VITAL study also found that high dose supplements of n-3 fatty acids are not effective in preventing heart attack, stroke, or death from cardiovascular disease.[78] However, as described in Chapter 3, "Optimal Nutrition," the VITAL study suggests that high dose supplementation might benefit some ethnic groups and those who have a low intake of fish. More research to confirm this is needed. In a following section, the role of drugs related to fish oils for the treatment of triglycerides over 500 mg/dl is presented.

The most recent meta-analysis that included the findings from VITAL found that daily marine omega-3 supplementation is moderately effective and provided a modest 3% to 8% reduction in CVD endpoints.[79] After an average of five years of use, omega-3 supplementation lowered rates of myocardial infarction, coronary heart disease death, total coronary heart disease, cardiovascular disease death, and total cardiovascular disease, but no benefits were found for stroke. The study also found that the higher the dose of omega-3 supplementation, the more pronounced were the CVD benefits.

Ultra low-fat (ULF) diets

As is described in Chapter 3, "Optimal Nutrition," Nathan Pritikin, Dean Ornish, and Caldwell Esselstyn Jr. found that a lifestyle intervention based on diet would usually halt the progression of coronary heart disease and even reverse it.[80] Other clinicians and researchers who advocate a very-low-fat whole-food plant-based diet include Connor,[81] McDougall,[82 83] Fuhrman,[84] Barnard,[85 86 87] Campbell,[88] Jenkins,[89] Greger[90] and Shintani.[91] Their patients have had similar beneficial health results from nutrition-based interventions.

Their studies have shown that although addressing all risk factors is important, a modified, healthier diet is among the most powerful lifestyle changes that can reduce the risk of CVD. The Ornish diet is ultra-low-fat (ULF) whole-food plant-based "beans and greens." Only about 10% of total calories are from fat, no saturated or trans-fats are allowed, and added sugars and refined grains are limited.

The diet consists of natural unrefined plant-based foods, fruits, vegetables, legumes, whole grains, soy, and cereals, avoids meat, refined grains, and refined grain products, minimizes non-fat dairy, or eliminates dairy, and eliminates added sugars, seafood, and most processed foods.[92] Esselstyn's advice is to not eat "anything with a face or a mother."[93] The ULF plant-based diet is high in fiber and low in rapidly absorbed simple sugars, so it has a low glycemic index.[94] Ornish has found that the addition of exercise and stress management additionally improves the outcomes of his lifestyle modification program.

Ornish's patients had more than a 90% reduction in the frequency of angina, on average, a 40% reduction in LDL cholesterol, measurable regression in the amount of their coronary artery stenosis, and improved blood flow to the heart.[95 96] Esselstyn's studies also showed that a nutrition-based intervention could stop and reverse the progression of very severe coronary artery disease without medicine or surgery.[97 98]

Vegan and vegetarian diets

The traditional diets of indigenous populations with low CVD risk typically have vegetarian or mostly plant-based dietary patterns. The notable difference from ULF eating is greater consumption of high-fat plant foods such as seeds, nuts, olive oil, and avocados. The Women's Health Study found that the fifth of those studied with the highest intake of fruits and vegetables was associated with a 20% to 30% reduction in risk of CVD compared to the fifth with the lowest intake.[99] Other groups with vegetarian diets, such as Seventh-Day Adventists, have a low incidence of CVD.[100] A study that included Seventh-Day Adventists found that people who consumed large amounts of meat protein and fat experienced a 60% increase in CVD, whereas consumption of large amounts of protein from nuts and seeds was associated with a 40% decrease in CVD.[101] A study in the *Journal of the American Heart Association* that compared four diets found that higher adherence to a healthy plant-based diet index was associated with a 19% lower risk of CVD mortality and an and 11% lower risk of all-cause mortality.[102]

Mediterranean, mixed, and balanced diets

A very-low-fat plant-based diet or vegetarian diet may be too restrictive for some of us to follow. If so, Mediterranean, mixed, and balanced diets should be considered as a good alternative that is easier to adhered to. Mixed and balanced diets are healthier variations of the typical diets consumed in the U.S. and other wealthy developed countries.[103 104] They include fat in the diet, but in the form of healthier polyunsaturated and monounsaturated fats, saturated and trans-fats remain restricted. Because they also allow a wider variety of foods than many diets, they are considered to be easier to adhere to.

Mediterranean eating improves cholesterol levels, insulin resistance, and the metabolic syndrome.[105] Foods that are emphasized include vegetables, fruits, nuts and seeds, beans and legumes, olive oil, selective dairy, whole grains, often fish and other seafood, limited consumption of meat, and sometimes consumption of moderate amounts of alcohol in the form of wine.[106] The Nurses' Health Study found that replacing 5% of calories from saturated fat with calories from unsaturated fat reduced the risk of coronary heart disease by 42%.[107 108 109] A meta-analysis of multiple such studies found a 10% reduction in coronary heart disease for every 5% substitution of unsaturated for saturated fats.[110]

A study found that high Mediterranean diet intake was associated with approximately a one-fourth relative risk reduction in CVD events compared to low Mediterranean diet intake.[111] The factors contributing to reduced risk included biomarkers of inflammation, glucose metabolism and insulin resistance, body mass index, blood pressure, and blood lipids. Adopting a Mediterranean diet has been found to reduce the risk of heart attacks,[112 113] but probably not as much as the results reported by Ornish.[114]

Mixed and balanced diets, such as the Dietary Approaches to Stop Hypertension (DASH)[115] diet, are diets modified to conform with authoritative dietary guidelines for healthier diets, such as the *Dietary Reference Intakes of the Institute of Medicine*, the *Dietary Guidelines for Americans*, and the *Dietary Recommendations of the World Health Organization.*[116] These authorities generally recommend an emphasis on plant-based foods and increasing the number of servings of fruits to two cups/day for a 2400 calorie diet, and vegetables to three cups/day for a 2400 calorie diet. A 2013 survey found that fewer than 15% of U.S. citizens had the recommended fruit intake, and 8.9% met the recommendations for vegetables.[117 118]

Regardless of which dietary pattern is chosen, it is important that lower saturated fatty acid consumption, for example from eating less red meat, be accompanied by increased consumption of healthy fats and higher-fiber whole plant foods rather than increasing consumption of refined carbohydrates, starches, and sugars.[119] Foods that are consistent with this recipe for cardioprotective cholesterol-lowering healthy eating include oats, barley, other whole grains, legumes, beans, nuts, all fruits, and soy foods.

Alcohol and cardiovascular disease

Some studies indicate that individuals who drink alcohol moderately (up to two drinks/day for men and one drink/day for women) experience a lower incidence of coronary heart disease than nondrinkers. Meta-analyses of cohort studies indicate that on a graph, there is a J-shaped relationship between alcohol consumption and all-cause mortality, with reduced risk for low-volume drinkers compared to abstainers and heavier drinkers.[120 121 122] One such analysis found an increased risk for abstainers and persons reporting more than three drinks per day and reduced risk for lighter drinkers due almost entirely to lower risk of death from cardiovascular disease.[123]

Experts caution that observational studies may overestimate the benefits of moderate alcohol consumption, and studies suggest that the J-shaped relationship between alcohol consumption and all-cause mortality is an artifact. People decrease their alcohol consumption as they age and become ill or frail or increase the use of medications. If these occasional or former drinkers are included in the abstainer category in prospective studies, it is suggested that it is not the absence of alcohol elevating their risk for coronary heart disease (CHD) but, instead, their ill-health. Meta-analytic results indicate that the few studies without this error found that abstainers and light or moderate drinkers are at equal risk for all-cause and CHD mortality.[124 125 126]

A 2016 analysis of 87 studies found that the apparent reduction of mortality among light to moderate drinkers disappeared when former drinkers were eliminated from the comparison group and the comparison group was limited to lifelong abstainers and occasional drinkers.[127] Furthermore, for cancer, cirrhosis, and many other diseases, there is a linear increase in risk with increasing ingestion of alcohol.[128]

The commonest heart arrhythmia, atrial fibrillation, is associated with an increased risk of stroke and death. A healthy lifestyle that features avoiding obesity, sedentary living, diabetes, and consumption of alcohol can help prevent its onset.[129 130] Moderate to heavy alcohol consumption is strongly associated with the occurrence of atrial fibrillation. However, even one drink a day is associated with a dose-dependent 8% increase in risk.

Although alcohol use has been advocated for its possible, but not fully proven beneficial effects on cardiovascular health, it is an intoxicating, addictive, toxic, carcinogenic drug and not a therapeutic agent. In the U.S. alcohol-associated annual deaths total about 88,000 or 9.8% of all deaths.[131] Alcohol-related costs to the U.S. were estimated at $249 billion in 2010.[132 133] According to Mozaffarian, drinking alcohol is not a sound strategy to reduce CVD risk because of alcohol-related accidents, homicides, and suicides, especially among younger adults, alcohol use has an overall net adverse effect on mortality.[134 135 136] The Chief Medical Officer of the U.K. found that there is no safe level of alcohol consumption.[137 138]

Sugar and cardiovascular disease

There is good evidence that excess sugar consumption contributes to the current U.S. epidemic of obesity, diabetes, and heart disease.[139 140] Although the human body can convert surplus calories in the form of each of the macronutrient categories (carbohydrates, proteins, fats, and alcohol) into fat, the biochemical pathways for metabolizing dietary fat, alcohol and the fructose found in almost all forms of added sugar, make it more likely that extra calories from these sources will end up stored as fat.[141] People with the metabolic syndrome are at high risk for CVD. Studies of children by Lustig and his colleagues have shown that sugar restriction can rapidly improve the unhealthy biomarkers that characterize the syndrome.[142]

Nearly one in 10 adults worldwide are now affected by diabetes, a condition that increases the risk of cardiovascular disease and harms not just the heart but also the kidneys, eyes, and peripheral circulation. Studies implicate excessive sugar intake as an independent cause of high diabetes rates and a contributor to the causation of cardiovascular diseases.[143] Consumption of sugar-sweetened beverages is associated with weight gain as well as type 2 diabetes.[144] The Health Professionals' Follow-Up Study found that participants in the top quartile of sugar-sweetened beverage intake (about 6.5 soft drinks per week) had a 20% higher relative risk of coronary heart disease than those in the bottom quartile.[145] The recommended daily consumption of added sugar is very low, with no more than 100 calories for women and 150 calories for men.

Preventing and reversing heart and other cardiovascular disease through physical activity

Exercise improves many factors that are associated with reduced risk of CVD by lowering blood pressure, increasing HDL-C, and reducing triglyceride and LDL-C levels.[146] The CDC estimates that being sedentary increases the risk of coronary heart disease by 1.5 to 2.4 times.[147] The Council on Clinical Cardiology and the Council on Nutrition, Physical Activity, and Metabolism report that the most physically active subjects studied generally have coronary artery disease rates half of those of the most sedentary groups.[148] [149] [150] A 2018 study found that those with below-average cardiorespiratory fitness were 40% more likely to die from any cause than those with above-average fitness and mortality was five times greater among those with low fitness compared to those with "elite" fitness.[151]

Although both moderate and vigorous activities are beneficial to health, vigorous activity is more beneficial and more cardioprotective.[152] [153] [154] One estimate is that running beats walking by a factor of 2:1 to 4:1 in mortality reduction at the same amount of physical activity as measured by metabolic equivalents.[155] Other, but not all, studies have also shown greater reductions in CVDs are associated with vigorous-intensity activities.[156] One study found that the greatest cardiovascular disease and all-cause mortality benefit occurred at three to five times the *2008 Physical Activity Guidelines for Americans* recommendation of 150 minutes of moderate and/or 75 minutes of vigorous physical activity per week. The study also found that there was no evidence of harm at 10 or more times the recommended minimum.[157]

Even low intensity activities that interrupt long sedentary periods are of benefit. A study over 4.9 years among older women that measured periods of inactivity with fitness trackers found that each hour of sedentary time was associated with a 12% higher risk for CVD, and when sitting time was uninterrupted, the risk could be as much as 54% higher.[158] Both total length of sedentary time and long uninterrupted bouts of sitting contributed to CVD risk, and both interruptions in bouts of sitting and reduced total sedentary time reduced risk.

Studies suggest that maintaining heart and blood vessel health requires physical activity four or five times a week—the usual changes with age will occur among sedentary people or, to some extent, among casual exercisers who work out only two or three times a week.[159]

Some studies have found that the combination of a healthier diet and exercise has a more profound influence on achieving a favorable blood lipid pattern that either diet or exercise alone.[160] Physical activity also helps to prevent obesity and diabetes, both of which increase the risk of cardiovascular disease. Additional information on the cardiovascular and other benefits of physical activity can be found in Chapter 9, "Benefits of Physical Activity."

Inflammation and cardiovascular disease

Chronic inflammation is an unhealthy condition. Elevation of C-reactive protein (CRP) is a sign of inflammation anywhere in the body, including in arterial walls. Elevated CRP may be a biomarker for CVD rather than a cause of it. Other heart attack risk factors such as abdominal obesity are associated with elevated CRP. In the presence of elevated LDL-C elevated CRP is associated with increased risk of heart attack or stroke. CRP can be reduced by physical activity, weight loss, quitting smoking, and taking lipid-lowering statin drugs.[161]

Controlling blood pressure to reduce the risk of stroke and heart attack

High blood pressure (BP), or hypertension, is among the most common cardiovascular risk conditions in the United States and a major cause of coronary heart disease, brain damage and dementia, congestive heart failure, stroke, loss of vision, and renal failure.[162,163] According to recent estimates, hypertension is present in approximately 100 million adults in the United States. The incidence of hypertension increases with age. It affects about two-thirds of adults aged 60 years or older, more than 75% of individuals aged 75 years or older, and the lifetime risk of developing hypertension exceeds 90% if a person lives long enough.[164,165,166] Hypertension is associated with 41% of all CVD deaths.[167,168,169]

It is well established that lowering blood pressure (BP) through diet and other lifestyle interventions, or with medications, substantially reduces the risk of CVDs. Although high blood pressure is very common, almost half of Americans with high blood pressure do not have their blood pressure under control according to the standard of a systolic BP <140 mm Hg (millimeters of mercury) and a diastolic BP <90 mm Hg. As is the case with high cholesterol, high blood pressure usually causes few symptoms, and unfortunately, many Americans with high blood pressure are neither aware of their hypertension nor taking antihypertensive medications.[170 171]

Most strokes result from a combination of high blood pressure and atherosclerosis. Two-thirds of those with a first heart attack and three-quarters of those with a first stroke have hypertension, commonly defined as a systolic over a diastolic reading of 140/90 mm Hg or higher.[172] A stroke occurs when the blood supply to the brain is disrupted either because an artery is narrowed or blocked with a blood clot or if a weak or damaged artery ruptures and causes bleeding in the brain, a hemorrhagic stroke. Stroke can cause the functions of a particular part of the brain to be impaired or stop altogether. Blood clots formed elsewhere in the body, such as in the heart during atrial fibrillation, can also travel to the brain and cause a stroke.

Smoking is an important risk factor for stroke. Smoking increases the risk of both heart attack and stroke by two to three times.[173] Studies have shown that, overall, Black Americans between ages 45 and 64 have two to three times the risk of stroke compared to white people. Among Black Americans, smoking doubles the risk of stroke.[174]

About 2% of all strokes and possibly up to 25% of those in young and middle-aged people are caused by a dissection (tear) in an artery that may be spontaneous, caused by falls, participating in sports, yoga moves, or chiropractic manipulations. The risk of stroke is also increased among people who have migraine headaches, especially among those who have associated symptoms (called an aura), such as blurry vision.[175] Substance misuse can also cause strokes, and with the increasing use of cocaine, methamphetamines, and marijuana, more strokes are occurring among young people.[176] Marijuana may accelerate heart rate, increase blood pressure, and cause agitation, seizures, hallucinations, strokes, and even death. The use of energy, weight-loss, and a variety of other dietary supplements, some of which contain substances that mimic amphetamines, are of concern. As is discussed in Chapter 5, "Vitamins and other Supplements," these products are not beneficial for health and may cause harmful effects on heart rate, blood pressure, and blood clotting, and they should be avoided.

How common are strokes, and what are the health effects of a stroke?

Stroke is both a leading cause of disability and pre-COVID-19, was the fifth most frequent cause of death, and according to the American Stroke Association, Americans paid about $73.7 billion in 2010 for stroke-related medical costs and disability.[177 178]

The CDC and the American Stroke Association summarize the scope of the problem:[179 180]

- Stroke kills more than 130,000 Americans each year—one out of every 19 deaths.
- Every year, more than 795,000 people in the United States have a stroke.
- About 185,000 strokes—nearly one of four—are in people who have had a previous stroke.
- The lifetime risk of stroke in North America is 22.4%.[181]
- About 87% of all strokes are ischemic strokes when blood flow to the brain is blocked.

The disabilities caused by a stroke can be devastating. A stroke can cause one or several of five types of disabilities: paralysis or problems controlling movement, sensory disturbances including pain, problems using or understanding language, problems with thinking and memory, and emotional disturbances. Brain damage caused by a stroke can include cognitive and sensory impairments, epilepsy, speech or communication disorders, visual disturbances, poor attention, behavioral problems, and poor quality of life.[182]

High blood pressure also causes brain damage that is subtler than a stroke. A study in the journal *Lancet Neurology* found that even among individuals in their 40s, those with any degree of increased blood pressure had damage to the structural integrity of the brain's white matter and decreases in the volume of its gray matter, injuries associated with cognitive decline.[183] The study found that the amount of brain injury worsened as blood pressure increased. Even the modestly increased blood pressure of prehypertension causes brain damage that is likely to contribute to cognitive decline and possibly eventually to dementia. Because vascular brain injury develops insidiously over time, by knowing and treating their high blood pressure at a young age, people can improve their late-life brain health. Because high blood pressure causes cumulative damage over long periods of time, time-averaged or "cumulative" BP is powerful predictors of coronary heart disease, heart failure, stroke, and vascular dementia.[184 185 186]

Several studies provide good evidence that elevated blood pressure in middle-life is associated with reduced cognitive function at older ages.[187 188 189 190] In one study, participants, who were on average, 56 years old, were followed for 20 years. Prehypertension or hypertension was present at baseline in 58% of white and 76% of Black American study participants.[191] Death was a major outcome related to having hypertension at the first evaluation, with fewer than 50% of individuals with systolic blood pressure (SBP) greater than 160 mm Hg surviving to an average age of 76 years.[192] Of those who survived, there was a modest but significant association between baseline SBP and the rate of cognitive decline. The higher the middle-life SBP, the greater the rate of decline. Individuals receiving hypertension treatment had substantially slower rates of cognitive decline compared with those who were untreated.

A source of brain damage made likely by chronic hypertension is a series of small strokes that may not be easily recognized when they occur, but the resulting cumulative brain damage can cause multi-infarct or vascular dementia, the second most common cause of dementia after Alzheimer disease. As is described in greater detail in Chapter 8, "Preventing Dementia," vascular damage to the brain may lead to Alzheimer disease.

Managing Hypertension to Reduce the Risk of Stroke

Elevated blood pressure, elevated blood cholesterol levels, and cigarette smoking are the most important risk factors for heart attack and stroke. The risk of stroke can be decreased by adopting a healthy lifestyle, and if needed, medical therapy such as antihypertensive drugs to help avoid the hazards of atherosclerosis and high blood pressure. By reducing blood pressure to a normal range, the risk of a stroke can be reduced by about 50% and the risk of a heart attack by 20%.[193]

Since there is no single condition that is associated with all of the increased risks of stroke and cardiovascular disease, the best strategy is to follow the guidance of the Lifestyle Checklist and simultaneously address multiple risk factors. Those that can be modified so as to decrease stroke risk include smoking, diet, high blood cholesterol, high blood pressure, diabetes, obesity, alcohol, stress, and lack of exercise. Avoiding abuse of substances such as cocaine, methamphetamines, various forms of marijuana, and the use of energy, weight-loss, and a variety of other dietary supplements is also important to decrease the risk of stroke.

Preventive measures to avoid a stroke from an arterial dissection (a tear) include the use of proper protective gear and avoiding falls when participating in sports, caution with yoga moves, and caution with chiropractic manipulations. People who have frequent headaches, or migraine headaches, especially those who have an aura, should have their headaches evaluated by their health provider and avoid the use of estrogen-containing oral contraceptives and any other drug that might increase the propensity for blood clots.

Among the several interventions to decrease the risk of stroke, controlling blood pressure is the most critical. In general, the lower blood pressure is, the healthier one's cardiovascular system is, and the lower the risk of stroke and heart attack is.[194] Although a blood pressure of 120/80 mm Hg or lower is considered a normal blood pressure, most but not all epidemiological studies and clinical trials suggest that cardiovascular risk increases in a linear fashion at any level of blood pressure above of 110/70 mm Hg.

About 30% of Americans have what was formerly called prehypertension or borderline hypertension with blood pressure between 121/81 and 139/89. Systolic blood pressures of 140 mm Hg or higher or diastolic pressures of 90 mm Hg or higher are considered hypertension (now called stage 2 hypertension), but there is considerable debate about the level of blood pressure that will benefit from treatment with drugs and what the target BP level should be for drug treatment.[195]

Blood pressure fluctuates throughout the day and is regulated by the interplay between the strength of heart contractions, for example, during exercise compared to at rest or during sleep. Blood pressure is also regulated by hormones and by the nervous system in that stress raises blood pressure and relaxation and sleep lower it. Other influences on blood pressure include how dilated your blood vessels are, how elastic your blood vessels are—atherosclerosis makes them stiffer, so peak pressures are higher, and how well your kidneys function to regulate sodium in the body—more sodium means greater blood volume and higher blood pressure.

Five to 10% of hypertension is termed secondary hypertension because it is caused by, or secondary to, a disease condition, a drug, or metabolic disorder. Kidney disease, a narrowing of the arteries that supply blood to the kidneys, a variety of adrenal gland tumors and other hormone disorders, sleep apnea, and certain drugs can cause medically treatable forms of secondary hypertension. Blood pressures should be measured after five minutes of rest, and they are often raised by the stress of visiting a doctor—so-called "white coat hypertension."

Ninety to 95% of high blood pressure in the U.S. is considered to be essential hypertension because it is related to lifestyle, diet, and the condition of the body's vasculature and not caused by a single disease condition or factor. Family history, genetics, and race influence the risk of hypertension, but an important factor is the typical American diet that is high in salt (sodium) and also low in foods that are high in potassium such as fruits and vegetables.

Physical inactivity, overweight, and obesity are lifestyle factors that make important contributions to hypertension, and they too can be modified. For some people, becoming physically active and losing weight can normalize blood pressure. But among lifestyle interventions to prevent and treat hypertension, the most effective is the adoption of a nutritional pattern that limits sodium in the diet. Essential hypertension can often be controlled with these lifestyle interventions. If that fails, hypertension is usually amenable to treatment with antihypertensive drugs that are available through a prescription from a health care provider. Most antihypertensive drugs are effective and have tolerable and often no noticeable side effects.

Limiting dietary sodium to manage high blood pressure

In general, the more sodium in an individual's diet, the higher an individual's blood pressure is. One such study, the Trials of Hypertension Prevention (TOHP), showed a linear 17% increase in cardiovascular disease risk per 1000 mg per day increase in sodium from levels starting at 1,500 mg per day.[196] The average of 3,500-4,000 mg of sodium a day in the typical American's diet far exceeds the American Heart Association (AHA) recommendation of a limit of 2,400 mg (5.8 gm salt), or even better a 1,500 mg of sodium (3.6 gm salt) per day for everyone including children.[197]

There is considerable individual variation in if and how much salt increases blood pressure. Some people are "salt resistant," the sodium content of their diet has little or no effect on their blood pressure.[198] Some research suggests that very low sodium consumption will increase the risks of death from CVDs and all causes, but most research supports the current recommendations to limit sodium.[199] [200] [201] [202] [203]

The Institute of Medicine (IOM) examined research on dietary sodium intake and health outcomes in the general U.S. population and among individuals with hypertension; prehypertension; those 51 years of age and older; Black Americans; and those with diabetes, chronic kidney disease, and congestive heart failure. The 2013 report from the Institute of Medicine concluded that existing evidence suggests that:[204]

- Consuming more than 2300 mg of sodium a day increases the risk of high blood pressure.
- There is not enough evidence to say that eating less than 2,300 mg of sodium a day benefits cardiovascular disease outcomes for the general population.
- In people with known cardiovascular disease, diabetes, or chronic kidney disease, there is some evidence that a diet of 1,500 to 2,300 mg of sodium a day may have negative health effects compared with higher-sodium diets. However, this evidence is not strong enough to say that these individuals should be treated differently than the general population.[205]

Since the release of the report, a study among individuals with chronic kidney disease (about 11% of U.S. population) suggests that reductions in sodium intake to the 2,300 mg/day level would have considerable benefit in preventing heart failure, myocardial infarction, and stroke.[206 207]

The IOM report led to confusing news reports with headlines like "Doubts About Restricting Salt" and "Study finds Low-Salt Diet Poses Health Hazard" that inaccurately suggest there is no health benefit from decreasing salt intake. Because most Americans consume far more than 2300 mg of sodium a day, a decrease in sodium intake to an average of 2,300 mg per day would be beneficial to most people. Some observers would say that there is not enough evidence that further decreasing sodium intake to 1500 mg a day has additional benefit for the prevention of cardiovascular disease—or is harmful.[208 209 210] However, a very careful analysis published in the *New England Journal of Medicine* in 2016 concluded that there is strong evidence that there is a strong linear dose-response effect of sodium reduction on blood pressure and CVD risk down to 1,000 mg/day.[211]

Because salt is added to so many processed foods, including canned foods, bakery goods, soups, snack foods such as chips, and fast foods such as pizza, it is difficult to limit intake of sodium. Note that 1 gram (gm) of table salt contains 413.19 milligrams (mg) of sodium. As a result, 90% of Americans exceed the 2,400 mg/day recommendation.[212] According to the AHA, reducing daily sodium intake to less than 1,500 mg per day is particularly important for persons who are age 51 and older and those of any age who are Black or have hypertension, diabetes, or chronic kidney disease. The 1,500 mg recommendation applies to about half of the U.S. population, including children, and the majority of adults.

For most people, there is little need to worry about not getting enough sodium. Even in the probably unlikely instance that it did turn out to be harmful, the CDC estimates that fewer than 1% of Americans reach the 1,500 mg daily limit—our food supply is just too loaded with sodium. In fact, one large international study of 17 countries found that, as measured by sodium excretion, only 4% of study subjects ingested sodium in the U.S. recommended ranges. Only 3.3% of those studied consumed sodium as low as 2,300 mg per day, and just 0.6% of those studied reached 1,500 mg per day.[213]

A low sodium diet is even more effective in lowering blood pressure when it is combined with measures to increase fitness through appropriate levels of physical activity,[214] attaining and maintaining a healthy weight and managing stress.[215] Alcohol and cigarettes also contribute to hypertension. More than one drink of alcohol a day can raise blood pressure, and the chemicals in cigarette smoke raise blood pressure and damage blood vessels.

Evidence-based guidelines for blood pressure targets

It is clear that avoiding high blood pressure is very important to health, but medical scientists are far from total agreement about what the healthiest blood pressure target should be at differing ages and in the presence or absence of CVD, diabetes, or kidney disease. Since the selection of an appropriate blood pressure goal is an important life-long consideration for most of us, the following discussion considers what optimal blood pressure targets are.

A long-standing and standard of high blood pressure was a systolic pressure of 140 mm Hg or higher and/ or a diastolic blood pressure of 90 mm Hg or higher. But in 2014, a committee of experts, the Joint National Committee (JNC 8), suggested less stringent goals for blood pressure and concluded: "There is strong evidence to support treating hypertensive persons aged 60 years or older to a BP goal of less than 150/90 mm Hg and hypertensive persons 30 through 59 years of age to a diastolic goal of less than 90 mm Hg; however, there is insufficient evidence in hypertensive persons younger than 60 years for a systolic goal, or in those younger than 30 years for a diastolic goal, so the panel recommends a BP of less than 140/90 mm Hg for those groups based on expert opinion. The same thresholds and goals are recommended for hypertensive adults with diabetes or nondiabetic chronic kidney disease (CKD) as for the general hypertensive population younger than 60 years."[216]

Many studies raised questions about the JNC 8 blood pressure guidelines that set higher blood pressure goals. They include epidemiologic studies demonstrating a linear relationship between blood pressure and cardiovascular risk. For each 20 mm Hg increase in systolic blood pressure (SBP), or 10 mm Hg increase in diastolic blood pressure (DBP), or both, greater than 115/75 mm Hg, there was a two-fold increase in mortality associated with stroke and coronary artery disease. This suggests that the lower the blood pressure, the lower the CVD risk.

Evidence against accepting the new higher targets for blood pressure came from the SHEP study that found that over five years, lowering of average SBP from 155 mm Hg to 143 mm Hg resulted in a 32% reduction in cardiovascular events.[217][218] Some randomized controlled trials have found that lowering blood pressure by as little as 10 mm Hg in patients with hypertension can reduce a person's lifetime risk for cardiovascular and stroke death by 25% to 40%.[219]

Among the studies cited for choosing lower blood pressure targets are those that show benefits from treating what was called "prehypertension," a systolic blood pressure of 120 to 139 mm Hg, and a diastolic blood pressure of 80 to 89 mm Hg. Treatment of patients with CVD and with prehypertension is associated with a decreased risk of cardiovascular morbidity and mortality. It is less clear if there are benefits from treating those with prehypertension who do not have CVD.[220 221]

Additional evidence supporting low blood pressure targets comes from the Systolic Blood Pressure Intervention Trial (SPRINT).[222] The trial compared the benefit of intensive treatment of systolic blood pressure to a target of less than 120 mm Hg with standard treatment to a target of less than 140 mm Hg among persons age 50 or older who had an increased risk of cardiovascular disease but without diabetes. Participants treated to achieve a systolic blood pressure of less than 120 mm Hg, as compared with less than 140 mm Hg, had a 25% lower relative risk of heart attack, stroke, and heart failure; a 43% lower rate of death from cardiovascular causes; and a 27% lower risk of death from any cause. An analysis of the older participants in the SPRINT trial with a SBP target of less than 120 mm Hg found a one-third lower rate of cardiovascular events and all-cause mortality, and the overall rate of serious adverse events was not different between treatment groups.[223]

The intensive treatment did have some drawbacks. There were significantly (30%) higher rates of some adverse events (falls, low blood pressure, fainting, electrolyte abnormalities, and acute kidney injury or acute renal failure) in the intensive-treatment group. Furthermore, even with intensive lifestyle modification and medical therapy, blood pressure will remain above target in many patients. This suggests the need for population-level initiatives such as reduced sodium content in food.[224 225 226 227]

Similar to the findings of the SPRINT trial, the Hypertension in the Very Elderly Trial (HYVET) evaluated patients over age 80 who lowered their blood pressure with an angiotensin-converting–enzyme (ACE) inhibitor. They reduced their risk of stroke by 30%, their risk of death from cardiovascular causes by 23%, their risk of death from any cause by 21%, and they had a 64% reduction in the rate of heart failure.[228]

After considering new studies and the controversies resulting from the JNC 8 guidelines, in 2017, the American College of Cardiology and the American Heart Association (ACC/AHA) produced new hypertension guidelines for diagnosis and treatment of hypertension.[229 230 231] The new definitions lower the thresholds for a diagnosis of hypertension (see Table 6.4. below). This increases in the proportion of adults in the U.S. defined as having hypertension from 32% to 46% and a substantial 31 million more adult Americans (to a total of more than100 million) being defined as hypertensive. Most of those newly categorized as being hypertensive will be advised to treat their condition by adopting a healthier lifestyle, but about 4.2 million more Americans will be advised to use drugs to treat their hypertension.[232 233]

Table 6.4. 2017 ACC/AHA Guidelines for Diagnosis and Treatment of Hypertension

Blood Pressure Category	**Diagnostic Criteria SBP (Systolic Blood Pressure mm Hg) DBP (Diastolic Blood Pressure mm Hg)**	**Treatment and Target**
Normal	SBP less than 120 DBP less than 80	Optimize Lifestyle
Elevated (formerly prehypertension)	SBP 120-129 and DBP less than 80	Optimize Lifestyle Target is normal BP
Stage 1 Hypertension (formerly prehypertension)	SBP 130-139 or DBP 80-89	If no CVD Optimize Lifestyle If diabetic or 10 yr. CVD risk reaches 10%, add drugs If CVD present, add antihypertensive drugs Target is less than 130/80
Stage 2 Hypertension	SBP 140 or higher or DBP 90 or higher	If no CVD Optimize Lifestyle If diabetic or 10 yr. CVD risk reaches 10%, add drugs If CVD present, add antihypertensive drugs Target is less than 130/80
Hypertensive Crisis	SBP 180 or higher and/ or DBP 120 or higher	Get immediate medical care and hospitalization

Are the newest blood pressure targets better?

The new blood pressure guidelines have not been universally accepted because the evidence for the benefits of treating mild hypertension and those individuals without established cardiovascular disease is less certain. So far, the American College of Physicians and the American Academy of Family Physicians are not changing their goals for people over age 60: SBP of 150 for those at average or low cardiovascular risk and a SBP target of 140 for those at high CVD risk.

It is not surprising that the latest guidelines on hypertension have not ended the controversies relating to blood pressure diagnosis and treatment goals. Writing in the *JAMA* prior to the release of the 2017 guidelines, Aram Chobanian noted that setting blood pressure goals is not an exact science.[234] More than 75% of persons aged 75 or older have hypertension, and the reduction of SBP is clearly beneficial, but the exact SBP goal is still unclear.

The authors of one study concluded that their findings contradict the commonly held "lower is better" hypothesis,[235] and that their findings support the recommendation to treat persons without cardiovascular disease who have a systolic blood pressure above approximately 140 mm Hg, but treatment would not be of benefit and may be even harmful in persons with lower systolic blood pressure levels.[236]

Evidence about the lack of benefits of intensive lowering of BP among the elderly comes from a randomized, controlled study, ACCORD.[237] It found no significant difference in the primary outcome (nonfatal myocardial infarction, nonfatal stroke, or death from cardiovascular causes) between the intensive care (SBP less than 120 mm Hg) and the standard care (SBP less than 140 mm Hg) treatment groups. There was an increased risk of adverse events in the group targeting SBP to less than 120 mm Hg (including elevations in serum creatinine and electrolyte abnormalities). However, the intensive care group did have a 40% decreased stroke incidence, and there was a nonsignificant reduction in CVD events.[238]

Additional caution about aggressive blood pressure lowering comes from a study of nearly 400,000 Kaiser healthcare system patients with hypertension, 19% of whom had ischemic heart disease, and 30% of whom had diabetes.[239] The study compared blood pressures with the risk of mortality and end-stage renal disease (ESRD) and found that the optimal BP for the lowest risk in this population was a SBP of 137 mm Hg and a DBP of 71 mm Hg.

The Kaiser study authors concluded that both higher and lower treated BP compared with 130 to 139 mm Hg systolic and 60 to 79 mm Hg diastolic ranges had worse outcomes and that their study adds to the growing uncertainty about BP treatment targets. The Kaiser study showed a significant J-shaped association between actual treated BP levels and adverse outcomes, that is to say, increased mortality at very low blood pressure levels. Individuals with very low blood pressures might be sicker and hence have higher mortality.[240] An editorial commentary on the study noted that this study provides more support for relaxing BP treatment targets.

A commentary in the *JAMA* concerning blood pressure targets for people with diabetes and hypertension noted that a recent meta-analysis including 74 trials and more than 300,000 participants found no benefit to antihypertensive therapy in trials with mean baseline systolic BP less than 140/90 mm Hg but strong evidence supporting treatment of patients with diabetes and BP of 140/90 mm Hg or higher with a goal to lower BP to less than 140/90 mm Hg.[241 242]

A 2018 article assessing the new guidelines in the *New England Journal of Medicine* was in favor of some elements of the new ACC/AHA guidelines, including increased use of home monitoring of blood pressure and individualized risk assessment.[243] The authors are less sanguine about one-size-fits-all blood pressure goals. In particular, they note that many elderly have stiff non-compliant blood vessels that elevate peak blood pressure readings, and they may have dizziness and poor mentation if their SBP approaches 140 mm Hg. They concluded that while a blood-pressure treatment target of less than 130/80 mm Hg makes sense for high-risk patients, for everyone else, it seems more reasonable to continue defining hypertension as a blood pressure of 140/90 mm Hg or higher.

This target was supported by a 2019 study published in the *JAMA* that considered the cardiovascular outcomes of having systolic BP less than 130 mm Hg, diastolic BP 80 mm Hg or greater compared to having the older definition of high blood pressure systolic BP less than 140 mm Hg, diastolic BP 90 mm Hg or greater.[244] The study goal was to determine if lowering the diastolic threshold for hypertension from 90 mm Hg to 80 mm Hg (the new 2017 ACC/AHA definition of isolated diastolic hypertension, IDH) was associated with improved cardiovascular outcomes. The study found that there was no significant association between IDH as defined by the 2017 guideline and atherosclerotic cardiovascular disease, heart failure, or chronic kidney disease.

However, in addition to the SPRINT trial, there is support for the new guidelines that lower the goal for blood pressure to below 140/90. A very large study using data from 1.3 million adults in an outpatient population found that the risk of CVD events was highest for systolic hypertension, but both systolic and diastolic hypertension independently predicted adverse outcomes.[245] An increased risk was found above either 130/80 mm Hg or 140/90 mm Hg. The study also found evidence of a J-shaped curve. The study authors concluded that their work supports recent guidelines that lowered blood pressure targets for high-risk patients.

In most epidemiological studies of hypertension, medically untreated individuals have a linearly progressive increase in CVD and mortality with higher BP levels, without any evidence of a J-shaped curve, that is to say, lower, rather than increased mortality, at very low blood pressure levels. For example, a nine year prospective study in China of more than 500,000 adults age 30 to 79 found that each 10 mm Hg increase in systolic blood was associated with a 30% higher risk of ischemic heart disease and stroke and an even greater risk of hemorrhagic stroke. Down to a systolic blood pressure of 120 mm Hg, there was no evidence of a J-shaped curve.[246]

A 2020 study with an average of 14.5 years of follow-up among 1,457 participants without CVD published in *JAMA Cardiology* found that beginning with a systolic blood pressure level of 90 mm Hg, there was a stepwise increase in the prevalence of atherosclerotic cardiovascular disease risk factors, including coronary artery calcium, and the risk of atherosclerotic cardiovascular disease. For every 10-mm Hg increase in systolic blood pressure, there was a 53% higher risk for atherosclerotic cardiovascular disease. This study also found no evidence of a J-shaped curve.

These observations have strengthened the argument that the "lower the blood pressure, the better the outcomes."

What is the bottom line on hypertension?

A review of the history of hypertension studies titled "Lessons in Uncertainty and Humility–Clinical Trials Involving Hypertension" pointed out that there is considerable variation in interpretation of the results of various trials and in the level of confidence placed in their findings.[247] In spite of uncertainty about blood pressure level goals, I suggest the following:

First, a primary objective should be the prevention of hypertension by the adoption of a healthy lifestyle according to the Lifestyle Checklist. This includes a healthy diet with limitation of sodium, getting to and staying at a normal weight, maintaining a high level of physical activity, and avoiding substance abuse, including the use of tobacco. Some individuals may also benefit from measures to manage stress.

Second, probably any systolic blood pressure above 110 mm Hg or diastolic blood pressure above 70 mm Hg increases the risk of cardiovascular disease but by very little at 120/80 mm Hg, a level considered normal. Lower is usually healthier, and 110/70 or 120/80 are worthy goals—but for some, perhaps many people, not obtainable easily or at all. Furthermore, several studies suggest that there is little risk from a blood pressure of up to 140/90 mm Hg.

Finally, if you need antihypertensive drugs to bring your blood pressure to a normal range, do not hesitate to take them. Even if you are on effective antihypertensive drugs, optimizing lifestyle will bring many additional health benefits.

My Story

Without treatment, I have what is now defined as stage 1 high blood pressure with SBP 130-140 and DBP 85-90. With 10 mg a day of Lisinopril, an angiotensin-converting enzyme (ACE) inhibitor that is available as an inexpensive generic, my typical SBP is 115-120, and DBP is 65-70. I don't add any salt to food, but I don't go out of my way to avoid sodium in my diet. I consider my daily antihypertensive regimen to be a success.

What about baby aspirin to prevent stroke and other CVDs? Is this a good idea?

For many years low-dose aspirin was considered to be a way to provide at least a small degree of protection against heart attacks and ischemic strokes because aspirin decreases the propensity of blood to clot. And one-quarter of people age 40 or older (about 29 million Americans) are taking a daily aspirin.[248] But low-dose aspirin (81 mg) increases the risk of cerebral hemorrhage and gastrointestinal bleeding, and it has become uncertain if there is a net benefit from aspirin therapy for people at average or even moderately elevated CVD risk.

The U.S. Preventive Services Task Force (USPSTF) advises aspirin therapy for primary prevention of CVD for people in their fifties who are at high risk of CVD (10% or higher risk of a heart attack or stroke over the next 10 years, based on the calculator, tinyurl.com/riskCVD) and who are not at increased risk for bleeding.[249] The Task Force also said that aspirin can be considered for people in their sixties who are at high risk of CVD, but cautions that their risk of bleeding is greater and aspirin's net benefit smaller. Because of inadequate evidence, the USPSTF made no recommendation for people under age 50 or over 70.

A 2016 meta-analysis from 11 trials of aspirin for primary CVD prevention, found that aspirin reduced the relative risk of nonfatal myocardial infarction by 22% and death by 6%, but was associated with a 59% increase in gastrointestinal bleeding and a 33% increase in hemorrhagic stroke.[250][251]

A 2019 meta-analysis considered a total of 13 trials with 164,225 participants without CVD.[252] Aspirin use was associated with significant reductions in cardiovascular events (60.2 vs. 65.2 per 10,000 participant-years) but an increased risk of major bleeding events (23.1 vs. 16.4 per 10,000 participant-years).

Three recent clinical trials suggest that taking aspirin for primary prevention of CVD is not beneficial or, at best, marginally beneficial. In the first trial, ARRIVE (Aspirin to Reduce Risk of Initial Vascular Events), no prevention of CVDs was found over the five year study period. Both patients on daily low-dose aspirin and those taking a placebo had similarly low rates of CVD (about 4%). Rates of gastro-intestinal bleeding (mostly mild) were also low, at 0.5% in the group on placebos, but higher in the aspirin group at 1%.[253]

A second study, ASCEND (A Study of Cardiovascular Events in Diabetes), measured CVD in diabetics, a group at elevated risk. After seven years, the study found that the group taking aspirin had a slightly lower rate of CVD events, 8.5%, compared to 9.6% in the placebo group, but this was counterbalanced by a higher rate of major bleeding events (4.1% vs. 3.2%).[254]

The third, a five year ASPREE (ASPirin in Reducing Events in the Elderly) study, found that low dose aspirin conferred no significant improvement in rates of CVD events, disability, or dementia. The aspirin group had a higher rate of major bleeding, including hemorrhagic strokes (3.8% vs. 2.7% in the control group).[255] [256] [257] The study authors concluded that the use of low-dose aspirin as a primary prevention strategy in older adults resulted in a significantly higher risk of major hemorrhage and did not result in a significantly lower risk of cardiovascular disease than placebo.

According to a review in the *University of California, Berkeley Wellness Letter*, "...in more recent years, many experts stopped recommending aspirin therapy to prevent first heart attacks and strokes (primary prevention) in most people, though they continue to strongly advise it to prevent recurrences (secondary prevention) in people who already have CVD." In 2019, the American Heart Association and the American College of Cardiology recommended against the use of low-dose aspirin in people older than 70 who do not have existing CVD or in anyone who has an increased risk of bleeding.

Taken together, these studies suggest that if you are at low are moderate risk of CVD taking low dose aspirin would provide little benefit and, like all medications, it should only be taken if prescribed by a health professional. An editorial in the *New England Journal of Medicine* that commented on the three aspirin trials concluded that "... the best strategy for the use of aspirin in the primary prevention of cardiovascular disease may simply be to prescribe a statin instead."[258]

In the presence of increased risk of stroke because of atrial fibrillation, and when other CVD risk factors are present, including age over 75, previous stroke, heart valve, and other cardiac disorders, anti-clotting drugs may be prescribed. In addition to aspirin, there are other antiplatelet or anticoagulant drugs to reduce the likelihood of heart attack or stroke by inhibiting blood clot formation. These drugs include warfarin (Coumadin, Jantoven), clopidogrel (Plavix) and prasugrel (Effient) and a group of newer anticoagulants that are easier to monitor (Eliquis, Pradaxa, Savaysa, Xarelto).[259] They are only taken when prescribed and supervised by a health professional.

Beyond a healthy lifestyle, treatment options for high cholesterol to prevent cardiovascular disease

This chapter has described how lifestyle changes can manage blood pressure and prevent CVDs. Although nearly everyone with a typical American lifestyle develops some degree of atherosclerotic cardiovascular disease, the medical establishment does not vigorously promote lifestyle interventions as a first choice to prevent and treat CVDs. Undoubtedly all doctors are well intended, but they lack training in preventive medicine because medical schools focus on curing rather than preventing disease. In addition, many doctors have insufficient time to educate patients about the Building Blocks of Health because the pressures of medical practice today push them to spend less time with more patients. So typical medical care often turns to drugs and surgery as a first choice rather than a valuable adjunct to behavior change. The treatments described below are valuable measures to supplement a healthy lifestyle.

Lipid lowering drugs to prevent and treat cardiovascular disease

An optimally healthy diet and other lifestyle changes such as weight loss may be able to bring about a healthy pattern of blood cholesterol without use of drugs and their associated side effects and expense. But if diet and other lifestyle changes do not work as well as needed, or are too difficult to be adhered to, therapy with statins and other drugs are a good treatment choice for decreasing LDL-cholesterol and the risk of CVDs.

Statins have been shown to reduce the risk of stroke and heart attack by about one-quarter to one-third. They are now taken by more than one-quarter of Americans age 45 and older. On average, statins bring about a 25% to 55% reduction in LDL-C, a 5% to 10% increase in HDL-C, and a 10% to 20% decrease in triglycerides. The more prolonged statin treatment is, the larger is the reduction in CVD events. The downward trend in cardiovascular disease in the U.S. is attributed in considerable part to the greatly increased use of statins.[260 261]

Studies have considered the benefits of statin therapy among healthy men and women with no previous history of CVD. One such study found a 31% reduction in myocardial infarction and CHD-related death.[262] A meta-analysis of 27 randomized trials among people of low risk (a five year risk of major vascular events lower than

10%) found that typical statin therapy reduced the risk of major vascular events by about 20%.[263] A meta-analysis review of statin therapy use among patients with no history of CVD found a 12% reduction in deaths and a 25% reduction in CVD events.[264] A similar study found that treatment with a statin (lovastatin) reduced the incidence of first major coronary events by 37% and myocardial infarction by 40%.[265] The JUPITER trial among healthy men and women with a median LDL-C of 108 mg/dl and elevated C-reactive protein found that aggressive lowering of LDL- C reduced the risk of myocardial infarction, stroke, and revascularization.[266 267 268]

In addition to the lipid-lowering effects of statins, they appear to improve the functioning of arteries so they can carry more blood during exercise and reduce inflammation as indicated by lowering C-reactive protein levels. Statins are usually trouble-free, but at times they cause muscle aches, especially at the higher doses needed for some people. There is also a small increased risk of developing diabetes, liver damage, upset stomach, and reports of an increased risk of short-term memory loss and confusion. A rare but serious side effect is muscle inflammation and damage (rhabdomyolysis) that causes the release of a protein (myoglobin) from muscle cells that can seriously impair kidney function.[269]

Although some individuals report memory problems with certain statins, use of a different statin may resolve the problem, and new data on the possible link between statin use and memory is reassuring. It suggests that statins may even provide some benefits for cognitive functioning. A six-year study found that statin ever-users and never-users had no significant difference in the rate of decline in either memory or global cognition.[270] The study also found a protective interaction between statin ever-use and the rate of decline in long-delayed recall performance for patients carrying the APOE-4 genotype, the genotype with a high risk of Alzheimer disease. A meta-analysis of 16 studies found no link between statin use and impaired cognition. The study also found that in studies lasting three to 25 years, statins were associated with a 29% decreased risk of dementia.[271]

Statins are not a substitute for a healthy lifestyle. There is evidence that statin treatment and increased fitness are each independently associated with lower mortality. A study published in *Lancet* found that over a 10-year period, the risk of death was 18.5% in people taking statins versus 27.7% in those not taking statins.[272] The mortality of the fittest of those on statins was 70% lower than the least fit statin users. The importance of fitness was shown by the finding that the fittest of the study subjects who were not using statins had lower mortality than the least fit statin users. The combination of statin treatment and increased fitness resulted in substantially lower mortality risk than either alone, reinforcing the importance of physical activity for all individuals, including those with high cholesterol.

Cholesterol treatment guidelines

Medical experts have many views about the use of statins, so a decision to start a statin or other lipid-lowering drug that will likely be taken for a lifetime is not straightforward and deserves a considerable discussion with your health care provider. In 2013 the American College of Cardiology and the American Heart Association (ACC/AHA) published a *Guideline on the Treatment of Blood Cholesterol to Reduce Atherosclerotic Cardiovascular Risk in Adults.*[273 274 275] The guideline endorsed use of statins because, among lipid-lowering medications, statins had the strongest evidence of improved patient health.[276] One estimate is that the treatment of 10,000 patients for five years with statins would cause one case of serious muscle injury (rhabdomyolysis), five cases of muscle inflammation (myopathy), 75 new cases of diabetes, and seven hemorrhagic strokes while averting about 1,000 heart attacks and other serious cardiovascular events among those with preexisting CVD, and averting 500 CVD events among those with elevated risk but without preexisting disease.[277 278]

The 2013 AHA/ACC guidelines have an appropriate emphasis on lifestyle changes to prevent CVDs. However, the recommendation called for abandoning specific goals for a healthy level of LDL-C and basing the decision to use statins on a 10-year risk assessment of heart attack or stroke. This was a change that many medical experts (including me) do not agree with.

In summary, the 2013 ACC/AHA guidelines recommended statins for the following groups:

- People age 40 to 75 with a 7.5% or higher risk of heart attack or stroke within ten years based on an online arteriosclerotic cardiovascular disease (ASCVD) risk estimator at http://tools.acc.org/ASCVD-Risk-Estimator/, and, http://www.cvriskcalculator.com
- People with a history of cardiovascular disease
- People age 21 or older with very high LDL-C, i.e., a LDL-C level of 190 mg/dl or higher
- People ages 40 to 75 with type 1 or type 2 diabetes

The Mayo Clinic also offers an online decision guide at https://statindecisionaid.mayoclinic.org

One study estimated that according to the 2013 ACC/AHA guideline, statins should now be prescribed for 56 million Americans.[279] The AHA estimates that 33 million of these individuals would be without overt cardiovascular disease but are over the 10-year 7.5% risk threshold. Some experts postulate that perhaps all of the more than 73 million adults in the United States who have elevated LDL-C should be considered for statin therapy.[280] An article in *Lancet*, "Statins for all by the age of 50 years?," suggests that adoption of a 10% or more cardiovascular risk threshold would classify 83% of men older than 50 years and 56% of women older than 60 years in Britain as needing a statin based on a 2003 Health Survey for England.[281] Many medical experts were supportive of the 2013 guidelines and assert that the benefits of statins outweigh any conceivable serious adverse effects.[282] But immediately after their release, articles appeared in the medical literature questioning their appropriateness. The question that was most frequently asked was: Would the new guidelines lead to the unjustified treatment of millions of people?

Articles were published in the *JAMA* titled, "More than a Billion People Taking Statins?"[283] and "Healthy Men Should Not Take Statins."[284] Their main arguments were that the decrease in mortality would be small, the formula overestimates risk, that the adverse side effects of statin use are significant, and that individuals with the highest risk have the most to gain.[285 286 287] Commentators also expressed concern that both doctors and their patients will be lulled into thinking that taking statins is all that is necessary to avoid CVD when adopting a healthy lifestyle is the most important way to prevent CVD.

Although some experts said the new guidelines were problematic because they overestimate risk, other critics argued that they underestimate risk because some (especially young) people with only moderately elevated LDL levels and no other risk factors would have a low short-term (10-year) risk and not be recommended to take statins even though they would be at a high lifetime risk of CVD.[288] Some experts advocated a return to target-based lipid guidelines.[289 290] *The University of California, Berkeley, Wellness Letter* noted, "We are hesitant to endorse the new guidelines. It is not clear that this approach—especially its emphasis on the risk calculator—will actually be more effective than the previous target-based guidelines."[291]

In 2016 the U.S. Preventive Services Task Force (USPSTF) released new statin guidelines for the primary prevention of cardiovascular disease (CVD) in adults.[292 293] Primary prevention refers to measures taken to prevent CVD among individuals without overt evidence of CVD. The recommendations are:

- Initiate use of low- to moderate-dose statins in adults aged 40 to 75 years without a history of CVD who have one or more CVD risk factors abnormal blood lipids, diabetes, hypertension, or smoking and a calculated 10-year CVD event risk of 10% or greater.
- Selectively offer low- to moderate-dose statins to adults aged 40 to 75 years without a history of CVD who have one or more CVD risk factors and a

calculated 10-year CVD event risk of 7.5% to 10%.
- Current evidence is insufficient to assess the balance of benefits and harms of initiating statin use in adults 76 years and older.

In a 2016 editorial in the *JAMA*, Greenland pointed out that including the USPSTF statement, five different guidelines for statin use have been published since 2013.[294] He notes that there is a lack of agreement on specific LDL-C targets of therapy and on specific treatment initiation thresholds, with the 2013 ACC/AHA guideline recommending the lowest threshold. All five of the guidelines uniformly advise that clinical judgment, along with thoughtful patient-clinician discussion, is indicated, regardless of the level of patient risk. All guidelines also emphasize the importance of lifestyle interventions to reduce risk in all patients, regardless of lipid-lowering drug use.

Greenland has what he calls several important take-home messages:[295]

- Ensure statin use by higher-risk patients. Every patient at age 40 years or older should be considered for possible statin therapy.
- Additional testing can inform the patient-physician discussion.
- Based on data from younger patients, it is reasonable to treat otherwise healthy individuals older than 75 years.
- Last, and perhaps most important, clinical judgment and patient input are critical components of the decision process, especially for older patients and those at a lower risk.

In an additional editorial comment on the USPSTF guidelines, Gurwitz and colleagues note that although compelling evidence exists supporting statins for secondary prevention in individuals younger than 75 years with clinical arteriosclerotic CVD, there is less evidence of their utility for primary prevention in older age groups.[296] In one study, a subgroup analysis of men and women aged 70 to 82 years, found that statin therapy had no statistically significant effect on the primary composite outcome (coronary death, nonfatal myocardial infarction, and fatal or nonfatal stroke).[297] In contrast, a meta-analysis of 28 clinical trials that included 14,000 people over age 75 found that statins reduced major CVD events similarly for all age groups—by about 20%.[298] But with increasing age, there was a trend towards smaller relative risk reductions in vascular event and mortality outcomes.

A 2020 study published in the *JAMA* found that initiating statin use among nearly 327,000 veterans at an average age of 81 was associated with 25% fewer deaths from all causes and 20% fewer CVD deaths.[299] All study subjects were free from CVDs at the start of the nearly 7-year study, 97% were men and 91% were white, so the relevance of the study to women, more diverse populations and those with preexisting CVDs is less certain than it is for white men. An editorial that accompanied the study concluded that although additional studies are needed, "These findings provide a compelling argument for the use of statins for primary prevention in older patients."[300]

In an editorial comment in *JAMA* on the new USPSTF guidelines, Redberg and Katz expressed reservations about use of statin therapy for primary prevention of CVD by older adults.[301] They pointed out that even though some studies have estimated that close to 20% of statin users have muscle problems, many of the trials did not ask about commonly reported statin effects, such as muscle pains and weakness, and only recorded myopathy—a rare side effect.[302] Redberg and Katz note that persons at low risk who have little chance of benefit have an equal chance of harms, and unfortunately, the evidence base for harms of statins is incomplete. Harms may include more obesity and more sedentary behavior because people on statins may mistakenly think they do not need to eat a healthy diet and exercise as they can just take a pill to give them the same benefit.[303] Their summary comment is, "Given the serious concerns about the harms of the reliance on statins for primary prevention, it is in the interest of public health and the medical community to refocus efforts on promoting a heart-healthy diet, regular physical activity, and not smoking."[304]

Risk assessment or targets for HDL-cholesterol?

A commentary from Navar and Peterson in the *JAMA* advocates use of statins but also expresses concern about sole reliance on a risk assessment formula to decide about use of statins for primary prevention.[305] They point out problems with the USPSTF recommendation guidelines with the example of a theoretical Mr. Young a 41-year-old man with hypertension and an unhealthy blood lipid profile: a total cholesterol level of 245 mg/dL; a LDL-C of 155 mg/dL; and a HDL-C of 50 mg/dL. According to the risk assessment formula, his estimated 10-year cardiovascular disease (CVD) risk is 2%, with an estimated lifetime CVD risk of 50%. Mr. Young has a high cholesterol and hypertension but is only at a relatively low risk in the short term from cardiac events because of his young age. Another example, Mr. Smith is a 63-year-old man with a lifetime risk factor profile similar to that of Mr. Young, except that his cholesterol levels indicate low risk, his total cholesterol is 160 mg/dL; LDL-C, 80 mg/dL; and HDL-C, 50 mg/dL. His estimated 10-year CVD risk is 10%, and his estimated lifetime CVD risk is 50%.[306]

Based on these patients' respective 10-year CVD risk estimates, the USPSTF recommendation statement would not suggest statin treatment for Mr. Young despite his elevated LDL-C level but would recommend therapy for Mr. Smith despite his "normal" or healthy LDL-C level. There is compelling evidence that early treatment can delay the onset of CVD later in life among adults with elevated cholesterol levels.[307] So waiting to treat Mr. Young until he is old enough to reach a 7.5% or higher 10-year CVD risk would be likely to expose him to many years of unhealthy elevated cholesterol levels. And it is entirely plausible that prolonged reductions in LDL-C with statin use would reduce the long-term risk of CVD. Navar and Peterson also note that in almost every trial to date, statins have been found efficacious in reducing CVD risk, so it is reasonable to consider offering statin therapy to younger populations. They suggest that clinicians "... practice the art of medicine and engage with patients in shared decision making regarding strategies for CVD prevention."[308 309]

One consideration about low targets for LDL-C and triglycerides is some evidence that low LDL-C levels are associated with an increased risk of hemorrhagic stroke. In a study among women, those with LDL-C lower than 70 mg/dl and in the lowest quarter of triglyceride levels were at twice the risk of hemorrhagic stroke compared to women with LDL-C of 100 to 129.9 mg/dl.[310] This finding must be balanced against the evidence that among patients with a prior ischemic stroke or transient ischemic attacks, use of high dose statins to lower HDL-C to a target of 70 mg/dl had a lower risk of a subsequent ischemic stroke and no statistically significant increased risk of hemorrhagic stroke.[311]

Commentators on the study that found that low HDL-C increased hemorrhagic stroke pointed out that it is important to consider the clinical relevance of the study.[312 313] Although the absolute hemorrhagic stroke risk per year in the highest risk group category was 0.04% per year (on average 0.02% per year higher), the reduction in risk of other CVDs from statin use may be greater. The Cholesterol Treatment Trialists' Collaboration showed that every 10 mg/dL lowering of LDL-C reduces the annual CVD-risk by 1.03%.[314] As always, keep in mind that twice the risk of a rare event, such as a hemorrhagic stroke compared to an ischemic stroke and other CVDs, is still a rare event.

New 2018 guidelines

In 2018, the American College of Cardiology, the American Heart Association (ACC/AHA) and ten additional professional organizations concerned with cardiovascular health released *2018 Cholesterol Clinical Practice Guidelines*.[315 316] The new guidelines for managing cholesterol are more complicated. They keep some features of the 2013 risk assessment framework, including a stress on lifestyle measures relating to diet, weight, blood pressure, and physical activity. The new guidelines continue reliance on the calculation of 10-year CVD risk for therapy recommendations, but for some patients with high CVD risk, they recommend a LDL-C target of 70 mg/dl or lower. They further personalize risk assessment and decisions about treatment, and they also emphasize that the lower a person's LDL-C the better for CVD health and include the option of adding non-statin drugs for people at high risk.

The following summary of the guidelines describes interventions based on the health status of individual patients—but don't rely on this summary for decisions relating to CVD prevention or therapy, your health care provider should be consulted. The 2018 guidelines are available at, https://professional.heart.org/statements.

The guidelines consider three groups to be at high CVD risk and therefore are candidates for statins and possibly additional cholesterol-lowering drugs:

- People with a history of CVD, such as a heart attack, angina, or stroke
- People ages 40 to 75 who have diabetes (which greatly increases CVD risk)
- People with very high LDL-C (above 190 mg/dl), often from familial hypercholesterolemia

For others, between the ages of 40 and 75, the guidelines recommend using a risk calculator, such as the ASCVD Risk Estimator Plus, (online at https://tools.acc.org/ASCVD-Risk-Estimator-Plus/#!/calculate/estimate/), or the 2013 American Heart Association/American College of Cardiology (AHA/ACC) risk calculator (online at cvriskcalculator.com/) to estimate 10-year risk of a major CVD event. The following treatment recommendations differ for various categories of risk.

Low risk

A person with a 10-year risk below 5% is considered to be at low risk and usually not a candidate for a statin. However, as already noted, avoiding many years of risk factors such as high cholesterol and high blood pressure suggests starting statin treatment for someone who is at low risk mainly because of their young age.

High risk (10-year risk above 20%)

Take a high-dose statin to reduce LDL by at least 50%.

Intermediate risk (10-year risk 7.5% to 20%) and borderline risk (10-year risk 5% to 7.5%)

Consider well known major risk factors such as smoking, hypertension, obesity, and inactivity; in addition, evaluate of other "risk-enhancing factors," including:

- Family history of premature CVD; for males, that means a heart attack or stroke before age 55; for females, before age 65
- Persistently elevated LDL-C (160 to 190 mg/dl)
- Persistently elevated triglycerides (175 mg/dl or above)
- Metabolic syndrome, characterized by three or more of the following: abdominal obesity, high blood pressure, high blood sugar, high triglycerides,

and low HDL-C

- Chronic kidney disease
- High-risk ethnicity (such as South Asian)
- Chronic inflammatory disorders (such as rheumatoid arthritis or psoriasis) or HIV/AIDS
- History of early menopause (before age 40) or pregnancy-related conditions that increase CVD risk, such as preeclampsia

Start treatment on the basis of this evaluation and after a discussion about the pros and cons of statins with a health care provider. Make a shared decision. If treatment is decided on, the goal is to reduce LDL cholesterol by at least 30% with a moderate-intensity statin. A coronary artery calcium (CAC) scan may help make the decision about treatment.

The treatment guidelines focus primarily on people ages 40 to 75 because almost all of the major clinical trials have involved that age group. They do advise people under 40 or over 75 with CVD, diabetes, or very high LDL-C to take statins. For others in these age groups, the benefits and risks of statin therapy should be considered on an individual basis.

The guidelines call for assessing adherence and percentage response to LDL-C lowering medications and lifestyle changes with repeat lipid measurement four to 12 weeks after statin initiation or dose adjustment, repeated at three to 12 months as needed.

Who should be taking a statin?

Making sense of all of the guidelines is not easy. All of the guidelines stress the importance of shared decision-making with a health care provider before embarking on long-term use of a statin drug. Since studies of the epidemiology of cardiovascular disease indicate that having a total cholesterol below 150 mg/dl and an LDL-C below 100 mg/dl, or better yet an LDL-C below 70 mg/dl is highly protective against most CVDs, attaining these targets is an effective way to reduce CVD risk. And if they can be reached through lifestyle modification, without statins or other drugs and their attendant risk of side effects, these targets are a worthy goal. The most important action to prevent CVD should always be to adopt a healthy lifestyle with normal weight and blood pressure, a healthy diet and plentiful physical activity. As a Viewpoint in the *JAMA* noted, "… the ACC/AHA[317] risk calculation leads to treatment as men become older even if they have no risk factors other than their unmodifiable age and sex. To many, it sounds absurd that there is no such thing as healthy aging and that everyone eventually will need some medication."[318]

But if a healthy lifestyle does not suffice to reach a LDL-C below 100 mg/dl, the available evidence demonstrates benefit from statin use, including for those who do not have markedly high blood cholesterol.[319 320] A recent a meta-regression analysis in *JAMA* suggests that the lower the LDL-C, regardless of the therapy used to lower it, the lower the relative risk of major vascular events.[321] If statins are needed to obtain the optimal blood lipid pattern associated with the lowest risk of CVD, the preponderance of evidence indicates that they should be used, even in those without overt CVD. Statins cause few adverse effects, lower rates of CVD by about 30%, and lower all-cause mortality by 10% to 15%.[322 323 324 325]

In spite of uncertainties about their use in individuals younger than 40 and older than 75, I recommend basing the decision to use statins mainly on the presence of risk factors, i.e., the presence of hypertension, obesity, physical inactivity, and especially on blood lipid levels. The risk calculator is certainly one factor to consider, but I favor aiming for the blood lipid level targets that are known to be associated with decreased CVD risk, i.e., an LDL-C of 70 mg/dl or lower, rather than on the10-year CVD risk formula. The *University of California, Berkeley Wellness Letter*, is also on record supporting blood lipid level targets rather than the projected 10-year risk of CVD events.[326] (Full disclosure: I serve on the editorial board of the *University of California, Berkeley Wellness Letter*.)

When to take non-statin drugs to lower LDL-C

In addition to statins, there are several other medications that reduce cholesterol and can be used either alone or in combination with statins. As with statin therapy, any decision about a non-statin drug calls for a discussion between patient and doctor to assess individual risk factors, the benefits and risks of treatment, patient preferences, and cost if a PCSK9 (proprotein convertase subtilisin–kexin type 9) inhibitor is being considered.

The 2018 ACC/AHA guidelines do not recommend routine use of non-statin drugs for people at borderline or intermediate cardiovascular risk since any additional benefit is likely to be marginal. If further lowering of LDL-C is warranted for them, increasing statin dosage is the preferred option.

The 2018 ACC/AHA guidelines advise that those with CVD or are at very high risk, to use additional non-statin LDL-C lowering medication. Some individuals at high CVD risk can't tolerate high-dose statins, and for others, high-dose statins don't lower LDL the recommended 50%. If their LDL cholesterol remains ≥70 mg/dl, the guidelines advise consideration of the addition of ezetimibe to statin therapy. Ezetimibe (Zetia), is one of a class of lipid-lowering compounds that selectively inhibits the intestinal absorption of cholesterol.[327] It can lower LDL-C an additional

20%.[328] Like statins, ezetimibe is now available as an inexpensive generic.

Vytorin contains a combination of ezetimibe and simvastatin (a statin). The Improved Reduction of Outcomes: Vytorin Efficacy International Trial (IMPROVE-IT) reported that adding ezetimibe to effective statin therapy in stable patients who experienced an acute coronary syndrome reduced LDL-C from 70 mg/dl to 54 mg/dl and reduced risk of atherosclerotic cardiovascular disease outcome at seven years from 34.7% to 32.7%.[329 330]

Another approach to inhibiting the intestinal absorption of cholesterol is through the use of bile acid sequestrants. They are absorptive resins usually taken as a powder or pill in combination with a statin or niacin. Typically, they lower LDL-C by 10% to 20%.[331]

If the addition of ezetimibe to a statin doesn't reduce LDL enough, and LDL-C remains ≥70 mg/dl, the ACC/AHA guidelines suggest that a PCSK9 inhibitor would be a "reasonable" adjunct. In 2003 it was discovered that gain-of-function mutations in the gene encoding PCSK9 caused familial hypercholesterolemia. The subsequent discovery that loss-of-function mutations in PCSK9 cause lower LDL-C led to the development of monoclonal antibodies that inhibit PCSK9 action and lower LDL-C and HDL-C. Two of the monoclonal antibodies in this relatively new treatment category, evolocumab (Repatha) and alirocumab (Praluent), have been extensively tested. In 2015, the FDA approved their use by patients as an adjunct to diet and maximally tolerated statin therapy for the treatment of adults with familial hypercholesterolemia or clinical atherosclerotic cardiovascular disease, who require additional lowering of LDL-C.[332]

A trial of evolocumab, injected subcutaneously every two weeks or monthly as an adjunct to standard lipid-lowering therapy, caused an additional 61% reduction in LDL-C levels.[333] A similar trial of alirocumab also lowered LDL-C by 61%.[334] A more recent trial among high-risk patients who were followed for an average of 2.2 years found an average decline in LDL-C of 59%, a decline in HDL-C of 51% and a decline in triglycerides of 16%. The main study endpoints, cardiovascular death, myocardial infarction, stroke, hospitalization for unstable angina, or coronary revascularization, occurred in 9.8% of evolocumab-treated patients as compared with 11.3% of patients who received a placebo; this corresponded to a 15% risk reduction.[335]

PCSK9 inhibition confers additional cardiovascular benefit beyond that achieved by usual lipid-lowering treatments, but the gain among the high-risk patients in the clinical trials is modest, and the cost is steep. Initially provided at about $14,000 per year, to treat 20 million Americans would add up to $280 billion a year and,

"...the cost of this single drug would match the entire cost for all other prescription pharmaceuticals for all diseases in the United States combined."[336] Recent price cuts of about 50% to these drugs may help them to have a role in treating some patients who do not respond well to other therapies, including those with statin intolerance.[337] Even with 2018 reductions in price, these are expensive drugs, and PCSK9 inhibitors have been approved only for people who have CVD or very high LDL-C.

In February 2020, the FDA approved a new drug, Nexletol (bempedoic acid), an oral, once-daily, non-statin for LDL-C lowering.[338] Nexletol is indicated as an adjunct to diet and maximally tolerated statin therapy for the treatment of adults with familial hypercholesterolemia or established atherosclerotic cardiovascular disease (ASCVD) who require additional lowering of LDL-C. In studies, Nexletol provided an average of 18% LDL-C lowering when used with moderate or high-intensity statins. The effect of Nexletol on the biomarkers of cardiovascular disease suggests benefits, but this has not yet been demonstrated by clinical trials.

Drugs for treating high triglycerides

On average, statins bring about a 25% to 55% reduction in LDL-C, a 5% to 10% increase in HDL-C, and a 10% to 20% decrease in triglycerides.[339] If triglycerides remain high (150 mg/dl or higher) even after using statins and adherence to the factors on the Lifestyle Checklist, (e.g. controlling diabetes and weight, a plant-based diet, exercise, eliminating alcohol), a variety of drugs can be considered. Two types of non-statin drugs target high triglycerides: fibrates and omega-3-acid ethyl esters.

Fibrates, either fenofibrate (various brands) or gemfibrozil (Lopid), are recommended for very high levels of triglyceride levels, 500 mg/dl or higher. They reduce triglyceride levels by 20% to 50% but also raise LDL-C by about 10%. A statin can be added to fibrates to counteract any increases in LDL-C.[340]

The omega-3 fatty acids found in fatty fish and fish oil interfere with the conversion of dietary fats into triglycerides. Three forms of omega-3-acid ethyl esters have been FDA approved for the treatment of high triglycerides that are at a level of 500 mg/dl or higher. Lovaza contains eicosapentaenoic acid (EPA) and docosahexaenoic acid (DHA). Epanova contains another form of omega-3 fatty acids. Vascepa contains only a purified form of EPA (icosapent ethyl).

The REDUCE-IT (Reduction of Cardiovascular Events with Icosapent Ethyl–Intervention Trial), studied patients on statins with high CVD risk, LDL-C levels controlled with statin therapy, but who had elevated triglyceride levels (135 to 500 mg/dl). It found that over five years, the risk of major adverse cardiovascular events was lower by 25% among patients who received 4 gm of Vascepa daily than among those who received a placebo.[341] Vascepa is the first FDA approved drug to both reduce triglycerides and reduce cardiovascular risk among patients with elevated triglyceride levels. It is approved as an add-on to maximally tolerated statin therapy. Patients must also have either established cardiovascular disease or diabetes and two or more additional risk factors for cardiovascular disease.

In clinical trials, Vascepa was associated with an increased risk of atrial fibrillation or atrial flutter (irregular heart rhythms) requiring hospitalization. Vascepa was also associated with an increased risk of bleeding events among patients who were also taking other medications that increase the risk of bleeding, such as aspirin, clopidogrel, or warfarin. Patients with allergies to fish or shellfish should be advised about the potential for allergic reactions. According to a review article in the *New England Journal of Medicine*, icosapent ethyl is a proprietary and highly purified form of EPA, and the findings from REDUCE-IT should not be generalized to assume that there will be benefits from dietary supplementation with fish oil.[342]

Surgery to prevent and treat cardiovascular disease

Although this book is focused on what individuals can do for themselves to prevent, and sometimes to treat various diseases, a mention of some other therapies that may be prescribed by your health care provider for CVDs may be helpful.

When a patient has greatly obstructed coronary arteries, a revascularization procedure may be undertaken with the goal of relieving angina or preventing a heart attack. The main surgical approaches are angioplasty and bypass surgery. Angioplasty (percutaneous coronary angioplasty or intervention—PCI) is carried out under local anesthesia. A cardiologist threads a balloon into the narrowed area of one or more coronary arteries and then inflates the balloon to compress plaques and widen the partially blocked area. It is usually carried out with the insertion of a permanent stent to keep the expanded portion of the artery open. In a small proportion of patients, less than one percent, the artery being operated on will block because of a blood clot, spasm, or tear. This can cause a heart attack or require emergency bypass surgery.

Even when angioplasties are successful in opening up an artery, narrowing or closure (restenosis) occurs after about six months in about 10% of patients with a drug-releasing stent, 15% of those with a bare-metal stent, and 30% of patients who do not have a stent inserted. Although angioplasty will often temporarily relieve the symptoms of angina, it is no more effective than intensive medical treatment in the prevention of heart attacks or extension of life expectancy.[343 344] Angioplasty is performed more than one million times a year in the U.S., and a number of studies suggest that it is overused. Leading medical societies, including the American

Heart Association and the American College of Physicians, recommend a combination of lifestyle and drug therapy as the best treatment and the best way to prevent heart attacks among those with stable coronary heart disease.

A surgical revascularization procedure, angioplasty or coronary artery bypass grafting (CABG) may be appropriate to prevent a heart attack when atherosclerosis has narrowed multiple coronary vessels or causes unstable angina—also called acute coronary syndrome.

A person may be developing unstable angina if they experience chest discomfort or pain that:

- Feels different, is more severe, comes more often, or occurs with less activity or while they are at rest.
- Lasts longer than 15 - 20 minutes.
- Occurs without cause (for example, while asleep or sitting quietly).
- Is not relieved by rest or respond well to the medicine nitroglycerin.
- Occurs with a drop in blood pressure or shortness of breath.

Unstable angina is a medical emergency that should be treated immediately because it is a warning sign of an impending heart attack. The use of angioplasty may prevent a heart attack. If an arteriogram reveals plaque that is so severe that angioplasty cannot be carried out or if there are blockages in all three major coronary arteries or the left main coronary artery, a coronary artery bypass graft (CABG) may be recommended. This is a major procedure that requires opening the chest and may also require placing the patient on a heart-lung machine that oxygenates and pumps blood while the operation is underway. The surgeon takes arteries or veins from other parts of your body and uses them to bypass coronary artery blockages or provide a source of arterial blood flow from an artery in the chest. If necessary, a patient may undergo one, two, three, or more bypass grafts.

More than 400,000 bypass surgeries are carried out each year at the cost of $100 billion. Only in a portion of patients receiving the procedure, high-risk patients with the most severe coronary disease, does CABG surgery reduce the risk of a heart attack and prolong life. CABG surgery carries important risks, and recovery takes six to 12 weeks. Major complications such as a heart attack or stroke occur in 2% to 10% of patients, and there is a 1% to 2% chance of death from the procedure. CABG surgery does reduce the incidence and severity of angina, but lifestyle changes often work just a well at a fraction of the cost and essentially no risk.

A final thought about health advice

Often, such advice does not call for enough lifestyle change. We are not asked to do enough. Modest lifestyle changes will bring about modest gains in health. A healthy lifestyle is not all or nothing, but the more items on the Lifestyle Checklist you can say yes to, the healthier you will become and remain.

Summary of the Essential Facts

Almost everyone with the typical American lifestyle develops some degree of atherosclerotic cardiovascular disease over time. But a healthy lifestyle can postpone cardiovascular illnesses and death by decades. It is important to develop healthy lifestyle habits in childhood and avoid a lifetime of eating an unhealthy diet with large amounts of added sugar, trans and saturated fat, and highly processed foods, control blood pressure, maintain a high level of physical activity, and avoid overweight and obesity.

CVD is largely preventable by putting into place the Building Blocks of Health by following the Lifestyle Checklist that addresses diet and lifestyle factors that account for over 90% of the risk of a heart attack:

- Smoking and vaping: Don't start or quit if you are a smoker.
- Blood cholesterol: Know your LDL-C and control LDL-C through optimal nutrition and use of statins and other drugs if needed. Aim for 70 mg/dl or lower.
- Hypertension: Know your blood pressure, avoid hypertension by limiting dietary sodium to 2,300 mg/day, and use of antihypertensive medicines if needed—lower is better. Aim for 120/80 mm Hg or at least below 140/90 mm Hg.
- Diabetes: Limit dietary sugar and avoid overweight and obesity.
- Overweight and obesity: Maintain a normal weight.
- Diet: Eat a whole food plant-based Mediterranean or ultra-low fat Ornish style diet.
- Physical activity: Meet the recommended 150 minutes a week of moderate intensity physical activity; in general, the more, the better.
- Alcohol consumption: Avoid entirely or at least have no more than one drink a day for both women and men.
- Psychosocial factors: Manage stress.

7
Preventing Cancer

Cancer is a complex disease, with more than 100 kinds of cancer affecting different parts of the body in many different ways. Many factors can influence the risk of getting cancer; the goal of this chapter is to help you to avoid cancer by adopting a healthy lifestyle and having appropriate screening tests.

My Story

Cancer is such a pervasive disease that it is a rare person who has not been touched by it. My first recollection about its reach was hearing that my glamorous and kindly aunt had ovarian cancer. Aunt Mim, who had no children of her own, appeared like a benevolent Santa every Christmas with toys for my brother, sister, and me. But suddenly, in her 40s, she was dying, and soon, I'm sure we were told, gone to heaven.

In college, a freshman-year roommate died suddenly from acute leukemia. And cancer changed my outlook on living when I was in medical school after being on the wards of Children's Hospital in Boston. As a prestigious teaching hospital, Children's was the destination for many children with cancer from New England and more distant places. Unfortunately, Children's Hospital was to be the final destination for many babies and delightful children. After that experience, I decided that no matter how long a life I was privileged to lead, I was one of the lucky ones; at least I got to grow up.

More recently, one of my most cherished colleagues and a sister-in-law have died young from breast cancer, and my mother-in-law has died from pancreatic cancer. Modern science has taught us how to prevent, treat, and cure many scourges, but with cancer, we still have very far to go.

What is cancer?

Cancer occurs when some of the cells in the body become abnormal and grow out-of-control. This happens when the DNA that regulates cellular growth undergoes changes called mutations that sometimes turn out to be harmful. DNA (deoxyribonucleic acid) is the genetic "blueprint" found in each cell of the body. Genes are the sub-units of DNA where mutations occur. Genes regulate the synthesis of the protein building blocks of the body that are needed for its growth, structure, and function. Genes determine inherited traits, such as hair and eye color. The genes that are inherited can already have flaws, or genes can undergo mutations that can increase susceptibility to or cause cancer and some other diseases.[1]

In a normal cell, when DNA is damaged, the cell may repair the damage, or the cell may die. When a cell becomes cancerous, the damaged (mutated) DNA is not repaired, the cell doesn't die at an appropriate time as it normally would, and the cell goes on making new abnormal and unneeded cells, all with the same damaged DNA. Usually, several mutations are needed before a cell becomes cancerous. Mutations alone are not enough to produce a cancer. The damaged cell must be stimulated by "tumor promoters." For example, estrogen is a promoter that stimulates the growth of breast cells.[2]

Unlike normal cells, cancerous cells keep growing and can invade normal tissues. When cancer cells spread and grow in places beyond the tissue where they originated, the new growths are called metastases. Many types of cancer form tumors, others, like leukemia, involve bone marrow and other blood-forming organs, and when the cancer cells circulate through the bloodstream, they too can grow in other tissues.

Untreated, cancer can grow slowly or rapidly, and, unfortunately, even when treated, cancer often causes serious illness and death by invading vital organs and interfering with bodily functions that are necessary for life. Benign tumors are growths that are not cancerous, but they can cause problems or even death if they grow large enough to impinge on and impair the function of healthy organs and tissues. Benign tumors do not grow into other tissues or metastasize, so they are much less likely to be life-threatening.

Causes of cancer and cancer prevention

The damage to DNA that leads to cancer can occur from a variety of external environmental causes, including ionizing radiation, exposure to carcinogenic (cancer-causing) chemicals, and infection with certain viruses and bacteria. Unhealthy conditions and behaviors, including smoking, alcohol consumption, obesity, an unhealthy diet, and physical inactivity, also increase the risk of cancer. Inheritance of certain genes also increases the risk of cancer.

Cancer causes you can control

The American Cancer Society (ACS) estimates that among Americans, as many as two-thirds of cancers result from things that we can control, with smoking linked to about one-third of all cancer deaths in the U.S. and another third of cancers linked to weight, diet, and lack of physical activity.[3]

Some studies suggest a smaller proportion of cancers can be prevented by lifestyle choices. An article in *JAMA Oncology* in 2016 estimated the proportion of cases of cancer and deaths from cancer that could be prevented by a healthy lifestyle based on data from the Nurses' Health Study and the Health Professionals Follow-up Study.[4] Study subjects were considered to be in a low-risk group if they: 1) were never or past smokers of less than a pack a day for five years; 2) did not drink alcohol or drank moderately (no more than one drink/day for women, two drinks/day for men); 3) had a BMI of at least 18.5 but lower than 27.5; and, 4) were physically active at least 75 vigorous-intensity or 150 moderate-intensity minutes a week. All others were in a high-risk group.

In the low-risk group, the incidence of cancer was 25% lower for women and 33% lower for men; and mortality was 48% lower for women and 44% lower for men than for those in the high-risk group. The study authors concluded that by quitting smoking, approximately 80% to 90% of lung cancer deaths could be avoided, and from 10% to 70% of deaths from other specific cancers could be prevented by a healthy lifestyle. They found that, among the health professionals studied, 20% to 40% of cancer cases, and about half of cancer deaths could be prevented through lifestyle modification.

A similar study published in the *British Journal of Cancer* concluded that 40% of cancers in the U.K. were related to life choices with about half of the preventable cancers linked to smoking, a quarter of the preventable cases linked to unhealthy diets, and the remaining preventable cases linked to obesity and alcohol.[5] A 2017 commentary in the *New England Journal of Medicine* provided the estimates of the potential for reduction in rates of specific cancers shown in Table 7.1[6] below.

An international study estimated the proportion of cancers worldwide that could be attributed to modifiable risk factors.[7] Of the seven million deaths from cancer worldwide in 2001, an estimated 2.43 million, or 35%, were attributable to nine potentially modifiable risk factors: obesity and overweight, low fruit and vegetable intake, physical inactivity, smoking, alcohol use, unsafe sex, and air pollution. In

Table 7.1. Potential Reductions in Cancer Mortality[8]

Disease	Intervention	Percent Reduction in Mortality
Lung cancer	Smoking cessation at age 50	62%
Cervical cancer	Screening and HPV vaccination	95% & 100%
Liver disease and cancer	Hepatitis B vaccination	90%
Breast and ovarian cancer	If BRCA1 & 2 positive, salpingo-oophorectomy[9]	53%
Breast cancer	If high risk, estrogen receptor modulators	50%
Hepatitis C	Treatment	50% (all-cause)
Endometrial cancer	Avoid obesity[10 11]	40%

high-income countries, such as the U.S., smoking, alcohol use, and overweight and obesity were the most important factors linked to cancer, and these lifestyle factors are likely to be the predominant preventable causes of cancer risk for an individual. With a healthy lifestyle, the risk of getting a cancer will be much lower, but chance mutations that accumulate with age and cellular replication are likely to be the greatest proportion of the overall cancer risk.[12]

Cancer causes you cannot control

The role of cellular mutations was considered in a 2015 study from Johns Hopkins University. It suggested that the most frequent cause of cancer is not susceptible to prevention because most cancers occur when DNA is damaged after random errors or mutations in the replication of DNA that occur when normal cells repeatedly reproduce as a person ages. The study found that those tissue types that undergo the most numerous divisions of cells give rise to human cancers millions of times more often than other tissue types. According to the study, the lifetime risk of cancers of many different types is strongly correlated with the total number of divisions of the normal self-renewing cells that maintain the health of that particular tissue. And only a third of the variation in cancer risk among tissues is attributable to environmental factors or inherited predispositions. The majority of cancers are due to "bad luck," that is, random mutations arising during DNA replication in normal, noncancerous stem cells.[13] Following this publication, a number of scientists have suggested that the Hopkins study greatly underestimated the role of external risk factors in the causation of cancer.[14 15 16 17]

In addition to random mutations, other factors that affect cancer risk that an individual cannot control are age, gender, and genetic makeup. It is estimated that 5% to 10% of all cancers are related to specific inherited genes that increase susceptibility to cancer. In the U.S., one out of eight women (12%) will develop breast cancer, but women who have inherited one of the BRCA1 and BRCA2 genetic mutations are about five times more likely to develop breast cancer—approximately 70% by age 80. Overall, about 5% to 10% of breast cancer cases are thought to be due to an inherited genetic mutation. Usually, inherited mutations that increase susceptibility to cancer have incomplete penetrance; this means that not everyone with the mutation will get cancer.

It may not always be possible to modify or avoid some external environmental factors that increase the risk of cancer, such as air pollution and workplace exposure to carcinogens. Bartenders and wait staff may be exposed to secondhand smoke; workers in chemical plants may be exposed, and workers in the funeral industry and hair and nail salons may be exposed to formaldehyde and other chemicals. Although environmental exposures may be important for people living in some places and working in some occupations, in general, these risk factors are considered to be responsible for a much smaller portion of cancers than other risk factors that individuals can control. The ACS estimates that only 6% of all cancer deaths are the result of exposure to environmental hazards. Other cancer experts have concluded that this number is underestimated because of widespread occupational and community exposures to the vast number of untested chemicals Americans now encounter.[18] For more information on environmental hazards, see Chapter 14, "Environmental Pollutants and Toxins."

Studies of risk perception confirm that we tend to worry more about risks over which we feel we have little control, such as air and water pollution, even if they do not pose nearly as much of a cancer risk as some other things over which we do have considerable control, like obesity and consumption of alcohol.[19] Unfortunately, we cannot eliminate all risk of developing cancer, but we can lessen our risk by getting certain vaccinations, avoiding some environmental exposures, and adopting the same healthy behaviors on the Lifestyle Checklist that markedly reduce the risk of cardiovascular and other diseases.

Healthy lifestyle choices include avoiding tobacco, avoiding overweight and obesity, limiting or better yet avoiding alcohol, engaging in regular physical activity, protecting skin from the sun, and avoiding or treating certain infections. Eating a whole-food, plant-based diet abundant in fruits and vegetables and fiber may also help prevent cancer. Even though recent studies suggest that the proportion of cancers we can prevent through the adoption of a healthy lifestyle may be lower than previously thought, reduction of exposure to important behavioral and environmental risk factors would prevent a substantial proportion of deaths from cancer.

And since it is not possible to prevent all cancers, getting the recommended cancer screening tests is essential for the early detection of pre-cancerous conditions and early cancers. Unfortunately, early detection of small cancers does not guarantee that they have not metastasized and that they are curable, but early detection usually greatly improves the chances of successful treatment and cure.

How common, costly, and risky is cancer?

Cancer is the second most common cause of death in the U.S., only slightly exceeded by deaths from cardiovascular diseases. In some U.S. states, cancer is the leading cause of death. Globally, cancer is the leading cause of death. Since 1950, U.S. heart disease death rates have declined by more than half, but cancer death rates have declined much more slowly in spite of an annual investment by the National Cancer Institute, other federal agencies, charities and pharmaceutical companies estimated at $116 billion in 2018.[20] In 2019, the National Cancer Institute alone spent an estimated $6.6 billion on cancer research, nearly three times more than the investment in cardiovascular disease research.[21]

The financial costs of cancer are high for both the person with cancer and for society as a whole. The National Institutes of Health (NIH) estimated the 2009 overall annual costs of cancer were $216.6 billion. Of this total, direct medical costs were $86.6 billion, and indirect mortality costs (cost of lost productivity due to premature death) were $130 billion[22] Annually, more nearly 1.8 million Americans will be diagnosed with cancer, and about 600,000 will die of cancer – that's more than 1,600 people a day.

The incidence of cancer refers to the number of new cases that develop in a certain place during a given period of time, such as a year. About one-half of all men and one-third of all women in the U.S. will develop cancer during their lifetimes. Fortunately, the odds of dying from cancer are much lower. One in four men and one in five women will die from cancer.

Cancer prevalence is the number of people who have ever been diagnosed with cancer who are still living at a specified point in time. Currently, two out of three people will survive at least five years after a cancer diagnosis. Excluding basal cell and squamous cell skin cancers and all non-invasive (in-situ) cancers other than bladder cancer, the National Cancer Institute estimates that (as of January 1, 2016), there were more than 15 million cancer survivors in the U.S.—either living with cancer or cancer-free[23] Nearly half of cancer survivors are 70 years of age or older. About three million are men living after a diagnosis of prostate cancer, and about three million are women who have had a breast cancer diagnosis. Breast and prostate cancers are examples of cancers with high prevalence because they are common, and because 90% of people with these cancers survive at least five years

Table 7.2. Cancer New Cases, Percent of Cases and Deaths in the U.S., 2010

Cancer Cases and Deaths in the U.S.

Estimated New Cases, 2010*		Estimated Deaths, 2010	
Male	Female	Male	Female
Prostate 217,730 (28%)	Breast 207,090 (28%)	Lung & bronchus 86,220 (29%)	Lung & bronchus 71,080 (26%)
Lung & bronchus 116,750 (15%)	Lung & bronchus 105,770 (14%)	Prostate 32,050 (11%)	Breast 39,840 (15%)
Colon & rectum 72,090 (9%)	Colon & rectum 70,480 (10%)	Colon & rectum 26,580 (9%)	Colon & rectum 24,790 (9%)
Urinary bladder 52,760 (7%)	Uterine corpus 43,470 (6%)	Pancreas 18,770 (6%)	Pancreas 18,030 (7%)
Melanoma of the skin 38,870 (5%)	Thyroid 33,930 (5%)	Liver 12,720 (4%)	Ovary 13,850 (5%)
Non-Hodgkin lymphoma 35,380 (4%)	Non-Hodgkin lymphoma 30,160 (4%)	Leukemia 12,660 (4%)	Non-Hodgkin lymphoma 9,500 (4%)
Kidney 35,370 (4%)	Melanoma of the skin 29,260 (4%)	Esophagus 11,650 (4%)	Leukemia 9,180 (3%)
Oral cavity & pharynx 25,420 (3%)	Kidney 22,870 (3%)	Non-Hodgkin lymphoma 10,710 (4%)	Uterine corpus 7,950 (3%)
Leukemia 24,690 (3%)	Ovary 21,880 (3%)	Urinary bladder 10,410 (3%)	Liver 6,190 (2%)
Pancreas 21,370 (3%)	Pancreas 21,770 (3%)	Kidney 8,210 (3%)	Brain & other nervous system 5,720 (2%)
All sites 789,620	All sites 739,940	All sites 299,200	All sites 270,290

*Excludes basal and squamous cell skin cancers and in situ carcinoma except urinary bladder.
Data from the National Cancer Institute.

Source: Swartzberg JE, Wolf JL. Preventing Cancer: Strategies to Reduce Your Risk. University of California, Berkeley Wellness Report. 2011.

after diagnosis. Some other common cancers, such as lung cancer, and less common cancers such as pancreatic and liver cancer, have low survivor rates with fewer than 20% of people surviving at five years after diagnosis.[24]

Tobacco tops the list of avoidable risks for cancer[25][26][27][28]

The Institute of Medicine estimates that 76% of Americans have at some time used tobacco, and 32% became dependent on it. Smoking has declined in the U.S. from about 42% of the adult population in 1965 to 15.5% in 2016, with about 17.5% of men and 13.5% of women smoking.[29] About 37.8 million American adults continue to smoke. Unfortunately, smoking cigarettes, cigars, nicotine dosing e-cigarettes, and hookahs, as well as using chew and snuff, remains common among American youth. Even though tobacco advertising targeting youths is restricted, and anti-smoking educational efforts are widespread, about 6% of high school seniors are smokers.

Smoking and other uses of tobacco are the leading causes of preventable deaths in the U.S. and worldwide.[30] About half of all Americans who keep smoking will die from a disease linked to smoking. Smoking cigarettes is linked to the deaths of more Americans than alcohol, car accidents, suicide, AIDS, homicide, and illegal drugs combined. Estimates of annual smoking-related mortality range from 437,000 to 556,000 and about 160,000 of these deaths are from many different forms of cancer. Up to one in five deaths in the U.S. each year are from illnesses related to tobacco use, and about 30% of cancer deaths are smoking-related. The non-cancer deaths caused by smoking are caused by a variety of diseases, predominantly cardiovascular diseases, and chronic obstructive pulmonary disease (COPD), a lung disease that includes emphysema and chronic bronchitis.

Cigarette smokers die younger than non-smokers. A study done in the late 1990s by the Centers for Disease Control and Prevention (CDC) found that smoking shortened male smokers' lives by 13.2 years and female smokers' lives by 14.5 years. Men and women who smoke are much more likely to die between the ages of 35 and 69 than those who have never smoked. Stopping smoking by age 40 reduces the loss of life from tobacco-related causes by about 90%. Quitting at any age is likely to reduce the risk of premature death.[31] [32]

Is vaping safer?

E-cigarettes are also known as electronic nicotine-delivery systems (ENDS) because the main experience for the user is from nicotine, an addictive substance. There is some evidence that e-cigarettes are better at helping smokers to quit than nicotine patches or lozenges.[33] There is a concern, especially for youth, that e-cigarettes lead to nicotine addiction and are a gateway to other addictions, including to smoking cigarettes.[34] [35] E-cigarettes have very high nicotine content, come in many flavors, and can be used discreetly. The CDC's National Youth Tobacco Survey reports rapid increases in e-cigarette use among youth.[36] The percent of high school seniors who use e-cigarettes increased from 1.5% in 2010 to 13% in 2017.[37] [38] An estimated 27.5% of high school students and 10.5% of middle school students vaped in 2019.[39]

The health risks of electronic cigarettes or "vaping" are not as well studied as the hazards of tobacco, and as a relatively new product, first marketed in the U.S. in 2007, there is much less information about their long-term effects. Serious injuries requiring burn and wound care, including skin grafts, have resulted from e-cigarette explosions.[40] The aerosols in the delivery system deliver ultrafine particles to the lungs and contain many toxins and known carcinogens, including formaldehyde and acetaldehyde and flavorings that have not been approved for inhalation.[41] A study found that daily use of e-cigarettes increased the odds of a heart attack by 1.7 times over the risk among never-users, and daily cigarette smokers had nearly triple the risk.[42] Recently there has been an epidemic of vaping associated with lung disease mainly from black market street bought devices that add THC (the psycho-active ingredient of marijuana) diluted in a lipid such as vitamin E acetate. Some of the lung injuries from these products have been serious, with users ending up on ventilators and others dying from lung failure. As of December 2019, hospitalized lung injury cases topped 2,500 and vaping deaths totaled over 50.[43]

Cancers caused by smoking tobacco

Tobacco smoke contains more than 7,000 chemical compounds, with some 250 known to be harmful and at least 69 known to be carcinogens. In addition, tobacco smoke contains radioactive polonium, a known carcinogen. Smokeless tobacco is not safe as it contains more than 3000 chemical compounds, including at least 28 known carcinogens. Because most of the carcinogens in tobacco smoke reach all parts of the body through the bloodstream, it is not surprising that the risk of many types of cancer is increased.[44 45] The risks of marijuana smoke are not as well established but there is reason to think that smoke from all sources carries risks to health.[46 47]

The body parts in direct contact with smoke have the greatest increase in the risk of developing cancer. Tobacco and alcohol, especially in combination, increase the risk for cancers of the mouth, larynx, and throat. Smoking increases the risk of cancers of the mouth and pharynx by eight times. One or two packs of cigarettes a day increase the risk of lung cancer about 20 to 25 times over that of non-smokers and accounts for 87% of lung cancer deaths in men and 70% in women.[48] Even secondhand smoke increases the risk of lung cancer by 20% to 30%.[49] Lung cancer is not the most frequent cause of cancer, but it is the leading cause of cancer death in both men and women, and it is one of the hardest cancers to treat. More women in the U.S. die from lung cancer than from breast cancer.

According to the CDC, the risk of these cancers is increased by tobacco use:[50]

- Acute myeloid leukemia
- Bladder
- Cervix
- Colon and rectum (colorectal)
- Esophagus
- Kidney and ureter

- Larynx
- Liver
- Nose and sinuses
- Oropharynx (includes parts of the throat, tongue, soft palate, and the tonsils)
- Ovary (a type called mucinous ovarian cancer)
- Pancreas
- Stomach
- Trachea, bronchus, and lung

Smoking causes other major health problems

The CDC has identified many important health problems other than cancer that smoking contributes to:[51]

- More than half of the deaths related to smoking are caused by diseases other than cancer, among them are heart disease, aneurysms, bronchitis, emphysema, and stroke.
- About 90% of deaths from chronic obstructive pulmonary disease (COPD) are caused by smoking.
- Smokers have a 50% to 80% increased risk of dementia.
- Cigarette smoking weakens the immune system, makes asthma and pneumonia worse and causes gum disease and loss of teeth.
- By harming men's sperm, smoking can reduce fertility and increase risks for birth defects and miscarriage.
- Male smokers may be more likely to have erectile dysfunction (ED) than non-smokers.
- Tobacco use by women is linked to reduced fertility and a higher risk of ectopic pregnancy, miscarriage, early premature birth, stillbirth, low birth-weight infants, birth defects and sudden infant death syndrome (SIDS).
- Women past childbearing years who smoke have a lower bone density (osteopenia and osteoporosis) than women who never smoked and are at greater risk for broken bones.
- Smoking can increase the risk for cataracts and age-related macular degeneration (damage to the part of the retina needed for central vision).
- Smoking is a cause of type 2 diabetes and can make it harder to control. The risk of developing diabetes is 30% to 40% higher for active smokers than non-smokers.
- Smoking causes general adverse effects on the body, including inflammation and impaired immune function.
- Smoking is a cause of rheumatoid arthritis.

A study published in 2015 indicates that the excess mortality caused by smoking is underestimated. It found additional smoking-related causes of mortality beyond the 21 formally established as increased by smoking, including two common types of cancer.[52] According to the study, approximately 17% of the excess mortality among current smokers was due to associations with causes that were not previously established as attributable to smoking. These included associations between current smoking and deaths from:

- Renal failure (relative risk, 2.0 times that of non-smokers)
- Intestinal ischemia (relative risk, 6.0)
- Hypertensive heart disease (relative risk, 2.4)
- Infections (relative risk, 2.3)
- Various respiratory diseases (relative risk, 2.0)
- Breast cancer (relative risk, 1.3)
- Prostate cancer (relative risk, 1.4)

The study found that among former smokers, the relative risk compared to non-smokers for each of these outcomes declined as the number of years since quitting increased.

The implications of these grim statistics are clear: Do not start smoking; it is a true addiction. And if you use tobacco quit now. Avoid secondhand smoke, and smokeless tobacco as their risks are proven, too. Although there is, so far, much less data on e-cigarettes and cancer, the dangerous cardiovascular effects of nicotine are sure to remain. Many people have relied on help from health providers, especially with the use of nicotine replacement therapy (NRT) and other drugs, but the large majority of ex-smokers were able to quit on their own, usually "cold turkey."[53] And if quitting proves to be impossible, there is good evidence among individuals who smoke 15 or more cigarettes per day that a 50% reduction in smoking significantly reduces the risk of lung cancer. A study found that those whose smoking decreased from 20 to 10 cigarettes per day had a 27% decrease in lung cancer risk.[54]

Quitting smoking does not eliminate all of the increased risks of contracting all smoking-related diseases compared to non-smokers, but the reductions are substantial. By one year after quitting, the risk for a heart attack drops 36% to 50%. Within two to five years after quitting smoking, the risk for stroke is probably about the same as that of non-smokers. Quitting smoking decreases the risk for cancers of the mouth, throat, esophagus, and bladder by half within five years. Ten years after quitting smoking, the risk for lung cancer drops by half.[55]

Alcohol

The Centers for Disease Control and Prevention (CDC) estimates that during each of the years 2006 to 2010, excessive alcohol use led to approximately 88,000 deaths, 2.5 million years of potential life lost, and a shortening the lives of those who died by an average of 30 years. Further, excessive consumption of alcohol was responsible for one in 10 deaths among working-age adults aged 20 to 64 years. The economic costs of excessive alcohol consumption in 2010 were estimated at $249 billion, or $2.05 a drink.[56 57 58 59 60] The top causes of these deaths are liver disease and motor vehicle crashes, but cancer is also linked to alcohol. Additional discussion of the links between alcohol and health can be found in Chapter 6, "Preventing Cardiovascular Disease."

Undoubtedly almost everyone knows that the use of tobacco products causes cancer, but many people seem unaware that drinking any amount of alcohol causes some harm to health and is a major contributor to cancer mortality. A study that estimated alcohol-attributable cancer mortality found that alcohol consumption resulted in an estimated 18,200 to 21,300 cancer deaths annually, or 3.2% to 3.7% of annual U.S. cancer deaths. Among women, the most cancer deaths attributed to alcohol are from breast cancer. Among men, upper airway and esophageal cancer account for the most cancer deaths attributed to alcohol. Alcohol-attributable cancers result in an estimated 17 to 19 years of potential life lost. One study found that daily consumption of even small amounts of alcohol was risky in that up to 20 grams of alcohol (about 1.5 drinks) accounted for 26% to 35% of alcohol-attributable cancer deaths[61]

Short-Term Health Risks of Alcohol[62 63]

Excessive alcohol use has immediate effects that increase the risk of many harmful health conditions—most often the result of binge drinking:

- Injuries, such as motor vehicle crashes, falls, drownings, and burns
- Violence, including homicide, suicide, sexual assault, and intimate partner violence
- Alcohol poisoning, a life threatening medical emergency caused by dangerously high blood alcohol levels
- Risky sexual behaviors, unprotected sex, sex with multiple partners, unintended pregnancy, sexually transmitted diseases, including HIV
- Miscarriage and stillbirth or fetal alcohol spectrum disorders among pregnant women

Long-Term Health Risks of Alcohol[64 65 66]

Over time, excessive alcohol use can lead to the development of chronic diseases and other serious problems including:

- High blood pressure, heart disease, stroke, liver disease, and digestive problems
- Cancer of the breast, mouth, throat, larynx, esophagus, liver, and colon and possibly stomach, prostate, and pancreas
- Learning and memory problems, including dementia and poor academic performance
- Mental health problems, including depression and anxiety
- Social problems, including lost productivity, family problems, and unemployment
- Alcohol dependence, or alcoholism

Some people mistakenly think that certain types of alcoholic drinks are safer than others. Although there may be other carcinogens in alcoholic beverages, evidence suggests that alcohol (ethanol) is the most important carcinogen and that the risk of cancer is related to the total amount of alcohol that is consumed over time, not the type of drink.

How alcohol increases the risk of cancer is not fully understood. Since alcohol is a poison that damages cells, it is theorized that the increased need to repair or replace cells exposed to alcohol increases the replication of cells, and that could lead to cancer-causing DNA mutations. Alcohol is especially toxic to those cells in the mouth and throat that are exposed to the highest concentrations of alcohol. Drinking and smoking together raises the risk of these cancers far more than the effects of either drinking or smoking alone. Alcohol seems to help the carcinogens in tobacco invade and damage the cells of the mouth, throat, and elsewhere in the digestive tract and may also impair the ability of these cells to repair damage to their DNA. Depending on the site of the cancer and the level of alcohol consumption, risk may be slightly elevated, or an eight times greater risk for a cancer of the mouth and oropharynx in heavy drinkers.[67] About 20%-30% of deaths from cancers of the oral cavity, pharynx, larynx, and esophagus can be attributed to alcohol consumption.[68]

In the colon and rectum, bacteria can convert alcohol into acetaldehyde, a chemical that has been shown to cause cancer in lab animals. Long-term, regular, and heavy alcohol use has been linked to liver inflammation and scarring and an increased risk of liver cancer—the fourth most common cause of cancer-related deaths. Even a few drinks a week is linked to an increased risk of breast cancer in women. Drinking less, or better yet, not drinking alcohol at all is probably an important way for women to lower their risk of breast cancer. Alcohol can add extra calories to the diet and contribute to becoming overweight or obese—a known risk for many types of cancer.

To minimize the risk of developing cancer, it is best not to drink. For those who do drink, the American Cancer Society's recommendation is to limit intake to no more than two drinks per day for men and one drink a day for women. The 2020 Dietary Guideline's Advisory Committee recommends that both men and women limit drinks to one on days alcohol is consumed. A drink of alcohol is defined as 12 ounces of beer, 5 ounces of wine, or 1½ ounces of 80-proof distilled spirits (hard liquor).

These daily limits do not mean it's safe to drink larger amounts on fewer days of the week since this can lead to accidents, and health, social, and other problems. Excessive drinking includes binge drinking, heavy drinking, and any drinking by pregnant women or people younger than age 21.

Binge drinking, the most common form of excessive drinking, is defined as consuming:

- For women, four or more drinks during a single occasion
- For men, five or more drinks during a single occasion

Heavy drinking is defined as consuming:

- For women, eight or more drinks per week
- For men, 15 or more drinks per week

Although alcohol use is associated with many types of cancer and other health risks, its consumption is sometimes justified by the fact that low-to-moderate alcohol intake has been linked to a lower risk of heart disease, but these benefits are not unequivocally established.[69] Lowering the risk of heart disease is not a compelling reason to drink alcohol. As is described in Chapter 6, "Preventing Cardiovascular Disease," there are much better ways to reduce heart disease risk, including avoiding smoking, eating a whole-food plant-based diet low in saturated and trans-fats, staying at a healthy weight, staying physically active, and controlling blood pressure and LDL-Cholesterol. It is likely that an individual who adheres to this healthy lifestyle will gain no cardiovascular benefit from alcohol consumption. And clearly, heavy consumption of alcohol increases the risk of cardiovascular disease.

Overweight, physical activity, diet, and cancer risk

The American Cancer Society states that in addition to quitting smoking, some of the most important things you can do to help reduce your cancer risk are:

- Get to and stay at a healthy weight throughout life, with a BMI of under 25.

- Be physically active on a regular basis.
- Make healthy food choices with a focus on plant-based foods.

Bodyweight and cancer

One estimate is that one out of every three cancer deaths in the U.S. is linked to excess body weight, poor nutrition, and/or physical inactivity. These factors are all related to each other and may all contribute to cancer risk, but of these factors, bodyweight or more accurately adiposity (fatness) seems to have the strongest evidence of a causal link to cancer. According to the American Cancer Society, excess body weight contributes to as many as one out of five of all cancer-related deaths. A large study involving more than one million participants concluded that the proportion of all deaths from cancer that is attributable to overweight and obesity in U.S. adults 50 years of age or older who do not smoke might be as high as 14% in men and 20% in women.[70] A 2017 study by the CDC assessed the incidence of 13 cancers among more than 630,000 people. The study found that more than 55% of all cancers diagnosed among women and 24% of cancers among men were associated with overweight and obesity.[71 72]

In a dose-response relationship, the risk of cancer increases with increasing body mass index (BMI) or abdominal fat. People who are overweight have a small increase in risk, whereas, among the extremely obese, cancer mortality from all sites is 70% higher than that of people of normal weight. And studies indicate that after both dietary interventions and bariatric surgery, there are fairly immediate reductions in cancer incidence following weight loss.[73]

The causal links between body weight and cancer are not well understood. They appear to vary for different cancers. Excess body fat might affect cancer risk through effects on immune system function, inflammation, increased levels of hormones, such as insulin and estrogen, that can stimulate cancer growth, and factors that regulate cell division.

Being overweight or obese is clearly associated by epidemiological studies with an increased risk of the following cancers:[74 75]

- Breast (in women past menopause)
- Stomach (gastric cardia)
- Colon and rectum
- Liver
- Gallbladder
- Ovary
- Endometrium (lining of the uterus)

- Esophagus
- Kidney (renal cell)
- Pancreas
- Brain (meningioma)
- Thyroid
- Multiple myeloma

Being overweight or obese probably raises the risk of other cancers, such as:

- Malignant melanoma
- Non-Hodgkin lymphoma
- Male breast cancer
- Leukemia
- Cervix
- Aggressive forms of prostate cancer

The increase in relative risk of cancer varies according to an individual's weight classification and specific cancer. Meta-analyses suggest that compared to normal-weight individuals, the relative risk of getting cancer is 1.2 to 1.5 greater for overweight and 1.5 to 1.8 greater for obesity. There is a much higher relative risk for cancer of the esophagus (4.8) and endometrium (7.1) among those of the highest weight.[76] A study of obesity and colon cancer found that overweight women (BMI, 25.0-29.9) had a 37% increase in risk, and obese women, with a BMI of 30 or greater, had a 93% increase in risk.[77] A 2018 study attributes 5.6% of worldwide cancers to diabetes and suggests that a BMI of above 25 is associated with twice as many cancers as diabetes.[78]

Physical activity and cancer

People who undertake moderate or vigorous physical activity are at a lower risk of developing several cancers, especially lung and colorectal, but also those of the breast, endometrium (lining of the uterus), and advanced forms of prostate cancer.[79] [80] A study of more than 49,000 patients over nearly eight years found that those in the highest fitness category decreased the odds of developing lung cancer by 77% and decreased the risk of developing colorectal cancer by 61% compared to those who were the least fit.[81] Among those diagnosed with lung and colorectal cancer, over the eight years, those with high fitness decreased the risk of subsequent death from lung cancer by 44% and from colorectal cancer by 89%.

Information on the association of physical activity with the incidence of common types of cancer comes from a 2016 meta-analysis of data from 12 prospective U.S. and European cohorts with self-reported physical activity.[82] The study compared moderate to vigorous intensity leisure-time physical activity with the incidence of 26 types of cancer among a total of 1.44 million study participants. The ratio of risk (Hazard Ratio) of developing a cancer for individuals with high vs. low levels of leisure-time physical activity was found to be lower among those with high physical activity for 13 cancers:

- Esophageal adenocarcinoma (Hazard Ratio 0.58)
- Liver (HR 0.73)
- Lung (HR 0.74)
- Kidney (HR 0.77)
- Gastric cardia (HR 0.78)
- Endometrial (HR 0.79)
- Myeloid leukemia (HR 0.80)
- Myeloma (HR 0.83)
- Colon (HR 0.84)
- Head and neck (HR 0.85)
- Rectal (HR 0.87)
- Bladder (HR 0.87)
- Breast (HR 0.90)

Leisure-time physical activity was associated with 27% higher risks of malignant melanoma (HR 1.27) and an unexplained and possibly insignificant 5% higher risk of prostate cancer (HR 1.05). The increased risk of malignant melanoma might be the result of sun exposure during outdoor physical activity.

Although the amount of physical activity needed to reduce cancer risk is uncertain, the consensus is that a good starting place is the *2018 Physical Activity Guidelines Scientific Report* recommendation for adults that calls for at least 150 minutes of moderate-intensity or 75 minutes of vigorous-intensity physical activity each week or an equivalent combination.[83] As described in more detail in Chapter 9, "Benefits of Physical Activity," moderate activities include brisk walking, biking, even housework, and gardening. Vigorous activities make you use large muscle groups, increase your heart rate, and make you out of breath.

Neither the type or amount of physical activity needed to reduce cancer risk nor the biological mechanism by which physical activity reduces cancer risk are well understood. Since physical activity contributes to reaching and staying at a healthy body weight, avoiding overweight and obesity may be an important way that physical activity reduces the risk of cancer.

Diet and cancer

Because cancer risk varies substantially between countries and groups of people with different dietary patterns, there have been many studies looking for links between diet and cancer. There are many over-the-top claims that "superfoods" with high levels of phytochemicals (a wide variety of chemical compounds that occur naturally in plants) and antioxidants are "cancer fighters," but much of the evidence linking food and cancer is not particularly strong.[84] Many retrospective studies suggest that high fat and red meat in diets are factors that increase the risk of cancer and that consumption of fruits, dietary fiber, vegetables, and especially the phytochemicals in fruits and vegetables, all contribute to reduced risk.

Soy, fruits and vegetables

There is some evidence that eating traditional soy foods such as tofu may lower the risk of cancers of the breast, prostate, or endometrium (lining of the uterus), and possibly other cancers. For example, a study suggests that plant-derived dietary phytoestrogens (compounds with weak estrogen-like activity found in peas, beans, soy products, and other foods) may decrease lung cancer risk.[85] And there is some but not particularly strong evidence suggests eating fruits and vegetables may somewhat lower the risk for cancers of the lung, mouth, throat (pharynx), larynx, esophagus, stomach, colon, and rectum. Unfortunately, the retrospective studies linking diet and cancer have methodological problems because of the difficulty in accurately recalling diets, and because over many years, people frequently change their diets.[86 87]

A prospective study considered four nutritional scores and overall, breast, prostate, and colorectal cancer risk.[88] The scores are the cancer-specific World Cancer Research Fund/American Institute for Cancer Research (WCRF/AICR) score, the Alternate Healthy Eating Index 2010 (AHEI-2010), a score based on adherence to the Mediterranean diet (MEDI-LITE), and the French National Nutrition Health Program-Guideline Score (PNNS-GS). A one-point increment of the WCRF/AICR score was significantly associated with a 12% decrease in overall cancer risk. The three other diets were associated with smaller reductions in overall cancer risk. The WCRF/AICR score performed best. Probably, because compared with other tested diet scores, it included a stronger penalty for alcohol, which is a major risk factor for several cancer sites.

A study based on the diet questionnaires submitted every four years by participants in the Nurses' Health Study (88,301 women, starting in 1980) and the Nurses' Health Study II (93,844 women, starting in 1991) found that women who ate more than 5.5 servings of fruits and vegetables each day had an 11% lower risk of breast cancer than those who ate 2.5 or fewer servings.[89] The study defined a serving as one cup of raw leafy vegetables, half a cup of raw or cooked vegetables, or half a cup of chopped or cooked fruits.

Red and processed meat

The current consensus, based increasingly on the few prospective studies that are the least susceptible to biases, is that high consumption of red meat and processed meat is associated with an increased risk of colorectal and possibly pancreatic, prostate, and stomach cancers. When meat is processed by smoking or by adding preservatives such as salt or sodium nitrite, the added compounds cause the increased risk. In 2015, the WHO's International Agency for Research on Cancer (IARC) Monographs Programme classified the consumption of red meat as probably carcinogenic, and processed meat was classified as carcinogenic to humans, based on sufficient evidence that the consumption of processed meat causes colorectal cancer. The IARC concluded that each 50-gram portion of processed meat eaten daily increases the risk of colorectal cancer by 18%.[90 91] Because of this increase in cancer risk and cardiovascular health risks, it is best to avoid bacon, sausage, lunchmeats, hams, hot dogs, and other processed meats.

Fish

Fish is a rich source of omega-3 fatty acids. Studies in animals have found that these fatty acids may stop cancer from forming or slow its growth, but it is not clear if they can affect cancer risk in humans. As was described in Chapter 3, "Optimal Nutrition," the well-designed VITAL clinical trial of high dose (1 g per day) supplementation with omega-3 fatty acids did not result in a lower incidence of major cardiovascular events or cancer than a placebo.[92]

Dietary Fiber

Studies suggest that dietary fiber from good sources such as beans, vegetables, whole grains, and fruits is linked with a lower risk of some types of cancer, especially colorectal cancer. Although a diet high in fruits, vegetables, and whole grains does not appear to be as strongly protective against cancer as was thought previously, these dietary components have benefits for protection against overweight, diabetes, and cardiovascular disease, and they may offer some protection against cancer. Vegetarian diets may lower cancer risk. Typically, they are low in saturated fat and high in fiber, vitamins, and phytochemicals, and do not include eating red and processed meats.[93] More research on fruits, vegetables, phytochemicals, dietary fiber, and cancer is needed, but it is still prudent to eat at least 2½ cups of a variety of colorful vegetables and fruits each day.

Nuts

Consumption of nuts has been found to be associated with reduced risk of cardiovascular disease, total cancer, all-cause mortality, and mortality from respiratory disease, diabetes, and infections. In a meta-analysis of 20 studies, a one-ounce (28 grams) per day increase in nut intake over those who ate little or no nuts was associated with a 29% decreased risk of coronary heart disease, a 21% decreased risk of CVD, a 15% lower risk of all cancers, and a 22% lower risk of all-cause mortality.[94] There is some doubt about the findings of this study because the intake of nuts is so small.

Although it cannot be considered definitive, a 2014 British study of 1,806 prostate cancer patients and 12,005 men without prostate cancer found that the more that diets contained tomato products and other plant-based foods, the greater the reduction in the risk of prostate cancer. Consuming 10 or more servings of tomatoes and tomato products per week was associated with an 18% reduced risk for prostate cancer.[95]

Food processing

Freezing and canning are food processing methods that provide the benefit of preventing spoilage and preserving nutritional value. But much processed food is high in added fat, sugar, and salt—all of which are deleterious to the food's nutritional value. For example, some fruits are packed in high sugar syrup, and some canned vegetables are high in sodium. High sugar intake can increase the consumption of calories, contribute to obesity, and indirectly increase cancer risk. Processed meat has been classified as carcinogenic to humans. Another example of food processing that is detrimental is the refining of grains, which both increases their glycemic index and greatly lowers the amount of fiber and other compounds that may reduce cancer risk.

There is some evidence that highly processed foods may raise cancer risk. A five-year study found that every 10% increase in ultra-processed foods (e.g., baked goods, processed meats, sugary cereals) was associated with a 12% greater risk for all cancers and an 11% increased risk of breast cancer.[96] No significant link with prostate or colorectal cancer was found.

Salt and pickling

Although diets that contain excessively large amounts of foods preserved by salting and pickling increase the risk of stomach, nasopharyngeal, and throat cancer, the levels of salt used in cooking and food processing in the U.S. do not appear to affect cancer risk.

Antioxidants, vitamins, and other dietary supplements

A diet rich in vegetables, fruits, and other plant-based foods may reduce the risk of cancer, but there is little proof that dietary supplements can reduce cancer risk, and some studies have found that certain supplements increased risk of cancer. As is described in more detail in Chapter 5, "Vitamins and Other Supplements," studies of a large variety of dietary supplements, including vitamins A, C, D, E, and folate, have not found that they lower cancer risk. Some studies have found an increased risk of cancer and other diseases among those taking supplements. For example, folic acid supplements may increase the risk of prostate cancer, advanced colorectal polyps, and possibly breast cancer. The best way to get all vitamins is by eating vegetables, fruits, and enriched whole-grain products. The role of vitamin D in cancer and other health issues is the subject of much research, but the Institute of Medicine concluded that outcomes related to cancer and other neoplasms, could not be linked reliably with calcium or vitamin D intake.[97]

The VITAL study described in Chapter 3, "Optimal Nutrition," was a high-quality, randomized, double-blind trial. It found that high doses of vitamin D (2000IU per day or three times the RDA) taken for 5.3 years did not reduce the risk of invasive cancers.[98] Treatment effects did not vary with baseline levels of vitamin D, so even people with low levels did not benefit. There was some indication that normal-weight participants may have had a lower cancer incidence and that starting after two years, those taking vitamin D had a lower death rate than those taking a placebo. These secondary endpoint results are less reliable and should be considered a finding that needs additional study.[99]

Although there is some evidence that calcium supplements reduce the risk of colorectal cancer, a high calcium intake, whether through supplements or food, has also been linked with an increased risk of prostate cancer. Men should try to get, but not exceed, recommended levels of calcium, mainly through food sources.

Coffee, tea, and cancer

There is no sound evidence that coffee, tea, or caffeine increases or decreases the risk of cancer.

Fat

The best studies have not found that fat intake increases cancer risk, or that lowering fat intake reduces cancer risk.

Genetically modified foods

Most soybeans and corn grown in the U.S. come from seeds that have been modified to resist herbicides, and in the case of corn, modified to make a natural insecticide. At present, there is no proof that the genetically modified foods currently on the market are harmful to human health or that they either increase or decrease cancer risk. However, some scientists suggest that additional studies are needed to assess possible long-term health effects. See Chapter 3, "Optimal Nutrition," for additional discussion of this subject.

Irradiated foods

There is no evidence that irradiation of foods used to kill harmful germs in or on foods to extend their shelf life causes cancer or has harmful health effects. The radiation of foods does not make them radioactive.

Non-nutritive sweeteners, sugar substitutes

Because of widespread use, many of these compounds, including aspartame, saccharin, and sucralose have been extensively studied and require approval by the FDA before they are allowed to be used for human consumption. At the moderate levels consumed in human diets, none of the sweeteners now in use show any increased cancer risk.

Olive oil, other edible oils

Olive oil and other oils used for cooking or salad dressings are not known to affect cancer risk other than possibly by increasing the likelihood of overweight and obesity—known cancer risks.

Organic foods

Organic foods are less likely to be contaminated by residues of pesticides and herbicides. Whether the consumption of organic foods carries a lower risk of cancer is uncertain. Eliminating or minimizing toxic residues by buying organically produced foods and by washing fruits and vegetables thoroughly before consuming them is a good idea and in keeping with the precautionary principle.

Food contaminants

Substances and compounds used in agriculture, animal farming, and food processing, sometimes end up contaminating food. Examples include growth hormones and antibiotics given to farm animals, trace amounts of pesticides and herbicides in plant-based foods, and compounds such as bisphenol A (BPA) or phthalates that enter food from packaging. Some of these compounds may influence cancer risk. Unintended contamination of food may also result in exposure to chemicals that may cause an increased risk of cancer. Examples include cadmium, mercury, and arsenic in rice. For many compounds, the effects on cancer risk are not clear, but there may be other good reasons to limit exposures, for example, to avoid developmental risks to a growing fetus. At the levels that contaminants are found in the food supply, lowering cancer risk is unlikely to be a major reason to avoid conventionally grown foods.

Food additives

Food additives are small amounts of substances that are added to color foods, prolong storage life, and improve flavor and texture. A number of food additives that have been used for years without apparent problems are classified as generally recognized as safe (GRAS). New additives undergo testing for cancer and other health effects in lab animals before being cleared by the U.S. Food and Drug Administration for use in foods.

Trans-fats

There is convincing evidence that trans-fats should be avoided because they raise blood cholesterol and greatly increase the risk of cardiovascular disease, but their effect on cancer risk has not been determined.

Turmeric, other spices

The effect of spices on cancer risk has not been determined.

High heat cooking

High-temperature frying, broiling, or grilling of high-protein foods, such as meat and fish, forms PAHs (polycyclic aromatic hydrocarbons) or HCAs (heterocyclic aromatic amines), compounds that in high doses cause many different kinds of cancer in laboratory animals. Observational studies have found that people who eat large amounts of barbecued, fried, or charred meat have increased risk of colorectal, pancreatic, and prostate cancer. However, it is not clear how much PHAs and HCAs contribute to the increase in cancer risk. The increased risk could be from a failure to eat abundant amounts of fruits and vegetables or other lifestyle behaviors that increase cancer risk. It is advisable to choose lower temperature cooking methods for meats such as braising, steaming, stewing, and microwaving to minimize possible cancer risk.

Infectious agents and cancer

A variety of viruses, bacteria, and parasites have been found to increase the risk of several types of cancer. In developing countries where many types of infections are highly prevalent, infections are linked to 15% to 25% of cancers. The proportion of new cancers in the U.S. that are ascribed to infectious agents is about 4%.[100]

There are several ways that infections can lead to a higher risk of cancer: by causing inflammation, by immune system suppression, or by damaging a cell's DNA and causing mutations. Although infections can raise a person's risk of cancer, most people with the infections that sometimes cause cancer never develop cancers.

Viruses

Viruses reproduce by entering a living cell, inserting their own DNA or RNA, and causing the cell to synthesize more viruses. This process can affect a normal cell's genes and may increase the risk of the cell becoming cancerous. Vaccines against several viruses have been developed to prevent a few human cancers. They must be given before the person is exposed to the cancer-promoting virus.

Human papillomaviruses (HPVs)

Human papillomaviruses (HPVs) cause almost all cases of cervical cancer.[101] They can also cause warts on the skin, mouth, genitals, and larynx and cause some cancers of the penis, anus, vagina, vulva, mouth, and throat. There are more than 100 types or strains of HPV, a virus that is spread by personal contact. More than 40 of them can be spread through sexual contact, and they are common in sexually active people. A dozen types are known to cause cancer. Although HPV infection is common, most people infected with HPV do not develop cancer.

Cervical cancer remains common worldwide but is much less frequent in the U.S. because of prevention through widespread screening with Pap tests. When a Pap test detects infected pre-cancerous cells, they can be removed or destroyed before they become cancerous. Frequently, treatment is not needed because the body's immune system controls the HPV infection and eliminates both the virus and the abnormal pre-cancerous cells. Testing for the presence and type of HPV strain can also guide treatment by revealing if one of the high-risk virus types is present in the cervix.

Vaccines against HPV[102]

Gardasil 9® protects against nine types of HPV. It usually prevents the cervical, vulvar, vaginal, and anal cancers caused by HPV, and genital warts caused by HPV. With two or three doses (depending on age), Gardasil 9® protects against the seven high-risk types of HPV responsible for more than 90% of cervical cancers and two other HPV types accounting for 90% of genital warts.[103] [104] It is approved and recommended for use in females age nine to 45 prior to their becoming sexually active and infected with HPV. Gardasil 9® also protects against two strains of HPV virus that cause genital warts and has been approved for use in boys and young men to prevent anal cancers, genital warts and to prevent them from passing on HPV to their sexual partners.[105]

Hepatitis B virus (HBV) and hepatitis C virus (HCV)

HBV and HCV are transmitted from person to person. HBV can be transmitted by blood, sharing needles, unprotected sex, and body fluids. The rate of transmission of HCV by unprotected sex and body fluids is low. Usually, transmission occurs through contact with blood, for example, by sharing unsterilized needles.[106] A small proportion of the cases of viral hepatitis caused by HBV and HCV become chronic and increase a person's risk for developing cirrhosis, liver failure, and liver cancer.[107] About 40% of liver cancers in the U.S. are linked to HBV or HCV infection.

Hepatitis B has become less of a problem in the U.S. because of the widespread use of the hepatitis B vaccine. Treatment of chronic hepatitis B does not eliminate the virus, but it can suppress HBV replication and bring about remission of liver disease before the development of cirrhosis and liver cancer. However, there is no HCV vaccine, and an estimated 3.2 million people in the U.S. have chronic HCV infection. It is estimated that 75% of them do not know they are infected. Treating chronic hepatitis C infection with drugs that have a high cure rate is now possible.

Human immunodeficiency virus (HIV) and acquired immune deficiency syndrome (AIDS)

Infection with HIV, the virus that causes acquired immune deficiency syndrome (AIDS), does not seem to be a direct cause of cancers.[108] But because HIV infection weakens the body's immune system, it increases a person's risk of getting several types of cancer, especially some linked to other viruses. HIV is spread through semen, vaginal fluids, blood, and breast milk from an HIV-infected person. HIV is not spread by insects, through water, or by casual contacts such as talking, shaking hands, hugging, coughing, sneezing, or from sharing dishes, bathrooms, kitchens, phones, or computers.

Known routes of HIV spread include:

- Unprotected sex (oral-least likely, vaginal, or anal-most likely) with an HIV-infected person
- Injections with needles or injection equipment previously used by an HIV-infected person
- Prenatal and perinatal (during birth) exposure of infants from mothers with HIV
- Breastfeeding by mothers with HIV
- Transfusion of blood products containing HIV (U.S. blood has been tested since 1985)
- Organ transplants from an HIV-infected person (donors are now tested for HIV)
- Penetrating injuries or accidents (usually needle sticks) in health care workers

HIV infects, weakens and destroys the immune system's helper T-cells and increases susceptibility to cancer. This leaves the body susceptible to the damage caused by other viruses such as HPV, and a weak immune system may not attack and destroy newly formed cancer cells. HIV infection has been linked to a higher risk of developing anal cancer, Hodgkin lymphoma, non-Hodgkin lymphoma, lung cancer, cancers of the mouth and throat, skin cancers (basal cell, squamous cell, and Merkel cell), Kaposi sarcoma, invasive cervical cancer, and central nervous system lymphoma. Taking anti-HIV drugs may reduce the risk of getting these cancers.

Less common cancers that are linked to viral infection[109]

Epstein-Barr virus (EBV) is a herpes virus that infects almost everyone in the U.S. before the age of 20. EBV causes the symptoms of infectious mononucleosis in some people. EBV remains in the body throughout life and increases a person's risk of getting rare cancers, including nasopharyngeal cancer and fast-growing lymphomas such as Burkitt lymphoma. Other rare cancers that are linked to viral infections, especially in people with weak immune systems, include Kaposi sarcoma, primary effusion lymphoma, multicentric Castleman disease, adult T-cell leukemia/ lymphoma (ATL) and Merkel cell skin cancer.

Bacteria linked to cancer

Helicobacter pylori (H. pylori)

About one in three adults have evidence that their stomach is infected with the bacteria H. pylori. It sometimes causes stomach ulcers and inflammation that, over time, may lead to stomach cancer, including some types of lymphoma of the stomach. Although more than half of all cases of stomach cancer are thought to be linked to H. pylori infection, most people infected with these bacteria never develop cancer. Although stomach cancer is the fourth most common cancer worldwide, it makes up only about 2% of cancers in the U.S. Individuals infected with H. pylori who have had ulcers should be treated with antibiotics to decrease the risk of gastric cancer.[110 111]

Chlamydia trachomatis

Chlamydia trachomatis is a very common sexually transmitted bacteria that can infect the female and male reproductive tract as well as other parts of the body. Because it frequently does not cause symptoms, it can persist undetected for years and may cause pelvic inflammatory disease and infertility. Chlamydia seems to interact with HPV in a way that promotes cancer growth and increases the risk of becoming infected with HIV.[112]

Parasites and cancer

Certain parasitic worms can also raise the risk of developing some kinds of cancer.[113] These organisms are not found in the United States, but they can infect people who live in or travel to other parts of the world. Liver flukes, from eating raw or undercooked freshwater fish, have been linked to increased risk of developing cancer of the liver bile ducts. S. haematobium, the cause of schistosomiasis, is a parasite found in the water of some countries in the Middle East, Africa, and Asia. Infection with this parasite has been linked to bladder cancer.

Ionizing radiation and cancer[114 115]

Near ultraviolet light and ultraviolet A (UV-A), both have about the same wavelengths. They, and visible light, infrared, microwave, radio waves, and low-frequency radio radiation are all examples of non-ionizing radiation. In contrast, far-ultraviolet light and UV-B, X-rays, gamma rays, and all particle radiation from radioactive decay are regarded as ionizing. Ionizing radiation carries enough energy to liberate electrons from atoms, thereby ionizing them. Ions can damage the DNA inside of cells and cause mutations that result in cancer, so exposure to all types of ionizing radiation increases cancer risk.

The sources of ionizing radiation can be natural, for example, from radon gas, or human-made from a nuclear accident or medical procedures such as routine X-rays and computed tomography X-ray (CT) scans. Atomic bomb survivors were found to have an increased risk of developing cancer at multiple sites in the body. The level of risk for cancer increases as the dose of radiation received increases. Since cancers from radiation may take years to develop, cancers may occur many years after exposure.

In the U.S., several federal agencies require employers to limit, monitor, and disclose radiation exposures. Depending on the workplace, the Occupational Safety and Health Administration (OSHA), the Nuclear Regulatory Commission, and the Department of Energy, set the safety standards for workplace radiation exposure.
For the majority of people, exposure to natural sources of radiation makes up most of the annual dose of ionizing radiation.[116] The two major sources of this natural radiation are cosmic rays and radionuclides originating from the earth's crust. Radionuclides are pervasive in the ground, rocks, building materials, and drinking water. About half of the annual dose of ionizing radiation from natural sources comes from the inhalation of the radon gas that arises from the decay of radium-226. It is estimated that the average person receives a dose of about 3 mSv per year of background radiation from naturally occurring radioactive materials and cosmic radiation from outer space. These natural "background" doses vary throughout the country and are greater for people living at high altitudes.[117]

Although there is probably no threshold below which ionizing radiation can be considered completely safe, most studies have not detected an increased risk of cancer among people exposed to low levels of radiation. Even so, scientists and regulatory agencies agree that even small doses of gamma and x-radiation probably increase cancer risk, although by a very small amount, so minimizing exposure to any dose of ionizing radiation is a good idea.

Radon and cancer[118 119 120]

Radon-222 is a colorless, odorless, radioactive gas, and, when inhaled, it is the source of about half of the background radiation that people in the U.S. are exposed to. After cigarettes, radon is the second most common cause of lung cancer in the U.S. Exposure to the combination of radon gas and cigarette smoke creates a greater risk for lung cancer than either exposure alone and most radon-related lung cancers occur among smokers.[121 122] Radon is normally found at very low levels in outdoor air and in drinking water from surface sources. Elevated radon levels have been found in a wide variety of places and in every state in the U.S. Because fresh air is usually not well circulated, radon can be found at higher levels in the air in houses and other buildings. Most exposure to radon comes from being indoors and from water from underground sources, such as well water.

The EPA estimates that nearly one out of every 15 homes in the United States may have elevated radon levels. Radon levels in a home can be checked with a do-it-yourself kit or by hiring a professional. Radon levels are usually highest in places closest to the soil or rock that is the source of the radon, such as the in the basement or crawl space. The EPA recommends testing all homes below the 3rd floor, even new homes. If the levels are high, various methods can be used to reduce radon levels, such as sealing cracks in floors and walls or increasing ventilation. For more information about radon testing, call the National Radon Hotline at 800–55–RA-DON or go to EPA.gov/radon.

Ultraviolet radiation and skin cancer[123]

Most skin cancer, the most common type of cancer, can be avoided by limiting exposure to ultraviolet (UV) rays from the sun or from man-made sources, such as indoor tanning beds. More than 3.5 million skin cancers are diagnosed each year in the U.S. Of the UV reaching the earth's surface, 95% is UVA, and 5% is UVB. UVB is 1000 times more potent than UVA, for example, in causing sunburn. Both UVA and UVB rays cause long-term skin damage and can contribute to skin cancer.

Ways to lower the chances of getting skin cancer are:

- Stay out of the sun when the sun is the strongest, between the hours of 10 a.m. and 4 p.m., even on hazy and cloudy days.
- Protect skin by wearing a hat, shirt, and sunglasses when in the sun. If light can get through your clothing, so can some UV. Both adult and children's sunglasses should be labeled "UV absorption up to 400 nm" or "Meets ANSI UV Requirements" and block at least 99% of UV rays. Those labeled "cosmetic" block about 70% of UV rays. Sunglasses without a label may not provide any UV protection. Be aware that UV protection comes from an invisible chemical in or applied to the lenses, not from the color or darkness

of the lenses.

- Use generous amounts of a "broad spectrum" sunscreen that protects against both UVA and UVB rays—most people do not use enough. Choose a sunscreen with a sun protection factor (SPF) of at least 15, (SPF 30 or higher is somewhat better) and reapply it every two hours. A higher SPF number means more UVB protection—it does not describe UVA protection. For example, when using an SPF 15 sunscreen, you get the equivalent of one minute of UVB rays for every 15 minutes in the sun. Remember, all sunscreens only provide partial protection, and sunless tanning products do not protect against UV damage.
- Don't use tanning beds or sun lamps because they emit UVA and usually also UVB rays. Tanning bed use has been linked with an increased risk of melanoma, especially if its use started before the age of 30.[124]
- Keep babies younger than six months out of direct sunlight and protect children from the sun using sunscreen, hats, and protective clothing.

A study found that some of the 16 ingredients used in four sunscreens sold in the U.S. are absorbed through the skin and can be measured in the bloodstream.[125] The FDA rates zinc oxide and titanium oxide as safe, but there is too little information to rate the other 12 chemicals that were absorbed. In the study, avobenzone, the most common ingredient used in sunscreens, and oxybenzone were both absorbed and persisted in the bloodstream. Oxybenzone has been found to be toxic to corals and is banned in some places. Because there is little research on the health effects of sunscreen ingredients, the health effects of the chemicals that are absorbed is not known.[126]

Early detection of skin cancer by visual inspection of the skin is usually not difficult but may require evaluation by a dermatologist and require a skin biopsy to make a diagnosis. If detected early, successful treatment is very likely for squamous cell and basal cell cancers, the commonest forms of skin cancer. Early detection also increases the likelihood of curing malignant melanoma, a more serious and sometimes fatal form of skin cancer.

Medical exposure to radiation and cancer[127]

In today's medical world where defensive medicine is frequently practiced, over a lifetime, substantial exposure to medical X-rays is common. The FDA estimates that exposure to 10 mSv from an imaging test would be expected to increase the risk of death from cancer by about one chance in 2,000. Studies of young women exposed to high doses of X-rays to the chest and spine have found an increased risk of breast cancer in later life. Studies comparing people with meningioma (a usually benign brain tumor) are more likely to have had frequent dental X-rays than those without the tumors.

A study in England of exposure to radiation from CT (computed tomography X-ray) scans found that children who received a dose of at least 30 mGy (the same as 30 mSv and about equal to 10 years of background radiation) to the bone marrow had three times the risk of leukemia compared to those who received a dose of 5 mGy or less. A dose of 50 mGy or more to the brain was linked to more than three times the risk of brain tumors. A single CT scan can easily exceed 150 or even 1500 times a conventional X-ray, and multiple CT scans can deliver a radiation dose equivalent to many years of background radiation.[128]

According to one calculation, if current overuse continues, it will lead to 3% to 5% of U.S. cancers.[129] However, some X-ray studies cause minimal exposures, for example, the approximate radiation dose from a chest X-ray is 0.1 mSv, the equivalent of 10 days of background radiation. A single dental X-ray is about the same as an average day's background radiation, and a bone density scan even less.

For a table of radiation dose comparing background radiation with medical procedures prepared by the ACR (American College of Radiology) and the RSNA (Radiological Society of North America),[130] go to https://www.radiologyinfo.org/en/info.cfm?pg=safety-xray

The increased risk of cancer from exposure to any single test is likely to be very small. And it is reassuring that most studies have not documented an increased risk of cancer after imaging tests that use X-rays. But radiation exposure is cumulative over a lifetime. So imaging tests that use radiation should only be undertaken when medically indicated, and the parts of the body that aren't being imaged should be shielded.

Another question that may be raised is the risk of radiation from the treatment of cancer. According to the American Cancer Society, "When considering radiation exposure from radiation therapy treatment for cancer, the benefits generally outweigh the risks. Overall, radiation therapy alone does not appear to be a very strong cause of second cancers."

Known and probable human carcinogens[131]

The leading causes of an increased risk of cancer are lifestyle factors that we can control, such as smoking, obesity, alcohol, and lack of physical activity. Another important cause is random genetic mutations or "bad luck." However, many people are more afraid of exposure to carcinogens—the substances and exposures in our environment that can lead to cancer. We tend to exaggerate risks that are not under our control, for example, carcinogens in drinking water, as was dramatized in the movie Erin Brockovich; even though these risks may be less important than risks we can do something about, like quitting smoking or not drinking alcohol.

There is no way to avoid exposure to all known or suspected carcinogens. We encounter ionizing radiation from natural sources, such as cosmic radiation from the sun, and we use common medicines and chemicals that are probable carcinogens. Carcinogens increase the risk of cancer, but their cancer-causing potential is quite variable. Often, exposure to carcinogens does not cause cancer, but some carcinogens may cause cancer after very small exposures, and others only after prolonged, high levels of exposure. Many times, it is difficult to find out if a substance will cause cancer in humans. Although, as a precaution, it is usually assumed that exposures that cause cancer at larger doses in laboratory animals can also cause cancer in humans, some chemicals have been classified as carcinogens erroneously.

When the evidence is conclusive, the substance is classified as a carcinogen. When the available evidence is compelling but not considered conclusive, the substance may be classified as a probable carcinogen. Because it is impractical to study all of the thousands of chemical entities that exist, often there just isn't enough information to know how to classify a specific chemical and, of carcinogen candidates, most are listed as being of probable, possible, or unknown risk.

The principal agencies responsible for determining the cancer-causing potential of various substances are the WHO's International Agency for Research on Cancer (IARC) and in the U.S. the National Toxicology Program (NTP), the Environmental Protection Agency (EPA) and several other U.S. federal agencies. The lists prepared by these agencies only include those agents that have been evaluated, and the lists do not present information about how likely it is that an agent will cause cancer.

IARC has evaluated the cancer-causing potential of more than 900 likely candidates, placing them into one of the following groups:

- Group 1: carcinogenic to humans
- Group 2A: probably carcinogenic to humans
- Group 2B: possibly carcinogenic to humans
- Group 3: unclassifiable as to carcinogenicity in humans
- Group 4: probably not carcinogenic to humans

The National Toxicology Program (NTP) Report on Carcinogens has placed about 240 substances and exposures into two groups of agents:

- Known to be human carcinogens

- Reasonably anticipated to be human carcinogens

The U.S. Environmental Protection Agency (EPA) maintains the Integrated Risk Information System (IRIS), an electronic database that contains information on human health effects from exposure to certain substances in the environment. The EPA uses a rating system similar to that of IARC:

- Group A: carcinogenic to humans
- Group B: likely to be carcinogenic to humans
- Group C: suggestive evidence of carcinogenic potential
- Group D: inadequate information to assess carcinogenic potential
- Group E: not likely to be carcinogenic to humans

Reports from the IARC and NTP have more detailed information and the American Cancer Society website lists many chemicals known or probable carcinogens at http://www.cancer.org/cancer/cancercauses/othercarcinogens/generalinformation-aboutcarcinogens/known-and-probable-human-carcinogens

A few of the known human carcinogens that many people are familiar with are:[132]

- Aflatoxins (from mold)
- Alcoholic beverages
- Asbestos (all forms) and mineral substances (such as talc or vermiculite) that contain asbestos
- Engine exhaust, diesel
- Infection with Epstein-Barr virus
- Fission products, including strontium-90
- Formaldehyde
- Outdoor air pollution and the particulate matter in it
- Pesticides
- Radon-222 and its decay products
- Tobacco
- Ultraviolet (UV) radiation, including UVA, UVB, and UVC rays
- Ultraviolet-emitting tanning devices
- X- and gamma-radiation

There is evidence that pesticides used in agricultural, commercial, home, and garden applications are associated with increased cancer risk. Pesticides include a diverse group of chemical structures, and their uses include for control of insect pests (insecticides), molds (fungicides), and unwanted plants (herbicides). Specific chemical entities have been identified that are likely to increase the risk of lymphoma, leukemia, multiple myeloma, prostate and breast cancers. The current approach to reducing the risk of cancer is to minimize or eliminate exposure (e.g., by protecting farmworkers and choice of organically grown food) and to continue research to better identify and eliminate the most dangerous pesticides.[133] See Chapter 14, "Environmental Pollutants and Toxins," for additional information.

Air pollution[134]

About one in every 28,000 Americans may develop a cancer due to outdoor air pollutants, and more than 2 million people live where the lifetime cancer risk is particularly high. When outdoor air quality is bad due to weather conditions, traffic, industrial accidents, or forest fires, it is best to spend time indoors and limit time outside during peak traffic. Individual actions that can help keep the air cleaner include carpooling or use of public transportation, reducing or better yet eliminating fireplace and wood stove use, avoiding the use of gas-powered lawn and garden equipment, and refraining from burning leaves or other materials.

Indoor air can be as polluted or more polluted than outdoor air. In addition to avoiding tobacco smoke, it is best to avoid cleaning products, mothballs, and manufactured wood products that can release potentially carcinogenic volatile organic compounds (VOCs). Plywood and other manufactured wood products can release formaldehyde. To limit exposure to these sources, open windows and doors often and use venting systems in bathrooms and kitchens. Avoid the use of fireplaces, wood stoves, incense, air fresheners, and scented candles. More on this topic can be found in Chapter 14, "Environmental Pollutants and Toxins."

Genetics and family cancer syndromes[135]

Only about 5% of cancers are linked to the inheritance of mutated genes. These abnormal genes are present in every cell in the body, including the cells without cancer. Since each parent provides one of the two copies of most genes, if both genes are normal, acquiring two mutations is less likely and would usually take more time than acquiring the one new mutation that would be needed to cause a cancer if one gene is already abnormal. Cancers caused by inherited gene mutations that increase cancer susceptibility tend to occur earlier in life. When cancers are of an uncommon type, if they occur at younger ages than is usual, in a sex that is not usually affected (for example breast cancer in a male) or also occur in a close relative, like a parent or sibling, they are more likely to be caused by a family cancer syndrome. The well-known actor Angelina Jolie brought worldwide attention to the Hereditary Breast and Ovarian Cancer (HBOC) syndrome when she chose to undergo a bilateral mastectomy to reduce her risk of cancer because she carried the BRCA1 gene.

The lifetime risk for women of developing breast cancer in the general population is about 12%. Women with BRCA1 gene mutations have a 50% to 70% chance of developing breast cancer and a 39% to 46% chance of developing ovarian cancer by age 70. Women with a BRCA2 gene have a breast cancer risk of 40% to 60% and an ovarian cancer risk of 11% to 27%.[136] The HBOC syndrome can also increase the incidence of fallopian tube cancer, primary peritoneal cancer, male breast cancer, pancreatic cancer, prostate cancer, and some other cancers.[137]

A recent study found that breast cancer risk for women under age 40 with mutations of a third gene PALB2 was higher than among the general population, with a 14% chance of developing breast cancer by age 50 and a 35% chance of developing the disease by age 70. The study also found that individuals with PALB2 mutations had more than twice the risk of ovarian cancer compared with the general population.[138] [139]

A different inherited syndrome, hereditary non-polyposis colorectal cancer (HNP-CC), or Lynch syndrome, greatly increases a person's risk for colon cancer, with the cancer often occurring before age 50. HNPCC also leads to a high risk of endometrial cancer, cancer of the ovary, stomach, small intestine, pancreas, kidney, brain, ureters, and bile duct. In another syndrome that increases the risk of colon cancer called familial adenomatous polyposis, hundreds of polyps are seen in the colon. Li-Fraumeni syndrome is another familial cancer syndrome that can lead to the development of a number of cancers, most often in childhood. The list of cancers includes sarcoma, leukemia, central nervous system cancers, cancer of the adrenal cortex, and breast cancer.

Reducing risks for specific cancers

Avoiding tobacco products and alcohol, being physically active, avoiding overweight or obesity, avoiding red and processed meats, and consuming a whole-food plant-based diet can reduce the risk of contracting many cancers. Listed below are other preventive measures specific to particular cancers.

Breast cancer

Don't smoke; avoid weight gain, overweight and obesity; don't drink alcohol, one drink a day can increase risk by 7% and two to five drinks a day by 40%; be physically active; eat a whole food plant-based diet that minimizes saturated fat, red and processed meat; avoid prolonged use of hormone therapy at menopause and exposure of the breasts to radiation, especially at a young age. Get screened for breast cancer according to guidelines for age, medical, and family history. See Chapter 13, "Sexual and Reproductive Health," for a discussion of the links between oral contraceptives and breast cancer.

Among women at heightened risk for breast cancer, the U.S. Preventive Services Task Force recommends consideration of drugs that have been shown to reduce the risk of breast cancer: tamoxifen, raloxifene, and the three aromatase inhibitors, anastrozole, exemestane and letrozole.[140 141] For most women, the absolute risk reduction is quite modest. For a woman with an estimated five-year risk of breast cancer of 1.66% or more, about average-risk for a 60-year-old woman, a 50% risk reduction over five years would correspond to an absolute risk reduction of 0.83% and treating 120 women for five years would prevent one case of breast cancer. A 2020 *JAMA* review of the use of drugs to reduce breast cancer risk recommended their use by women with a five year breast cancer risk of 3% or greater because of an absolute risk reduction of about 7 to 9 fewer invasive breast cancers for every 1000 women treated over five years. The study authors noted that tamoxifen is the only medication that has been studied and approved for use in premenopausal women and that for postmenopausal women, tamoxifen or raloxifene are the first-line options. Raloxifene is associated with lower rates of significant harms, but tamoxifen has stronger evidence of long-term benefit.[142]

Tamoxifen, raloxifene, and aromatase inhibitors do not bring about much reduction in breast cancer mortality or overall mortality, likely because they reduce the risk of the more treatable cancers. The benefits of risk-reducing medications must be balanced against their harms, including venous thromboembolism for women taking tamoxifen and raloxifene. Use of the Breast Cancer Surveillance Consortium Risk Calculator can help identify women who might benefit from the long-term use of these medications.[143]

Cervical cancer

To reduce the risk of cervical cancer, get vaccinated against human papillomaviruses (HPVs) before becoming sexually active, use condoms to avoid unprotected sex, and follow the American Cancer Society (ACS) guidelines for regular cervical cytology screening.

Colorectal cancer

To reduce the risk of colorectal cancer, avoid red meat and processed meat intake and consume high levels of fiber. One estimate is that with a healthy lifestyle and diet (avoiding obesity, physical inactivity, alcohol consumption, early adulthood cigarette smoking, and red meat consumption), as much as 70% of colon cancer can be avoided.[144] Follow the ACS guidelines for regular colorectal screening, especially if a family history is present or if polyps have been detected previously. Aspirin has been found to decrease the risk of colon cancer; one estimate is that regular long-term (at least five years) use of aspirin reduces the risk of all gastrointestinal cancers by 8% to 15%.[145 146 147] However, the regular use of aspirin is associated with an increased risk of serious adverse events, including a 37% increase in the risk of gastrointestinal bleeding and a 38% increased risk of hemorrhagic stroke.[148] See Chapter 6, "Preventing Cardiovascular Disease" for additional discussion of the use of aspirin.

Endometrial (uterine) cancer

Be physically active, avoid being overweight or obese, and avoid taking estrogens. Follow the ACS guidelines for regular cytology screening.

Lung cancer

More than 85% of lung cancers result from smoking tobacco. Avoid tobacco use, secondhand smoke, and radon exposure. Smokers should avoid using high-dose beta-carotene vitamins because they increase lung cancer risk among smokers. See Chapter 5, "Vitamins and Other Supplements."

Mouth, larynx, throat, and esophagus cancers

Avoid all forms of tobacco, alcohol, and especially the combination of the two. Avoid obesity and the associated acid reflux that increases the risk for cancer in the lower esophagus and at the junction of the esophagus and stomach. Heat damage from very hot beverages and foods may also increase the risk of mouth and esophagus cancers.

Ovarian cancer

Family history is a risk factor for about 10% of ovarian cancers, and recent studies suggest that even short-term use of hormone replacement therapy (HRT) among women over age 50 increases risk. A meta-analysis of 52 separate studies published in *Lancet* found one additional case (i.e., an increase from about five to six cases over ages 50 to 64) among every 1000 women taking HRT for five years compared to non-users. In ex-users, risks decreased the longer ago hormone therapy use had been discontinued, but risks during the first few years after stopping HRT remained appreciable.[149 150] However, critics of the study point out that a 10 year, double-blind prospective study on hormone therapy that reported no new cases of ovarian cancer was not part of the meta-analysis and that elimination of low incidence studies might significantly skew the data and limit the validity of the meta-analysis.[151]

Pancreatic cancer

Pancreatic cancer may soon overtake colon cancer and become the second most common cause of cancer death in the U.S. Avoiding smoking that doubles risk, avoiding alcohol, avoiding obesity, avoiding impaired glucose tolerance (pre-diabetes) and type 2 diabetes can all decrease the risk for pancreatic cancer.

Prostate cancer

Very low-fat plant-based diets may lower the risk of prostate cancer and slow its progression if cancer is already present.[152] Dairy foods, vitamin E supplements, and diets high in calcium may raise prostate cancer risk.

Stomach cancer

Avoid a high intake of salt, salt-preserved foods, processed meat, and obesity to prevent the gastric reflux that has been linked to obesity. Individuals with ulcers or stomach cancer who are infected with H. pylori should be treated with antibiotics. A high intake of fresh fruits and vegetables is linked with a lower risk of stomach cancer.

Factors that are unlikely to significantly alter the risk of cancer

When it comes to causes of cancer, there is much that we don't know, especially about factors that may have a minor influence on risk, either increasing it or decreasing it. A number of issues that are of concern to people but are not likely to be important causes of cancer are discussed in this section. Keep in mind that it is best to pay attention to, and as far as possible, eliminate known causes of increased risk of cancer rather than focusing on something that has not been demonstrated to affect risk one way or the other and probably is not an important cause of an increased risk of getting cancer.

Injuries

With the rare exception of cancers arising from burn scars (usually squamous cell carcinomas), injuries, including broken bones, have not been linked to cancer.

Stress

Research has not found a link between a person's personality, stress, or mental health and cancer risk.

Microwaves, radio waves, and other types of radiofrequency radiation (RF)

Near ultraviolet, visible light, infrared, microwave, and low-frequency radio frequency (RF) are examples of non-ionizing radiation. RF radiation comes from both natural sources and from broadcasting radio and television signals, transmitting signals from cordless telephones, cellular phones, cell phone towers, radar, Wi-Fi and Bluetooth, microwave ovens, and airport millimeter-wave full-body scanners. RF radiation does not cause cancer by damaging DNA in cells the way ionizing radiation does. Although there has been concern that some forms of non-ionizing radiation might have biological effects that could result in cancer, there is little evidence that this occurs.

Most animal and laboratory studies have found no evidence of an increased risk of cancer with exposure to RF radiation. Studies of people who may have been exposed to RF radiation at their jobs (such as people who work around radar equipment) have found no clear increase in cancer risk. If RF radiation is absorbed in large enough amounts by materials containing water, such as food, fluids, and body tissues, it can produce heat. This is the way that microwave ovens work. Exposure to high-intensity microwaves could lead to burns and tissue damage, but microwaves from ovens are contained within the oven, there is no evidence that they pose a health risk.

The millimeter-wave scanners used in airports for security screening do not use any high-energy radiation such as x-rays, and the amount of RF radiation used is less than that from a cell phone. According to the FDA, these scanners have no known health effects.

Cell phones are in widespread use throughout the world, and although they are considered safe, there is still debate about whether they cause brain or other cancers. Cordless phones operate at about 1/600 the power of cell phones, so they are much less likely to be a concern in terms of health effects. Among the studies that have looked at the possible link between cell phones and cancer are case-control studies in which past cell phone use was compared in patients with brain tumors (cases) to people without brain tumors (controls). Although the Interphone study published in 2010 showed a possible link to glioma among the heaviest users, there was no overall increase in brain tumors, a finding consistent with most other studies. Since then, Swedish studies found an increased risk of malignant brain tumors among 10 year or longer users and a three-fold increased risk of glioma among 25-year users.

Other studies carried out in Denmark, the U.K., and France generally found no association between long-term cell phone use and brain tumors, although the French study did find an increased risk among the heaviest users.[153] It has been argued that the laws of physics provide evidence that cell phone use cannot cause cancer because cell phone radiation is just too weak to break chemical bonds; the radiation is 480,000 times weaker than UV rays.[154]

The American Cancer Society has summarized cell phone studies as follows:

- In most studies, patients with brain tumors do not report more cell phone use overall than the controls. This finding is true when all brain tumors are considered as a group, or when specific types of tumors are considered.
- Most studies do not show a "dose-response relationship," which would be a tendency for the risk of brain tumors to be higher with increasing cell phone use.
- Most studies do not show that brain tumors occur more often on the side of

the head, where people hold their cell phones.
- A few studies have found a possible link. For example, several studies published by the same research group in Sweden have reported an increased risk of tumors on the side of the head where the cell phone was held, particularly with 10 or more years of use. It is hard to know what to make of these findings because studies by other researchers have not had the same results, and there is no overall increase in brain tumors in Sweden during the years that correspond to these reports.

According to the National Cancer Institute (NCI): "Studies thus far have not shown a consistent link between cell phone use and cancers of the brain, nerves, or other tissues of the head or neck. More research is needed…." According to the FDA, which regulates the safety of radiation-emitting devices such as cell phones in the U.S.: "The majority of studies published have failed to show an association between exposure to radiofrequency from a cell phone and health problems." All of this inconclusive data suggests that if there is a risk from cell phone use, it is small. However, the studies do not include children, and although there is little data for pregnant women, a recent study suggests that the risk of miscarriage may be tripled by exposure to cell phone and other non-ionizing radiation.[155]

If you are concerned, use a wired headphone or use the speaker feature to minimize exposure since the intensity of emissions declines rapidly with distance from the source. The advice from the *University of California, Berkeley Wellness Letter* is, "One undisputed danger posed by cell phones is using them for any purpose while driving. The National Safety Council estimates that 20% of crashes (1.1 million a year) in the U.S. involve cell phones."[156]

Power lines, electrical devices, and extremely low frequency (ELF) radiation[157 158 159 160 161 162]

Extremely low frequency (ELF) radiation has even lower energy than other types of non-ionizing radiation like radiofrequency radiation, visible light, and infrared. Generating, transmitting, distributing, and using electricity all expose people to ELF radiation. Some sources include power lines, household wiring, and anything using electricity. This can include anything from refrigerators and vacuum cleaners to television sets and computer monitors.

The possible link between ELF radiation and cancer has been studied both in lab animals (exposed to strong magnetic fields) and in people. Studies in rats and mice have found no increase in the risk of any type of cancer, and most human studies of adults have not found links between ELF magnetic fields and cancer. Some studies that looked at the effect of ELF electric fields on childhood leukemia did not find a link, but others suggest a small increase in risk for children at the highest exposure levels compared to those with the lowest exposure levels. One estimate is that 1%

to 4% of childhood leukemia cases could be attributed to exposure to ELF radiation.[163]

The U.S. Federal Communications Commission (FCC) has said radiofrequency emissions from antennas used for cellular transmissions result in exposure levels on the ground that are typically thousands of times below safety limits. Therefore, there is no reason to believe that such towers could constitute a potential health hazard to nearby residents. The International Agency for Research on Cancer (IARC) has classified ELF magnetic fields as "possibly carcinogenic to humans." It also has stated that ELF electric fields are "not classifiable as to their carcinogenicity to humans."

In 1999, the National Institute of Environmental Health Sciences (NIEHS) described the scientific evidence suggesting that electromagnetic field (EMF) exposures pose a health risk as "weak," but stated that it was enough to "warrant limited concern." The NIEHS recommends that people concerned about their EMF (and ELF radiation) exposure find out where their major EMF sources are and move away from them or limit the time spent near them. Moving even an arm's length away from a source will dramatically lower exposure. For example, although being directly under a power line exposes you to its highest strength field, that exposure is often only in the range of what you could be exposed to when using certain household appliances.

The amount of energy given off by both CRT and flat screens is far below government exposure thresholds. No evidence supports a link between ELF radiation from television and computer screens and health problems. Still, some displays are designed to minimize the magnetic fields that they give off. These are labeled as being "TCO 99" or "TCO 03" compliant.

Early Detection of Cancer

To find cancer early, while it's small, less likely to have metastasized and is likely to be easier to successfully treat and cure, you should: 1) know and look for the signs and symptoms of cancer and, 2) have the recommended cancer screening exams. Some common cancers or pre-cancerous conditions can be detected and treated before symptoms appear. A variety of screening tests can also help determine if health-related symptoms and signs are caused by a cancer.

Signs and symptoms of cancer

Signs are manifestations (like weight loss) that can be detected by an individual and someone else. A symptom is something (like weakness or pain) that is felt or noticed by the person who has it. Both can be indications of injury, illness, or disease. For the detection of cancer, a good rule is not to ignore signs and symptoms, especially if they are of a long duration or are getting worse.

Since cancer can affect almost any part of the body, it can cause a wide variety of signs and symptoms. Sometimes even a very small tumor can cause symptoms. Cancers of the pancreas and ovary are examples of tumors that frequently cause few symptoms until they have grown large and metastasized. A cancer may also cause symptoms such as fever, fatigue or weight loss that are neither specific to any part of the body nor unique to cancer because many other health conditions can cause the same signs and symptoms. Signs and symptoms that warrant further investigation include unexplained weight loss, fever, fatigue, pain, change in bowel habits or bladder function, sores that do not heal, white patches inside the mouth or white spots on the tongue, unusual bleeding or discharge, persistent cough or hoarseness, thickening or lump in the breast or other parts of the body, indigestion or trouble swallowing, and a recent change in a wart or mole or any new skin change.

Cancer screening

During periodic routine health exams, in addition to obtaining a patient's history, health care providers may carry out a physical examination that could help detect cancers of the breast, thyroid, oral cavity, skin, lymph nodes, testes, and ovaries. If a sign, symptom, or finding on the physical exam warrants it, more tests may be indicated.[164] Often a biopsy is the only way to be sure whether or not cancer is present.

Although screening tests have the potential to extend lives or even prevent a death from cancer, they can also have drawbacks. They may be costly in time and resources, stressful, physically harmful, and misleading with false positives leading to unneeded biopsies and other tests. They may also result in false negatives that provide a false sense of security. Because new information is constantly being obtained through research, screening recommendations are likely to change frequently. Cancer experts often have legitimate disagreement about which screening tests are appropriate, how frequently to test, and at what ages they should be used. Furthermore, screening that is appropriate for one person's health circumstances is often different from that for another person. It is advisable to consult with your health care provider about which screening tests should be undertaken and on what schedule based on each person's individual circumstances.

General information about cancer screening is presented below, but it is important to consult your health care provider and follow up-to-date cancer screening recommendations—they change when there is new scientific information. A good guide can be found in the document, *American Cancer Society Guidelines for the Early Detection of Cancer* available at http://www.cancer.org/healthy/find-cancer-early/.

Screening for breast cancer[165]

Breast cancer screening options include mammograms, family history, genetic testing, and MRIs. There is considerable controversy about the most appropriate ages and frequency for mammograms, and decisions should be individualized according to family history and other risk factors after a consultation and discussion with a health care provider. Mammography may miss some cancers and result in false-negatives. False-positives can lead to unnecessary anxiety, additional testing, and unnecessary biopsies.

Some breast cancers can develop and spread rapidly between mammograms, so early detection does not work well to prevent illness and death from them. Other breast cancers, called ductal carcinoma in situ (DCIS) may stay small and local, but there is no good way to know if they would not cause problems, so these cancers are also treated.[166] Recently there has been a movement to follow up routine mammography screening among women with dense breasts with MRI studies because tumors are more difficult to detect in dense breasts. This practice detects more cancers but also increases the risk of biopsies when cancer is not present, and it is not known if the cancers needed to be found and treated to prevent illness and prolong life.[167] Advocacy groups such as the Susan G. Kommen Foundation have generally advocated more frequent screening than the National Institutes of Health or the U. S. Preventative Services Task Force (USPSTF), expert bodies that have expressed concern about overtesting, overdiagnosis and overtreatment.[168]

One reason screening recommendations may differ is that better evidence is needed to help women make screening decisions. For example, some breast cancer experts do not think it is certain that annual rather than biannual screening decreases breast cancer mortality. Some data suggests that annual screening may be more appropriate for premenopausal women because earlier diagnosis will help this group of women who are more likely to have tumors with less favorable prognostic characteristics.[169]

A key component of both ACS and USPSTF recommendations is that screening decisions should be individualized to reflect a woman's values and preferences as well as breast cancer risk.[170] However, considering the high level of publicity, emotion, and fears about cancer (especially about breast cancer), evidence-based decision-making may be difficult for medical practitioners and even more so for individual women. As Rosenbaum has noted in commenting on decisions about mammography, "...it is as much our job to figure out how to best help our patients lead healthier lives as it is to honor their preferences."[171]

A simplified version of the 2015 ACS recommendations for women at average risk is:[172]

- Women ages 40 to 44 should have the choice to start annual breast cancer screening with mammograms if they wish to do so. The risks of screening, as well as the potential benefits, should be considered.
- Women age 45 to 54 should get mammograms every year.
- Women age 55 and older should switch to mammograms every two years, or, have the choice to continue yearly screening.

The American College of Obstetrics and Gynecology (ACOG), as of June 2017, has a different recommendation for women at average risk:[173]

- ACOG recommends that women and their obstetrician/gynecologists engage in a dialogue that includes a discussion of the woman's health history, the benefits and harms of screening, and the woman's concerns, priorities, values, and preferences about the potential benefits and harms of screening.
- Annual or biannual mammograms beginning at age 40 until at least age 75 with the decision to discontinue screening mammography based on a shared decision-making process informed by the woman's health status and longevity.

Additional resources are available at http://www.acog.org/Womens-Health/Breast-Cancer-Screening.

The U. S. Preventative Services Task Force also has a different recommendation:

- For women at average risk begin routine screening at age 50
- Biennial screening mammography for women aged 50 to 74 years

USPSTF recommendations say: "While screening mammography in women aged 40 to 49 years may reduce the risk for breast cancer death, the number of deaths averted is smaller than that in older women and the number of false-positive results and unnecessary biopsies is larger. The balance of benefits and harms is likely to improve as women move from their early to late 40s," and notes that "In addition to false-positive results and unnecessary biopsies, all women undergoing regular screening mammography are at risk for the diagnosis and treatment of noninvasive and invasive breast cancer that would otherwise not have become a threat to their health, or even apparent, during their lifetime (known as 'overdiagnosis'). Beginning mammography screening at a younger age and screening more frequently may increase the risk for overdiagnosis and subsequent overtreatment."[174]

The USPSTF recommends counseling, risk assessment, and after evaluation, the testing of women with a personal, or family history, or ancestry (e.g., Ashkenazi Jewish ancestry where risk is one in 40), of breast, ovarian or peritoneal cancer associated with BRCA1/2 gene mutations. The USPSTF recommends against routine risk assessment, genetic counseling, or genetic testing for women whose personal or family history or ancestry is not associated with potentially harmful BRCA1/2 gene mutations.[175 176]

The International Agency for Research on Cancer (IARC) concluded that there was sufficient evidence that mammography reduces breast cancer mortality in women ages 50 to 69 and 70 to74, but limited evidence for women ages 40 to 44 and better but still limited evidence for women 45 to 49 years of age.[177]

Two letters to the editor of the *New England Journal of Medicine* commenting on the IARC working group report disagreed with their findings. One author pointed out that in European countries, reductions in breast cancer mortality were greater among women not screened than among those who were screened. He concluded that screening resulted in overdiagnosis, the detection of cancers that will not cause death or symptoms.[178] The other author disputed the IARC finding that mammography would decrease breast cancer mortality among women in the 70 to 74 age group.[179]

It is not surprising that when a Swiss Medical Board's report on mammography was made public in 2014, its recommendation to limit mammography programs was highly controversial.[180 181] It acknowledged that systematic mammography screening might prevent about one death attributed to breast cancer for every 1000 women screened, even though there was no evidence to suggest that overall mortality was affected. At the same time, it emphasized the harm — in particular, false-positive test results and the risk of overdiagnosis. The board, therefore, recommended that no new systematic mammography screening programs be introduced and that a time limit be placed on existing programs.

Additional evidence in favor of mammography reducing the risk of fatal breast cancer comes from a large Swedish study published in the journal *Cancer* in 2020.[182] In Sweden, the mammography screening recommendation is every 18 months beginning to at age 40 and every 24 months for those aged 55 to 69. The study of 549,091 women found a 41% lower incidence of breast cancer that was fatal within 10 years in women participating in screening compared with women not screened and a 25% reduction in the incidence of advanced disease. The study could not rule out the possibility that women who underwent screening had healthier behaviors that could account for the reductions in breast disease that were observed. A 2017 study among Dutch women published in the *British Medical Journal* found little evidence that mammography screening reduced advanced breast cancer or mortality.[183] However, several experts concluded that the evidence from the Swedish study indicates that screening saves lives.[184]

A study modeled the cost of the common practice of annual mammography compared to USPSTF guidelines of less frequent screening.[185] The estimated cost of annual screening of 85% of the population of women would be $10.1 billion compared to $3.5 billion for screening according to the USPSTF's recommendations, guidelines that the authors of the study consider to be based on scientific evidence and most likely to maximize patient benefit and minimize harm. The cost savings would be enough to double the annual budget of the National Cancer Institute.

According to the ACS, research does not show a clear benefit of physical breast exams done by either a health professional or by an individual, so regular clinical breast exams and breast self-exams are no longer recommended. Still, the ACS suggests that women should be familiar with how their breasts normally look and feel and report any changes to a health care provider right away.

For more information on breast cancer screening consult the ACS document *Breast Cancer: Early Detection* (http://www.cancer.org/cancer/breastcancer/moreinformation/breastcancerearlydetection/breast-cancer-early-detection-toc); the (2016) *Final Recommendation Statement, Breast Cancer: Screening of the U. S. Preventative Services Task Force* (http://www.uspreventiveservicestaskforce.org/Page/Document/RecommendationStatementFinal/breast-cancer-screening1); and the *Journal of the American Medical Association Patient Page* (http://jama.jamanetwork.com/article.aspx?articleid=2463258).[186]

Screening for colorectal cancer[187 188]

A 2020 draft recommendation of the USPSTF is that beginning at age 45 the initiation of these tests that find polyps and cancer:

- Flexible sigmoidoscopy every five years*, or
- Colonoscopy every 10 years, or
- Double-contrast barium enema every five years*, or
- CT colonography (virtual colonoscopy) every five years*
  * If the test is positive, a colonoscopy should be done.

A different schedule may be indicated based on previous findings, personal or family history. Colonoscopy is considered the "gold standard" of testing, the other tests are less reliable, but they have the advantage of being less invasive. An annual fecal occult blood test, or an annual immunochemical test (FIT), or an annual stool DNA test that can detect abnormal DNA from cancer or polyp cells may be helpful in detecting polyps and cancer.

The American Cancer Society provides information on colorectal cancer screening at http://www.cancer.org/cancer/colonandrectumcancer/moreinformation/colonandrectumcancerearlydetection/colorectal-cancer-early-detection-toc.

Screening for cervical cancer[189 190 191]

Based on increasing evidence, the trend in recommendations for cervical cancer is less frequent screening. Current guidelines call for cervical cancer screening with a cytology (Pap) test every three years beginning at age 21 up to age 65. Because women frequently clear HPV infections without treatment, women under age 21 should not be tested. The trend is to replace the Pap test with HPV testing that can detect the presence of the high-risk cancer-causing strains of HPV. Depending on age, a history of cervical cancer or findings of cervical pre-cancer, HPV testing, and a different screening schedule may be indicated.

In 2018 the U.S. Preventive Services Task Force recommended screening for cervical cancer every three years with cervical cytology alone in women aged 21 to 29 years and screening every three years with cervical cytology alone, every five years with DNA testing for high-risk HPV (hrHPV) alone, or every five years with hrHPV in combination with cytology (co-testing) in women aged 30 to 65 years. The USPSTF recommends against screening for cervical cancer in women younger than 21 years, against screening for cervical cancer in women older than 65 years who have had the adequate prior screening and are not otherwise at high risk for cervical cancer, and against screening for cervical cancer in women who have had a hysterectomy with removal of the cervix and do not have a history of a high-grade precancerous lesion or cervical cancer.[192] As with all cancer screening recommendations, ongoing research will help identify better cervical cancer screening recommendations, so check with your health care provider for up-to-date information and a discussion of how it best fits your own situation.[193]

The American Cancer Society offers a cervical cancer guide at http://www.cancer.org/cancer/cervicalcancer/detailedguide/index.

Screening for endometrial (uterine) cancer

Women should know that post-menopausal or any unexpected vaginal bleeding or spotting can be symptoms of endometrial cancer that should be evaluated by their health care provider. Based on symptoms and history, endometrial biopsies may be indicated.

The American Cancer Society offers an endometrial cancer guide at http://www.cancer.org/cancer/endometrialcancer/detailedguide/endometrial-cancer-detailed-guide-toc.

Screening for ovarian cancer

Similar to women with lung and pancreatic cancers, women with ovarian cancer may have few symptoms, so they are typically diagnosed in late stages, resulting in poor outcomes. Only 20% of patients with ovarian cancer are diagnosed with stage I disease; their five-year survival rates are greater than 90%. For women diagnosed with stage III or IV ovarian cancer, five-year survival rates are approximately 17% to 39%. In 2017 the U.S. Preventive Services Task Force (USPSTF) updated recommendations on screening for ovarian cancer and reiterated the recommendation against screening for ovarian cancer in asymptomatic women at average risk who are not known to have a high-risk hereditary cancer syndrome.[194 195 196] The task force concluded that there is no current test for the early detection of ovarian cancer suitable for widespread population use in women that could reduce ovarian cancer mortality.

Screening for lung cancer[197 198 199]

Lung cancer is the leading cause of cancer-related mortality in the U.S., with 159,000 deaths in 2014. Survival is greatly increased by early diagnosis and is underused by the heavy smokers for whom it is indicated. X-ray screening has a very high likelihood of false-positive results and has not been demonstrated to save lives when carried out among individuals at average risk. So routine screening is not indicated except for individuals who are at high risk of lung cancer due to cigarette smoking with at least a 30 pack-year smoking history and are either still smoking or have quit smoking within the last 15 years.

The American Cancer Society offers information on lung cancer prevention and screening at http://www.cancer.org/cancer/lungcancer-non-smallcell/moreinformation/lungcancerpreventionandearlydetection/lung-cancer-ped-toc.

Screening for prostate cancer

Prostate cancer is the second leading cause of cancer-related deaths among men. Indications of prostate cancer can be detected by testing for blood levels of prostate-specific antigen (PSA) and by a digital rectal exam. Further testing may include a biopsy. Although screening can help find many prostate cancers early, like breast cancer screening, PSA screening is an area of contentious debate, and medical science is still evaluating the evidence about whether the benefits of screening and treatment outweigh the side effects and other risks.

Opponents of screening maintain that the risk of harm outweighs the modest benefits and, therefore, that PSA screening should be uniformly discouraged. They argue that the PSA does not detect cancer, only that a man may have it; that the biopsies that detect cancer cannot reliably differentiate cancers that would never cause a problem (about one-third to one-half of prostate cancers) from potentially life-threatening cancers; that PSA testing has led to large numbers of men treated for clinically insignificant disease; and in some important studies no decrease in all-cause death rates, just fewer deaths from prostate cancer. Opponents of testing also point out that the side effects of treatment such as urinary and bowel incontinence and impotence are serious and cause long-lasting detriments to quality of life.

Proponents of prostate cancer screening argue that screening is responsible for approximately 45% to 70% of the decline in age-adjusted prostate cancer mortality observed in the U.S. over the past two decades and that PSA levels, family histories and other risk factors such as race should guide screening decisions.[200][201][202][203][204]

A 2014 evaluation of PSA test recommendations published in the *JAMA* suggested that harms could be reduced and outcomes could be improved by considering PSA testing every other year, and a high PSA threshold for biopsies.[205] The review also suggested that active surveillance or watchful waiting may be the optimal treatment strategy for men with lower-risk prostate cancers, particularly with a lower PSA level at diagnosis or a biopsy Gleason score of lower than 7, (the Gleason score is a 1-10 measure of how aggressive a prostate cancer is). Active surveillance includes serial PSA tests, physical examinations, and biopsy with treatment administered at a sign of more aggressive disease. Watchful waiting is observation with only palliative treatment offered when disease progresses.

The 2017 recommendation statement from the U. S. Preventative Services Task Force (USPSTF) notes that the largest trial to show a benefit of prostate cancer screening found that slightly more than one man per 1000 offered screening avoided death from prostate cancer, after an average follow-up of 13 years.[206][207] There is also evidence that three men per 1000 offered screening may avoid incurable metastatic disease after an average follow-up of 12 years.[208]

A 2017 review in the *New England Journal of Medicine* pointed out: "That there is still no clarity about the usefulness and desirability of routine PSA-based screening after 25 years and two large trials suggests that its net benefit is unlikely to be more than marginal, whereas the harms are proven and substantial."[209]

Guidelines for screening have been promulgated by several professional groups. The American Cancer Society recommends that starting at age 50, men should talk to a health care provider about the pros and cons of testing so they can decide if testing is the right choice for them. If you are Black or have a father or brother who had prostate cancer before age 65, you should have this talk with a health care provider starting at age 45.[210]

In 2018 the U.S. Preventive Services Task Force (USPSTF) recommended that for men aged 55 to 69 years, the decision to undergo periodic PSA-based screening for prostate cancer should be an individual one and should include discussion of the potential benefits and harms of screening with their clinician.[211] The USPSTF recommends against PSA-based screening for prostate cancer in men 70 years and older.

The American Urological Association (AUA)[212] recommends shared decision making for men aged 55 to 69 years. For men electing to be screened, an interval of two years or more may be preferable to annual screening. The AUA recommends against PSA screening in men younger than 40 years, against routine screening between ages 40 and 54 years for men at average risk, and against routine screening in men older than 70 years or any man with less than a 10-year to 15-year life expectancy."[213] In 2018 the AUA released the following statement: "We agree with the USPSTF that Black American men and men with a family history of prostate cancer are at an increased risk of developing the disease, and that they should discuss with their physicians the benefits and risks of testing in order to make a shared, informed decision."[214]

A large trial evaluating the value of PSA screening was reported on in 2018.[215][216] In the cluster-randomized trial in the U.K., men aged 50 to 69 years had a single PSA screening test or usual care, with an estimated 10-15% of men getting a PSA test. Over a 10-year period, the one-time screening increased the detection of low-risk prostate cancer cases but was not associated with a significant difference in cumulative prostate cancer mortality.

Writing in the *JAMA* in 2018, H. Ballentine Carter recommends that first, physicians should offer screening primarily to patients for whom the evidence of benefit is strongest, i.e., those aged 55-69 years.[217] And since older age is associated with more aggressive prostate cancer, a very healthy older man with the prospects of extended life might benefit from PSA testing. Nevertheless, routine screening of average-risk men 70 years and older should be rare, because older men are more likely than younger men to experience the harms of screening, diagnosis, and treatment. Second, a 2- to 4-year PSA testing interval, rather than annual testing, could reduce false-positive test results and overdiagnosis without substantially sacrificing the benefits of screening. Third, a family history of cancer mortality related to adenocarcinoma (including prostate cancer) and Black American race may identify men with more to gain from screening compared with a man at average risk.

A 2020 article in the *New England Journal of Medicine* noted that increased PSA screening contributed to a decline in the incidence of and deaths from metastatic prostate cancer but did not reliably translate into increased longevity.[218] And while a few people receive substantial benefit from extensive PSA screening, many more are exposed to over-diagnosis and over-treatment with needless biopsies and operations. The authors suggest raising the PSA threshold for referral to urology and likely biopsy from 4 to 10 ng/mL and careful evaluation by urologists of PSA level trends and other factors, such as a Gleason scores, to guide decisions about treatment or active surveillance.

A 2020 study in the *New England Journal of Medicine* considers that with the increased emphasis on active surveillance and better detection, the balance of benefits and harms of screening is more favorable for screening than is generally appreciated.[219] This is because PSA screening avoids incurable metastatic prostate cancer disease and mortality and new methods of active surveillance diminish the harms of overdiagnosis.

The field of prostate cancer screening is evolving rapidly with biopsies guided by MRI, ultrasound, and the development of new genetic tests to help identify aggressive cancers.[220]

Screening for skin cancer

The most serious form of skin cancer is melanoma. They constitute less than 5% of skin cancers but cause an estimated 75% of skin cancer deaths.[221] Melanoma are usually pigmented lesions. Any skin change, including those to a wart, mole, or freckle that changes color, size, or shape, or that loses its sharp border may be a melanoma and should be evaluated by a health care provider, preferably a dermatologist. If found early and it has not grown deep into the skin, melanoma can be treated successfully. The five-year survival rate (percentage of people who live at least five years after diagnosis) at this stage is around 97%. After melanoma has metastasized, the five-year survival rate is less than 20%.

According to the American Cancer Society, the most important warning sign of melanoma is a new spot on the skin or a spot that is changing in size, shape, or color.[222] Another important sign is a spot that looks different from all of the other spots on your skin (known as the ugly duckling sign). If you have one of these warning signs, have your skin checked by a dermatologist.

The ABCDE rule is another guide to the usual signs of melanoma. Be on the lookout and tell your doctor about spots that have any of the following features:

- A is for Asymmetry: One half of a mole or birthmark does not match the other.
- B is for Border: The edges are irregular, ragged, notched, or blurred.
- C is for Color: The color is not the same all over and may include different shades of brown or black, or sometimes with patches of pink, red, white, or

blue.

- D is for Diameter: The spot is larger than 6 millimeters across (about ¼ inch—the size of a pencil eraser), although melanomas can sometimes be smaller than this.
- E is for Evolving: The mole is changing in size, shape, or color.

Some melanomas don't fit these rules. It's important to tell your doctor about any changes or new spots on the skin, or growths that look different from the rest of your moles.

Other warning signs are:

- A sore that doesn't heal
- The spread of pigment from the border of a spot into the surrounding skin
- Redness or a new swelling beyond the border of the mole
- Change in sensation, such as itchiness, tenderness, or pain
- Change in the surface of a mole, such as scaliness, oozing, bleeding, or the appearance of a lump or bump

Although attention to visual signs of skin cancer has been recommended, there is doubt about the value of visual inspection for screening for skin cancer. The U.S. Preventive Services Task Force (USPSTF) found that evidence to assess the net benefit of screening for skin cancer with a visual skin examination is limited.[223] [224] Even doctors find it difficult to tell the difference between melanoma and an ordinary mole. The lack of clear cut evidence of the value of skin inspection suggests that it is important to consult a dermatologist to evaluate any areas of skin that concern you, to inspect areas that may be hard for an individual to see, and when indicated, to biopsy lesions to make definitive diagnoses.

To see examples of normal moles and melanomas, visit the Skin Cancer Image Gallery at:http://www.cancer.org/cancer/skincancer/galleries/skin-cancer-images.

Thyroid neoplasia

For years thyroid tumors classified as cancers were treated with surgical excision of the thyroid (total thyroidectomy), multiple radioactive iodine treatments, and a lifetime of daily doses of thyroid hormone. This is appropriate care for some aggressive thyroid cancers but not for the most common type, papillary thyroid cancer. Recently an international group reclassified papillary thyroid cancers as a non-malignancy because they have almost no likelihood of metastasis. The new name for the condition is "noninvasive follicular thyroid neoplasm with papillary-like nuclear features" or NIFTP.[225]

When the US Preventive Services Task Force (USPSTF) released its latest recommendation, it advised against routine screening for thyroid cancer among asymptomatic adults, reaffirming a position it has held since 1996. The USPSTF update says that such screening leads to "overdiagnosis and overtreatment" of relatively slow-growing (indolent) tumors, the sort that the reclassification addresses.[226 227]

Genetic counseling and testing[228]

If cancer is diagnosed in a close relative, especially if it is of an uncommon type or occurs at a younger than usual age, the cancer is more likely to be caused by a family cancer syndrome. It then may be desirable to carry out genetic testing to look for gene mutations that might put a person at heightened risk of getting cancer and other diseases. A negative result may help relieve anxiety or uncertainty. A positive result can help a person decide to undertake preventive measures. This might include taking medicines (chemoprevention), preventive (prophylactic) surgery, lifestyle changes, increased awareness of cancer signs and symptoms, and possibly earlier, more extensive and more frequent screening so as to find disease earlier, when treatment is more likely to be successful.

The American Cancer Society cautions about genetic testing: "The test can tell what might happen, but it cannot tell what will happen. On the other hand, a negative result does not mean you have no risk of getting the disease... A positive genetic test result can also affect other family members. More family members may need to be tested. Sometimes family secrets are revealed as a result – paternity, adoptions, or other difficult issues may come up. Having a gene or passing a gene on to children can bring out feelings of guilt or anger."

The issue of privacy may be a concern in that employers and insurance companies might get and use genetic information to discriminate against a person by not hiring or promoting them. The Genetic Information Nondiscrimination Act (GINA) law forbids most employers from doing this. GINA also bars health insurers from turning down people or charging higher premiums for health insurance based on genetic information or the use of genetic counseling and testing. The law also bars these insurers from asking for or requiring genetic tests.

Summary of the essential facts

- Avoid tobacco, vaping, and secondhand smoke. It is never too late to quit.
- Avoid overweight and obesity.
- Be physically active.
- Eat a whole-food plant-based diet high in fiber, fruit, and vegetables (at least 2½ cups a day).
- Avoid refined grains and added sugar.
- Eliminate or at least limit red meats.
- Eliminate processed meats.
- Avoid high heat cooking of high-protein foods (poultry, meat, fish).
- Do not drink alcohol or at least limit it to one alcoholic drink a day or less.
- Protect your skin from the sun.
- Limit CT Scans and X-rays.
- Test for radon.
- Avoid hazardous workplace exposures.
- Avoid indoor and outdoor air pollution .
- Get girls and boys vaccinated against HPV.
- Have regular check-ups and up-to-date recommended cancer screening tests.

This chapter owes much to information made available by the American Cancer Society (ACS), and the reader is encouraged to consult the ACS website at http://www.cancer.org for easy to understand information about cancer prevention and treatment. For questions about cancer, you can call the American Cancer Society anytime, day or night, at 1-800-227-234.

8
Preventing Dementia

According to a survey, dementia is second only to cancer as the most dreaded illness in the United States.[1] Undoubtedly any sign of cognitive decline can raise fears of incipient dementia and become a source of anxiety among people who have normal age-related memory lapses. A decline in thinking, learning, and judgment skills due to aging is nearly universal. Beginning as early as our late 40s and 50s, almost everyone experiences some degree of memory loss. As brain processing speed slows, we become slower to retrieve information and slower to learn new things.

Early cognitive decline seldom interferes with normal living. It may progress to mild cognitive impairment (MCI) that is characterized by minimal occupational impairment, increased difficulty with complex tasks, greater problems with memory or attention compared to others of the same age.[2] MCI is not Alzheimer disease or dementia, but it makes it four times more likely that a person will progress to dementia. MCI is estimated to affect far more people than those with dementia, perhaps 10% to 20% of Americans older than age 65. A review of the management of MCI suggests there is value in interventions focused on aerobic exercise, mental activity, and cardiovascular risk factor control. So far, no drug has proven to be effective.[3]

Many people have normal age-related memory lapses, and others have reversible cognitive issues secondary to stress, depression, or lack of sleep. But to make the diagnosis of dementia requires a finding of significant impairment of at least two of the following mental functions:[4]

- Memory
- Communication and language
- Ability to focus and pay attention
- Reasoning and judgment

- Visual perception

Alzheimer disease

Alzheimer disease (AD) and dementia from other causes is a leading cause of disability and death. In individuals over 71 years of age, the prevalence of dementia in the U.S. is estimated to be nearly 14%, with 10% attributed to Alzheimer disease and 4% to other causes such as vascular disease. The prevalence of dementia increases from 5% of those ages 71 to 79 to 37% of those over 90.[5] According to the Alzheimer Association, 5.4 million Americans are living with the disease today, and that number could rise as high as 16 million by 2050.[6]

People with the apolipoprotein E4 (ApoE4) gene (and a few other rare genes) are at high risk of Alzheimer disease. About 25% of Americans have a single copy of the ApoE4 gene and a lifetime Alzheimer risk of 30%. The 2% to 3% with two copies have a lifetime risk of between 50% and 90%. This can be compared to a risk of 9% to 10% for most people who are without any copies of the ApoE4 gene. The greatly increased risk of Alzheimer disease with either one, or worse yet with two copies of the ApoE4 gene, suggests that genetic testing should be considered, especially if a family member has Alzheimer and, even more urgently, if it occurs at a young age.

Although considered the sixth leading cause of death, many death certificates will list other diseases such as urinary tract infection, pneumonia, or generalized organ failure as the cause of death when AD has caused the deterioration of basic bodily functions or other health problems that led to the terminal illness. One recent study estimates that the number of deaths caused or contributed to by AD is six times higher than previously thought, and therefore, AD is possibly the third leading cause or contributing cause of death with as many as 503,000 U.S. deaths in 2010.[7]

Nearly 20% of Medicare dollars are spent on people with Alzheimer disease and other dementias. The Alzheimer Association projects that in 2050, treatment may require as much as one of every three Medicare dollars. Total payments for health care, long-term care, and hospice for patients with dementia were estimated to be $236 billion in 2016 with the potential to grow to more than $1 trillion in 2050.[8]

The brain pathology of Alzheimer disease is characterized by extracellular plaque deposits of the protein fragment beta-amyloid and intracellular twisted strands or tangles of the protein tau, inflammation, brain nerve cell damage, and nerve cell death. A theory, espoused by Dale Bredesen and others, is that the damaging beta-amyloid deposition is a response of the brain attempting to protect itself from three metabolic and toxic threats:[9]

- Inflammation, from infection, diet (e.g., trans-fats), or other causes
- Decline and shortage of supportive nutrients, hormones, and other brain supporting chemicals
- Toxic substances such as metals or biotoxins, produced by microbes such as molds

Bredesen considers AD to be the result of a lack of brain nourishing factors and a surfeit of toxic factors, many of which relate to modern lifestyles that lead to brain damage. His recommended approach to prevention and treatment of Alzheimer disease is to identify which of the many contributors to the three classes of threats to brain health are afflicting an individual, to minimize or better yet remove the threats, and to increase brain supporting factors.

My UCSF colleague Edward Blonz, has advanced a theory that the genesis of AD is a lack of adequate brain cell nourishment with energy resources. He considers that an age-related decline in the ability of glucose to cross the blood-brain barrier creates metabolic stress that shifts the normal, benign processing of amyloid-protein precursors toward pathways associated with the production of the amyloid-plaques and the tau-containing neurofibrillary tangles that are characteristic of the disease.[10] The implication of this hypothesis is to focus research on developing various methods to maintain adequate brain energy resources. For example, ensuring the health of the vascular system through maintaining physical fitness may improve the ability of glucose to cross the blood-brain barrier, and a high fiber diet may make it easier for other nutrients to cross the blood-brain barrier.

Vascular dementia

Vascular dementia is secondary to multiple small strokes or atherosclerosis that compromises flow in blood vessels and injures brain tissue. Vascular dementia often causes gradual changes in cognition as damage accumulates. Pathological studies show that many individuals have mixed dementia with the brain changes of more than one type of dementia presenting simultaneously. Research is now focused on the role of the vascular system in preventing amyloid deposition and Alzheimer disease because blood vessels have an essential role in bringing nourishment and oxygen to and removing toxins from the brain. There is some evidence that anemia is associated with an increased risk of AD.

Prevention of Alzheimer disease

Healthy lifestyle behaviors can help slow age-related cognitive decline and help prevent Alzheimer disease and other causes of dementia. Preventive interventions should address the multiple factors that increase risk. They include being physically active, avoiding cardiovascular disease risk factors such as high blood pressure and unhealthy diets, preventing diabetes by avoiding overweight and obesity, avoiding alcohol and smoking, managing depression, getting enough uninterrupted sleep, and possibly cognitive training.[11] One estimate is that about one-third of AD cases worldwide could be prevented by measures like these.[12]

More than 100 clinical trials with more than 200 drugs have been studied so far in largely unsuccessful attempts to reverse or at least halt the progress of Alzheimer.[13] Prevention seems to be a more promising approach. Although some individuals may have one of the 20 AD linked genotypes, including various apolipoprotein E (notably ApoE4) genetic variations, that can increase susceptibility by five or even 15 times, a healthy lifestyle seems to provide some protection. This potential is shown by the fact that among identical twins with the same genotype but different lifestyles, the onset of AD may differ by as much as 15 years.

Lifestyle and dementia

The Caerphilly Collaborative Cohort Study assessed the association of five lifestyle factors with various health indicators among men aged 45 to 59 over 30 years.[14] The five factors were:

- Not smoking
- Low body weight (BMI 18 to 25)
- Regular exercise (at least one-half hour walking or equivalent, e.g., 2 miles of walking or 10 miles of biking a day)
- Plant-based diet (at least three servings of fruit and/or vegetables a day)
- Low alcohol intake (one glass of wine a day or less)

The study found that of those studied, just 5% had "healthy" behavior defined as adhering to four or five of the healthy behaviors. They had about a 60% lower incidence of dementia than the 39% of men who were defined as "unhealthy" with no or just one of the five healthy behaviors.[15 16] After the exclusion of men with early-onset dementia, of the five behaviors, exercise was found to have the strongest correlation with avoidance of dementia.

The Finnish Geriatric Intervention Study to Prevent Cognitive Impairment and Disability (FINGER) was a randomized controlled trial based on the theory that multiple factors are involved in the causation of Alzheimer disease.[17 18] It carried out the simultaneous modification of vascular and lifestyle-related risk factors that have been found to be associated with dementia risk in observational studies: an intensive 2-year Mediterranean style diet, supervised exercise, cognitive training, and cardiovascular risk monitoring. The study assessed changes in cognition with a comprehensive neuropsychological test battery and compared the intervention group to a control group that got general health advice and cardiovascular monitoring. The study found that both groups improved cognitive performance, but the intervention group benefited 25% more than the control group. The authors of the study concluded that their trial suggests that a multifactorial intervention could improve or maintain cognitive functioning in at-risk older people.

A study from the U.K. found that both high genetic risk and absence of healthy lifestyle factors (not smoking, regular physical activity, healthy diet, and moderate alcohol consumption) were associated with increased risk of developing dementia.[19] Those with the lowest lifestyle scores had a 34% higher risk of dementia compared to those with the best. A low lifestyle score, together with high genetic risk, tripled the risk of dementia compared to those with low genetic risk and the healthiest lifestyles. Having the highest genetic risk increased the risk of dementia by 91% over those at low genetic risk. A favorable lifestyle decreased the risk of dementia among those with high genetic risk by about one-third.

Physical activity and dementia

Studies suggest that physical activity and cardiovascular fitness are important to protect the brain against Alzheimer disease, age-related cognitive decline, and the commonest vascular causes of dementia— atherosclerosis and mini-strokes.[20 21] Although the significance of the findings is uncertain, studies suggest that long periods of sitting are associated with decreased blood flow to the brain—getting up for a walk every 30 minutes or so can counter this.[22 23]

Experiments with laboratory animals have found that exercise has a beneficial effect on brain health. They show that exercise induces the growth of new brain cells, including in the hippocampus, a brain region that is essential for memory and learning. Studies of lab mice, bred to be predisposed to develop Alzheimer disease, found that compared to those who were sedentary, the mice that exercised on running wheels had reduced levels of beta-amyloid plaque.[24]

A randomized controlled study of exercise training demonstrated that loss of hippocampal volume in late adulthood (usually about 1% a year) is not inevitable and can be reversed with moderate-intensity exercise. One year of aerobic exercise was sufficient for the increased hippocampal volume that is a marker for improved memory function.[25] A long-term study of nearly 19,500 healthy people found that at age 70, only 0.8% of study participants were affected with dementia.[26] But by age 85, this proportion increased to 14.8%. After an average follow-up of 25 years, the study found that those who were most physically fit, based on an exercise treadmill test when the study began, were about one-third less likely to develop dementia than those who were the least fit. The authors of the study were careful to point out that their findings do not prove that staying fit will prevent dementia, but the study does suggest a strong association between maintaining high physical fitness and preventing dementia.

Another study evaluated 2,257 physically capable retired men in Hawaii between the ages of 71 and 93.[27] The research found that men who walked less than 400 meters (a quarter-mile) a day were almost twice as likely to develop Alzheimer or other forms of dementia as men who walked more than two miles daily. In a similar study, women aged 70 years and older who participated in higher levels of physical activity scored better on cognitive performance tests and showed less cognitive decline than women who were less active.[28] Women who walked at an easy pace for at least 90 minutes per week (13 minutes a day) had higher cognitive scores than those who walked less than 40 minutes per week (6 minutes a day). Women with the highest levels of physical activity had significantly less cognitive decline than women with the lowest levels of physical activity.

Another study has shown that not only does physical activity slow age-related mental decline but that it can improve cognition.[29 30] The study found that previously sedentary people over age 60 who walked rapidly for 45 minutes three days a week could significantly improve their mental-processing abilities. The study indicates that aerobic exercise creates new neurons and connections. A 2016 study found that the most physically active elderly had less age-related loss of brain volume than those who were sedentary.[31] A higher volume of gray matter was found among the most active participants in the study, those who had about 500 calories a day of extra energy expenditure.

A study of the fitness records of 30,000 Norwegians found that after 10 years, people who remained fit throughout the period were 40% to 50% less likely to develop dementia than those who started out and remained unfit.[32] Those men and women who entered middle age out of shape and then gained fitness also equally reduced their later risk of dementia—more evidence that it is never too late to start and benefit from exercise.

Most studies on the link between exercise and cognitive health have focused on aerobic activities such as running. To see if weight training would have similar results, a study compared brain scans of three groups of women with existing brain white matter lesions.[33] One group undertook twice a week resistance training, a second group did once a week resistance training, and a third group just worked on balance and stretching twice a week. At the end of a year, the twice a week weight training group improved physical functioning such as walking speed and had less progressive shrinkage and other signs of damage to their brain white matter than the other two groups.

A meta-analysis review of 18 previous studies of exercise on cognition published in the journal *Psychological Science* noted the following benefits:[34]

- Exercise programs involving both aerobic exercise (walking, running, swimming, cross-country skiing, bicycling) and strength training produced better results on cognitive abilities than either one alone.
- Older adults benefit more than younger adults do from physical activity, possibly because older adults have more to gain as age-related declines become more prevalent.
- More than 30 minutes of exercise per session produced the greatest benefit, a finding consistent with many existing guidelines for adults.

One question is, how intense and how long does exercise have to be to gain cognitive benefits? There is recent evidence from one study that even 10 minutes of very easy exercise improves immediate brain functioning, as seen in scans and performance on memory tests.[35] A different study found that a single 30-minute workout of moderate intensity (70% of maximum effort) also immediately increased brain activity in areas needed to recall memories of common knowledge, also termed semantic memory.[36]

Another study contrasted the cognitive benefits of steady walking on a treadmill for 50 minutes three times a week with interval training that consisted of 4 rounds of high-intensity walking on an inclined treadmill for 4 minutes, followed by 3 minutes of easy walking.[37] The incline walking was intense enough to boost heart rates to 90% of each person's maximum. After only 12 weeks, the high-intensity interval walkers showed significant improvements in both physical endurance and memory. This study is consistent with many others that show that the greater the intensity of physical activity, the greater the gains of physical and cognitive fitness.

However, not every study of physical activity has shown benefits to cognition. A 24-month trial to determine whether a physical activity program results in better cognitive function, lower risk of mild cognitive impairment (MCI) or dementia, or both, compared with a health education program, did not result in improvements in cognitive function.[38]

The *2018 Physical Activity Guidelines Advisory Committee Scientific Report* concluded that there is moderate evidence for an association between greater amounts of physical activity and better cognition, including performance on academic achievement tests; better performance on neuropsychological tests, such as those involving processing speed, memory, and executive function; and decreased risk of dementia.[39]

Studies suggest that physical activity is a moderately effective way to improve brain health. Regular aerobic exercise increases blood flow to the brain and helps to support the formation of new neural connections. Physical exercise has been shown to improve attention, reasoning, and components of memory. Aerobic exercise training can be expected to bring about a slowing of loss or modest gains in cognitive performance.

Multiple factors increase the risk of dementia.

Diabetes, alcohol, smoking, and other cardiovascular disease risk factors, not just physical fitness, also influence the risk of cognitive decline and dementia. A study among veterans measured physical fitness with a treadmill test at the average age of 60 and determined cognitive status based on medical records at an average of 10 years later, at which time 5.8% of the study sample were evaluated to have some form of cognitive impairment.[40] Those scoring six or lower metabolic equivalents on their treadmill fitness test had a more than four times greater risk of cognitive impairment, including Alzheimer disease than those with scores of 12 or higher.

The risk of cognitive impairment dropped 8% with every 1-point increase in exercise capacity. Smoking, that increased the risk of cognitive impairment by 44%, age and high cholesterol were identified as risk factors for cognitive decline. The greater the number of risk factors, age, high BMI, smoking, and low fitness, the greater the risk of cognitive impairment. At 15 years of follow-up, of those without any risk factors, very few had dementia or cognitive impairment, whereas, among those with four risk factors, about one-third had dementia or cognitive impairment.

Diabetes is a risk factor for dementia

Diabetes is a known risk factor for dementia, and higher glucose levels increase the risk of dementia in people without diabetes.[41] The mechanism by which diabetes affects cognition is not fully understood, but there is some evidence that vascular disease secondary to diabetes may be the main culprit rather than an increase in the plaques and tangles found in Alzheimer disease.[42 43 44 45] A 2017 study found that overweight and obese participants with type 2 diabetes had more severe and progressive abnormalities in brain structures and cognition during early-stage type 2 diabetes compared with normal-weight study subjects.[46]

Alcohol is a risk factor for dementia

Heavy alcohol consumption impairs cognitive performance with both immediate and long-term deleterious effects on the brain's anatomy, neurological, and psychological functioning. Although there are some studies that suggest that moderate alcohol consumption, especially red wine, provides some protection against Alzheimer disease, existing data do not support the practice of initiating or maintaining consumption of alcohol as a way to prevent dementia.[47 48 49 50 51]

A 2017 study in the British Medical Journal reinforces the evidence that for brain health, it is best to avoid all alcohol consumption.[52] The study assessed the alcohol consumption and cognition of 550 British civil servants over 30 years and found that the amount of alcohol that can be consumed without brain damage is lower than previously thought, and there is no cognitive advantage to any level of drinking. The study considered links between various levels as defined by units of alcohol use, cognition, and brain structure. The study defined a unit as 10 ml of pure alcohol. About two units are in a large beer, 9 per bottle of wine, and one in a 25 ml hard liquor shot.

Alcohol use was found to be associated with impaired white matter microstructure, and reduced right-sided hippocampal volume in a dose-dependent manner. Even men who drank moderately, defined as 14 to 21 units of alcohol a week, were three times more likely to have hippocampal atrophy than abstainers. Very light drinking, 1-6 units a week, conferred no protection relative to abstinence. Higher alcohol consumption was associated with reduced white matter integrity and a faster decline in verbal fluency.

The study found that alcohol use by 24.6% of women and 40.3% of men over the 30 year period of the study averaged 14 units (112gm) or greater per week placing a high proportion of the study group at three times the odds of hippocampal atrophy and, on average, and compared to abstainers, suffering a 17% greater decline in verbal fluency over 30 years. A commentary on the study estimated that alcohol-related brain damage accounts for possibly 10% of early-onset dementia and potentially 10% to 24% of dementia cases in nursing homes.[53 54]

Cardiovascular disease is a risk factor for dementia

Being obese, smoking, high blood pressure, high cholesterol, and diabetes are well known cardiovascular risk factors. Their presence in mid-life is associated with an increased risk of the amyloid plaques associated with dementia later in life.[55]

A study published in the *JAMA* in 2017 considered the links between brain amyloid and the following cardiovascular risk factors: body mass index ≥30, current smoking, hypertension, diabetes, and total cholesterol ≥200 mg/dl.[56 57] The study found that over an average of nearly 24 years, compared to those with no midlife vascular risk factors, the odds of elevated brain amyloid with one vascular risk factor present was 88% higher and with two or more vascular risk factors the risk was nearly tripled at 2.88 times. The strongest association between risk factors and brain amyloid was found among study subjects who were obese at midlife. They were twice as likely to have elevated brain amyloid in later life as those of normal weight. Late-life vascular risk factors were not associated with late-life brain amyloid deposition. The study authors concluded that their findings are consistent with a role for vascular disease in the development of Alzheimer disease.

Additional evidence of the role of CVD in dementia comes from a study in the *JAMA* that found that people with optimal cardiovascular risk factors are at substantially reduced risk for dementia.[58 59 60 61] In the study, people ages 65 and older who did not have dementia or cardiovascular disease underwent neuropsychological testing for dementia every two or three years for an average of almost nine years. The seven optimal risk factors/metrics were those found by the American Heart Association to be associated with optimal cardiovascular health:

- Not smoking
- Healthy weight, body mass index (BMI) less than 25
- Regular physical activity
- Healthy diet, eating fish twice a week or more and fruits and vegetables at least three times a day
- Total cholesterol (untreated) below 200 mg/dL
- Fasting blood sugar (untreated), below 100 mg/dL
- Blood pressure (untreated), below 120/80 mm Hg.

On average, the presence of each optimal factor was associated with a 10% lower risk of developing dementia. Over the course of the study, the incidence rate of dementia per 100 person-years was 1.56 for those with no to two optimal risk factors, 1.23 for those with three or four optimal factors, and 0.83 for those with five to seven optimal factors. Only 7% of people had five to seven optimal factors, but their incidence of dementia was about half that of those with no to two optimal risk factors. The researchers controlled for education, socioeconomic status, and the presence of the APOE-4 gene that increases dementia risk.

The study authors concluded that "In this cohort of older adults, increased numbers of optimal cardiovascular health metrics and a higher cardiovascular health score were associated with a lower risk of dementia and lower rates of cognitive decline. These findings may support the promotion of cardiovascular health to prevent risk factors associated with cognitive decline and dementia."

Even among young adults with a mean age of 25, cardiovascular health factors affect brain vascular structure, function, and brain tissue integrity, as visualized with magnetic resonance imaging.[62] Already at this young age, optimal cardiovascular health was associated with better cerebral perfusion and fewer subclinical brain lesions—thus emphasizing the importance of avoiding cardiovascular risk factors.

Cardiac health is also linked to Parkinson's disease, a condition characterized by problems with disruption of movement, disruption of cognitive functions, and often dementia. About 1 million Americans are living with Parkinson's disease. A study in South Korea considered if the presence of the metabolic syndrome was linked to Parkinson's disease.[63] The metabolic syndrome is defined as the presence of three or more of the following: abdominal obesity, high blood pressure, high blood sugar, high triglycerides, and low HDL-C. The analysis indicated that individuals with metabolic syndrome had a 24% higher risk of incident Parkinson's disease, and each metabolic syndrome component was positively associated with Parkinson's disease risk.

The role of blood lipids

Observational studies of statin use to lower LDL-C have shown a decreased risk of Alzheimer disease. In contrast, randomized controlled treatment trials of statins to treat established AD have been uniformly negative.[64,65] In a small group of study subjects at high risk of CVD, higher LDL-C and lower levels of HDL-C were associated with greater brain amyloid levels independently of APOE genotype. This finding suggests that healthy HDL-C and LDL-C levels can protect against the deposition of brain amyloid just as they protect against cardiovascular disease.[66]

The role of hypertension

The American Heart Association recognizes that chronic arterial hypertension is a well-established risk factor for vascular and Alzheimer dementia.[67] It disrupts the structure and function of cerebral blood vessels, leads to inadequate blood perfusion and damage of white matter regions critical for cognitive function, and may promote Alzheimer disease pathology.[68,69,70]

Chronic hypertension can cause a series of small strokes that may not be recognized. The resulting cumulative brain damage can cause multi-infarct or vascular dementia that is second only to Alzheimer disease as the most common cause of dementia, and vascular damage to the brain may lead to or contribute to Alzheimer disease.

Because vascular brain injury develops insidiously over a long time, diagnosing and treating high blood pressure at a young age could improve late-life cognitive health.

Research based on data from the Framingham Heart Study found that among individuals in their 40s, those with prehypertension or any degree of increased blood pressure had damage to the structural integrity of the brain's white matter and decreases in the volume of brain gray matter.[71] The study found that the higher the blood pressure, the greater the amount of brain injury, cognitive decline, and probably the risk of dementia.

A meta-analysis of 14 randomized clinical trials with an average duration of 4.1 years found that blood pressure lowering with antihypertensive agents was associated with a lower rate of development of dementia or cognitive impairment at 7.0% of those treated compared to 7.5% of patients in a control group, a difference that was statistically significant.[72]

A study with long-term (24 year) follow-up found that individuals with mid-life hypertension have increased risk for dementia and that mid-life hypertension that is followed by late-life low blood pressure was associated with even greater risk for dementia.[73] The SPRINT/MIND trial found that over 5 years, intensive (systolic blood pressure target less than 120 mm Hg,), rather than standard blood pressure lowering (SBP less than 140 mm Hg.) in adults age 50 or older did not decrease the risk of probable dementia, but it did significantly reduce by 19% the risk of mild cognitive impairment—a frequent precursor of dementia.[74] The same study found intensive blood pressure treatment resulted in a small decrease in dementia associated white matter brain lesions but a small decrease in total brain volume—a sign of brain atrophy.[75] Editorial comment on this result was that earlier, midlife management of blood pressure may be optimal, and later blood pressure lowering interventions require careful monitoring for the potential cognitive harm associated with late-life low blood pressure.[76]

The role of obesity

Obesity, especially abdominal obesity, is another cardiovascular risk factor that is associated with an increased risk of Alzheimer disease. A normal BMI at midlife may delay the onset of Alzheimer disease.

An analysis of data from nearly 1,400 participants in the Baltimore Longitudinal Study of Aging found that being overweight or obese at age 50 may lead to earlier onset of Alzheimer disease.[77] Over the nearly 14-year study duration, about 10% of the group developed Alzheimer disease, and each unit increase in midlife body mass index (BMI) accelerated the onset of Alzheimer disease by 6.7 months.

Researchers studied 6,583 people age 40 to 45 in northern California who had their abdomens measured.[78] At age 73 to 87 (an average of 36 years later), 16% of the participants had been diagnosed with dementia. The study found that those who were overweight or obese according to BMI but did not have a large abdomen were 1.8 times more likely to develop dementia than those of normal weight and abdomen size. Those who were overweight and had a large abdomen were 2.3 times more likely to develop dementia than people with a normal weight and abdomen size. People who were both obese and had a large abdomen were 3.6 times more likely to develop dementia than those of normal weight and abdomen size.

The role of nutrition

Although many studies find that a healthy diet decreases the risk of dementia and cognitive decline, other long-term studies do not.

U.S. cohort studies have found significantly slower cognitive decline with consumption of two or more daily servings of vegetables, with the strongest associations observed for six or more weekly servings of green leafy vegetables.[79 80 81] Studies have found that high consumption of dietary saturated and trans-fats increases the risk of Alzheimer disease. In one study, persons in the upper fifth of saturated-fat intake had 2.2 times the risk of incident Alzheimer disease compared with persons in the lowest fifth.[82] The study authors concluded that a high intake of unsaturated fats may be protective against Alzheimer disease, whereas intake of saturated or trans-fats may increase risk.

A study that included data from 10 countries found that high amounts of meat in the diet had the highest correlations with increased Alzheimer disease prevalence.[83] Consumption of foods high in added sugar and high-fat dairy products was also found to be associated with increased risk. Foods that were protective against AD included fruits, vegetables, grains, low-fat dairy products, legumes, and fish.

Alpha-linolenic acid (ALA) is found in some green vegetables, vegetable oils, nuts, and seeds. The body converts ALA into EPA and DHA, the omega-3 fatty acids that are found in oily fish. Omega-3s in foods may provide some benefit for the preservation of cognitive function, whereas omega-3 fatty acids in the form of fish oil supplements (a $1 billion industry in the U.S.), do not appear to be effective.[84 85 86 87] Many other dietary supplements make unsupported claims that they promote brain health. Although they have annual sales of more than $3 billion, they have not been scientifically proven to be protective and may cause harm.[88]

A systematic review that included four prospective studies of Alzheimer disease risk from the Columbia Aging Project (following older adults for various time intervals between 1992 through 2006) found that decreased risk of Alzheimer disease was associated with the Mediterranean dietary pattern.[89 90] In the Columbia study, reduced risk ranged from 34% to 40% for nondemented persons in the highest third of adherence compared with the lowest.[91] An 11% reduction in the risk of mild cognitive impairment converting to Alzheimer disease was observed for each unit increase in the Mediterranean diet score.[92] A study among a Scottish cohort also found that greater adherence to a Mediterranean style diet resulted in a lower rate of brain atrophy over a three-year period.[93]

The Mediterranean-DASH Intervention for Neurodegenerative Delay (MIND) diet was designed with the objective of supporting cognitive health. It is a hybrid diet incorporating basic components from the Mediterranean diet and Dietary Approaches to Stop Hypertension (DASH) diet.[94] It was developed with modifications based on reviews of the literature on nutrition and brain aging to identify the nutrients, foods, and dietary patterns most likely to support brain health and reduce the risk of dementia.[95 96 97 98 99] Since studies do not find a strong association between the consumption of fruits and prevention of cognitive decline, the MIND diet designers did not specify daily fruit servings as do the DASH and Mediterranean diets. However, the MIND diet includes berry consumption because of the finding of positive associations between intake of blueberries and strawberries and slower cognitive decline that was found in the Nurses' Health Study.[100]

MIND study authors note that: "Similar to the Mediterranean and DASH diets, the MIND diet score emphasizes natural plant-based foods and limited intakes of animal and high saturated fat foods but uniquely specifies the consumption of berries and green leafy vegetables, and does not specify high fruit consumption (three to four servings per day in the DASH and Mediterranean diets), high dairy (2+ servings per day in DASH), high potato consumption (2 servings per day in the Mediterranean), or greater than one fish meal per week (more than 6 meals/week in the Mediterranean)."[101]

In one study, the MIND diet was more predictive of slower cognitive decline than either the Mediterranean or DASH diets. The MIND diet score was associated with a slower rate of cognitive decline, equivalent to 7.5 years of younger age among the participants in the top third of MIND diet scores compared with the lowest third.[102] In a study specifically focused on Alzheimer disease, it was found that the MIND and Mediterranean diets were comparable.[103] Similar data has come from a study of older adults from 11 European countries. It found that self-reported frequent consumption of fruits and vegetables was associated with improved health outcomes, including mental health and cognitive functioning.[104]

A study of dementia published in the *American Journal of Clinical Nutrition* in 2020 followed 2,801 men and women for an average of 20 years.[105] At the start of the study, the participants averaged age 59 and were free from dementia. Over the duration of the study 158 participants developed Alzheimer disease, and 35 developed other forms of dementia. The study found that individuals with the highest (>60th percentile) intakes of flavonols, anthocyanins, and flavonoid polymers had a 42% to 76% lower risk of dementia relative to individuals with the lowest intakes (≤15th percentile), depending on the type of flavonoid consumed.

Flavonoids are naturally occurring bioactive pigments found widely in plant-based foods. Common sources of flavonoids include anthocyanin-rich blue berries, strawberries and red wine, flavanone-rich citrus fruits and juices, flavan-3-ol-rich teas and dark chocolate, flavone-rich parsley and celery, flavonol-rich onions and apples, and isoflavone-rich soy products.

Other studies, including a major long-term (25-year) prospective study, did not find a significant association between diet, dementia risk, and cognitive decline.[106] The study evaluated diet with a score based on six components for which the highest intake is seen to be ideal (vegetables, fruits, whole grains, nuts and legumes, long-chain omega-3 fatty acids, and polyunsaturated fatty acids excluding omega-3 fatty acids) and four components for which avoidance or the lowest intake is seen to be ideal (sugar-sweetened drinks and fruit juice, red and processed meat, trans-fat, and sodium); and one component for which moderate consumption was thought to be ideal (alcohol intake).

The study found that diet quality assessed during midlife was not significantly associated with subsequent risk for dementia. The study authors noted that other studies, especially those with long follow-up of 15 years or longer, did not find a significant association between diet, dementia risk, and cognitive decline. Their conclusion was that whether a healthy diet plays a role in shaping cognitive outcomes in combination with other healthy behaviors, or in subgroups at increased risk for dementia, remains unclear.

The role of sugar and artificial sweeteners

The 2020 Dietary Guidelines Advisory Committee recommended that adults consume less than 6% of their total daily calories from added sugar, but most Americans consume far more. Much of the excess sugar is in the form of sugar-sweetened beverages (SSBs) such as soft drinks, fruit drinks with added sugar, and 100% fruit juice. The Framingham Heart Study used a self-report to estimate the dietary intake of SSBs and evaluated brain health with neuropsychological testing (assessing verbal memory, processing speed, and other executive functions) and brain imaging (to assess hippocampal and total brain volume).[107] The study found that high consumption of SSBs among participants (average age of 54 years) was associated with the brain pathology markers of early-stage Alzheimer disease: poorer memory, smaller overall brain volume, and a smaller hippocampus—an area of the brain important for learning and memory.

Compared to those with no consumption of SSBs, those who drank 1 to 2 SSBs per day had brain volume changes equivalent to 1.5 additional years of brain aging, and those who drank more than 2 SSBs per day had the equivalent of 2 years of brain volume aging. Compared to those with no consumption, those who drank 1 to 2 SSBs per day had Logical Memory Delayed scores equivalent to 5.8 additional years of brain aging, and those who drank more than 2 SSBs per day had scores equivalent to 11 additional years of brain aging. The magnitude of these effects was attenuated when adjustments for physical activity and healthy nutrition were made.

The investigators noted that although their findings are consistent with animal studies, because their research was an observational study at a single point in time, it could not be considered conclusive with regard to cause-and-effect. Even so, the results of the study suggest that minimizing dietary intake of sugar may guard against the brain atrophy and memory impairment associated with accelerated brain aging and Alzheimer disease.

This data about SSBs and brain health suggests that it might be a good idea to substitute artificially sweetened diet soda for SSBs. But a 2012 study found that artificially sweetened soft drinks were also associated with an increased risk of stroke.[108] The study found that people who had any recent consumption of diet drinks, regardless of the amount per day, were about 16% more likely to have a stroke as those with no consumption of diet drinks. These findings were also attenuated somewhat when the data were adjusted for hypertension and additional CVD risk factors.

A 2017 follow-up Framingham Heart Study also found that people who drank diet soda were more likely to develop stroke and dementia compared to those who did not.[109] In contrast to the previous study on SSBs, the investigators found no correlation between SSB intake and stroke or dementia. Compared to those who did not drink diet drinks, they found that people who drank one to six diet drinks a week had a 1.41 times, but not a statistically significant increase in all-cause dementia. Those who drank a greater amount, one or more diet soda per day, were 2.47 times more likely to develop dementia. These findings were attenuated somewhat when the data were adjusted for additional CVD risk factors, including diabetes and blood lipid status.

After adjustments for age, sex, education, caloric intake, diet quality, physical activity, and smoking, higher recent and higher cumulative intake of artificially sweetened soft drinks were associated with an increased risk of ischemic stroke, all-cause dementia, and Alzheimer disease dementia. When comparing daily consumption of one or more diet drinks cumulative intake to none per week, the hazard ratios were 2.96 (the 95% confidence interval was large, 1.26–6.97) for ischemic stroke and 2.89 (the 95% confidence interval was large, 1.18–7.07) for Alzheimer disease.

Although the researchers adjusted their data for age, smoking, diet, and other factors, they could not completely control for preexisting conditions like diabetes, which may have developed over the course of the study and is a known risk factor for dementia. People with diabetes, as a group, consume more diet soda, so some of the correlation between diet soda intake and dementia may be due to diabetes, as well as other vascular risk factors and not related to diet soda consumption.

Vitamins and dietary supplements

Consumption of various dietary supplements, including vitamins, particularly B-vitamins, has been proposed as a way to prevent and treat dementia. There is some evidence only that high dose B vitamins may slow cognitive decline.[110] Currently, only a deficiency in vitamin B12 can be reliably linked to Alzheimer disease and cognitive decline in the U.S. population.[111] [112] Although many foods are fortified with B vitamins, vitamin B12 deficiency is found among the elderly occurring in 3%, and borderline deficiency in up to 20% of persons age 50 and older. B12 deficiency is usually the result of increased prevalence of atrophic gastritis that limits stomach acid production and because of other digestive conditions like celiac and Crohn's disease that interfere with absorption of vitamin B12 in the small intestine. B12 deficiency can also occur among long-term vegans since animal products are the only source of naturally occurring vitamin B12.[113] [114] [115]

Because the body can store a substantial amount of vitamin B12, the development of deficiency can be a slow, insidious process that takes years to develop. B12 deficiency causes anemia, fatigue, cognitive impairment, and psychiatric disturbances such as depression, as well as degeneration of the spinal cord, and peripheral nerve damage that results in symptoms such as numbness and tingling. Injected or orally administered synthetic vitamin B12, a form that is easily absorbed, can reverse the symptoms of the neurologic syndrome, including the cognitive disturbances, but the nerve damage from the vitamin B12 deficiency syndrome is irreversible if left untreated.

The role of sleep

The glymphatic system that eliminates the brain's waste products, such as the beta-amyloid associated with Alzheimer dementia, functions mainly during sleep.[116] Although it is not possible to definitively say if poor sleep is the cause or the result of the small brain infarcts (microinfarcts) that are linked to dementia, there is a strong association between sleep disturbance and dementia. There is evidence that untreated sleep apnea, a cause of disrupted sleep, is associated with mild cognitive impairment and Alzheimer disease 10 years sooner than its occurrence among those without the disorder.[117] In one study, autopsies of the one-quarter of men with the lowest oxygen levels during prior sleep tests were almost four times more likely to show microinfarcts in the brain, compared to men with the highest oxygen levels. Men who spent less time in slow-wave sleep—the deep, restorative stage of sleep—tended to show more atrophy in their brain tissue.[118]

Mental workouts–do they work?

The brain retains some degree of plasticity and forcefully taxing it can, to some extent, protect as well as revive declining skills. Video games are being considered as a quick way to help aging brains get better at tasks like noticing visual stimuli and rapidly shifting the focus of their attention. Purveyors of brain training services probably promise more than they can deliver. The currently hyped commercial cognitive training tools that promise to stave off mental decline are not certain to provide benefits. Even so, they have estimated sales of over $1.3 billion per year. A meta-analysis of research suggests that training works to provide long-term improvements in the skills undertaken, but the gains do not carry over into other areas. In other words, playing Sudoku or doing crossword puzzles makes you better at Sudoku or crosswords but doesn't improve math or memory skills.[119 120 121]

Some studies are more encouraging. An analysis of 51 studies of brain-training found no improvements in memory or other mental skills in cognitively healthy older people from home-based computerized cognitive training. The analysis did find that group-based computerized cognitive training (CCT) is somewhat effective—its overall effect on cognitive performance in healthy older adults is positive but small—and it is ineffective for executive functions and verbal memory.[122]

One study of 10 years duration followed three separate groups with an average age of 74 who were trained in memory, or reasoning, or speed of processing. Five years after the initial training, each of the groups still demonstrated improvements in the skills in which they had trained, but the gains did not carry over into other areas. Each cognitive intervention resulted in less decline in self-reported difficulty with activities of daily living compared with the control group. Reasoning and speed training, but not memory training, resulted in improved targeted cognitive abilities for 10 years.[123]

Another encouraging study was carried out by my colleagues at UCSF. They demonstrated that a specially designed home computer driving game called NeuroRacer improved both multitasking and cognitive control among adults age 60 to 85 with effects persisting for six months. The more difficult the game was, the more positive the cognitive results. In contrast to many other studies, the benefits of this training extended to untrained cognitive functions such as sustained attention and working memory. These findings provide hope for the possibility of finding new ways to improve the cognitive functioning of the aging brain.[124]

Clive Thompson, a *New York Times Magazine* writer, emphasizes that there is much hype and controversy in the brain training field, but some recent developments show promise. Several companies are seeking approval from the Food and Drug Administration to market their games as therapeutic for cognitive health.[125]

So, what is the bottom line on brain training? A group of 30 scientists issued a consensus statement.[126] They note that "Any mentally effortful new experience, such as learning a language, acquiring a motor skill, navigating in a new environment, and, yes, playing commercially available computer games, will produce changes in those neural systems that support the acquisition of the new skill. For example, there may be an increase in the number of synapses, the number of neurons and supporting cells, or a strengthening of the connections among them. This type of brain plasticity is possible throughout the life span, though younger brains seem to have an advantage over the older ones."

But the experts caution with a summary statement: "We object to the claim that brain games offer consumers a scientifically grounded avenue to reduce or reverse cognitive decline when there is no compelling scientific evidence to date that they do. The promise of a magic bullet detracts from the best evidence to date, which is that cognitive health in old age reflects the long-term effects of healthy, engaged lifestyles. In the judgment of the signatories below, exaggerated and misleading claims exploit the anxieties of older adults about impending cognitive decline. We encourage continued careful research and validation in this field."[127]

What can we learn from superagers?

At age 80 or older, superagers have superior episodic memories that are as good as those of average middle-aged adults.[128] [129] They have been shown to have slower than average age-related whole-brain cortical volume loss.[130] As Lisa Feldman Barrett has pointed out, we don't know the best ways to increase our chances of becoming a superager, but the best answer so far is to work hard at something.[131] Both vigorous physical exercise and strenuous mental effort seem to be important. But there is a downside. It takes hard work, and hard work comes with discomfort, fatigue, and frustration. Feldman Barrett says that "Superagers are like Marines: They excel at pushing past the temporary unpleasantness of intense effort. . . . You must expend enough effort that you feel some 'yuck.' Do it till it hurts, and then a bit more . . . . All brain tissue gets thinner from disuse. If you don't use it, you lose it." So, by all means, do something that taxes your brain in productive ways, the harder, the better. Whatever activities you force your brain to engage in, you will get better at them.

Keep in mind that physical activity and other aspects of a healthy lifestyle are more important to brain health than mental gymnastics to avoid cognitive decline and dementia. We know that staying physically active, getting plenty of sleep (see Chapter 15, "More Advice About Healthy Living," for more on sleep), avoiding diabetes by limiting sugar intake and overweight, avoiding misuse of alcohol and tobacco, consuming a low saturated fat whole-food plant-based diet, and keeping blood lipids and blood pressure in healthy ranges are important to brain health. All these health-supporting factors are found on the Lifestyle Checklist.

What is next?

The failure of almost all drugs to prevent decline or improve cognitive function has promoted rethinking of the approach to Alzheimer disease. One theory that is being explored is that with aging and cardiovascular risk factors, the integrity of blood vessels and the blood-brain barrier weakens, and pathogens (bacteria and viruses) cause brain inflammation and the deposition of amyloid.

Infection of the brain or elsewhere in the body with herpes simplex virus (HSV), herpesvirus (HHV) and other microbes has been linked to Alzheimer disease.[132] However it is not known whether neuroinflammation is a cause, rather than a consequence, of the amyloidosis, tau deposition, and ultimately neurodegeneration seen in AD.

Research has found that the gradual damage with normal aging correlates very strongly with the changes in blood vessels in the hippocampus and parahippocampal gyrus, areas heavily involved in memory and learning. Blonz suggests focusing research on developing various methods to maintain adequate brain glucose and other energy resources.

As it is with many diseases, the best hope for coping with Alzheimer disease seems to be in prevention. Establishing and maintaining a healthy metabolism, including physical activity, good nutrition, and other measures to improve cardiovascular health, seems to be crucial to prevention.[133][134] A study published in *Lancet* in 2020 indicates that modifying 12 lifestyle risk factors might prevent or delay up to 40% of dementias. The modifiable factors are excessive alcohol consumption, head injury, air pollution, low education, hypertension, hearing impairment, smoking, obesity, depression, physical inactivity, diabetes, and infrequent social contact.[135]

Summary of the essential facts

Some decline in memory and cognitive function with age is normal. Reversal of dementia is very difficult, only partially successful or impossible after it is well established, so prevention through measures that preserve brain health is crucial.[136][137][138]

These measures improve all aspects of health and also protect against age-related cognitive impairment, Alzheimer disease, and the vascular causes of dementia:

- Adhere to the guidelines of the Lifestyle Checklist.
- Consider testing for ApoE4 and other genes that heighten risk.
- Be physically active, the more vigorous, the better (40% lower risk).
- Take on hard and challenging mental work.
- Avoid cardiovascular disease risk factors, high blood pressure, high LDL-Cholesterol.
- Consume a whole food plant-based (Ornish or Mediterranean or MIND) diet.
- Prevent insulin resistance and diabetes (50% increased risk).
- Avoid overweight and obesity.
- Limit alcohol, better yet to avoid brain damage don't drink any amount of alcohol .
- Do not use mind-altering drugs they are brain-damaging.
- Do not smoke (50% to 80% increased risk).
- Manage depression and anxiety.
- Get enough sleep.
- Stay socially connected.
- Protect your head from injury.
- Rule out vitamin B12 deficiency, stress and other reversible causes of dementia
- Do not rely on brain training to avoid cognitive decline.
- No known dietary supplement improves cognition and brain health, save your money.

9
Benefits of Physical Activity

Probably everyone thinks that it is good to exercise. But most of us are not familiar with the science that shows that physical activity provides important health benefits. The reasons people exercise include controlling weight; improving personal appearance; improving muscle strength, balance, fitness and athletic ability for participation in sports; feeling better and more energetic, and just having fun at the gym, playing sports, or hiking out of doors. As is described in Chapter 8, "Preventing Dementia," being physically active is also one of the best ways to support brain health and avoid dementia. As one evolutionary anthropologist put it, after two million years of evolution, unlike our ape cousins, humans require high levels of physical activity to be healthy.[1]

And why do we use the term physical activity rather than exercise? Physical activity is muscle contraction that increases energy expenditure above that at rest— the body's basal level. Exercise is defined as a subcategory of physical activity that is planned, structured, repetitive, and purposive for the improvement or maintenance of one or more components of physical fitness. Sport is another subcategory of physical activity.[2]

Science confirms that physical activity is good for health and longevity. In 2007, the Department of Health and Human Services (DHHS) appointed a scientific committee called the Physical Activity Guidelines Advisory Committee to assess the scientific information on physical activity and health. The committee's report, the *Physical Activity Guidelines Advisory Committee Report*, 2008[3] formed the basis of the *2008 Physical Activity Guidelines for Americans*.[4] A decade later, a new 2018 Physical Activity Guidelines Advisory Committee has issued a report, *2018 Physical Activity Guidelines Advisory Committee Scientific Report*.[5] This report formed the basis for the *2018 Physical Activity Guidelines for Americans*.[6] The information in this chapter is based on these reports and research from additional sources.[7]

My Story

Undoubtedly, we all have an exercise history. Perhaps, it is just avoiding exercise. I ran the 100 and 220 dashes in junior high school and played pick-up squash in college, but I was not particularly physically active until my late 30s. I don't recall my exact motivation for taking up jogging; it probably was because I was feeling unfit, sluggish, and packing a few extra pounds. After a lot of daily runs, many 10K races, and six marathons, I learned the importance of progressing slowly to avoid injuries and that physical activity helped me to feel good, have energy, control weight, and look better. For the last decade, my back has given me trouble when running, so I alternate daily cycling over a 16-mile route and walking on a 4-mile route. I am an ardent believer in the merits of physical activity.

A physical activity report card for Americans

In 2016 only 26% of men, 19% of women, and 20% of adolescents report performing sufficient physical activity defined as at least 150 minutes of moderate-intensity aerobic (endurance) physical activity and two days per week of muscle-strengthening (resistance) activity for adults and at least 60 minutes of moderate-intensity aerobic physical activity and three days per week of muscle-strengthening activity for youth.[8] An estimated $117 billion in U.S. annual health care costs and about 10% of premature mortality are associated with inadequate physical activity.[9] Moving more and sitting less will benefit everyone.

According to the 2015-2016 National Health and Nutrition Examination Survey (NHANES), 25.7% of adults reported sitting for more than eight hours per day, and 44.6% were inactive.[10] Among U.S. adults, average sitting time increased from about five hours a day in 2007 to about six hours a day in 2016.[11] Figure 9.1 below, reproduced from the *2018 Physical Activity Guidelines Advisory Committee Scientific Report*,[12] shows that based on a standard of 150 minutes of moderate to vigorous physical activity a week, half of Americans are still either inactive or insufficiently active.

Epidemiological studies indicate that sedentary behavior harms health.[13 14 15] A systematic review of 27 studies found that sedentary children and adolescents are more likely to be obese and have unfavorable measures of blood pressure, total cholesterol, self-esteem, social behavior, physical fitness, and academic achievement.[16] For adults, the study found "strong evidence of a relationship between sedentary behavior and all-cause mortality, fatal and non-fatal cardiovascular disease (CVD), type 2 diabetes, and metabolic syndrome." In addition, there is moderate evidence for increased incidence of ovarian, colon and endometrial cancers.

Fig. 9.1. Distribution of Self-Reported Volume of Moderate-to-Vigorous Physical Activity, 150 Minutes per Week Increments, U.S. Adults, 2015

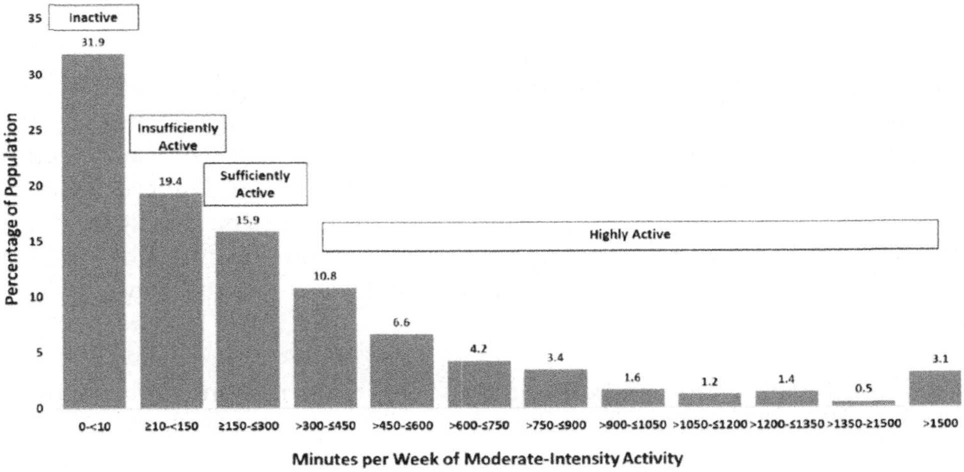

Source: Adapted from data found in the National Health Interview Survey, 2015.

By observing our fellow humans, we probably realize that the biological age of our bodies does not always correspond closely to our chronological age. One measurement of biological age is average leukocyte (white cell) telomere length. Telomeres are protective buffers at the ends of chromosomes. Young people's cells generally have longer telomeres than those of older people because, over time, with each cell division, the telomere ends become shorter.

A study compared changes in telomere length in middle-aged men and women who did not exercise with those started on a supervised program of either aerobic exercise (brisk walking, jogging, or high-intensity training) or resistance training with weights.[17] The aerobic trainers lengthened their telomeres, whereas the weight trainers did not, even though they too gained aerobic fitness compared to when they were inactive. This suggests that different forms of physical activity may provide different benefits.

Evidence that exercise can keep our body's cells biologically younger comes from a study of individuals who persisted with high levels of physical activity for as many as 50 years.[18] The athletes in their 70s were found to be biologically about 30 years younger than their chronological age as judged by both the study of capillaries and enzymes in their tissue samples, and by their aerobic capacity—a key health marker for all-cause mortality. Their aerobic capacities were about 40% higher than that of inactive people the same age. Gretchen Reynolds, writing on physical activity and health in the *New York Times*, noted that there is evidence that a decade after fitness training, health benefits persist, even among those who stop exercise, as measured by blood pressure and insulin sensitivity, but not with regard to maintaining aerobic capacity.[19]

Nielsen television survey data indicates that U.S. adults watch an average of more than five hours of TV a day.[20] A study of young adults in China found that independent of physical activity and energy intake, each one-hour increase in average daily television watching was associated with a modest decrease in mean telomere length, signifying approximately a 1.2 to 1.8 years increase in biological age.[21] The difference in telomere length for a three-hour a day increase in television watching would be roughly comparable to the difference in telomere lengths between smokers and non- smokers.[22]

There is substantial variation between U.S. states in the proportion of Americans who are physically inactive. Of course, there are many variables that could affect health and longevity, but the average life expectancy in the four states (Colorado, Oregon, Utah, Washington) with 15% to less than 20% of adults inactive was about age 80. This can be compared to a life expectancy of age 75 to 76 in the seven states (Alabama, Arkansas, Kentucky, Louisiana, Mississippi, Oklahoma, Tennessee) where 30% or more of adults were inactive.[23]

Humans evolved to be active

According to Daniel Lieberman, a professor of biological sciences at Harvard, an important reason that we are sedentary is that humans have been selected by evolution to exercise only as much as they must to survive.[24] According to this theory, a prominent adaptation has been for humans to develop prowess at running—for example, humans have an Achilles tendon, an adaptation useful mainly for running, and chimpanzees, our closest living relatives, do not. Running proficiency is a trait essential for persistence hunting, still practiced in the Kalahari Desert, where small bands of hunters chase animals until their prey collapse from overheating and exhaustion. However, because during millions of years of evolution, the energy provided by food was often scarce, human anatomy and physiology were also selected to avoid unnecessary exertion and conserve energy for survival and reproduction. "No hunter-gatherer goes out for a jog, just for the sake of it, I can tell you from personal experience," says Lieberman. In food-scarce environments, "They go out to forage, they go out to work, but anything else would be unwise, not to mention maladaptive."[25]

One report on Lieberman's work commented that "humans were born to run— but as little as possible."[26] Most human anatomical and physiological systems evolved to require stimuli from physical activity to adjust functional capacity up or down in response to the demands placed on them. Our bodies evolved to be adept at down-regulation of biological systems to slow metabolism and conserve energy whenever possible. We did not evolve to stay healthy in an environment with plentiful food and little need for physical activity. Because selection never operated to cope with the long-term effects of chronic inactivity, mechanisms for conserving energy expenditure now result in diseases. Without adequate stimuli from physical activity, the result is poor health, including disuse atrophy of muscles, obesity, diabetes, weakening of bones and osteoporosis, cardiovascular diseases, and even cognitive decline and dementia.

According to Lieberman, there is no evolutionary-determined dose or type of physical activity that will optimize health. "...because humans evolved to be active for play or necessity, efforts to promote exercise will require altering environments in ways that nudge or even compel people to be active and to make exercise fun." Lieberman thinks that one way to make exercise fun is to make it social. Other steps to encouraging physical activity include having physical-education (PE) requirements at schools and colleges and to making it easy in workplaces and communities. When I was a freshman at Harvard, there was an exercise requirement, but it was done away with in the 1970s, even though there is plentiful evidence that physically active college students are happier and do better with their studies. The bottom line is that as a society and as individuals, we need to fight back against two million years of human evolution, telling us to take it easy when we can.[27] Sloth really is a deadly sin.[28]

Physical activity improves health

Physical activity provides a variety of benefits that help individuals sleep better, feel better, and perform daily tasks more easily. Greater amounts of regular moderate-to-vigorous physical activity reduce the risk of many of the most common and expensive diseases or conditions in the U.S. Physical activity can lower blood pressure,[29] improve blood lipid patterns[30], lower risk for heart disease, stroke, and other cardiovascular diseases;[31 32] reduce the risk of the metabolic syndrome, increase bone density, and reduce the risk of osteoporosis;[33 34 35] reduce the risk of breast, colon, endometrial, esophageal, kidney, stomach, lung cancer, and other cancers;[36 37] help prevent or relieve anxiety and depression;[38 39] and help weight loss and maintenance of normal weight. Especially when both resistance and aerobic physical activity are combined, physical activity improves glucose tolerance and insulin sensitivity and reduces risk of developing type 2 diabetes.[40] Falls with injuries among the elderly are less common among individuals who are or become more physically active.

Summary of major findings from the 2018 Physical Activity Guidelines Advisory Committee Scientific Report[41]

- Strong evidence demonstrates that moderate-to-vigorous physical activity improves the quality of sleep.
- Physical activity promotes immediate improvements in brain executive function—the ability to plan, organize, self-monitor, and inhibit or facilitate behaviors, initiate tasks, and control emotions.
- Physical activity improves cognition, including memory, processing speed, attention, and academic performance.
- Regular physical activity reduces the risk of clinical depression and reduces depressive symptoms.
- Regular physical activity reduces symptoms of anxiety.
- Regular physical activity improves perceived quality of life.
- Physical activity improves physical function among individuals of all ages, enabling them to conduct their daily lives with energy and without undue fatigue.
- Greater amounts of moderate-to-vigorous physical activity are associated with preventing or minimizing excessive weight gain in adults, maintaining weight within a healthy range, and preventing obesity in adults and children ages three to 17 years.
- Physically active women are less likely to gain excessive weight or develop diabetes during pregnancy or develop postpartum depression.
- Greater amounts of physical activity reduce the risk of dementia and improve cognitive function.
- Regular physical activity provides health benefits to children as young as ages three to five years.
- Regular physical activity reduces the risk of falls and fall-related injuries among older adults.
- Regular moderate-to-vigorous physical activity reduces the risk for cancers of the breast, colon, bladder, endometrium, esophagus, kidney, lung, and stomach.
- Regular physical activity can reduce the risk of developing a new chronic condition, including osteoarthritis, hypertension, and type 2 diabetes, reduce the risk of progression of chronic conditions, and improve quality of life and physical function.

Some benefits happen immediately.

A single bout of moderate-to-vigorous physical activity will reduce blood pressure, improve insulin sensitivity, improve sleep, reduce anxiety symptoms, and improve cognition on the day that it is performed. Most of these improvements become even larger with the regular performance of moderate-to-vigorous physical activity. Other benefits, such as disease risk reduction and physical function, accrue within days to weeks after adopting a new physical activity routine.

The benefits of physical activity can be achieved in a variety of ways.

The target range of physical activity suggested in the 2008 Scientific Report was 150 to 300 minutes (500 to 1,000 MET-minutes) per week of moderate-intensity physical activity. METs are metabolic equivalents, one MET is the amount of oxygen consumed and calories burned at rest. The 2018 Scientific Committee endorsed the validity of this target range. Since 2008, more science documents the value of reducing inactivity even if the 150 to 300 minutes a week target of moderate-intensity physical activity is not achieved.

A summary of the *2018 Physical Activity Guidelines Advisory Committee Scientific Report* major findings about physical activity targets and schedules is:

- For individuals who perform no or little moderate-to-vigorous physical activity, replacing sedentary behavior with light-intensity physical activity reduces the risk of all-cause mortality, cardiovascular disease incidence and mortality, and the incidence of type 2 diabetes.
- For individuals whose amount of moderate-to-vigorous physical activity is below the current public health target range of 150 to 300 minutes a week of moderate-intensity physical activity, even small increases in moderate-intensity physical activity provide health benefits. There is no threshold that must be exceeded before benefits begin to occur.
- For individuals below the target range, substantial reductions in risk are available with relatively small increases in moderate-intensity physical activity.
- Individuals already within the physical activity target range can gain more benefits by doing more moderate-to-vigorous physical activity.
- Bouts, or episodes, of moderate-to-vigorous physical activity of any duration, may be included in the daily accumulated total volume of physical activity.
- Some physical activity is better than none.
- For most health outcomes, additional benefits occur as the amount of physical activity increases through higher intensity, greater frequency, and/or longer duration.
- Most health benefits occur with at least 150 minutes a week of moderate-intensity physical activity, such as brisk walking. Additional benefits occur with more physical activity.
- Both aerobic (e.g., walking, running, swimming, cross-country skiing,

bicycling) and muscle-strengthening physical activity is beneficial.
- Health benefits occur for children and adolescents, young and middle-aged adults, older adults, and those in every studied racial and ethnic group.
- The health benefits of physical activity occur for people with disabilities.
- The benefits of physical activity far outweigh the possibility of adverse outcomes.

New York Times writer Gretchen Reynolds, at the end of 2014, summed up research on the benefits of physical activity as follows: "In various experiments, physical activity was found to lessen and even reverse the effects of aging on human skin; protect against age-related vision loss; improve creativity; lower people's risk of developing heart disease even if they had multiple risk factors for the condition; increase the numbers of good bacteria in athletes' guts; raise exercisers' pain tolerance; and alter, in desirable ways, how our DNA works."[42]

There are favorable benefits from physical activity that relate not just to health but also to our personal goals and sense of wellbeing. They include maintenance of a desirable weight, getting and keeping an attractive athletic body appearance and a body composition with a greater lean mass, higher levels of energy and endurance, and the psychological benefits of a good mood and higher self-esteem. High levels of physical activity help us to look better, feel better, and function better.

A word of warning: If these descriptions of the positive benefits of physical activity have inspired you to start or intensify an exercise routine, please read the cautions in this chapter about getting started. Especially if you are over the age of 30, or have any health condition, or are taking medication, make sure that you have a checkup and clearance from your medical care provider and remember that to avoid injuries and other problems, it is important to warm up, increase the amount of physical activity slowly, and cool down.

Physical activity and mortality

The 2008 Physical Activity Guidelines Advisory Committee's review concluded that there is good evidence that physically fit and habitually physically active adults are healthier and less likely to die prematurely than those who are sedentary.[43 44 45 46] According to an article in *Scientific American*, "...being physically active is the single most important thing that most of us can do to improve or maintain our health."[47] The epidemiology of participation in sport strongly suggests that participants derive health benefits and reduce mortality.[48]

One estimate is that people who are physically active for about seven hours (420 minutes) a week have a 40% lower risk of dying early than those who are active for less than 30 minutes a week. The recommended two hours and 30 minutes (150 minutes) a week (21.4 minutes a day) of moderate-intensity aerobic activity (e.g., brisk walking at about 100 steps per minute) lowers the risk of premature death. One estimate is that 250,000 deaths per year in the United States, approximately 12% of the total, are attributable to a lack of regular physical activity.[29 50 51]

A recent study at the Cleveland Clinic considered the risk of death compared to cardiorespiratory fitness.[52] Over an average of 8.4 years, study subjects with below-average cardiorespiratory fitness were 40% more likely to die of any cause than those with above-average fitness. All-cause mortality was five times greater among those with low fitness compared to those with "elite" fitness. The study authors concluded that "Cardiorespiratory fitness is inversely associated with long-term mortality with no observed upper limit of benefit. Extremely high aerobic fitness was associated with the greatest survival and was associated with benefit in older patients and those with hypertension."

In some studies, moderate recreational activities were found to confer the same health benefits as more vigorous activities.[53] An 11-year study of 5,700 older men in Norway (ages 68 to 77), published in the *British Journal of Sports Medicine*, found that irrespective of whether the activity was light or vigorous, those who exercised for 30 minutes six days a week experienced a mortality reduction of 40% and lived around five years longer than those who were sedentary. The authors of the study concluded that increased physical activity was as beneficial as giving up smoking in reducing all-cause mortality.[54]

A cohort study in the United Kingdom assessed physical capability with three objective measures of physical capability: grip strength, chair rise time for 10 rises, and standing balance time up to 30 seconds. Those who could not complete any of the three tests had death rates more than 12 times higher than those who were able to complete the tests. The adjusted hazard ratio of all-cause mortality for participants in the lowest vs. highest quintiles (fifth) of physical capability was 3.68.[55 56]

Analysis of the records of 55,137 runners maintained by the Cooper Institute found that the risk of dying from any cause was 30% lower among runners compared to non-runners, and the benefits were about the same regardless of the duration or speed (intensity) of running. The runners had a lower risk of dying than those who engaged in less strenuous activities such as walking.[57] A follow-up study found that runners had a 25% to 40% reduced risk of premature mortality and lived approximately three years longer than non-runners.[58] Improvements in life expectancy leveled off at about four hours of running per week.

The benefits of even a small amount of low-intensity physical activity are striking.

The largest difference in health and longevity would appear to be between being sedentary and any level of physical activity. Many, but not all, studies find that higher levels of activity, both duration, and intensity, add additional benefits with a dose-response pattern: greater intensity of physical activity lowers mortality more than less intense physical activity. The harder the workout, the greater the health benefits.[59] For example, a Finnish study of twins designed to minimize genetic variability found that over a 17-year time span, compared to a twin who was sedentary and reported no leisure-time physical activity, on average, the occurrence of death was 29% lower for a twin who was an occasional exerciser and 43% lower for twins who were conditioned exercisers.[60]

Fig. 9.2. Relationship of Moderate-to-Vigorous Physical Activity to All-Cause Mortality

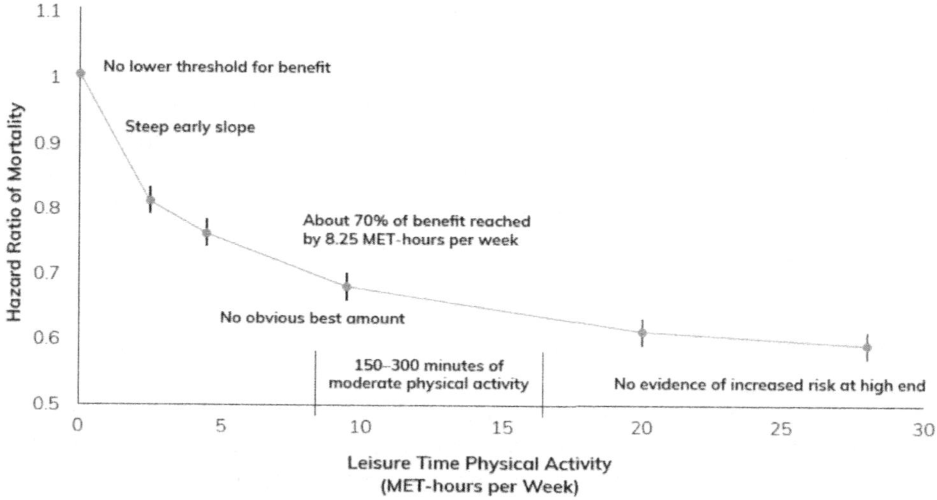

Source: Adapted from data found in Moore SC, Patel AV, Matthews CE. Leisure time physical activity of moderate to vigorous intensity and mortality: a large pooled cohort analysis. PLoS Med. 2012;9(11):e1001335. doi:10.1371/journal.pmed.1001335.

Source: 2018 Physical Activity Guidelines for Americans

As is shown in Figure 9.2, above, from the *2018 Physical Activity Guidelines for Americans,* the risk of death declines with increasing levels of physical activity.

A study conducted in Taiwan found that compared to inactive study subjects, those with an average of 15 minutes a day of moderate-intensity physical activity reduced their all-cause mortality by 14%, with 35 minutes a day the reduction was 20%, with 60 minutes a day the reduction was 29%, and with 90 minutes a day, the reduction was 35%.[61] Two hours a week of vigorous-intensity activities provided health benefits similar to four hours a week of moderate-intensity physical activities. The study confirms that even small increases in physical activity offer important health benefits.

Because people in many countries are spending the majority of their day sitting, and this is linked to an increased risk for many chronic diseases and premature death,[62] a study was undertaken among middle-aged and older men and women to consider how much sitting is too much and if light-intensity physical activity improves longevity.[63] In contrast to many studies that rely on self-reporting to obtain objective data, the study combined data from eight studies in which more than 36,000 participants wore a motion sensor for between four and seven days in total. Over a six-year period, the study found a strong association between total physical activity of any intensity, even light chores, and a decreased risk of dying. The study found that per 1,000 participants, 23 individuals died in the most active 25% of participants compared with 130 deaths per 1,000 participants in the least active 25%—more than a five-fold difference between groups.

The study also estimated how much time being physically active was associated with a maximally reduced risk of death. For moderate to vigorous intensity activity about 24 minutes per day (168 minutes per week) and five hours a day of light exercise was associated with the greatest risk reduction—more than this did not seem to lower the risk further. High amounts of sitting and other sedentary time above 9.5 hours per day was associated with an increased risk of death. In contrast, sitting levels below this threshold did not seem to be strongly linked to a difference in risk.

In another study of light physical activity among 5861 women with an average age of 78, those in the highest quartile of light physical activity, as measured by accelerometers and averaging six hours a day, had a 42% lower risk of heart attack or coronary death and a 22% reduced risk of cardiovascular disease events compared with those in the lowest quartile who averaged three hours a day of light physical activity.[64]

Additional data on the value of light physical activity comes from the Women's Health Study.[65] It measured daily average step counts among older women in their 70s and then checked subsequent deaths four to five years later. The study found that the least active women averaged about 2,700 steps a day, and higher averages of steps per day reduced deaths up to a plateau of about 7,500 steps a day. Just reaching 4,500 steps a day was associated with being 40% less likely to have died in the follow-up period than those taking about 2,700 steps a day, and walking faster or slower did not seem to affect mortality.

One study has noted that there is no scientific basis for the notion that 10,000 steps a day is best for health and that there is limited information on how many daily steps are needed for health.[66] Walking a mile requires 2000-2200 steps depending on stride length. The commonly cited goal of 10,000 steps a day seems to have come from the brand name of a Japanese pedometer, Manpo-kei, that translates to "10,000 steps meter."

A 2020 study published in the *JAMA* found that a greater number of steps per day was significantly associated with lower all-cause mortality.[67] The adjusted hazard ratio (see Chapter 16, "Understanding Scientific Data," for definition of hazard ratio) for 8000 steps/day vs. 4000 steps/day was 0.49. The reduction in mortality with an increasing number of steps plateaued at about 12,000 steps per day. This relationship is shown in Figure 9.3, that compares mortality rates to steps per day adjusted for study participants characteristics and health according to age, diet quality, sex, race-ethnicity, BMI, education, alcohol consumption, smoking status, diabetes, stroke, coronary heart disease, heart failure, cancer, chronic bronchitis, emphysema, mobility limitation, and self-reported general health. The effect was prominent for cardiovascular deaths but also was significant for cancer deaths. There was no significant association between step intensity and all-cause mortality after adjusting for the total number of steps per day.

Fig. 9.3. U. S. All-Cause Mortality and Daily Step Count

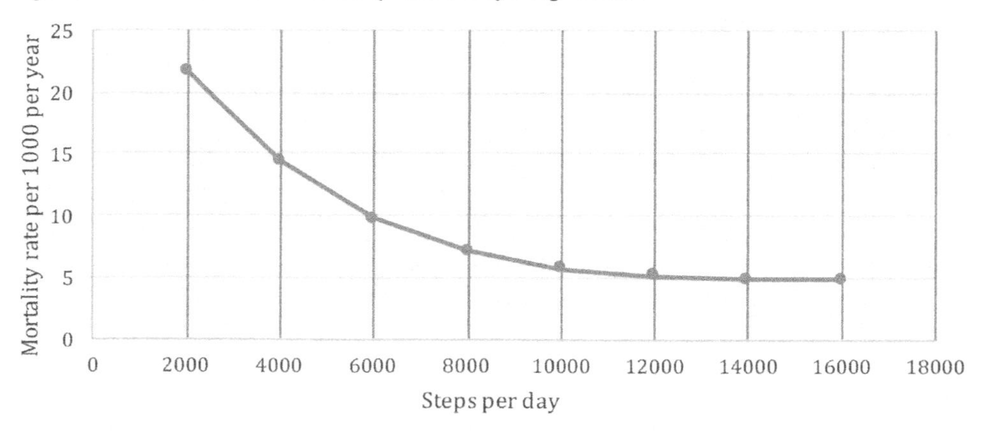

Source: Saint-Maurice PF, Troiano RP, Bassett DR, et al. Association of Daily Step Count and Step Intensity with Mortality Among US Adults. JAMA. 2020;323(12):1151–1160. doi:10.1001/jama.2020.1382

It has recently been said that sitting is as bad for your health as smoking. It is not. One estimate is that those with the longest duration of sitting have excess annual mortality of 190 per 100,000 people compared to those who sit the least.[68] The heaviest smokers can have an annual risk difference of 2,000 per 100,000 compared to never smokers— a ten times greater absolute risk than that for the most sedentary behavior.

A study of middle-aged and older Australians found that compared with those who reported no moderate to vigorous physical activity, those reporting 10 to 149, 150 to 299, and 300 or more minutes/week of moderate to vigorous physical activity had adjusted hazard ratios for all-cause mortality of 0.66, 0.53, and 0.46, respectively.[69]

Other studies have shown greater reductions in the mortality rate from vigorous-intensity activities than from moderate activities.[70] A study among people age 40 and older found that the total duration of moderate-to-vigorous physical activity was associated with reduced mortality risk.[71] It did not matter if the physical activity was in bouts of five minutes, 10 minutes or of any duration. Daily totals of more than 40 minutes were associated with a reduction in the death rate of more than 50%. The *2018 Physical Activity Guidelines Advisory Committee Scientific Report* concluded that strong evidence demonstrates that decreased cardiovascular disease mortality and decreased all-cause mortality is proportional to the amount of physical activity. This is a dose-response relationship.

One obvious question is, does starting to exercise later in life after being mostly sedentary reduce mortality? The answer is, yes. The NIH-AARP Diet and Health Study, with 315,000 participants, found that over about 13 years, those who reported engaging in moderate to vigorous physical activity since their teens or 20s had about a one-third lower risk of death—mostly from lower rates of CVD but also from less cancer.[72] Additional good news is that the study found that those who became physically active between the ages of 40 and 61 also had a 35% lower mortality rate. This study provides evidence that it is never too late to start exercising. Yet another finding of the study was that those who were physically active as teens or young adults, and then became sedentary in middle age, lost the longevity benefits of exercise. It may never be too late to start, but you have to keep at it to retain the benefits.

How much is too much? Can you get too much exercise?

The *2008 Physical Activity Guidelines for Americans* recommended a minimum of 75 vigorous-intensity (7.5 metabolic-equivalent hours per week) or 150 moderate-intensity minutes per week of aerobic activity for substantial health benefit and suggested additional benefits accrue from doing more than double this amount. However, it has not been entirely clear if there is an upper limit of health and longevity benefit or if harm could occur with greatly increased levels of physical activity.

Using self-reported physical activity data from more than 650,000 individuals in six studies in the National Cancer Institute Cohort, a study compared individuals reporting no leisure-time physical activity to those with various multiples of the recommended minimum to quantify the dose-response association between leisure-time physical activity and mortality and define the upper limit of benefit or harm associated with increased levels of physical activity.[73] The study found a 20% lower mortality risk among those performing some physical activity but less than the recommended minimum of 7.5 metabolic-equivalent hours per week, a 31% lower risk at one to two times the recommended minimum and a 37% lower risk at two to three times the minimum. A ceiling for mortality benefit occurred at three to five times the physical activity recommendation; however, compared with the recommended minimum, the additional benefit was a modest 8% improvement (from 31% to 39%). There was no evidence of harm at 10 or more times the recommended minimum. A similar dose-response relationship was observed for mortality due to cardiovascular disease and cancer.

In summary, the study found the lowest risk of mortality among those who engaged in 450 to 750 minutes of physical activities a week (an average of one to 1.8 hours a day) of moderate- or half that amount of vigorous-intensity physical activities and no excess risk, but no mortality gain at 10 or more times the minimum. The authors concluded that meeting the *2008 Physical Activity Guidelines for Americans* minimum by either moderate- or vigorous-intensity activity was associated with nearly the maximum longevity benefit.

However, as is described in the section below on physical activity and cardiovascular disease, there is some evidence from studies of ultra-marathoners that it is possible to "overdose" on exercise, and exceedingly high levels of physical activity might harm health.

Physical activity, fitness, and aging

The body's ability to take in and use oxygen, the VO2 maximum capacity, is considered the gold standard for measuring cardiorespiratory fitness. Higher VO2 correlates well with biological age, as indicated by telomere length. A study found that sedentary older study subjects had 40% shorter telomeres than those from either sedentary or physically active young study subjects. In one study, compared to older sedentary people, telomere length only decreased by 10% in older runners. This study, and many others, indicate that exercise and fitness have an anti-aging effect at the molecular level.[74][75][76] A study measured the muscle enzymes and capillaries of fit life-long exercisers who were in their 70s. It found that the exerciser's muscles were similar to those of people 30 years younger.[77] Studies of resistance training have found that cardiovascular events such as heart attack and stroke were substantially lower among those who lifted weights, even if the workouts were occasional.[78]

If cardiovascular fitness correlates with health and longer life, it may be useful for individuals to determine their fitness age, and then implement proven ways to improve fitness. To assess fitness age without access to an exercise laboratory, scientists tested more than 5,000 Norwegian adults and devised an algorithm for a non-exercise test of fitness (NET-T) to calculate aerobic capacity based on a person's sex and measurement of resting heart rate, waist size, and exercise routine.[79] The test can be found at: https://www.worldfitnesslevel.org/#/.

My Story

I took the test and found that my estimated fitness age was 18 years younger than my chronological age. My 80 minutes a day of biking or walking seems to be paying off.

In a study of more than 55,000 Norwegian adults using the non-exercise test, good cardiorespiratory fitness was associated with decreased all-cause and CVD mortality in men and women below 60 years of age.[80] Another study of 4,200 Senior Olympics qualifiers age 50 to 100 that used the non-exercise test methodology found that "While the athletes' average chronological age was 68, their average fitness age was 43, a remarkable 25 years less."[81]

A similar study examined the association of the validated fitness algorithm with all-cause and CVD mortality among 32,319 adults aged 35-70 years who took part in eight health surveys for England and Scotland between 1994 and 2003.[82] After adjusting for potential confounders, including diabetes, hypertension, smoking, social class, alcohol, and depression, a higher fitness score according to the fitness algorithm was associated with a lower risk of mortality from all-causes (15% lower in men and 12% lower in women) and from CVDs (25% lower in men and 27% lower in women).

Another study of highly active and fit older male and female cyclists age 55–79 years found much variation in fitness between individuals of the same age, but on average, that their physical functioning on a wide variety of measures, such as balance, reflexes, metabolic markers, and memory, remained fairly stable—and close to those found among 30 year-olds.[83] Although some declines with age were observed, including loss of muscle mass and strength and decreased maximal rate of oxygen consumption (VO2max), the expected decline in many markers of aging had not occurred. A follow-up study of the cyclists found that there was little loss of muscle mass and strength in those who exercise regularly.[84 85] The cyclist's body fat and cholesterol levels also did not increase with age, and the men's testosterone levels remained high. The T-cells in their immune systems, although showing signs of senescence and being less robust, were more numerous than would have been found in a sedentary population of similar age.

Another similar study was undertaken to determine if repeated exposure to ultra-endurance aerobic exercise is beneficial or detrimental. The study found that ultra-marathon athletes had 11% longer telomeres than healthy controls. The investigators concluded that the magnitude of this difference translates into about 16 years difference in biological age and that regular engagement in ultra-endurance aerobic exercise attenuates cellular aging.[86] Studies of muscle biopsies carried out at the Mayo Clinic found that exercise can reverse some of the deleterious changes in muscle cells and improve their functioning.[87] In contrast to even moderate activity, sedentary behavior is a risk factor for the physical frailty that is a strong risk factor for disability and death.[88] A recent editorial in the *JAMA* noted that "Activity may be the best treatment for aging."[89]

Regular physical activity strengthens bones and muscles, improves the ability to carry out daily activities, and prevents falls

Healthy bones, healthy joints and strong muscles are essential to remaining physically active and avoid losing the ability to do everyday activities such as climbing stairs or grocery shopping. Physical inactivity contributes to the frailty experienced by the elderly that leads to falls, injuries such as hip fracture, and inability to lead a normal self-sufficient life. Research shows that doing aerobic, muscle-strengthening, and bone-strengthening physical activity of at least a moderately-intense level can slow the loss of bone density that comes with age. The recommended 150 to 300 minutes per week of at least moderate-intensity aerobic activity lowers the risk of hip and other fractures. Muscle-strengthening activities help increase or maintain muscle mass and strength.[90]

Although it may be counter-intuitive, because it may seem that damaged joints would only improve with rest, regular physical activity helps improve arthritis and other conditions affecting the joints. Research shows that 130 to 150 minutes a week of moderate-intensity, low-impact aerobic activity can improve pain management, ability to carry out everyday tasks, and quality of life.

Physical activity can reduce the risk of heart and other cardiovascular diseases

Physical inactivity greatly increases the risk of heart attack, stroke, metabolic syndrome, and other cardiovascular diseases.[91] The CDC estimates that being sedentary increases the risk of coronary heart disease by 1.5 to 2.4 times.[92] Exercise training improves many metabolic factors that are associated with reduced risk of cardiovascular disease including lower blood pressure, increased high-density lipoprotein cholesterol (HDL-C), reduced serum triglyceride, lower LDL-Cholesterol levels, and possibly, increased numbers of larger safer LDL-C molecules and decreased numbers of small more dangerous LDL-C molecules.[93]

The Council on Clinical Cardiology and the Council on Nutrition, Physical Activity, and Metabolism have concluded that both epidemiological studies of occupational and leisure-time physical activity, and objective measures of exercise capacity such as treadmill performance, have consistently documented a causal relationship between physical activity and a reduced incidence of coronary artery disease (CAD) events. Studies find that the most physically active subjects generally have CAD rates half of those of the most sedentary group.[94 95 96]

Independent of the volume of activity, engaging in some vigorous activity is more beneficial to health than moderate physical activity—higher-intensity activities provide more cardioprotection.[97 98 99] One investigator has suggested that two minutes of moderate physical activity may not be equivalent to one minute of vigorous activity, and that running beats walking by a factor of between 2:1 to 4:1 in mortality reduction at the same volume of physical activity as measured by metabolic equivalents.[100]

A meta-analysis to evaluate the association between cardiorespiratory fitness and coronary heart disease or all-cause mortality, evaluated data from 33 eligible studies.[101] Over a follow up of 1.1 to 26 years, study participants with low cardiorespiratory fitness were found to have had a 70% higher risk for all-cause mortality and a 56% higher risk for coronary heart disease/cardiovascular events than study participants with high cardiorespiratory fitness.

A study of more than 30,000 Australian women born in the 1920s, 1940s, and 1970s in the *British Journal of Sports Medicine* found that physical activity reduced the risk of heart attack, stroke, metabolic syndrome and other cardiovascular diseases.[102] It considered physical inactivity, excess weight, smoking, and high blood pressure. Among the four factors studied, up to age 30, smoking was the most important contributor to heart disease. From age 30 until the late 80s, low physical activity levels were responsible for higher levels of risk than any of the three other risk factors. The potentially important role of nutrition and blood cholesterol levels was not evaluated in the study.

At one time, marathoners and other long-distance runners thought that their high levels of physical activity made them "heart attack proof." Unfortunately, if other cardiovascular risk factors are present, such as the high LDL-C from a typical high saturated fat, high sugar, high sodium American diet, the cardioprotective effects of exercise may not be enough to prevent cardiovascular disease.[103] Marathon runners are much less likely to get heart attacks than those who are less physically fit, but a few marathoners do get heart attacks. The fact that vigorous physical exertion can simultaneously increase the short-term risk of sudden death, usually due to underlying coronary artery disease, rare types of enlarged hearts and electrical conduction defects, yet also offer protection from the risk of cardiovascular disease in those who regularly exercise is sometimes called the "paradox of exercise."[104]

A review of 30 studies on prolonged exercise and heart health was reassuring in that the authors concluded that there is no level of exercise that is dangerous or too much for a healthy heart, but a medical evaluation is warranted if a person has known heart disease, heart symptoms, or a family history of sudden death.[105]

There is some evidence from studies of ultra-marathoners that excessive long-term endurance exercise may induce adverse heart remodeling and scarring, but most studies indicate that the greater the amount of exercise, the lower the risk of cardiovascular disease.[106 107 108 109] Evidence of a reduction in CVD mortality comes from studies of top-level athletes who engage in high levels of vigorous-intensity exercise, including Olympic marathoners and Tour de France cyclers. A meta-analysis of 10 studies found a CVD-related mortality rate that was 27% lower than for the general population.[110 111]

But as Gretchen Reynolds, writing in the *New York Times* has pointed out, "... precisely how much exercise might be needed in order to avoid heart disease has remained very much in question."[112] Reynolds cited a study that contrasted the heart disease risk differences between mail service office workers who sat most of the day with mail carriers who walked most of their workdays. The study subjects wore activity monitors, and cardiovascular risks were assessed by metabolic syndrome categorization and a measure of 10-year prediction of cardiovascular risk. The study found that time spent in a sedentary posture was associated with higher coronary heart disease risk and larger waist circumference. For every hour beyond five that workers sat each day, they added about two-tenths of a percentage point to their predicted likelihood of developing heart disease. The study found that almost any amount of standing and walking reduced heart disease risk, but the greater the volume of physical activity, the greater the benefit. Mail carriers who walked for more than three hours a day, covering at least 15,000 steps (about seven miles), or spent >7 hours per day upright, generally had normal body mass indexes, waistlines, and low-risk metabolic syndrome profiles.[113 114]

Some studies have found that the combination of a healthier diet and exercise has a more profound influence on achieving a favorable blood lipid pattern that either diet or exercise alone.[115] As described in Chapter 6, "Preventing Cardiovascular Disease," in one study, over a 10-year period, the fittest of those on statins had a

70% lower mortality than the least fit statin users, but the fittest of the study subjects who were not using statins had lower mortality than the unfit statin users.[116] Physical activity also helps to prevent obesity and diabetes, both of which increase risk of cardiovascular disease.

So clearly, an aerobic physical activity that improves endurance is associated with decreased CVD, but what about resistance training with weights? Additional evidence is needed, but one study found a 50% lower incidence of cardiovascular events, such as heart attack, stroke, or death, among those who weight trained occasionally compared to those who never did.[117]

Physical activity can reduce the risk of certain cancers.

Compared to people who are not active, it is well established that people who are physically active have a lower risk of colon and breast cancer. As is described in more detail in Chapter 7, "Preventing Cancer," a meta-analysis of 12 prospective studies found that higher levels of leisure-time physical activity were associated with a lower incidence of many common types of cancer, including endometrial cancer and lung cancer.[118] The study compared moderate to vigorous intensity leisure-time physical activity with incidence of 26 types of cancer and found that high vs. low levels of leisure-time physical activity were associated with lower risks of 13 cancers including esophageal adenocarcinoma, liver, lung, kidney, gastric cardia, endometrial, myeloid leukemia, myeloma, colon, head and neck, rectal, bladder and breast. The study authors concluded that leisure-time physical activity was associated with lower risks of many cancer types regardless of body size or smoking history. Research also shows that getting regular physical activity helps cancer survivors improve their physical fitness and have a better quality of life.

The 2018 Physical Activity Guidelines Scientific Advisory Committee evaluated 45 systematic reviews, meta-analyses, and pooled analyses comprising hundreds of epidemiologic studies with several million study participants. The Committee determined that strong evidence linked highest versus lowest physical activity levels to reduced risks of many types of cancer, with risk reductions ranging from approximately 10% to 20%.

Regular physical activity seems to reduce the risk of mental decline and dementia

Among those over 71 years of age, the prevalence of dementia in the U.S. is estimated to be nearly 14%, with 10% attributed to Alzheimer's disease and 4% to vascular disease and other causes. As is described in greater detail in Chapter 8, "Preventing Dementia," cardiovascular fitness appears to help protect against both

Alzheimer disease and the common vascular causes of dementia, mini-strokes, and atherosclerosis.[119 120] Other studies have found that physical activity, both aerobic activities and weight training, slow age-related mental decline, and improve cognition. The most physically active elderly have less age-related loss of brain volume than those who are sedentary.[121 122]

A meta-analysis review of 18 studies of the effect of exercise on cognition published in the journal *Psychological Science* concluded that exercise programs involving both aerobic exercise and strength training produced better results on cognitive abilities than either one alone. Older adults benefit more than younger adults. More than 30 minutes of exercise per session produce the greatest benefit.[123]

A study among veterans that measured physical fitness with a treadmill test found that those scoring six or lower metabolic equivalents on their fitness test had a more than four times greater risk of cognitive impairment, including Alzheimer disease, than those with scores of 12 or higher.[124]

Physical activity can improve mental health and mood

The risk of depression is lower for physically active adults who perform the recommended levels of aerobic or a combination of aerobic and muscle-strengthening activities. Regular physical activity also appears to reduce symptoms of anxiety and depression for children and adolescents. Although less well-proven, many people find that physical activity improves the quality of sleep, reduces anxiety, and improves mood.[125] According to Sanchis-Gomar et al., "Health is a state of physical, mental, and social well-being and not merely the absence of disease or infirmity. In this regard, vigorous intensity exercise is usually performed in groups or social networks, which improves emotional, intellectual, social, and spiritual well-being; sleep and mood; interest in sex; stress relief; energy and stamina; and mental alertness."[126 127]

A 25-year study found that at all ages, the greater the physical activity, the less likely those studied were to have symptoms of depression.[128] When evaluated five years later, sedentary people who began a three-times a week regimen had a lower mean number of symptoms and an estimated 19% reduction in the odds of depression. A meta-analysis review of 39 randomized clinical trials to study if exercise is associated with improvements in depression found that in most studies, exercise was associated with a reduction in depression scores.[129] The review concluded that the effect was only small or moderate and that well-designed clinical trials were needed.

Physical activity helps control weight

In 1977 Covert Bailey wrote a best-selling book, *Fit or Fat*, pointing out that the "overweight" problem people have is really a problem of too little muscle mass and too much fat or adiposity.[130] We are "overfat" when too high a proportion of our total body weight is made up of fat. Weight is gained when the calories expended by the body, including those used during physical activity, are less than the calories you take in through food and drink. Research shows that physical activity can help attain and maintain a normal weight.[131][132] However, as is described in more detail in Chapter 4, "Weight Control," exercise is an inefficient way to lose weight compared to the restriction of calories.

As fitness improves, muscles become more sensitive to the effects of insulin, and lower levels of insulin are needed to keep blood sugar in a normal range and help avoid the overshoot of insulin that leads to low blood sugar, excessive hunger, and overconsumption of food. Increased physical activity, especially when resistance and aerobic exercise are combined, reduces diabetics' need for insulin, and may prevent the progression of pre-diabetes.[133]

When losing weight, as much as one-third of the weight loss can come from the muscle that it is desirable to keep, rather than from the fat we want to lose. Exercise when dieting is one strategy to counter and minimize this. In one study, dieting walkers and weight trainers both lost about 20 pounds, but the weight-trainers lost only two pounds of muscle compared to the walkers—they lost four pounds.[134] Both groups lost more fat than dieters who did not exercise.

Another dietary strategy to retain and build muscle mass during both dieting and weight-training is to consume a plentiful supply of protein. An analysis of 17 clinical trials of people over age 60 (average age 73) found that consuming 10 to 35 grams of extra protein per day significantly increased lean muscle mass and leg strength in men but not much in women.[135] A review of 49 studies found that weight-trainers consuming 1.6 grams of protein a day per kilogram of body weight had modestly larger increases in muscle size and strength than those consuming lesser amounts.[136] Higher amounts than 1.6 gm/kg of protein were not beneficial. Benefits did not differ according to the protein's form (liquid or solid), or the source (plant or animal), or the time of day it was ingested. For a 70-kilogram (154 pound) man, 1.6 gm/kg of protein would be 112 grams a day of protein, precisely double the USDA nutrition goal recommended 56 grams a day for men. The USDA recommendation for women is 46 grams a day. This is not a difficult goal to reach from plant and animal sources. A cup of beans contains 15-18 grams of protein, a chicken breast 43 grams, yogurt 10 to 20 grams per cup, and an 8-ounce glass of fat-free milk contains approximately 8.5 grams of protein—nearly 40% of the total calories of skim milk.

For most people, an important long-term solution to the problem of being "overfat" is to both decrease the calories consumed and increase the calories expended by becoming more physically active. Increasing physical activity builds muscle and, assuming no increase in calories ingested, "burns" fat calories. The *Guidelines* suggest that the equivalent of 150 minutes of moderate-intensity activity a week should be considered a minimum to help to maintain a normal weight. Some people will need much more exercise to maintain a low level of body fat. For most people, getting to and staying at a healthy weight requires both regular physical activity and healthy nutrition without excess calories.

The National Runners and Walkers Health study has found that study participants who were runners had lower body mass indices and lower waist circumferences than the walkers, even though energy expenditures did not differ very much. Age-related weight gain was attenuated by running in both sexes and by walking in women.[137] One possibility relating to the difference between walkers and runners is that the more intense exercise of running helps to control appetite. One study on a small number of subjects indicated that compared to walkers, runners have higher levels of the appetite-suppressing hormone peptide YY and are less interested in food after running than walkers are after walking.[138]

There is some evidence that you can more efficiently burn fat if you exercise on an empty stomach rather than after a meal. In one study, twice as much body fat was mobilized from muscle and other body sites after exercise on an empty stomach than after a high-calorie shake.[139] Rather than deriving energy from the recent meal, the body's stores of glucose, glycogen, and fat were mobilized.

To achieve or maintain a healthy weight, the *Guidelines* suggest meeting the minimum level of physical activity. And if this does not suffice, either gradually increase the level of physical activity (toward the equivalent of 300 minutes a week of moderate-intensity aerobic activity), or reduce caloric intake, or both, until your weight-control goals are met. By regularly checking body weight, you can find the amount of physical activity that works for you.

For weight control, vigorous-intensity activity is far more time-efficient than moderate-intensity activity. For example, an adult who weighs 165 pounds (75 kg) will expend an additional 280 calories over baseline from a brisk 5-mile walk of 75 minutes duration at four miles an hour (these calories are in addition to the calories normally used by a body at rest). That person can expend the same number of additional calories in one-third the time (25 minutes) by running 2.5 miles at a 10 minutes-per-mile pace.

The Harvard Medical School provides a table that lists the calories burned in 30 minutes for people of three different weights according to activity, including walking, sports, and everyday household activities. It is available at: https://www.health.harvard.edu/diet-and-weight-loss/calories-burned-in-30-minutes-of-leisure-and-routine-activities.

Physical fitness

The *2008 Physical Activity Guidelines for Americans*[140] use the term "physical activity" to refer to bodily movement that enhances health. This is a different lens than considering physical activity that aims for athletic fitness. Baseline activity refers to the light-intensity activities of daily life, such as standing, walking slowly, and lifting lightweight objects. People who do only baseline activity are considered to be inactive.

The *2008 Guidelines* asserted that very short (less than 10 minutes) episodes of moderate- or vigorous-intensity activity, such as climbing a few flights of stairs were not long enough to count toward meeting the recommended *Guidelines for Physical Activity*. New research, described in the *2018 Physical Activity Guidelines Advisory Committee Scientific Report*, on high-intensity training of very short duration, and studies that used activity trackers that measured total minutes per day of moderate or vigorous physical activity, show that a health effect occurs with just about any duration of an activity.[141 142] In general, shorter, more frequent physical activities are equivalent to less frequent activities of longer duration if the total time is the same. The health benefits of a workout of 30 minutes on five days a week are the equivalent of 50 minutes on three days a week.

One 6-year study based on accelerometer readouts found that replacing just 30 minutes of sedentary time with an equal amount of light activity was associated with a 14% reduced risk of mortality.[143] The study found that replacement of sedentary time with moderate to vigorous activity was related to 50% mortality risk reduction, and there was a 42% reduced risk of mortality when light physical activity was replaced by moderate to vigorous activity.

There is evidence from a 15-year observational study in the U.K. that one or two (probably weekend) workouts are just as beneficial to avoid premature death as is the same total amount of physical activity three or more times during a week.[144] Many of the study subjects were men, about half of whom engaged in vigorous exercise just once a week. The study found that men and women who exercised in bouts of less than 10 minutes duration were 29% less likely to die prematurely from any cause than those who never worked out. The lead author of the study noted that "Reductions in risk were similar in the weekend warriors and the regularly active." Gretchen Reynolds, writing in the *New York Times*, noted that this is good news for about one-third of Americans who only work out on weekends.[145]

Physical activity–getting started

The following section includes excerpts updated and modified from the *2008 Physical Activity Guidelines for Americans*. It provides advice about options for physical activity, getting started safely, how much to do, and how often.

Brisk walking, jogging, cycling, and lifting weights are examples of health-enhancing physical activity. Some people, for example, postal carriers and construction workers, may get enough physical activity on the job to meet the *Guidelines*. Any physical activity provides some health benefits, but research has found that most benefits will accrue for adults from a minimum of 150 minutes (two hours and 30 minutes) a week of moderate-intensity, or 75 minutes (one hour and 15 minutes) a week of vigorous-intensity aerobic physical activity, or an equivalent combination of moderate- and vigorous-intensity aerobic activity.

Walking is an example of moderate-intensity aerobic activity, and jogging or running is an example of vigorous-intensity aerobic activity. For additional and more extensive health benefits, the *Guidelines* recommend that adults should increase their moderate-intensity aerobic physical activity to 300 minutes (five hours) a week, or 150 minutes a week of vigorous-intensity aerobic physical activity, or an equivalent combination of moderate- and vigorous-intensity activity. The bottom line is that more physical activity confers additional health benefits.

Aerobic activity (also called an endurance activity or cardio activity) requires sustained use of the body's large muscles. Examples are brisk walking, running, bicycling, jumping rope, and swimming. They are vigorous enough to substantially increase oxygen demand and cause a person's heart to beat faster than usual during a workout but do not exceed that ability of heart and lungs to keep up with the muscle's increased demand for oxygen. Aerobic capacity is measured in terms of maximal oxygen uptake (VO2max) during maximal exertion.

Aerobic physical activity has three components:

- Intensity, or how hard a person works to do the activity;
- Frequency, or how often a person does aerobic activity; and
- Duration, or how long a person does an activity in any one session.

Research has shown that the total amount of physical activity is more important for achieving health benefits than is any one of its three components: frequency, intensity, and duration.

Anaerobic exercise is vigorous exercise, like a 100-yard dash, that causes muscles to go into oxygen debt. In anaerobic exercise, the heart, lungs, and blood supply to the muscles cannot keep up with their need for oxygen, and the exercise will, therefore, be of relatively short duration.

Muscle-strengthening activity features multiple repetitions of resistance training that causes the body's muscles to work or hold against an applied force or weight. These activities involve weights, elastic bands, body weight, machines for resistance, and calisthenics. The *Guidelines* call for muscle-strengthening and bone-strengthening activities on two or more days a week as these activities provide additional health benefits. The effects of muscle-strengthening activity are limited to the muscles doing the work, so it's important to work all the major muscle groups of the body: legs, hips, back, abdomen, chest, shoulders, and arms.

Muscle-strengthening activity also has three components:

- Intensity or how much weight or force is used relative to how much a person is able to lift;
- Frequency, or how often a person does muscle-strengthening activity; and
- Repetitions, or how many times a person lifts a weight (analogous to duration for aerobic activity).

Bone-strengthening activity is sometimes called weight-bearing or weight-loading activity. These activities produce an increase of force on the bones that promotes bone growth and strengthening. The needed force on bones is commonly produced by impact with the ground. Examples of bone-strengthening activity include jumping, running, brisk walking, and weight-lifting exercises. Bone-strengthening activities can also be aerobic and muscle strengthening. Excellent aerobic activities such as cycling and swimming do not do nearly as much for skeletal health as do weight-bearing exercises such as walking and running.

Getting started

Inactive adults or those who don't yet do 150 minutes of physical activity a week should work gradually toward this goal. To reduce the risk of injury, it is important to increase the amount of physical activity gradually over a period of weeks to months. The initial amount of activity should be at a light or moderate intensity for short periods of time, with the sessions spread throughout the week. For example, an inactive person could start with a walking program consisting of five minutes of slow walking several times each day, five to six days a week. The length of time could then gradually be increased to 10 minutes per session, three times a day, and the walking speed could be increased slowly.

Muscle-strengthening activities should also be gradually increased over time. Initially, these activities can be done just one day a week, starting at a light or moderate level of effort. Over time, the number of days a week can be increased to two, and better yet, more than two. Each week, the level of effort (intensity) can be increased slightly until it becomes moderate to high.

To reduce the risk of injuries and other adverse events, people should:

- Protect themselves by using appropriate gear and sports equipment, looking for safe environments, following rules and policies of venues and sports, and making sensible choices about when, where, and how to be active.
- Be under the care of a health care provider if they have chronic health conditions or symptoms.

Active adults often need to increase their aerobic activity to exceed the minimum level, move toward 300 minutes a week, and also do muscle-strengthening activities on at least two days each week. Substituting vigorous-intensity aerobic activity for some moderate-intensity activity both helps achieve greater fitness and saves time. Using the 2-to-1 rule of thumb, doing 150 minutes of vigorous-intensity aerobic activity a week provides about the same (and possibly more) benefits as 300 minutes of moderate-intensity activity. Undertaking a variety of activities probably reduces the risk of overuse injury.

Highly active adults should maintain their activity level and are also encouraged to do a variety of activities to ensure all major muscle groups are strengthened.

Key guidelines for older adults

The key guidelines for adults also apply to older adults. In addition, the following guidelines are just for older adults:

- When older adults cannot do 150 minutes of moderate-intensity aerobic activity a week because of chronic conditions, they should be as physically active as their abilities and conditions allow.
- Older adults should do exercises that maintain or improve balance if they are at risk of falling.
- Older adults should determine their level of effort for physical activity relative to their level of fitness.
- Older adults with chronic conditions should understand whether and how their conditions affect their ability to do regular physical activity safely.

If you answer "yes" to one or more of these questions, you shouldn't start exercising without first consulting your physician or health care provider.

- Do you smoke cigarettes?
- Are you overweight by more than 10–20 pounds?
- Are you 35 years old or older?
- Have you ever had a heart attack?
- Is there a history of heart disease in your family? Did either of your parents have a heart attack in their fifties or sixties (or earlier)?
- Have you ever had an abnormal electrocardiogram (ECG)?
- Have you ever thought that your heart was beating too fast?
- Do you have arthritis?
- Is your range of motion limited in any of your joints?
- Do you have any chronic illnesses?

A cardiovascular and musculoskeletal exam can reveal whether you have any problems that might limit your participation in whatever activity you choose. If you're afraid of getting hurt, the good news is that moderate-intensity aerobic activity, such as brisk walking, is generally safe for most people.

Start slowly. Cardiac events, such as a heart attack, are rare during physical activity. But the risk does go up when you suddenly become much more active than usual. That's one reason it's important to start slowly and gradually increase your level of activity.

If you have a chronic health condition such as arthritis, diabetes, or heart disease, consult your health care provider to find out if your condition limits, in any way, your ability to be active and make a physical activity plan that matches your abilities. It is important to avoid being inactive because the health benefits of physical activity far outweigh the risks of getting hurt.

Ways to understand and measure the intensity of aerobic activity

There are two ways to track the intensity of aerobic activity: absolute intensity and relative intensity.

Absolute intensity is the amount of energy expended per minute of activity. A MET (metabolic equivalent) stands for the amount of oxygen you consume and the number of calories you burn at rest. The energy expenditure of light-intensity activity, for example, is 1.1 to 2.9 METs. Moderate-intensity activities expend 3.0 to 5.9 METs. Walking at three miles per hour or 100 steps per minute has an intensity of three to four METS. The energy expenditure of vigorous-intensity activities is six or more METs. Walking 130 steps per minute is considered vigorous physical activity. Running at a 10 minutes per mile pace is equivalent to 10 METs. It is also possible to use watts, a measure of power as an objective gauge of energy output. Various fitness machines will provide an indication of watts expended at any moment during a workout. A beginner cyclist might average 70 to 75 watts whereas a Tour de France professional could reach an average of 350 to 375 watts over an hour. The ability to produce watts per body weight of a person is one measure of fitness.

Relative intensity is the level of effort required to do an activity. Less fit people generally require a higher level of effort than fitter people to do the same activity. Relative intensity can be estimated using a scale of 0 to 10, where sitting is 0, and the highest level of effort possible is 10. Moderate-intensity activity is a 5 or 6. Vigorous intensity activity is a 7 or 8.

When using relative intensity, people pay attention to how physical activity affects their heart rate and breathing. As a rule of thumb, a person doing a moderate intensity aerobic activity can talk, but not sing, during the activity. A person doing a vigorous intensity activity cannot say more than a few words without pausing for a breath.

Target heart rate and estimated maximum heart rate

One way of monitoring physical activity intensity is to determine whether a person's pulse or heart rate is within the target zone during physical activity.

For moderate-intensity physical activity, a person's target heart rate should be 50% to 70% of his or her age-related maximum heart rate. Although the science underlying calculation of maximum heart rate is not strong, this maximum is commonly estimated based on the person's age using the following formula: subtracting the person's age from 220. For example, for a 50-year-old person, the estimated maximum age-related heart rate would be calculated as 220 - 50 years = 170 beats per minute (bpm). The 50% and 70% levels would be:

50% level: 170 x 0.50 = 85 bpm, and
70% level: 170 x 0.70 = 119 bpm

Thus, moderate-intensity physical activity for a 50-year-old person will require that the heart rate remains between 85 and 119 bpm during physical activity.

For vigorous-intensity physical activity, a person's target heart rate should be 70% to 85% of his or her maximum heart rate. For example, for a 35-year-old person, the estimated maximum age-related heart rate would be calculated as 220 - 35 years

= 185 beats per minute (bpm). The 70% and 85% levels would be:

70% level: 185 x 0.70 = 130 bpm, and
85% level: 185 x 0.85 = 157 bpm

Thus, vigorous-intensity physical activity for a 35-year-old person will require that the heart rate remains between 130 and 157 bpm during physical activity.

Table 9.1. Examples of moderate and vigorous intensity physical activity

Examples of Different Aerobic Physical Activities and Intensities
Moderate Intensity • Walking briskly (3 miles per hour or faster, but not race-walking) • Water aerobics • Bicycling slower than 10 miles per hour • Tennis (doubles) • Ballroom dancing • General gardening
Vigorous Intensity • Racewalking, jogging, or running • Swimming laps • Tennis (singles) • Aerobic dancing • Bicycling 10 miles per hour or faster • Jumping rope • Heavy gardening (continuous digging or hoeing, with heart rate increases) • Hiking uphill or with a heavy backpack

Muscle-strengthening activity

Muscle-strengthening activities provide additional benefits not found with aerobic activity, including increased bone strength and muscular fitness. Muscle-strengthening activities can also help maintain muscle mass during a program of weight loss.

Muscle-strengthening activities make muscles do more work than they are accustomed to doing. That is, they overload the muscles. They should involve all the major muscle groups and should be done at least two days a week. One set of eight to 12 repetitions of each exercise is effective, although two or three sets is likely to be more effective. Short rest intervals of 30 to 90 seconds between sets seem best for building muscle endurance, and longer, two to five minutes rest intervals are recommended for building strength. Reps should be performed to the point at which it would be difficult to do another repetition without help. The development of muscle strength and endurance is progressive over time. Increases in the amount of weight or the days a week of exercising will result in stronger muscles.

Flexibility and balance activities

Flexibility is considered to be an important part of physical fitness, especially for some types of physical activity. Stretching exercises are effective in increasing flexibility and improving cardiovascular health. It is unclear whether they reduce the risk of injury. Time spent doing flexibility activities by themselves does not count toward meeting the aerobic or muscle-strengthening *Guidelines*.

Balance training activities are movements that safely challenge postural control. If practiced regularly, they improve the ability to prevent falls, whether walking, standing, or sitting. Standing on one foot, walking heel-to-toe, the balance walk, and using a wobble board are examples of balance training activities.

Warm-up and cool-down

A warm-up or cool-down involves doing an activity at a slower speed or lower intensity. A warm-up before activity allows a gradual increase in heart rate and breathing at the start of the episode of activity. A cool-down after activity allows a gradual decrease at the end of the episode. Time spent doing warm-up and cool-down may count toward meeting the aerobic activity *Guidelines* if the activity is at least moderate intensity (for example, walking briskly as a warm-up before jogging). A warm-up for muscle-strengthening activity commonly involves doing exercises with lighter weight.

Some athletes use icy water to cool down after a workout in the belief that it improves recovery and enhances fitness gains. The science behind this practice is weak. Recent research found that the biopsied muscle fiber size increases were greater among athletes who rested after weight training than those of athletes who underwent a post-workout cold soak.[146]

Adults can meet the *Physical Activity Guidelines* in all sorts of ways and with many types of physical activity. The choices of types and amounts of physical activity depend on personal health and fitness goals.

The beneficial effects of increasing physical activity: it's about overload, progression, and specificity

Overload is the physical stress placed on the body when physical activity is greater in amount or intensity than usual. The body's structures and functions respond and adapt to these stresses. For example, aerobic physical activity increases the efficiency and capacity of the lungs, heart, circulatory system, and exercising muscles. In the same way, muscle-strengthening and bone-strengthening activities overload muscles and bones and lead to adaptations that make them stronger.

Progression is closely tied to overload. Once a person reaches a certain fitness level, he or she progresses to higher levels of physical activity by continued overload and adaptation. Small, progressive changes in overload help the body adapt to the additional stresses while minimizing the risk of injury.

Specificity means that the benefits of physical activity are specific to the body systems that are doing the work. For example, aerobic physical activity largely benefits the body's cardiovascular system.

Beyond physical activity for health: getting physically fit

Research has documented the important health benefits of 150 or better yet 300 hours of moderate intensity physical activity a week. This level of physical activity contributes to fitness. But what about getting more highly fit with the goal of improving athletic performance? What sort, how often, how intense, and what duration should physical conditioning exercises for this purpose be? And what is the best schedule for someone who is sedentary and just embarking on a fitness program?

Good advice on getting athletically fit is found in the science-based books on aerobics by exercise physiologist, Kenneth Cooper. They provide a practical guide to fitness that was developed by Cooper for the United States Air Force. He studied the often-poor performance of soldiers at oxygen intensive exercises such as long-distance running, swimming, and bicycling. Cooper evaluated sustained performance in terms of a person's ability to use oxygen, or aerobic capacity and proposed that the combined capacity of lungs, heart and blood vessels to deliver oxygen to the body was the best index of overall physical fitness.

In his book, *Aerobics*, first published in 1968, Cooper presented a series of scientifically-proven exercise programs to improve physical performance.[147] He described the training effect that brings about biochemical and anatomic bodily changes that improve the body's ability to use oxygen. He found that not only do the muscles used in locomotion get stronger, but so does the heart and the muscles used in respiration. As fitness improves, circulation and oxygen transfer are facilitated by lower blood pressure and an increased number of oxygen-carrying red blood cells.

Research carried out by Cooper, and other exercise physiologists showed that to get the training effect needed to improve fitness, exercise must be of sufficient intensity, duration, and frequency. To help the average person get the exercise needed for a training effect, Cooper devised a points scale based on the oxygen requirements of a wide variety of aerobic exercises according to their length and duration. For example, walking or running two miles in 40 minutes or longer just barely begins to cause a training effect and is awarded one point whereas running the same two-mile distance in between 23:59 and 20 minutes gets a point score of seven. To reach what Cooper considers to be a minimum standard of fitness requires the accumulation of 30 points a week using running, walking, swimming, bicycling, or other aerobic exercises in any combination.

Dr. Cooper emphasizes that prior to beginning any fitness program or taking a fitness test, it is essential to get a medical checkup and clearance, especially if you are over age 30. To help guide initial intensity and speed of progression when starting a fitness program, Cooper has devised exercise schedules based on age and level of fitness based on the fitness tests he has devised, a 12-minute run for distance, or a run of 1.5 miles for speed. Cooper also emphasizes the importance of warming up before exercise and cooling down after.

A critical lesson from the experience of many people seeking to improve their fitness is to progress slowly. It is a mistake to rush a conditioning program. A gradual increase in intensity and duration over at least six weeks to attain a minimum level of fitness is needed, and gradual progression of intensity, duration, and frequency over many months thereafter is advisable. For example, Jeff Galloway recommends a 30-week schedule as the minimum required for someone to be able to go from an average of running two miles a day to be able to finish a marathon.[148]

Training with high-intensity physical activity

Considerable recent research is focused on the health and training effects of very short duration high-intensity physical activity and the idea that we can rely on a few high-intensity intervals as our only exercise and still improve our health and fitness. High-intensity training (HIT), also called high-intensity interval training (HIIT), requires repeated periods of maximum effort. This seems to be the most efficient way to promote aerobic fitness and may improve exercise performance to the same extent as traditional endurance training. Research on high-intensity interval training (HIT or HIIT) has shown that repeated brief periods of maximum effort exercise lead to the same muscle cell adaptations, fitness gains, and improved cardiovascular function as prolonged low-intensity exercise, but in a much shorter time.[149 150 151] The 2018 Physical Activity Guidelines Scientific Advisory Committee concluded that there is "moderate evidence to indicate that HIIT can effectively improve insulin sensitivity, blood pressure, and body composition in adults. These HIIT-induced improvements in cardiometabolic disease risk factors are comparable to those resulting from continuous, moderate-intensity aerobic exercise. They are more likely to occur in adults with overweight and obesity."[152]

The optimal time periods for maximum effort and recovery are not yet well established. Martin Gibala, a professor of kinesiology at McMaster University in Hamilton, Ontario, is one of the scientists who originated the HIT regimen. He suggests that "a minute of hard effort followed by a minute of gentle recovery is effective."[153] However, it is not clear if a relatively few (16-30) minutes of high-intensity exercise a week will confer the same health benefits as 75 minutes of vigorous exercise or 150 to 300 minutes of moderate intensity physical activity over a week as is recommended by the *Guidelines*. One potential drawback of short, intense sessions is that they don't burn many calories and may not be as effective for weight loss and maintenance as exercise schedules of longer duration. Another potential drawback is the possibility of injury from the high level of stress placed on the musculoskeletal and cardiovascular system.

One recent study evaluated twice weekly extremely short high-intensity training, consisting of 10 × 6-second sprints with a one-minute recovery between each sprint.[154] Metabolic health (measured by an oral glucose tolerance test), aerobic capacity (measured by incremental time to exhaustion on a cycle ergometer), and physical function (evaluated by a get-up and go test, sit to stand test and loaded 50-meter walk) were determined before and after training. Following eight weeks of HIT there was a significant improvement in aerobic capacity (8% increase in VO2 max), physical function (11% and 27%), and a reduction in blood glucose response (6% reduction). The authors of the study concluded that the study demonstrated the potential of HIT as a training intervention to improve skeletal muscle function and glucose clearance as we age and that HIT needs to be performed only twice a week to see major improvements in aerobic capacity, functional capacity and metabolic health in an untrained middle-aged population. They suggest that HIT, lasting no more than 11 minutes, may be used as a time-efficient method of reducing the risk of disease and functional decline in middle age.

One problem with many HIT regimens is that many adopters don't enjoy the high effort required in high-intensity interval workouts and soon abandon the programs. To address this problem, researchers in Denmark devised what they call a 10-20-30 training program.[155] The essential features of it are, that after a warm-up, exercise aerobically (run, row, or cycle) gently for 30 seconds (at about 30% of maximum intensity), accelerate to a moderate pace for 20 seconds (at about 60% of maximum intensity) and then go all out as hard as you can for 10 seconds (at 90–100% of maximum intensity), then repeat each 30 second, 20 second and 10 second session five times with no pause between sessions, take a two-minute rest and repeat five more times. Each session, when repeated five times, takes five minutes, and with a two-minute rest, the workout requires only 12 minutes. For those already in excellent shape, a third or even a fourth five-minute exercise period can be added. The creators of this workout regimen recommend that it should be limited to two or three times a week and followed by a rest day or a light workout.

In a study of the 10-20-30 training concept over a seven-week period, a group of recreational runners replaced their usual training sessions with three weekly 10-20-30 training periods of five minutes duration repeated three or four times interspersed by two minutes of rest.[156] A control group continued with their usual endurance training. The study found that even though the study participants had about a 50% reduction in training volume as measured by weekly mileage, VO2max was elevated by 4% and performance in a 1,500-m and a 5-km run improved by 21 and 48 seconds, respectively. Furthermore, the 10-20-30 training led to a marked reduction in systolic blood pressure as well as a lowering of total cholesterol and LDL-cholesterol.

Gretchen Reynolds asked Dr. Gibala, the professor of kinesiology who has studied and popularized HIT, "Is one minute the shortest possible HIIT workout or will I be writing about a 30-second workout soon?" Dr. Gibala responded, "I think one minute may be the limit. We are still looking for the exact sweet spot in terms of how little intense effort people can do and still get significant health and fitness benefits. So far, it looks as if three repetitions of 20-second intervals is the lowest effective load. But we are still experimenting. Stay tuned."[157]

The *University of California, Berkeley Wellness Letter* recently described and analyzed low-volume high-intensity interval training, the fitness regimen popularized as the 7-Minute Workout.[158] They note that there are many versions of the 7-Minute Workout accessible on websites and apps. They all feature high-intensity calisthenics with (in contrast to some HIT regimens) very little time, about 10 seconds, between each of perhaps 12 different calisthenics.[159] They concluded that there is some evidence that these workouts, when performed three to four times a week for several weeks, provide as much or more conditioning and cardiovascular benefit as a traditional 30-minute workout. The *Wellness Letter* advised those who want to try low-volume high-intensity interval training to make sure the workout is intense, that it includes a variety of exercises, and to alternate upper-body and lower-body exercises. They also suggest that it is important to use proper form to avoid injury and caution that even fit people may find these workouts challenging. They also advise individuals who are elderly, obese or have a heart condition to check with their physician prior to initiating any of the 7-Minute Workout programs.

Summary of the Essential Facts

- Regular physical activity reduces the risk of many adverse health outcomes including premature death; overweight and obesity; high blood pressure; unhealthy blood lipid patterns; dementia; heart disease, stroke and other cardiovascular diseases; metabolic syndrome; osteoporosis; breast, colon and other cancers; anxiety and depression; and type 2 diabetes.
- Regular physical activity provides beneficial health outcomes, including helping control weight and improving muscle strength, balance, fitness, athletic ability, and personal appearance.
- Any physical activity is better than none.
- Most health benefits occur with at least 150 minutes a week of moderate-intensity physical activity, or 75 minutes a week of vigorous-intensity physical activity, and these totals can be accumulated on any schedule.
- Depending on personal health and fitness goals, you can meet the *Physical Activity Guidelines* in all sorts of ways and with many types of physical activity.
- Both aerobic (e.g., brisk walking, running, swimming, cross-country skiing, bicycling) and muscle-strengthening physical activities are recommended, and together they are more beneficial than either alone.
- For most health outcomes, additional benefits occur as the amount of physical activity increases through higher intensity, greater frequency, and/or longer duration.
- If you are over the age of 30, or have any health condition, or are taking medication, make sure that you have a checkup and clearance from your medical care provider prior to undertaking a new physical activity regimen.
- To avoid injuries and other problems, it is important to warm up, increase the amount of physical activity slowly, and cool down.

10
Stress and Mental Health

The U.S. health system gives much attention to screening, diagnosis, and treatment of overt mental illness, and much less to preventing mental health problems and the enhancement of mental health. The focus of this chapter is on improving the quality of life and the prevention of mental health problems through healthy living. As with all of the health conditions dealt with in this book, the reader is advised to seek professional help from a reputable well-trained health care provider when any form of physical or mental illness occurs.

Defining mental health

According to the World Health Organization (WHO), good mental health is "a state of well-being in which the individual realizes his or her own abilities, can cope with the normal stresses of life, can work productively and fruitfully, and is able to make a contribution to his or her community."[1]

One formulation of mental health indicators is that they encompass three domains: emotional well-being (including perceived life satisfaction), psychological well-being (such as having a purpose in life and positive relationships), and social well-being (for example, social acceptance and a sense of community).[2 3 4] The presence of attentive and loving parents, siblings, and other caregivers in early life is especially important to foster good mental health. The social conditions that support good mental health include the conditions that lead to the satisfaction of basic human needs such as adequate housing, personal safety and safe neighborhoods, jobs with fair wages, high-quality education, equity in life opportunities, and access to high-quality health care.[5]

Mental illness is defined as "health conditions that are characterized by alterations in thinking, mood, or behavior (or some combination thereof) associated with distress and/or impaired functioning."[6] It is estimated that in any given year, one in five children and one of four adult Americans will develop a mental health disorder that goes beyond normal emotional ups and downs, and that begins to interfere with daily life. Common mental health illnesses include mood disorders, such as depression and bipolar (manic-depressive) disorder, substance use disorder, and anxiety disorders, such as panic disorder and social anxiety disorder. It is estimated that about 10% of people in the U.S. have some form of anxiety disorder at any time.[7 8 9]

Mental health problems occur across the entire lifespan. Because the young human brain remains more plastic and continues to develop through about age 24, therapeutic interventions in childhood that address mental health disorders improve the chances of favorable mental health outcomes. Interventions are most effective when tailored to the specific needs of those at the developmental stages of infants, toddlers, school-age children, adolescents, transitional age youth (18-24), adults, and geriatric patients.

By age 29, more than half of Americans will have had an impairing and clinically significant psychiatric illness, such as an anxiety disorder, a psychotic disorder, a substance use disorder, or major depressive disorder.[10] In 2015, nearly 18% of adults in the U.S. reported having a mental, behavioral or emotional disorder, and 3% of people age 12 or older and 7% of people age 18 to 25 reported the use of an illicit drug.[11] Mental health and substance misuse disorders are a leading cause of disease burden, rivaling cancer, and cardiovascular disease. In contrast to other wealthy countries, the U.S. has had higher rates of death from unintentional poisonings, the majority of which were due to drug overdoses.[12 13] Unfortunately, as the Centers for Disease Control and Prevention (CDC) notes, "it is estimated that only about 17% of U.S. adults are considered to be in a state of optimal mental health."[14 15]

Mental health problems are costly

Mental health issues are among the top 10 reasons for disability in the U.S. In 2013, the *New York Times* reported that the U.S. spends about $150 billion annually on direct medical costs to care for an estimated 11.5 million U.S. adults with a debilitating mental illness.[16] Indirect costs to the U.S. economy are equally important, with a cost of about $193 billion annually in lost earnings. In addition, an increased need for public services like food stamps and subsidized housing may require government outlays of another $140 to $160 billion a year. The *Times* author concluded that, all together, our cumulative mental-health issues — depression, schizophrenia, and bipolar disorder, among others — are costing the U.S. economy about a half-trillion dollars—more than the government spent on all of Medicare during the 2012 fiscal year.

Stress—what it is and what health problems does it cause?

Psychological stress has important implications for both physical and mental health. The human body has systems that trigger protective physiological responses to acute stressors, such as being in a threatening or dangerous situation or maybe just rushing to catch a bus. In these "fight or flight" circumstances, the body releases a surge of hormones, mainly epinephrine (adrenaline) and cortisol. These hormones increase the heart rate, increase glucose levels in the bloodstream, elevate blood pressure, and prepare the body for action. And when the stressful event is over, the body's physiology quickly returns to normal.

Our bodies are less well equipped to deal with the protracted mental stress that results from issues such as financial troubles, relationship problems, traffic jams, stressful jobs, and the other chronic stresses of modern living.[17]

Stress can result from experiencing a single traumatic event such as a car accident or a single sexual assault, or there may be ongoing trauma from domestic violence, recurrent child sexual abuse, or community violence. Chronic stress can be related to an event such as a divorce or death of a family member or societal prejudices concerning individual characteristics such as race, ethnicity, gender, sexuality, national origin, immigration status, cultural practices, accent, religion, dress, and age among others. Perceived unfairness in school admissions, hiring practices, position advancement, and other social situations can also be a source of a traumatic event or chronic stress.

Everyone has worries, but when they become pervasive, and out of control, the constant stress may cause symptoms such as fatigue, difficulty sleeping, nightmares, and irritability. Early childhood chronic stress and trauma, rather than a single event, can lead to adverse anatomical and neuroendocrine changes in the brain. Among the harmful effects of prolonged, unrelieved stress and elevated stress hormones is an increased risk of many physical health problems, including hypertension, heart disease, obesity, irritable bowel syndrome, anxiety, cognitive impairment, including memory problems, and depression.[18] For example, the Baltimore Memory Study carried out by Johns Hopkins researchers found that high levels of the stress hormone cortisol were linked to poor cognitive performance in older individuals.[19]

Trauma and stressor-related disorders

Reactive attachment disorder (RAD) is a serious condition in which an infant or young child doesn't establish healthy attachments with parents or caregivers. It may develop if the child's basic needs for comfort, affection, and nurturing aren't met, and loving, caring, stable attachments with others are not established.

Childhood trauma, abuse, or neglect without a caring adult to make the experiences less traumatic can also result in disinhibited social engagement disorder (DSED). This is an attachment disorder in which a child may actively and inappropriately approach and interact with unfamiliar adults.

Post-traumatic stress disorder (PTSD) is a form of chronic psychological stress that affects as many as 5% of people who experience a traumatic event such as an accident, violent crime, or wartime combat. It is characterized by intrusive and distressing memories of the trauma, hyper-vigilance, and diminished ability to relate to loved ones and cope with normal life activities. A combination of medications and psychotherapy is the most effective treatment.

Depression

Some people seem to be born to be happy and cheerful despite life's misfortunes. They are energetic, productive, and have a joyous temperament, that in an extreme form, is called hyperthymia. In contrast, some people are always down, they suffer from a chronic, often lifelong, mild depression called persistent depressive disorder (PDD) that was formerly called dysthymia, and no matter how fortunate they are, go through life with depressed mood and pessimism.[20 21] A very high proportion (perhaps 90%) of people with a persistent depressive disorder are subject to episodes of more severe depression, a mood disorder, and the most common type of mental illness.

Symptoms of depression include feelings of sadness and hopelessness, irritability, apathy, sleep problems, decreased energy, changes in appetite, inability to concentrate, feelings of worthlessness, and thoughts of death or suicide.[22] If many of these symptoms are present in a child more than one week or for more than two weeks in an adult, the person experiencing them may be among the 5% to 8% of the U.S. population suffering at least one episode of major depression each year and a lifetime risk of 16% to 19%.[23] Depression is a leading cause of disability, and depression increases the risk of illnesses such as asthma, heart attack, and stroke.[24 25]

There is a genetic component to depression. It is more likely if a parent or an identical twin had a mood disorder. Depression may be triggered by stressful life events such as childbirth (postpartum depression), a divorce, the death of a spouse, or developing a serious illness such as cancer or a heart attack. Seasonal affective disorder or SAD is a form of depression associated with the seasonal decline in daylight hours. Depression also may be associated with misuse of alcohol and other drugs and with a variety of neurological and other illnesses.

Bipolar disorder, formerly called manic depression, causes extreme mood swings that include emotional highs (mania or hypomania) and lows (depression).[26 27] Episodes of mood swings typically begin in the teen ages or the early 20s and may occur rarely or multiple times a year. When a person's mood shifts from depression to mania, they may feel euphoric and full of energy. Mood swings can affect sleep, judgment, behavior, the ability to think clearly, and cause significant distress and difficulty in life. Getting help and treatment with medications and psychological counseling from a mental health professional with expertise in bipolar disorder can help get the disorder under control.

Managing stress and avoiding depression

Adopting a healthy lifestyle can preserve and improve mental health as well as physical health. In the course of everyone's life, events bring anxieties, fears, and stresses. Managing stress requires the use of effective coping mechanisms. The following strategies have been found to help cope with stress and improve mood and self-image.[28 29]

Avoid misusing drugs and alcohol

Drugs and alcohol may temporarily make you feel better, but they usually lead to more problems and stress. At the 35-year point in the long-term Harvard Mastery of Stress Study, it was found that neurosis and depression tended to follow misuse of alcohol, rather than to cause it.[30]

Eat a healthy diet

A meta-analysis of 41 studies found that a healthy diet, in particular, a traditional Mediterranean diet that avoids processed meats and emphasizes fruit, vegetables, whole grains, and nuts, is associated with a reduced risk of depression.[31] The study authors suggested that the reason for the association is because, "...a number of factors have been proposed to cause diet-induced damage to the brain, including oxidative stress, insulin resistance, inflammation, and changes in vascularization, as all these factors can be modified by dietary intake and have been associated with the occurrence of depression."

The potential benefits of diet for depression are not yet fully understood, and the effects are probably modest and not likely to be a sole way to prevent or treat depression. Rather, adding lifestyle interventions addressing smoking cessation, physical activity, and diet quality may supplement usual psychological and pharmacological treatments.[32] It is worth noting that dietary supplements are not helpful in the prevention or treatment of major depressive disorders.[33 34]

Be physically active

Many individuals report and studies confirm that physical activity is a stress reliever.[35] A study found that when measured objectively, greater physical activity was associated with the prevention of depression.[36] Effects began when in a 24-hour period a person replaces sedentary behavior with 15 minutes of vigorous activity such as running; or more than 1 hour of moderate physical activity (e.g., fast walking); or some combination of light activity (e.g., standing, stretching, easy chores) and more vigorous activity.

A meta-analysis of 33 clinical trials, published in *JAMA Psychiatry*, found that resistance exercise training was associated with a significant reduction in depressive symptoms.[37] Long-term studies show that the more physically active people are, the less likely they are to be depressed, and if they start to exercise, their risk of depression declines.[38] Measuring this relationship is complicated by the fact that depressed individuals are less likely to exercise.[39] Although exercise has been documented to provide a modest improvement in stress-induced mood disorders, such as depression, the studies show that it is less effective than psychotherapy and drug treatment.[40] (See Chapter 9, "Benefits of Physical Activity," for additional details on the links between physical activity and mental health.)

Try relaxation techniques

Many people find that guided imagery, progressive muscle relaxation, yoga, tai chi, meditation, and biofeedback are good antidotes to stress. These and other mindfulness techniques can be learned from a variety of sources, including mental health professionals. Herbert Benson has studied the physical effects of meditation and documented that a variety of techniques have the same calming effect, including the lowering of blood pressure.[41] Dean Ornish advocates yoga for the relief of stress as a feature of his program for healthy living.[42]

Get enough sleep

Studies of interventions to treat insomnia have led to reductions in depression. Sleep is important not only to reduce stress and avoid depression but also for overall health, avoiding accidents, and being productive at work. Lack of sleep makes you "dumb and dangerous." See Chapter 15, "More Advice About Healthy Living," for more information on the importance of sleep.

Connect socially and share your feelings

You can get social-support help with stress-induced mood disorders by avoiding isolation, spending time with other people, and staying connected to your familial roots and culture. Getting support from your community, friends, family, a counselor, a doctor, or a clergyperson and sharing your problems can lighten your mental burdens.

Maintain or re-establish your normal routine

Familiar activities such as meals with family and friends, reading, watching TV, playing with a pet and exercising are examples of routines that are conducive to mental equanimity.

Stay active

Work or fun activities can help take your mind off your problems. Hobbies, sports, games, and volunteering are examples of ways you can stay active.

Seek professional help

If stress is overwhelming and unmanageable or leading to depression or anxiety, it is probably time to seek help from a mental health professional such as a clinical psychologist or psychiatrist. Mental health care providers offer three general types of therapy: insight into your situation, support and advice about how to change your situation or behavior, and medications.

Insights from a long-term study

The Harvard Mastery of Stress Study has followed the life course of a sample of Harvard college undergraduates since 1948 and through age 80. One striking finding was the importance of psychological support in childhood to health. After 35 years, the study subjects identified in midlife as suffering from illnesses such as coronary artery disease, hypertension, duodenal ulcer, and alcoholism, gave their parents significantly lower ratings on perceived parental caring.

Among study participants, twice as many (91%) who had diagnosed diseases in midlife felt that they did not have a warm relationship with their mothers as compared to the 45% of participants who felt they had a warm relationship. A similar association was found for fathers. Only 25% of subjects who rated both their mothers and fathers high in parental caring had diagnosed diseases in midlife. The study concluded, "Since parents are usually the most meaningful source of social support for much of early life, the perception of parental caring, and parental loving itself, may have important regulatory and predictive effects on biological and psychological health and illness."[43]

George Vaillant, the Harvard Mastery of Stress Study director, identified seven major factors that predicted physical and psychological healthy aging. Education, having a stable marriage, not smoking, not abusing alcohol, getting some exercise, maintaining a healthy weight, and employing mature adaptations (sometimes called defenses) to life stresses.[44 45]

In *The Atlantic*, Joshua Wolf Shenk summarized Vaillant's research:[46]

> Of the 106 Harvard men who had five or six of these factors in their favor at age 50, half ended up at 80 as what Vaillant called "happy-well" and only 7.5 percent as "sad-sick." Meanwhile, of the men who had three or fewer of the health factors at age 50, none ended up "happy-well" at 80. Even if they had been in adequate physical shape at 50, the men who had three or fewer protective factors were three times as likely to be dead at 80 as those with four or more factors. . . . Good sibling relationships seem especially powerful: 93 percent of the men who were thriving at age 65 had been close to a brother or sister when younger.

Preventing suicide

Suicide is associated with mental illness. Those who have chronic mood disorders such as depression or psychosis are 10 to 20 times more likely to commit suicide. About 7% of men and 1% of women diagnosed with depression die by suicide, and two-thirds of people committing suicide are depressed. The risk of suicide is 20 to 30 times higher than rates among the general population in people with untreated bipolar disorder (manic-depression).[47 48] Misuse of alcohol and pain and opioid use disorders are also linked to suicide and unintentional opioid overdose, as are relationship problems and adverse life events.[49 50] According to the CDC, between the years 2000 and 2016, suicides in the U.S. increased by 30%.[51] In 2017, of 47,173 deaths caused by suicide, 23,854 involved firearms, and 6,247 of these were among individuals age 15 to 24.[52]

An important risk factor for suicide in the United States is access to firearms. Guns were used in 51% of completed suicides in 2013.[53] Self-injury with a gun is fatal 84% of the time. This contrasts with an average of only 4% success by all other means. Suicide by suffocation/hanging is 69% fatal, and falls are 31% fatal, but together they account for fewer than half the number of deaths that guns claim each year. There is strong evidence that access to firearms in the home is associated with a significantly increased suicide risk and that reducing gun access for people at risk will reduce suicide. A study of gun ownership in California found that male handgun owners were seven times more likely and female handgun owners 35 times more likely to die by suicide with a firearm compared to firearm deaths among non-owners of handguns.[54]

Cognitive-behavioral therapy is an effective evidence-based intervention for the prevention of suicide.[55] Other promising preventive approaches include community-level awareness and education activities, strengthened mental health care, and addiction treatment because opioid use is associated with increased risk of suicide as well as accidental overdose deaths.[56 57]

If you or someone you know has suicidal thoughts, there is a new national crisis hotline number: 988. This 3-digit number will connect callers to the National Suicide Prevention Lifeline (accessed directly at 800-273-TALK or 800-273-8255) and route them to a local crisis center, staffed by trained crisis workers. The service is free, confidential, and available 24 hours a day, seven days a week. This hotline can also be used by anyone who would like to talk about life stresses or an emotional issue.

Treating depression

Depression should not be neglected. Although about one-third of patients with depression recover spontaneously, early intervention with professional mental health care can help avoid the continuation of the mental suffering of depression and increase the chances of remission.[58] Proper early treatment will help bring about remission of the symptoms of depression in 60% to 80% of cases. Treatment also decreases the risk of associated physical illnesses such as stroke, heart attack, and suicide.[59 60 61]

The main options for treating depression and bipolar disorder are antidepressant medications, psychotherapy, including cognitive behavioral therapy, and electroconvulsive (shock) therapy. Antidepressant drugs are often the first choice for treatment for depression. About one-third of people get full remission, one-third improve, and one-third, especially older people with major depressive disorder, do not respond to initial treatment. The effects of antidepressant drugs take 4 to 8 weeks to become evident and up to 16 weeks for a full benefit. It is often necessary to switch between various antidepressant drugs and classes of drugs to reach the best balance between benefits and side effects.[62]

Recently, new therapies for depression, including transcranial direct-current stimulation[63 64] and infusion of ketamine anesthesia or ketamine analogs is being explored.[65 66] Ketamine treatment is notable in that relief is immediate but not long-lasting, and side effects such as confusion and hallucinations are significant. A ketamine analog, esketamine, administered with a nasal spray 1 to 2 times a week, is effective alone and for use as an adjunct to oral antidepressants.[67] Although esketamine may cause short term side effects, including high blood pressure, nausea, dissociation, vertigo, and dizziness, it has been approved by the FDA for use under carefully controlled conditions of medical supervision.

These treatment modalities can be used alone or in any combination. Light therapy can be used to treat the depression caused by a seasonal affective disorder (SAD). Some research studies have shown that for mild to moderate depression, combination therapy using both medication and psychotherapy is more effective than either therapy alone. Combination therapy may also prevent or delay recurrences of depression. In addition, adopting a healthy lifestyle that helps deal with stress may help prevent depression (e.g., staying socially connected, avoiding substance misuse, getting exercise, etc.) and may hasten recovery from depression.

Anxiety disorders[68]

Anxiety is a normal response to life stresses. It is normal to have worries and get upset from time to time, but for some people, the level of anxiety gets out of control resulting in irrational fears and incessant worry that interfere with work and social activities. Anxiety may also cause heart palpitations, muscle tension, sleep problems, and other physical symptoms.

One form of anxiety manifests itself in the form of panic attacks, sudden 10 to 30-minute episodes characterized by a feeling of being out of control, confusion, fear of dying or losing one's mind, accompanied by physical symptoms such as a racing heart, sweating, dizziness, and feeling faint. Panic attack can be associated with many disorders from time to time or may be an isolated event. Panic disorder is diagnosed when there is a recurrent fear of panic attacks, and a person alters their behavior as a result.[69]

Other manifestations of an anxiety disorder include various phobias, including social anxiety disorder. Phobias are persistent, irrational fears, and avoidance of the things or activities that cause them. Examples include fear of closed spaces and fear of insects or animals such as mice. Social anxiety disorder, or social phobia, affects 7% of the U.S. population. It is characterized by a constant fear of social situations because of possible humiliation or embarrassment, feeling anxious or panicky before a social interaction, and a persistent fear of interacting with or talking to strangers.

Self-care for anxiety can include stress-reducing activities such as yoga and muscle relaxation, getting enough sleep, exercise, and avoiding caffeine and alcohol.[70] Treatment of anxiety disorders with cognitive behavioral therapy, with or without antidepressant drugs (selective serotonin reuptake inhibitors), is the preferred initial treatment strategy, but new drugs, deep brain stimulation, and other treatments provide alternatives for patients whose condition does not respond.[71]

Obsessive-compulsive disorder (OCD)[72]

Obsessive-compulsive disorder (OCD) usually starts in the teens or early 20s. It affects 1% to 3% of adults and is characterized by obsessions (recurrent repetitive thoughts, images, and impulses) and compulsive, often repetitive behaviors that interfere with normal activities and relationships. People with OCD recognize that their obsessions and compulsions are not rational and are unnecessary but cannot be resisted. OCD may lead to depression and benefits from psychotherapy and medications.

Attention deficit hyperactivity disorder (ADHD)

Attention deficit hyperactivity disorder (ADHD) is one of the most common childhood disorders, with symptoms such as difficulty staying focused and paying attention, difficulty controlling behavior, and hyperactivity. The average age of onset is seven years old. ADHD can continue through adolescence and adulthood and affects 9% of American children age 13 to 18 years old. Boys are at four times greater risk than girls. ADHD also affects about 4% of American adults age 18 years and older. Persons with ADHD may be predominantly inattentive or both hyperactive-impulsive and inattentive.[73]

The causes of ADHD are not well understood, but many studies suggest that genes play a significant role. Other factors, including premature birth, environmental factors such as exposure to lead, exposures in utero from the use of cocaine, alcohol, and smoking during pregnancy, brain injuries, delayed brain development, nutrition, and the social environment, might contribute to ADHD. Sugar does not cause ADHD or make symptoms worse. A possible link between ADHD and the consumption of certain food additives such as artificial colors or preservatives has long been suspected, but more research is needed to establish this as a causal relationship.

The impulsivity of teens with ADHD can lead to increases in behaviors that are risky and dangerous to health. Teenagers with ADHD get three times as many speeding tickets and are four times more likely to be involved in a car accident than their non-ADHD affected peers.[74] Because long-term deleterious consequences for work performance and social relationships in adulthood are very important, it is urgent to identify ADHD and intervene as early as possible.

Medication is the primary treatment modality for ADHD. It is combined with parenting interventions and psychotherapy for the consequences of ADHD, such as low self-esteem. Two types of medication are approved by the FDA for treatment of ADHD, stimulants (amphetamines and methyphenidate), and nonstimulants (atomoxetine, clonidine, and guanfacine).[75] Stimulant medications help reduce the frequency or severity of ADHD symptoms and improve cognitive functioning for many people. They may depress appetite, make sleep difficult, and rarely, stimulants cause more serious side effects such as raising blood pressure and heart rate. For some patients with ADHD, an alternative non-stimulant medication, such as guanfacine, is prescribed for its calming effect on anxious/traumatized children. Antidepressants are sometimes used to treat adults with ADHD.[76]

Autism Spectrum Disorder

Children with autism spectrum disorder (ASD) have a broad range of symptoms, skills, and levels of impairment or disability.[77]

ASD is characterized by:

- Persistent deficits in social communication and social interaction
- Restricted, repetitive patterns of behavior, interests, or activities
- Symptoms must be present in the early developmental period (typically recognized in the first two years of life)
- Symptoms cause clinically significant impairment in social, occupational, or other important areas of current functioning

The Centers for Disease Control and Prevention (CDC) estimates that about 1 in 68 children have been identified with ASD. ASD is almost 5 times more common among boys (1 in 42) than among girls (1 in 189). The exact cause of ASD has not been determined, but research suggests that both genes and environment play important roles.

Other conditions that children with ASD may have include:

- Sensory problems: They may either overreact or underreact to certain sights, sounds, smells, textures, and tastes.
- Sleep problems: Trouble falling asleep or staying asleep or have other sleep problems.
- Intellectual disability: Many children with ASD have some degree of intellectual disability. When tested, some areas of ability may be normal, while others—especially cognitive (thinking) and language abilities—may be relatively weak.
- Seizures: One in four children with ASD has seizures, often starting either in early childhood or during the teen years.
- Gastrointestinal problems
- Co-occurring Mental Disorders: Children with ASD are at higher risk of

developing mental disorders such as anxiety disorders, attention deficit hyperactivity disorder (ADHD), or depression.

ASD treatments

While there's no proven cure yet for autism spectrum disorder (ASD), treating ASD early, with intensive behavioral therapy during the toddler or preschool years, can significantly improve cognitive and language skills in young children with ASD. Using school-based programs and getting proper medical care can greatly reduce ASD symptoms and increase a child's ability to grow, learn new skills, and function better in daily life.

One type of widely accepted treatment is applied behavior analysis (ABA). The goals of ABA are to shape and reinforce new behaviors, such as learning to speak and play, and reduce undesirable ones. ABA, which can involve intensive, one-on-one child-teacher interaction for up to 40 hours a week, has inspired the development of other, similar interventions that aim to help those with ASD reach their full potential. Some medications can help reduce symptoms that cause problems for a child in school or at home.

Psychosis

The National Alliance on Mental Illness (NAMI) describes psychosis as: "An episode of psychosis is when a person has a break from reality and often involves seeing, hearing and believing things that aren't real." Approximately 3 in 100 people will experience an episode of psychosis during their lives.

Young adults are at an increased risk of experiencing an episode of psychosis because of the hormonal and structural changes in the brain that occur during puberty, but a psychotic episode can occur at any age. Psychosis is not a specific illness; rather, it is a symptom. A psychotic episode can be the result of a mental illness such as schizophrenia, physical illness, or injury, especially those involving the brain; substance use such as LSD and various "designer drugs;" trauma, for example, a violent assault; or extreme stress.[78 79]

A person with psychosis or a psychotic break cannot tell what is real. The National Institute of Mental Health notes that symptoms of a psychotic episode can include incoherent speech and disorganized behavior, such as unpredictable anger, but psychosis typically involves one of two major experiences:[80]

- Hallucinations: Seeing, hearing, or physically feeling things that aren't

actually there. The commonest example is hearing voices that may tell you to do something.
- Delusions: Strong, sometimes bizarre beliefs that are irrational, not true, and not part of the person's culture. For example, thinking you have special powers or are on a special mission, or having paranoid delusions that others are trying to harm you.

Psychosis can also manifest as impaired thought process with disorganized thinking in the absence of delusions or hallucinations.

In contrast to a short-term psychosis or "break," schizophrenia is a chronic, severe, and disabling brain disorder that has the prominent symptom of psychosis.[81] Schizophrenia affects about 1% of Americans. Adolescent-onset schizophrenia is uncommon; childhood-onset schizophrenia is rare. More often, symptoms such as hallucinations and delusions start between ages 16 and 30. Symptoms may include delusions, hallucinations or disorganized speech, and an impaired ability to function.

Common signs and symptoms of schizophrenia are:[82]

- Delusions: False beliefs that are not based in reality occur in most people with schizophrenia.
- Hallucinations: Seeing or hearing things that don't exist but seem real. Hearing voices is the most common hallucination.
- Disorganized thinking: Cognitive symptoms such as a poor ability to understand information and use it to make decisions and trouble focusing or paying attention. Cognitive problems can make it very difficult to begin and sustain planned activities, lead a normal life, and earn a living. These symptoms they can cause great emotional distress.
- Disorganized or abnormal motor behavior: This may include agitation or useless and excessive movement.
- Abnormal emotions: A person may appear to lack emotion, not make eye contact, not change facial expressions, speak in a monotone, or not add hand or head movements that normally occur when speaking. Also, the person may have a reduced ability to engage in everyday activities or lack the ability to experience pleasure.

Schizophrenia is thought to be caused by several factors, including abnormal brain anatomy and chemistry, but exact causation is not fully understood. It is known that schizophrenia is heritable, and, compared to the general population, it is ten times more likely to afflict people who have a first-degree relative with the disorder, such as a parent, brother, or sister. An identical twin of a person with schizophrenia has a 40% to 65% chance of developing the disorder.[83]

A combination of factors can help predict which young people are at high risk of developing schizophrenia. They include social isolation and withdrawing from others, an increase in unusual thoughts and suspicions, and a family history of psychosis. In young people who develop schizophrenia, this stage of the disorder is called the "prodromal" period.[84]

Predicting which adolescents with prodromal features will develop psychosis is not straightforward, and the majority of "high-risk" individuals never go on to develop a psychotic disorder. According to a director of the U.S. National Institutes of Mental Health:

> Very recently, the North American Prodrome Longitudinal Study (NAPLS) has improved prediction. Combining different types of information—cognitive testing, clinical features (e.g., unusual thoughts, suspiciousness, a decline in social functioning), a history of traumatic events, and a family history of psychosis—over 70 percent of those identified as high risk went on to develop psychosis. For the first time, we can accurately detect risk for psychosis in someone with prodromal symptoms, and the accuracy appears equal to or better than our predictions of heart disease or dementia. The bad news is that we don't yet have an intervention proven to prevent psychosis in those at risk. . ..[85][86][87]

Early identification and treatment may help get symptoms of childhood and adult-onset schizophrenia under control. Early treatment is also crucial in helping limit psychotic episodes, which can be extremely frightening to an adult or to a child and his or her parents.

Mind altering-drugs–marijuana

Marijuana and other psycho-active drugs can cause symptoms and behavior changes similar to those caused by mental health issues. As of August 2019, thirty-three states and the District of Columbia permitted some form of marijuana consumption for supposed medical reasons. Although federal law still considers marijuana (also known as cannabis) an illegal drug, many of these same states and the District of Columbia have also decriminalized possession of small amounts of marijuana and have legalized it for recreational use—a step that other states are considering. In fact, about two-thirds of the U.S. population now lives in a state with relaxed marijuana laws.

The legal trends on the regulation of marijuana use and possession are also fostered by the argument that marijuana is relatively harmless, especially compared to tobacco and alcohol, and that legal bans on use are futile, in that 30 million Americans use marijuana every year and 44% of teens have tried it at least once.[88] However, regular use among teens is much lower than ever use, with 6% of 12th graders reporting using marijuana daily in 2018.[89]

States that changed their laws still prohibit use by anyone younger than 21. Studies in four states over a time period of up to 8 years are reassuring in that use of marijuana changed little in the first few years after the laws were enacted. But there are some warning signs of trouble. For example, edible products containing marijuana put children at risk. Between 2005 and 2011, states that decriminalized marijuana saw a 30% increase per year in calls to poison control centers for children age 9 and younger who consumed marijuana products. Also, the number of drivers in fatal motor vehicle crashes who tested positive for marijuana in Colorado increased after medical marijuana became commercially available there in 2009.

Short-term and long-term effects of marijuana[90]

Although the public favors legalization and 60% of high school seniors do not think that regular marijuana use is harmful, marijuana does have a plethora of adverse short-term and long-term effects. Like nearly all use of drugs, self-medication is not a good idea. Most of the effects of marijuana are caused by the impact on the brain of the main active chemical in marijuana, THC (delta-9-tetrahydrocannabinol). Older studies of the risk of marijuana may be less relevant because, through selective plant breeding, the concentration of THC in marijuana has been increased nearly three times compared to supplies that were available as recently as 1995.

Short-term effects of marijuana

When someone smokes or eats marijuana, THC enters the bloodstream and binds with cannabinoid receptors in the brain. When these receptors are in the parts of the brain that govern sensory perception and pleasure, it causes the marijuana "high." THC also binds with receptors in other parts of the brain that affect thinking, memory, coordination, and concentration, and frequently causes unfavorable side effects, including:

- Difficulty with thinking and problem solving
- Problems with memory and learning, including problems studying, learning new things, and recalling recent events. These problems can last for days after use.

- Loss of coordination
- Distorted perception
- An increase in appetite
- Feeling lightheaded or drowsy
- A decrease in inhibitions that can lead to unsafe behavior such as risky sex or driving or possibly a propensity for violence
- Hallucinations (when taken in high doses)
- Delusions (when taken in high doses)
- Psychosis (when taken in high doses)

Loss of coordination and distorted judgment and perception can make driving unsafe. According to the National Institute on Drug Abuse (NIDA), studies in various locations found that approximately 4% to 14% of drivers who sustained injury or death in traffic accidents tested positive for THC. The NIDA also noted several studies that found that marijuana use more than doubles a driver's risk of being in an accident. This can be compared to the overall risk of a vehicular accident that increases by a factor of 5 with a blood alcohol level of 0.08%, the legal limit in most countries.

A new danger from marijuana use has emerged when adulterated vaping apparatus is used to inhale vaporized THC infused oils. The result has been multiple cases of compromised respiration, with some users ending up on ventilators and some dying from respiratory failure. It is still not entirely clear what has caused acute respiratory failure after vaping, but the inhalation of oils causing lipid pneumonia is likely.

Long-term effects of marijuana

Effects of long-term or heavy use include:

- Addiction (in about 9% of users overall or 2.7 million Americans, 17% of those who begin use in adolescence, and 25% to 50% of those who are daily users)
- Altered brain development including impaired neural connectivity
- Poor educational outcome, with an increased likelihood of dropping out of school
- Cognitive impairment, with lower IQ among those who were frequent users during adolescence
- Diminished life satisfaction and achievement (determined on the basis of subjective and objective measures as compared with such ratings in the general population)
- Symptoms of chronic bronchitis, but a risk of lung cancer has not been established

- An association with increased risk of anxiety, depression and chronic psychosis disorders (including schizophrenia) in persons with a predisposition to such disorders, but causality has not been established
- Long-lasting changes in brain function that can jeopardize educational, professional, and social success.

Especially young, developing brains are likely more susceptible to harm from marijuana than adult brains. In another study reported by the NIDA, researchers followed people from ages 13 to 38. They found that heavy users of marijuana in their teens who continued frequent use into adulthood had a significant drop in IQ, even if they quit. Effects can also be unpredictable when marijuana is used in combination with other drugs, but it is known that marijuana and alcohol potentiate the harmful effects of each of the drugs. If a person is committed to trying marijuana, they should at least wait until they're older than age 25 when their brains are fully developed.

Marijuana addiction

Many people erroneously think marijuana is not addictive. About 9% of people who use marijuana become dependent on it. The number increases to about one in six among those who start using it at a young age, and to 25% to 50% among daily users. By comparison, cocaine, a schedule 2 substance with supposedly less abuse potential than a schedule 1 drug like marijuana, causes 17% of those who use it to become addicted, and 23% of heroin users become addicted. Nicotine's addiction potential in tobacco is even worse, affecting an estimated 32% of smokers, many of whom go on to die from lung cancer, heart disease, and other tobacco-linked causes. While most people who smoke marijuana do not go on to use other drugs, long-term studies of high school students show that few young people use other illegal drugs without first trying marijuana.

People who use marijuana may also experience a withdrawal syndrome when they stop using the drug. It is similar to what happens to tobacco smokers when they quit—people report being irritable, having sleep problems, and weight loss—effects that can last for several days to a few weeks after drug use is stopped.

Currently, no medications exist for treating marijuana addiction. Treatment programs use behavioral therapies, and a number of programs are designed specifically to help teenagers who misuse marijuana. In addition to reaching out to talk to a parent, school guidance counselor, or other trusted adult, there are also anonymous resources, such as the National Suicide Prevention Lifeline (1-800-273-TALK) and the Treatment Referral Helpline (1-800-662-HELP). The Treatment Referral Helpline is provided by the Substance Abuse and Mental Health Services Administration. It refers callers to treatment facilities, support groups, and other local organizations that can provide help for their specific needs. Treatment centers can also be located by going to www.samhsa.gov/treatment.

What about the medical uses of marijuana?

Marijuana has not been approved by the U.S. Food and Drug Administration (FDA) to be used as a medicine. The uncertain purity and dosages of smoked and edible marijuana are not likely to be consistent with good pharmacologic medical practice. And most users of "medical" marijuana have no relevant medical condition that merits its use.

However, a comprehensive evaluation of the potential benefits of marijuana carried out by the National Academies of Sciences, Engineering, and Medicine considered medications containing synthetic THC to be of value in treating severe pain, spasticity, nausea in cancer patients undergoing chemotherapy, and to stimulate appetite in patients with wasting syndrome—severe, involuntary weight loss—due to AIDS.[91 92 93] These studies found that cannabinoids were associated with an increased risk of short-term adverse events included dizziness, dry mouth, nausea, fatigue, sleepiness, euphoria, vomiting, disorientation, drowsiness, confusion, loss of balance, and hallucination.

A 2019 review of the medical use of marijuana in the *JAMA* concluded that. "... most studies of the efficacy of cannabinoids on pain are for neuropathic pain, with relatively few high-quality studies examining other types of pain. At best, there is only inconclusive evidence that cannabinoids effectively manage chronic pain, and large numbers of patients must receive treatment with cannabinoids for a few to benefit, while not many need to receive treatment to result in harm."[94 95]

As noted by Volkow and colleagues in the *New England Journal of Medicine*,

> ...the effects of a drug (legal or illegal) on individual health are determined not only by its pharmacologic properties but also by its availability and social acceptability. In this respect, legal drugs (alcohol and tobacco) offer a sobering perspective, accounting for the greatest burden of disease associated with drugs, not because they are more dangerous than illegal drugs but because their legal status allows for more widespread exposure. As policy shifts toward legalization of marijuana, it is reasonable and probably prudent to hypothesize that its use will increase and that, by extension, so will the number of persons for whom there will be negative health consequences.[96]

There is a reasonable concern that the trajectory of a burgeoning marijuana industry could mimic that of tobacco, with the industrial production of readily available low-cost products, false claims of benefits and risk, and marketing to youth. There is also concern that under an onslaught of lobbying to protect corporate interests, regulation will lag, as it did with tobacco. The marijuana industry already has an advocacy organization—the National Cannabis Industry Association—to protect and advance its corporate interests.

CBD—a nonintoxicating component of marijuana

Consumption of cannabidiol, or CBD, is a new wildly popular fad being touted as a miracle cure for a wide variety of ailments. CBD is one of more than 100 biologically active components called cannabinoids that are in the cannabis plant. It is not psychoactive, so it will not get you "high." Even though it is promoted as a way to relieve pain, anxiety, insomnia, depression, and even as treatments for serious diseases like diabetes, cancer, schizophrenia, and multiple sclerosis, scientists know only that it has a variety of neurological and anti-inflammatory effects, but there is almost no evidence that it improves human health.[97]

The Food and Drug Administration considers CBD to be a drug, so it can't be marketed as a food or in drinks or as a dietary supplement. In spite of lack of data and a plethora of unproven claims, as of April 2019, 47 states, Puerto Rico and the District of Columbia have passed laws making CBD legal for medical and other uses.

Usually sold suspended in oil, alcohol (as a tincture), or vaporization liquid, it is good to keep in mind that CBD products are essentially unregulated, so their safety and quality are questionable.[98] One study found that 70% of 84 CBD products purchased online were mislabeled with regard to the amount of CBD, and 20% of them contained THC.[99]

The FDA has approved only one drug containing CBD based on clinical trials that found it reduced seizures in children with rare and severe forms of epilepsy. The drug Epidiolex is a 99% pure form of CBD that contains less than 1% THC. Adverse effects include elevated liver enzymes indicative of possible liver damage in 13% of patients and other side effects in about 10% of patients included, sleepiness, decreased appetite, diarrhea, fatigue, weakness, rash, sleep problems, and malaise. Epidiolex also caused blood abnormalities and an increase in suicidal ideation. The FDA approved guidelines for the use of Epidiolex caution that bilirubin levels and liver function tests should be obtained prior to starting treatment, and at one month, three months, and six months, as well as at one month following a dosage change. In summary, the CBD Epidiolex has a significant adverse effect profile, and the long-term effects of CBD use are not known.

CBD may harm health either because of these known or unknown direct effects of the drug or, because as is the situation with unproven claims for dietary supplements, turning to CBD for medical therapy may keep some patients from accessing appropriate, proven therapies to treat serious and even fatal diseases. Until CBD is proven by research now underway to be useful for the prevention of disease and improvement of health, and better data on its safety profile is available, it is best to avoid CBD.

Opioids and other mind-altering drugs

In addition to cannabis, ecstasy, LSD, PCP, mescaline, peyote, psilocybin, psilocin, cocaine, methamphetamines, and a variety of opioids, opium, morphine, heroin, oxycodone (OxyContin), hydrocodone (Vicodin), fentanyl, meperidine (Demerol), oxycodone and acetaminophen (Percocet), codeine, etc., are mind-altering drugs that have a spectrum of risks and some benefits—especially in the case of opioids for control of pain. Using these drugs may lead to confusion, euphoria, hallucinations, and other undesirable side effects that impair physical and mental health and day-to-day functioning. Unless medically indicated, they should be avoided.

In Chapter 2, "Lifestyle Checklist," I noted that a rapidly increasing epidemic of deaths from poisoning caused by prescription and illicit drug overdoses, mostly from opioids, was estimated to have reached more than 68,500 in 2018 and to have become one of the top ten causes of death.[100] The wider use of synthetic opioids, mainly fentanyl and its even more dangerous analogs such as carfentanil, are key drivers of the epidemic.[101]

Between 1995 and 2010, opioids prescribed for older adults increased by a factor of nine. Of course, there are legitimate uses of opioids for acute and chronic pain, but the risk of habituation and dependence is a severe adverse effect of their use. Opioid overdoses may start with a first opioid exposure from a prescription, from illegal sources, or from experimentation with a medication prescribed to a friend or relative.[102] Both prescribers and patients should strive to avoid the use of opioids and employ nonopioid drugs for mild or moderate acute pain.

When acute moderate or severe pain necessitates the use of opioids, prescribers should limit the course to the lowest dose and shortest duration possible, and patients should recognize that physical dependence develops quickly, especially after the fifth day of use. The risks of opioid use are mainly related to dose. They include sedation, depression, constipation, reduced libido, motor-vehicle collisions, sleep-disordered breathing, and accidental overdose. Excessive dose escalation in the management of chronic pain should be avoided except during end-of-life care.

The prescribing of opioids for chronic pain is not supported by strong evidence. Over time, the efficacy of pain control declines to the point that other less addicting and less dangerous drugs work just as well.[103 104] Patients should also recognize that discontinuing opioids after habituation to them may be difficult, very unpleasant, and is best undertaken under the supervision of a physician who can provide counseling and a variety of drugs to help to taper off of opioids.

The drugs used to limit withdrawal symptoms and treat habituation with opioids include methadone and buprenorphine.[105] Methadone is used mainly for higher levels of opioid dependence. Methadone is an opioid, a schedule 2 controlled substance that requires dispensing from a specialized clinic. Buprenorphine is also an opioid that can be used alone or in combination with naloxone, an opioid antagonist. It is used mainly for treating lower levels of opioid dependence. It has improved the treatment of opioid dependence for some patients because it causes less analgesia and euphoria but ameliorates withdrawal symptoms. It has less potential for addiction and has a better safety profile because buprenorphine causes less respiratory depression than methadone. Buprenorphine is a schedule 3 controlled substance so it can be provided from an individual physician's office.

Summing up

Clearly, mental health has a major influence on the quality of life, physical health, and health care costs. Mood disorders, anxiety, psychosis, and many other mental health conditions are major sources of unhappiness and disability. To prevent mental health problems and enhance mental well-being there are some things we can't do, like ensuring warm and caring parents or altering our genetic propensity to mental problems, and many things we don't fully understand, such as how to prevent psychosis in those at high risk.

But there are things under our control that we can do to foster good mental health. They include avoiding misuse of drugs and alcohol, getting enough exercise, employment of relaxation techniques, getting enough sleep, staying socially and physically active, and socially connected. The Harvard Mastery of Stress Study identified additional factors that predicted healthy physical and psychological aging that we can influence through our own behavior: having a stable marriage, being well educated, maintaining a healthy weight, and employing mature adaptations to life stresses.

It would be wonderful if all of us were happy and mentally healthy all of the time, but this is not the situation for most of us. You should not hesitate to seek professional help from a reputable well-trained health care provider when any form of mental illness occurs.

11
Preventing Infectious Disease

Worldwide, infections are a very common cause of human disease and death.[1] Clean water, sanitary handling of food, control of insect and animal sources of infection, use of vaccinations, and antibiotics have made infectious diseases usually less common causes of illness and death in the U.S. Still, even before the coronavirus pandemic, infections were among the top ten most frequent killers. And with 281,000 deaths by December 5, 2020, COVID-19 is already a leading cause of death in the U.S. in 2020.[2]

Infectious diseases are illnesses caused by germs or other pathogens. These organisms include bacteria, viruses, fungi, parasites, protozoa, and helminths (worms). They are acquired by exposure to other infected people, from insect and animal bites, by ingesting contaminated food or water, or by being exposed to organisms in the environment. An infection occurs when a pathogen overcomes the body's immune defenses and gets established somewhere in or on the body. An infection can occur almost anywhere but typically affects the skin or the respiratory, gastrointestinal, or urogenital systems. Most infections provoke an immune response and clear up after a few days.[3]

Despite much progress in preventing and curing infectious diseases, they are still with us. New causes continue to emerge, and some well-known and well-controlled infectious diseases such as measles have re-emerged as threats. Natural genetic variations in bacteria and viruses allow new strains of unknown and known pathogens, such as influenza and coronaviruses, to evolve and cause disease because our immune system has not previously encountered them. Increased contact with reservoirs of disease in wild animals such as monkeys and bats is also a source of new human infections. The viral cause of HIV/AIDS and the coronavirus now sweeping the world are likely to have been transmitted to humans from infections in wild animals.

Widespread and often unnecessary, use of antimicrobial drugs (antibiotics) in both humans and industrial-scale animal farming has led to the development of antibiotic-resistant pathogens. An estimated 21 million pounds of medically important antibiotics are used in food animals every year—three times the amount sold for use in humans.[4] This has made many infectious diseases, such as tuberculosis, malaria, and MRSA (Methicillin-Resistant Staphylococcus aureus), that were once susceptible to antibiotic drugs, much more difficult to control and cure. In 2019 the CDC estimated that antibiotic-resistant infections lead to 2.8 million infections from at least 18 different pathogens and more than 35,000 deaths a year.[5] In 2017, nearly 223,900 people in the United States required hospital care for C. difficile, and at least 12,800 people died. Since 2009 fungal infections with the yeast Candida auris have emerged, and some infections are resistant to all antifungal agents. Infections with some strains of Candida auris result in death rates up to 60%.[6]

Recently, decreased acceptance of vaccination has resulted in the re-emergence of previously well-controlled and, at times, fatal diseases such as whooping cough (pertussis) and measles. About 1 per 100 cases of whooping cough among babies six months old or younger is fatal, but the death rate is still about 1 per 1,500 cases among those who are older. Up to 30% of children who get measles have complications, and about 1 per 1000 cases are fatal. More than 200 different agents cause infectious diseases. Among those that are more serious than the common cold and are common to the U.S. and other developed countries are listed in Table 11.1.

Table 11.1. Infectious diseases that are common in the U.S.

Chickenpox	Influenza (Flu)	Rocky Mountain Spotted Fever	Streptococcus
Chronic Fatigue Syndrome	Infectious Mononucleosis	Rubella (German Measles)	Tetanus
COVID-19 (SARS-CoV-2)	Lyme Disease	Salmonella Infections	Toxic Shock Syndrome
Diphtheria	Malaria	Severe Acute Respiratory Syndrome (SARS) (SARS-CoV-1)	Tuberculosis
E. coli	Meningitis	Sexually Transmitted Diseases (multiple organisms)	Viral Hepatitis
Giardiasis	Mumps	Shingles (Herpes Zoster)	West Nile Virus
HIV/AIDS	Pneumonia	Staphylococcus	Whooping Cough (Pertussis)

Epidemic and pandemic diseases

A disease outbreak is called an epidemic when the number of people who become infected in a country or setting rises well beyond what is usual. A pandemic infects many more people and entails spread to a much wider geographical area, often worldwide. The Commission on a Global Health Risk Framework for the Future estimated the expected economic losses from potential pandemics could amount to about $60 billion per year. The coronavirus epidemic has already cost the world economy trillions of dollars, so the Commission's estimate has been vastly exceeded.[7]

The WHO lists the following infectious diseases as being epidemic and pandemic:[8 9]

- Airborne diseases: influenza (seasonal, pandemic, avian), severe acute respiratory syndrome (SARS), Middle East respiratory syndrome coronavirus (MERS-CoV), COVID-19 (SARS-CoV-2)
- Vector-borne diseases: yellow fever, chikungunya, Zika fever, West Nile fever
- Water-borne diseases: cholera, shigellosis, typhoid fever
- Epidemic meningitis
- Rodent-borne diseases: plague, leptospirosis, hantavirus, Lassa fever, rickettsia (murine typhus)
- Hemorrhagic fevers: Ebola virus disease, Marburg virus disease, Crimean-Congo hemorrhagic fever, Rift Valley fever
- Other zoonotic diseases: Nipah virus infection, Hendra virus infection

Other infectious diseases include those caused by:

- Protozoa
    - Chagas disease
    - Human African trypanosomiasis (sleeping sickness)
    - Leishmaniases
- Bacteria
    - Buruli ulcer
    - Leprosy (Hansen disease)
    - Trachoma
    - Yaws
- Helminths
    - Cysticercosis/Taeniasis
    - Dracunculiasis (guinea worm disease)
    - Echinococcosis
    - Foodborne trematodiases
    - Lymphatic filariasis

    - Onchocerciasis (river blindness)
    - Schistosomiasis
    - Soil-transmitted helminthiases
- Virus
    - Dengue and Chikungunya
    - Rabies

The headlines about Ebola, Zika, SARS, MRSA bacteria, West Nile Virus, MDR TB (multidrug-resistant tuberculosis), and flesh-eating bacteria (necrotizing fasciitis) have been replaced by nonstop news about the coronavirus pandemic. And infections such as those caused by the influenza virus and other causes of pneumonia and food poisoning are still with us. They are common infections that can be quite serious and often are fatal. The continuing risk of infectious diseases makes it imperative that we take care of our health by getting recommended vaccinations and practicing good hygiene, especially in the midst of the coronavirus epidemic.

COVID-19

By December 2020, the known global infections with the coronavirus SARS-CoV-2 had topped 66 million, caused more than 1.5 million deaths, and cases are occurring in all or nearly all countries.

The nature of COVID-19 disease, a novel coronavirus SARS-CoV-2, made it especially likely to become a pandemic. It is a respiratory virus that is highly infective person to person either from airborne droplets from a cough or sneeze, or, but much less likely, from touching shed virus particles on surfaces where they might live more than 72 hours. Another characteristic that heightens the risk of COVID-19 spread is the shedding of infectious virus particles before symptoms appear during an incubation period of 2 to 14 days and during the up to 80% of infections that are asymptomatic or mild cases. In contrast, SARS-CoV-1 (the coronavirus that causes a severe acute respiratory syndrome, or SARS) was more easily dealt with because it was not highly transmissible until an individual had symptoms.

An infectious agent's R_0 describes the average number of new infections that a contagious person can cause in a population that was not previously exposed to the agent. An R_0 greater than one for a virus suggests that without measures to prevent transmission, the number of people infected is likely to grow, whereas an R_0 of less than one suggests that transmission is likely to die out. Community spread of COVID-19 without contact with known infected individuals is occurring in many countries. Estimates are still being refined, but the R_0 for COVID-19 is expected to be around 2–3. For comparison, measles is highly contagious with an R_0 of 12-18 and Ebola less so with an R_0 of 1.5-2.5.

Information so far suggests that much COVID-19 illness is mild. A report out of China in the *New England Journal of Medicine* suggests serious illness, principally viral pneumonia, occurs in 16% of cases.[10] Of about 1,000 patients seen at Chinese hospitals, 5.0% were admitted to the intensive care unit (ICU), 2.3% needed mechanical ventilation for acute respiratory distress, and 1.4% died from respiratory failure. Older people and people with health conditions such as heart disease, lung disease, and diabetes are at greater risk of serious illness. Other data from China and elsewhere suggest that the death rate among hospitalized patients age 80 or older may reach 15%-30%, whereas children seem to mostly be spared from symptomatic COVID-19 disease.

The case fatality rate appears to be higher than severe seasonal influenza, which has a case fatality rate of approximately 0.1% but lower than SARS (10%) or MERS (36%). A variety of existing and experimental antiviral drugs are being studied as a treatment for COVID-19, but their efficacy, or lack thereof, has not yet been determined.

Predicting the course of COVID-19

In the short term, the spread of COVID-19 infections can be prevented to some extent by containment—the testing, identification, and isolation of cases and their contacts. Given the high efficiency of transmission, community spread is occurring and requires mitigation strategies, including social distancing (really physical distancing), avoiding poorly ventilated spaces, wearing masks to protect the wearer and prevent transmission to others, isolating and caring for ill persons, and minimizing large gatherings of people at markets, sporting events, and schools. In addition to physical distancing and the wearing of masks, personal and environmental hygiene are called for.

Although these measures are known to be effective, epidemiologists project that until a vaccine is widely administered, up to half of the 7.8 billion people on the planet could ultimately become infected, and millions could die. Lock-down procedures, shelter at home directives, and the wearing of masks have slowed the spread of the outbreak in many places. Even so, many countries are suffering a severe disruption of economic activity, hardship, and increased deaths through neglect of other endemic health problems as the resources of healthcare systems have become stretched thin and diverted to cope with the COVID-19 outbreak.

Longer-term, as occurred with other infectious disease outbreaks, better knowledge about prevention and treatment methods, and the needed resources to implement them, will become available. But this may be slow in all countries, especially in those where health systems are weak. It may turn out that some existing antiviral drugs are effective, and new, highly effective antiviral drugs may be developed, but this will take time. Treatment of cases with hyperimmune globulin from recovered persons and monoclonal antibodies may be possible, but these sophisticated therapies are likely to be impractical for developing countries and other low resource settings. Prevention of COVID-19 infection with immunization is now possible, but it will take time to disseminate and administer the vaccines. Fortunately, the efficacy of the new vaccines appears to be very high at 95%, as it is for measles. Widespread infection or immunization of 60% to 70% of people could lead to herd immunity that will limit the number of people at risk of getting new infections.

A lesson from the COVID-19 outbreak is to emphasize the importance of investing in robust public health systems. This must include research on the animal reservoirs of infectious agents that may infect humans and limiting human contact with them. Reservoirs of concern include "wet markets" of live animals, the hunting of "bush meat" in Africa, and farms with pigs and other domestic animals treated with antibiotics that lead to antibiotic-resistant infectious agents.

Common infections

Just about any part of the human body can become infected. We are all familiar with colds and other respiratory infections, gastrointestinal and urinary tract infections, but less common infections in other tissues such as bone, the valves and interior of the heart (endocarditis), and the brain also occur.

Every year, about 5% to 20% of U.S. residents acquire an influenza virus that infects the nose, throat, and lungs. The Centers for Disease Control and Prevention (CDC) estimates that influenza has resulted in between 9 million and 45 million illnesses, between 140,000 and 810,000 hospitalizations and between 12,000 and 61,000 deaths annually since 2010.[11] The virus that causes the COVID-19 disease is SARS-CoV-2, and like the influenza virus, SARS-CoV-2 is spread mainly between persons in households and public settings by the droplets made when infected people cough, sneeze or talk. Many people with influenza are hospitalized each year with complications such as bacterial pneumonia, ear infections, sinus infections, dehydration, and worsening of chronic medical conditions, such as congestive heart failure, asthma, or diabetes.[12]

The WHO estimates that worldwide there are a million new sexually transmitted infections (STIs) every day. The CDC estimates that there are nearly 20 million new sexually transmitted infections every year in the U.S., with half occurring among young people ages 15 to 24. Sexually transmitted infections are described in Chapter 13, "Sexual and Reproductive Health."

Skin infections are very common and can be caused by a wide variety of agents. Among them are:[13]

- Bacterial: cellulitis and impetigo, often caused by Staphylococcus
- Viral: shingles, warts, and herpes simplex
- Fungal: athlete's foot and yeast infections
- Parasitic: body lice, head lice, and scabies

Healthcare-associated infections (HAI), mainly those acquired in hospitals, are a serious infectious disease problem. A CDC survey estimated that on any given day, 3.2% of hospital patients have at least one healthcare-associated infection.[14] The study made a rough estimate that there were 687,200 HAIs in U.S. acute care hospitals in 2015. Common infections were pneumonia and ventilator-associated pneumonia, gastrointestinal illness, urinary tract infections often associated with catheters, bloodstream infections, and surgical site infections from inpatient surgery. A previous similar study in 2011 estimated that about 75,000 hospital patients with HAIs died during their hospitalizations.[15]

Preventing infection

Preventing all infections is not possible, but the risk of infection can be minimized by sanitary day-to-day behavioral practices.

Cover up and wear a face mask

To minimize spreading germs, it is better to cough and sneeze into a tissue or your sleeve, not your hand. If you are ill, or taking care of someone who is ill, or are in public during an outbreak of respiratory diseases such as the coronavirus, wearing a face mask that covers both your mouth and nose. A face mask or covering will provide some, but not perfect protection for you and others. The amount of protection provided by masks of various types is still being investigated but it is clear that they significantly decrease transmission of COVID-19. Infection with a low number of SARS-CoV-2 particles will increase your chance of a mild or inapparent case of COVID-19.

Physical distancing and ventilation

Social distancing (really physical distancing) of 6 feet or more can curb the spread of a respiratory virus, including the coronavirus. Avoiding long periods of exposure and closed-in, poorly ventilated spaces also helps limit the spread of respiratory pathogens.

Stay home when you have an infectious disease

Isolate yourself when you have an infectious disease. You may infect your colleagues, members of the public, and slow your own recovery. If you have a fever, skip your exercise regimen.

Wash your hands often

Use soap, rub hands for at least 20 seconds and use a clean towel. The use of anti-bacterial soaps are not recommended; they are no better than regular soap at preventing infections. But if washing with soap and water is not possible, an alcohol-based hand sanitizer is a reasonably good substitute. It is especially important to wash after coughing, sneezing, or blowing your nose, using the bathroom or changing diapers, before eating, when cooking or serving food, touching frequently touched areas or contaminated items, such as face masks, after contact with a sick person, or touching an animal or pet. As much as possible, avoid touching the front of your face mask, your nose, mouth, and eyes with your hands.

Handle and prepare food safely

Food can carry germs. For example, raw eggs may carry salmonella. Wash hands, utensils, and surfaces often when preparing any meal. Be especially careful with raw meat; use a separate cutting board for meat and cook meat well to kill germs. Some authorities suggest always to wash fruits and vegetables. Cook and keep foods at proper temperatures. To prevent the growth of bacteria, keep food hot or cold because germs grow best at room temperature. Don't leave food out—refrigerate it promptly.

Clean and disinfect commonly used surfaces

Bacteria and viruses live on surfaces. The COVID-19 virus can persist on a surface for up to 72 hours. Cleaning surfaces with soap and water is usually adequate. However, you should disinfect your bathroom and kitchen regularly and other areas if someone in the house is ill. You can use an EPA certified disinfectant (look for the EPA registration number on the label), bleach solution, or rubbing alcohol.

Don't share personal items

Avoid sharing personal items that can't be disinfected, like toothbrushes and razors. Avoid sharing towels. To avoid needle-stick injuries, disposable needles should not be shared, should only be used once and then placed in a sharps disposal container. The container can then be disposed of the according to community guidelines.

Avoid touching wild animals

You and your pets should avoid going near or touching living or dead wild animals that can carry germs or may be infested with fleas (they can jump on you), ticks, or lice that can cause infectious diseases such as Lyme disease. If you are bitten, talk to your doctor about the need for specialized treatments. Make sure that your pet's vaccinations are up-to-date.

Practice safe sex

Get tested for sexually transmitted diseases (STDs), and have your partner tested. To avoid STDs, use condoms or abstain. If you have HIV or are at risk of exposure to HIV, talk to your doctor about treatment and pre-exposure prophylaxis (PrEP).

Be a smart traveler

The risk of getting an infectious disease may be heightened when traveling, particularly when traveling to developing countries where the standards of sanitation for food and water may be less stringent. If you travel to a place where water safety is questionable, use a safe water source such as boiled or bottled water for drinking and brushing your teeth. Remember that not all bottled water is safe. Some investigation may be required to discern a reliable source of drinking water. Don't trust that the ice in your drink is from a safe source. International soft drink brands and beers are generally safe. When in developing countries, stick to foods that have been cooked, and avoid raw vegetables and unpeeled fruits.

Respect others and don't fly when you are ill. Because you are in a confined space, you are more likely to infect other passengers. Look up what you need to do for your health before travel. The CDC website has recommendations for specific countries. Depending on your destination, you should follow recommendations to update immunizations, and you may need special immunizations. You may need to take prophylactic drugs such as antimalarials. Insect repellents may be advisable in some travel settings.

Use antibiotics sensibly

Take antibiotics only when prescribed. Unless otherwise directed, or allergic to them, the usual advice is to take all prescribed doses of your antibiotic, even if you begin to feel better before you have completed the medication. Remember that most antibiotics are ineffective against viral diseases. Inappropriate overuse of antibiotics can lead to drug-resistant germs, and you may become allergic to the antibiotic and not be able to use it later on when you need it.

Immunization to prevent infections

The development of vaccination to prevent infectious disease is among the most important medical and public health advances that prevents illness, suffering, long-term disability, and death. Good hygiene and sanitation also prevent the spread of disease, but the germs that cause disease are still with us, and without vaccination, they would make many more people sick. The CDC estimates that over two decades, between 1994 and 2013, childhood vaccination prevented 322 million illnesses, 21 million hospitalizations, 732,000 deaths, and saved $295 billion in direct medical costs.[16]

Vaccines can prevent many but certainly not all infectious diseases. Based on extensive research, medical practitioners have developed schedules for vaccinations in childhood, for adults, and some for special situations like pregnancy and travel where you may be exposed to infectious diseases seldom or never found in the U.S. Make sure you and your family are up-to-date on your vaccinations. The CDC has detailed information about vaccination and recommended schedules on their website.[17] If your regular health care provider does not offer the vaccine you need, many communities will have an adult immunization and travel clinic. The CDC website (http://wwwnc.cdc.gov/travel/destinations/list) includes advice about infectious diseases for travelers listed by country.[18]

How vaccination works

When a disease-causing microbe (virus, bacteria, or a parasite like malaria) gets into your body, your immune system recognizes the invader and mobilizes to destroy it. Often this response works well, but it can be too slow and weak to prevent illness. Vaccines consist of killed or modified microbes, parts of microbes, or microbial DNA that do not cause illness but stimulate the body to mobilize the immune system as though an infection occurred. If re-exposure to the infectious agent occurs, the immune system will more quickly and strongly respond to stop the infection. Vaccines are very effective, and most childhood vaccines produce immunity about 90% to 100% of the time.

Vaccines also prevent outbreaks of disease and save lives when a high proportion of a community is immunized against a contagious disease. Even those members of the community who are not vaccinated get some protection against that disease because there is little opportunity for an outbreak. This helps those who are not eligible for certain vaccines—such as infants, pregnant women, or people with a weak (immunocompromised) immune system. This phenomenon is known as community or herd immunity. If too many people opt out of vaccination, not only are they at risk of illness, but the benefits of herd immunity are also lost.

How safe are vaccines?

Vaccines are not free from side effects, or "adverse effects," but most are very rare or very mild—for example, a sore arm or low-grade fever—and they go away within a few days. More serious side effects, like allergic reactions, are rare. Studies have shown a small increased risk for febrile seizures among children during the first to second week after the first vaccination with measles, mumps, rubella (MMR), and varicella (MMRV) vaccine, and not after the acellular pertussis vaccine, DTaP, or after varicella (chickenpox) vaccine.

It should be kept in mind that brief febrile seizures can happen with any condition that causes a fever, and they do not cause any permanent neurological damage. Up to 5% of young children will have at least one febrile seizure, usually associated with getting sick. Causes include common childhood illnesses like colds, the flu, an ear infection, or roseola. Getting a child vaccinated as soon as recommended prevents many more febrile seizures than are caused by vaccination because vaccination protects young children against measles, mumps, rubella, chickenpox, influenza, pneumococcal infections, and other diseases that can cause fever and febrile seizures.

Some adverse health problems following vaccination may be due to coincidence—not the vaccine. Based on flawed research, it has been claimed that autism was caused by vaccination. Although this link has been disproved, some people, including some celebrities, still promote this misinformation. Parents who refuse vaccination for their children leave them at risk of serious illness and even death.

What to do if someone has a reaction to a vaccine[19]

If a reaction to a vaccine occurs: Call a doctor. If the reaction is severe, call and take the person to a doctor or hospital emergency department immediately. Tell your doctor what happened, when it happened, and when the vaccination was given. Ask your doctor, nurse, or health department to file a Vaccine Adverse Event Reporting System (VAERS) form or call VAERS yourself at 1-800-822-7967.

The Food and Drug Administration requires that vaccines be tested for safety before they enter the market, and their performance is continually evaluated to identify any risks that might appear over time. Under the National Childhood Vaccine Injury Act of 1986, Congress established the National Vaccine Injury Compensation Program (VICP) to provide compensation to people injured by vaccines. Anyone who thinks they or a family member, often a child, has been injured can file a claim.

Who should be vaccinated?

Because of low levels of vaccine-preventable diseases in the U.S., lack of knowledge about the importance of vaccination, and unrealistic fears about the risks of vaccination, some people are reluctant to get vaccinated or have their children vaccinated. Paul Offit has described the development of an anti-vaccination epidemic based on misinformation and "irrational beliefs" about the risk of vaccination.[20] Unfortunately, many of the viruses and bacteria that cause illness still circulate in the U.S. Recent outbreaks of measles, mumps, and pertussis (whooping cough) among children who were not vaccinated are a vivid example of why it's important that children, especially infants and young children, teenagers, and adults, receive recommended immunizations on time.

Who should not get vaccinated?

Some people should not get certain vaccines or should wait to get them. For instance, children with compromised immune systems, as occurs with some cancer treatments, often need to wait to be vaccinated. Be sure to tell your health care provider if you have health problems or known allergies to medications or food. If a person has had a severe allergic reaction to a vaccine, the following dose is not recommended. However, a person with a mild, common illness, such as a cold with a low-grade fever, does not have to wait to be vaccinated. For more information on who should not get vaccinated, visit the CDC website.[21]

Vaccination recommendations

The CDC has specific vaccination recommendations for children, college ages, and young adults ages 19 through 24, adults, and seniors. There are also recommendations for catching up on immunization if the recommended schedule has not been adhered to.

For example, the CDC recommends vaccinations to protect children against 16 infectious diseases, including measles, mumps, rubella (German measles), varicella (chickenpox), hepatitis A, hepatitis B, diphtheria, tetanus, pertussis (whooping cough), Haemophilus influenza type B (Hib), polio, influenza (flu), and pneumococcal disease.

Vaccinations specifically recommended for young adults include meningococcal conjugate vaccine (MenACWY), Tdap vaccine (against tetanus, diphtheria, and pertussis, or whooping cough, unless immunized as a preteen or teen), HPV vaccination (see Chapter 7, "Preventing Cancer"), and seasonal flu vaccine.

Some vaccines are recommended only for travelers to places where the diseases occur. There are other vaccines, such as against anthrax, that are usually reserved for high-risk groups of people such as those in the military. Smallpox has been eliminated globally, and vaccination against smallpox is no longer needed.

Vaccination recommendations for adults

The recommended schedule of vaccination for an adult varies considerably depending on factors such as age, likely occupational, household or travel exposures, previous vaccinations or lack of prior vaccination, and an individual's health status. For example, the U.S. Preventive Services Task Force (USPSTF) recommends that pregnant women should be screened for hepatitis B virus and urinary tract infection. U.S. government recommendations for adults by age group, medical condition, and other indications can be found at https://www.cdc.gov/vaccines/schedules/downloads/adult/adult-combined-schedule.pdf. After consulting the detailed recommendations, the following immunizations should be considered:[22 23]

- Influenza vaccination (annually)
- COVID-19 (when available)
- Tetanus, diphtheria, and acellular pertussis (Td/Tdap) vaccination
- Varicella vaccination
- Human papillomavirus (HPV) vaccination
- Herpes Zoster vaccination (Shingrix, for all adults aged 60 years or older)
- Measles, mumps, rubella (MMR) vaccination (Adults born before 1957 are generally considered immune to measles and mumps)
- Measles component
- Mumps component
- Rubella component
- Pneumococcal (13-valent pneumococcal conjugate vaccine [PCV13] and 23-valent pneumococcal polysaccharide vaccine [PPSV23]) vaccination
- Meningococcal vaccination
- Hepatitis A vaccination
- Hepatitis B vaccination
- Haemophilus influenzae type b (Hib) vaccination
- For those with a weakened immune system, inactivated vaccines generally are acceptable (e.g., pneumococcal, meningococcal, and inactivated influenza vaccine; and live vaccines generally should be avoided)

Vaccination recommendations for seniors

With age, the body's immune system becomes weaker as do the protective effects of prior vaccinations. You're more likely to get diseases like the flu, pneumonia, and shingles — and to have complications that can lead to long-term illness, hospitalization, and even death.[24] Revaccination against the following infectious agents is recommended for persons over the age of 65:

- Influenza—annually (Flu)

- Herpes Zoster (Shingrix)
- Diphtheria
- Tetanus
- Pertussis (Whooping Cough)
- Pneumococcal disease (Pneumonia)

Summary of the essential facts

- Cover up coughs and wear a mask during epidemics caused by airborne transmission of pathogens.
- Physical distance and avoid poorly ventilated spaces if recommended.
- Stay home when sick.
- Wash your hands often.
- Choose, handle and prepare food safely.
- Clean and disinfect commonly used surfaces.
- Don't share personal items.
- Avoid touching wild animals.
- Practice safe sex.
- Be a smart traveler.
- Use antibiotics sensibly .
- Get vaccinated to stay healthy.

Good hygiene and self-care when sick is not enough to stay healthy and prevent infectious diseases. Vaccination is also essential to stay healthy—do not fear it—vaccination could save your life. Recommended vaccinations and vaccination schedules are updated frequently, so consult the Centers for Disease Control and Prevention for up to date information. Additional information can be found at http://www.cdc.gov/vaccines/default.htm

12
Preventing Osteoporosis

Osteoporosis defined

Osteoporosis or "porous bone" is a common condition of the skeletal system characterized by low bone mass and the deterioration and weakening of bone tissue.[1 2 3 4 5] Osteopenia is the mild loss of bone density and strength that precedes osteoporosis. Osteoporosis leads to an increased risk of bone fractures typically in the wrist, forearm, humerus (upper arm), femur (hip), and spine. Osteoporosis is very common. Worldwide, 1 in 3 women over 50 will experience osteoporotic fractures, as will 1 in 5 men.

According to the International Osteoporosis Foundation, osteoporosis and low bone mass are estimated to be a major public health threat for about 50 million American women and men aged 50 and older, and each year there are an estimated 10 million new fractures associated with osteoporosis in the U.S.[6] About half of white women in the U.S. will have an osteoporosis-related fracture in their lifetime.[7] In women over 45 years of age, osteoporosis accounts for more days spent in hospitalization than many other common diseases, including diabetes, myocardial infarction, and breast cancer.

Falls contribute to fractures. For example, 90% of hip fractures are the result of falls, and nearly half of those with a hip fracture have previously broken another bone. A third of people over age 65 fall annually, with approximately 10% to 15% of falls in the elderly resulting in a fracture. It is estimated that almost 60% of those who fell the previous year will fall again.[8]

Bone is made up mainly of collagen (connective tissue) and mineralized calcium. The skeletal system is not static, and bone is remodeled throughout life. In a continuous process, existing bone is resorbed, and new bone is formed in response to the demands placed on it. Bed rest and sedentary behavior promote bone resorption, and weight-bearing and high impact physical activity promote bone formation. During childhood and teenage years, new bone is formed, and bones become larger, heavier, and denser. Bone formation outpaces resorption until about age 30 when peak bone mass, defined as maximum bone density and strength, is reached.

Calcium and vitamin D are important to bone health because of their role in skeletal formation, maintenance, and prevention of osteoporosis. Adequate calcium consumption and weight-bearing physical activity strengthens bones, optimizes bone mass, and may reduce the risk of osteoporosis later in life. After about age 30, bone resorption slowly begins to exceed bone formation. Osteoporosis can occur when bone resorption occurs too quickly or when new bone formation occurs too slowly. Among women, bone loss is most rapid in the first few years after menopause.

The strength of bone is related to both the quantity of bone as measured by bone mineral (calcium) density (BMD) and also to the quality of bone structure that relates to its collagen, architecture (trabecular network pattern), micro-architecture, and bone mineral quality.[9] The importance of factors other than BMD or the amount of bone is shown by the fact that older individuals often have a much higher risk of poorly structured weaker bones and higher fracture risk than young people with the same BMD. In other words, the difficult-to-measure structural aspects of bone quality are as important as bone density as determinants of strong bones. The disconnect between bone density and bone strength has been shown by the finding that several drug treatments that increase bone density by only 1% to 6% can decrease fracture risk by 35% to 50%.[10]

Prevention of osteoporosis

Because osteopenia and osteoporosis are so common, everyone should be concerned with prevention.[11, 12] Many conditions associated with an increased risk of the development of osteoporosis are known, and many people with osteoporosis have several risk factors, but others who develop the disease have no known risk factors.[13, 14] Some risk factors are related to lifestyle, but others cannot be modified. Since it takes about 15 years for 10% of patients with mild osteopenia to progress to osteoporosis, the first step for those with osteopenia should be to address the risk factors that can be changed. And these same lifestyle factors should be addressed if osteoporosis is present.[15]

Risk factors you cannot change

Gender
Women are more likely to develop osteoporosis than men. Women have less bone tissue and lose bone faster than men, especially shortly before and for a few years after menopause.

Age
The risk of osteoporosis increases with advancing age; bones gradually become less dense and weaker with age. Age-related bone loss averages 0.1% to 1% per year, and those over age 65 are most at risk.

Body size
Being small-boned or underweight increases risk.

Ethnicity
White and Asian women are at highest risk. Black American and Hispanic women have a lower but still significant risk.

Family history
Heredity may play a role in susceptibility to osteoporosis. People whose parents have a history of fractures also seem to have reduced bone mass and may be at increased risk for fractures.

Risk factors you can change

Weight-Bearing Physical Activity
A sedentary lifestyle is an important risk for osteoporosis. Weight-bearing and high impact exercise are important for osteoporosis prevention and treatment. Examples include walking, hiking, jogging, playing basketball, playing soccer, climbing stairs, weight training, playing tennis, and dancing. Adequate weight-bearing physical activity early in life is also important to reach peak bone mass. In addition to strengthening bone, physical activity increases muscle strength, coordination, and balance, all factors that reduce the risk of falls and other accidents that cause fractures.

Recommended physical activity guidelines for adults are described in Chapter 9, "Benefits of Physical Activity." Adults should engage in at least 30 minutes of moderate physical activity most, but preferably all, days of the week. Children should engage in at least 60 minutes of moderate physical activity most, but preferably all, days of the week. Adequate levels of calcium intake can maximize the positive effect of physical activity on bone health during the growth period of children, an important time to maximize bone mass through physical activity. Some young females, particularly those training intensively for athletic competition, exercise too much, eat too little, and consequently experience amenorrhea. This increases their risk for low bone mass and fractures, especially overuse (stress) fractures.[16] Although another vulnerable time for women is just before and after menopause, with exercise, postmenopausal women can maintain or increase bone mineral density.[17 18 19]

Smoking

Smoking can lead to lower bone density and a higher risk of fracture, and this risk increases with age.[20]

Alcohol intake

Regular consumption of as little as 2 to 3 ounces a day may cause skeletal damage and increase the risk of bone loss and fractures, even in young women and men. The risk of vertebral and hip fractures in men increases greatly with heavy alcohol intake, particularly with long-term intake. People who drink heavily are at increased risk of fractures both because of bone loss and increased risk of falling.[21 22 23 24]

Nutrition, protein, calcium, and vitamin D

Most calcium in the American diet comes from milk, milk products, and foods with high levels of animal protein. National nutrition surveys show that many people consume less than half the recommended amount of calcium. However, the U.S. recommendation for calcium is set high. Vegetarians absorb and retain more calcium from food than do non-vegetarians, and there is little evidence that calcium intakes below the Dietary Reference Intake cause health problems for vegetarians. Calcium deficiency in vegetarians is rare.

Food sources of calcium include non-fat dairy products, such as milk and yogurt, but it is often not recognized that excellent sources of calcium are plant-based. They include dark green, leafy vegetables, such as broccoli, collard greens, bok choy, spinach, turnip greens, kale, okra, Chinese cabbage, dandelion greens, and mustard greens. Other good sources include sardines and salmon with bones; tofu; almonds; and foods fortified with calcium, such as fruit juices, cereals, soy beverages, calcium-set tofu, and breads. Although most people can get adequate calcium from food, a calcium supplement may be recommended by a health professional. (See Chapter 5, "Vitamins and Other Supplements," for more on calcium and vitamin D.)

Too much vitamin A

High doses of vitamin A may increase bone resorption and decrease formation.

Vitamin A may also harm bone by diminishing the ability of vitamin D to increase intestinal calcium absorption. Studies find that excessive preformed vitamin A (retinol) intake from food or supplements, but not beta carotene (found in fruit and vegetables), is linked to an increased risk of osteoporosis and hip fracture rates among women. One study found that a daily intake of 1,500 μg or more of vitamin A doubled the risk of osteoporosis and hip fractures in women aged 28 to 76.[25] An 18-year study published in the *JAMA* found that among postmenopausal women, the risk of hip fracture was almost doubled among women with retinol intakes of about 2000 μg per day or higher compared with those with intakes of less than about 500 μg/day.[26] One International Unit (IU) = 0.3 micrograms (μg) of retinol. It is best to avoid intake of preformed vitamin A (retinol) of 650 μg or 2000 IU or greater per day.

Sex hormone abnormalities

Abnormal absence of menstrual periods (amenorrhea), low estrogen level (after menopause), and low testosterone levels in men predispose to osteoporosis.

Anorexia nervosa

This eating disorder is characterized by an irrational fear of weight gain and avoidance of normal amounts of food. Because the onset of anorexia nervosa frequently occurs during puberty, when there should be maximal bone mass accrual, adolescent girls and boys with anorexia nervosa are at high risk for reduced peak bone mass.[27 28]

Certain medications

The medications that can contribute to bone loss include long-term use of glucocorticoids (steroid medications), long-term treatment with certain antiseizure drugs, gonadotropin-releasing hormone (GnRH) drugs used to treat endometriosis, excessive use of aluminum-containing antacids, certain cancer treatments, and excessive thyroid hormone.

Nutrition and osteoporosis

Calcium needs change over one's lifetime, with the greatest needs during childhood, adolescence, pregnancy, and breastfeeding. Postmenopausal women and older men may also need to consume more calcium. Ingestion of high levels of salt, sugar, caffeine, alcohol, and exposure to nicotine increases calcium loss. Studies show that fruit and vegetable intake is positively associated with increased bone density in men and women.[29 30 31 32 33]

There has been concern that excessive consumption of animal protein creates a heavy acid load in the blood that requires mobilization of calcium from bone to neutralize it and increases the loss of calcium in the urine.[34] However, a longitudinal study and a review of 61 studies found that higher intakes of protein from plant or animal sources did not have adverse effects on bone health in premenopausal women. However, some analyses suggest that low vegetable protein intake is associated with lower bone mineral density.[35 36]

A 2017 meta-analysis that included 16 randomized controlled trials and 20 prospective cohort studies concluded that there were no adverse effects from high protein intake on bone, and only the lumbar spine showed moderate evidence to support a protective benefit from high protein intake. The authors noted that the studies were so diverse that confounding could not be excluded and that additional studies were needed to clarify dietary protein's role in bone health.[37]

Osteoporosis is common in the U.S., even with relatively high consumption of milk and other calcium-rich dairy products. Although consumption of milk is advocated as a way to avoid osteoporosis, studies about the usefulness of milk in the prevention of osteoporosis have found conflicting results.[38 39 40 41] For example, a 20-year study conducted in Sweden found that women who drank more than three glasses of milk a day were more likely to suffer a broken bone and were at twice the risk of dying at the end of the study than those who drank less. A similar but less pronounced trend was found in men. However, an opposite pattern was found for fermented milk products, such as yogurt, suggesting a role of the sugars in milk.[42]

An inadequate supply of calcium from a diet low in calcium and vitamin D over a lifetime also contributes to the development of osteoporosis.[43 44 45] Studies in children and adolescents have shown that supplementation with calcium, dairy calcium-enriched foods, or milk enhances the rate of bone mineral acquisition. Many studies show that low calcium intake appears to be associated with low bone mass, rapid bone loss, and high fracture rates. Some studies show that vitamin D supplementation can reduce rates of bone loss and also fracture rates in older male and female adults, and the elderly. In institutionalized elderly women, this combined calcium and vitamin D supplementation reduced hip fracture rates. For example, the Nurses' Health Study found that older women who consumed at least 500 IU of vitamin D were one-third less likely to suffer a broken hip than women who got less than 200 IU per day.[46]

Other studies have found that calcium and vitamin D supplementation has little effect on fracture risk. A trial randomly assigned more than 36,000 postmenopausal women between the ages of 50 and 79 to receive 500 mg of elemental calcium as calcium carbonate with 200 IU of vitamin D3 twice daily or matching placebos for an average of seven years. Annualized rates of hip, total, and site-specific fractures were the same for each of the groups, and the calcium with vitamin D supplementation increased the risk of kidney stones (renal calculi) by 17%.[47]

Some of the differences in results of studies of vitamin D supplementation and fractures may relate to the dose of vitamin D. A meta-analysis that included five randomized controlled trials (RCTs) for hip fracture and 7 RCTs for nonvertebral fracture risk found that a vitamin D dose of 700 to 800 IU/day reduced the relative risk of hip fracture by 26% and any nonvertebral fracture by 23%. No significant benefit was observed for RCTs with 400 IU/day vitamin D. The study authors concluded that oral vitamin D supplementation between 700 to 800 IU/d appears to reduce the risk of hip and any nonvertebral fractures in ambulatory or institutionalized elderly persons and a vitamin D dose of 400 IU/d is not sufficient for fracture prevention.[48] However, a 3-year study of high-dose vitamin D at 4000 IU/day or 10,000 IU/day compared to the usual dose of 400 IU per day found that the higher doses resulted in lower bone density and provided no advantage over the 400 IU/day.[49]

A 2013 review by the U.S. Preventive Services Task Force (USPSTF) suggests that routine use of vitamin D and calcium supplementation by postmenopausal women is not of proven value for the primary prevention of fractures in non-institutionalized postmenopausal women.[50] The USPSTF did not address the value of higher doses of calcium and vitamin D, nor did they discuss younger women or individuals with osteoporosis.

A 2017 meta-analysis of 33 randomized trials reported in the *JAMA* included participants receiving vitamin D, calcium, or both. Compared to those receiving a placebo, there was no difference in the risk of fractures among these community-dwelling (not institutionalized) adults age 50 or older.[51] A 2018 analysis of data from 81 randomized controlled trials found that regardless of the dose, vitamin D supplements do not help prevent fractures or increase bone mineral density—even among postmenopausal women with osteoporosis.[52] A 2019 meta-analysis noted the inconsistent findings of randomized controlled trials (RCTs) assessing the effects of both vitamin D and calcium vs. placebo.[53] The meta-analysis of RCTs found no benefit for the risk of fracture from supplementation with vitamin D alone. The meta-analysis of the RCTs of daily supplementation with vitamin D and calcium demonstrated a marginally significant reduction in the risk of any fracture of 6% and a hip fracture of 16%.

Studies of extra calcium intake are inconclusive. Some show a protective effect, others show no benefit, and still, others show an increased risk of fractures. U.S. surveys have found no link between bone density and calcium consumption.[54] Long- term prospective studies from seven countries show no important reduction in fractures with increasing consumption of calcium.[55] In fact, rates of hip fracture tend to be high in countries with a high intake of calcium and low in countries with

low intake.[56] The bottom line on calcium is that with a healthy diet, it is usually not necessary to worry about calcium consumption or take calcium supplements.
As is shown in Table 12.1. the Recommended Dietary Allowances for calcium, (covering requirements of at least 97.5% of the population), range from 700 to 1300 mg/d for life-stage groups at least one year of age.

Table 12.1. Recommended Calcium Intakes

Life-stage group	mg/day
Infants 0 to 6 months	200
Infants 6 to 12 months	260
1 to 3 years old	700
4 to 8 years old	1,000
9 to 13 years old	1,300
14 to 18 years old	1,300
19 to 30 years old	1,000
31 to 50 years old	1,000
51- to 70-year-old males	1,000
51- to 70-year-old females	1,200
70 years old	1,200
14 to 18 years old, pregnant/lactating	1,300
19 to 50 years old, pregnant/lactating	1,000

Source: Food and Nutrition Board, Institute of Medicine, National Academy of Sciences, 2010.

The safe upper limit for calcium is:

- 1,000 mg/day for infants 0 to 6 months
- 1,500 mg/day for infants 6 to 12 months
- 2,500 mg/day for children 1 - 8 years
- 3,000 mg/day for children and teens 9-18 years including pregnant and breastfeeding teens
- 2,500 mg/day for adults 19-50 years including pregnant and breastfeeding women
- 2,000 mg/day for adults age 51 years and older

Symptoms and detection[57 58 59]

Osteoporosis is often called a silent disease because bone loss occurs without symptoms. People may not know that they have osteoporosis until their bones become so weak that a sudden stress from a bump or fall causes a hip (femur) to fracture or a vertebra to collapse. Collapsed vertebrae may initially be felt or seen in the form of severe back pain, loss of height, or spinal deformities such as stooped posture (kyphosis).

Osteoporosis is detected by measuring bone mass with a bone mineral density (BMD) test. The most widely used BMD test is a dual-energy x-ray absorptiometry or DXA. With a very low exposure to radiation, it can measure bone density at the hip and spine. BMD tests can identify osteoporosis, help estimate the risk of future fractures, and measure response to osteoporosis treatment. The U.S. Preventive Services Task Force (USPSTF) recommends that women should begin screening at age 65 or younger if a risk assessment indicates, (i.e., low body weight, parental history of hip fracture, smoking), but the evidence is insufficient to assess the balance of risks and harms of screening for osteoporosis to prevent osteoporotic fractures in men.[60 61] Other expert groups recommend that all postmenopausal women and men over 50 should be screened with DXA. Still, other expert groups say men at age 70 should begin screening. There are no "official" recommendations about how frequently DXA screening should be carried out. One recommendation is to screen every two to five years if osteopenia (mild loss of bone density) is present, and every two years for people with osteoporosis.[62]

DXA testing is expressed as a T-score that compares an individual's BMD to a young woman in her twenties or as a Z-score that uses the average for your age, gender, and race/ethnicity for comparison. T-scores are expressed as a negative number that is a measure of standard deviation (variance from an average) below normal. A T-score of -1 to -2.5 is classified as osteopenia, and a T-score of -2.5 and below is classified as osteoporosis. About one-third of women ages 50 to 65 and two-thirds of women over 65 fall into the osteopenia category. By the time women reach age 75, about half of them will have a BMD that places them in the osteoporosis category.[63]

There is no discrete cutoff between a finding of disease or no disease in measures of BMD using DXA technology. T-scores do not measure bone quality, so a low T-score in a young woman may represent a negligible risk of a fracture compared to an elderly woman with the same T-score.[64] In general, there is a continuum of fracture risk, with risk highest among individuals with low BMD values. There is debate about whether osteopenia should be considered a predictable aspect of aging and concern about the potential for overtreatment based on the diagnosis. One reason for this concern is that although they are at increased risk, many people with osteopenia do not go on to full-blown osteoporosis or have a fracture.

To help guide the decision about taking bone-strengthening drugs, the USPSTF recommends the use of one of 5 different tools. Four of these (the Osteoporosis Self-Assessment Tool [OST], the Osteoporosis Risk Assessment Instrument [ORAI], the Osteoporosis Index of Risk [OSIRIS], and the Simple Calculated Osteoporosis Risk Estimation [SCORE]) were specifically designed to identify individuals with a BMD T-score of –2.5 or lower. The FRAX (Fracture Risk Assessment Tool), a more complex computer-based country-specific fracture risk assessment tool, was designed to estimate 10-year probabilities of hip and major osteoporotic fracture.

The FRAX considers your age, health history, T-score, if you have had a previous fracture and other factors to calculate your risk of a fracture in the next ten years. Guidelines on the use of the FRAX suggest that treatment be considered if the 10-year risk of a hip fracture is 3% or higher or if the risk of a major osteoporotic fracture (e.g., hip, vertebra, humerus, or wrist) is 20% or higher. As is the situation with the use of BMD to assess fracture risk, the FRAX has limitations because patient-provided data may be inaccurate, presence of other diseases and conditions may not be accounted for, and some significant variables including physical activity, balance, calcium and vitamin D intake and use of tobacco and alcohol may not be fully accounted for in the model. The FRAX is available at https://www.sheffield.ac.uk/FRAX/tool. A similar risk calculator is available from The Foundation for Osteoporosis Research and Education at riskcalculator.fore.org.

Because it is simpler and as accurate as the other screening tools, a recent review of screening strategies for postmenopausal women younger than 65 recommends using the Osteoporosis Self-Assessment Tool (OST) before BMD testing.[65]

Treatment of osteoporosis

The decision to start a medication to halt or reverse bone loss should be made only after a thorough medical evaluation and with expert medical advice. Some experts consider that there are too many unanswered questions about their value to advise people with osteopenia to start bone-strengthening drugs, especially those with a low FRAX score. However, most fractures among women occur to those with osteopenia, and a new study suggests that the treatment of osteopenia is advisable. A 6-year study of women with osteopenia (T score between -1 and -2.5) found that treatment with IV zoledronate at 18-month intervals reduced the risk of fracture by 37%.[66]

If osteoporosis is present, most experts consider it a mistake to let fears about the rare side effects of bone-strengthening drugs deter initiation of them. A woman's risk of a fracture at some time in her life is 50%, and when indicated, drug treatment can reduce that risk by half.[67]

More than 20 medications are available for the prevention and/or treatment of osteoporosis.[68] Studies have consistently shown that, depending on the drug and the patient population, treatment reduces the risk of vertebral fracture by 30% to 70%, nonvertebral fractures by 15% to 20%, and hip fractures up to 40%. Among the possible drug therapies are bisphosphonates (usually the first choice for drug treatment); estrogen agonists/antagonists (also called selective estrogen receptor modulators or SERMS); calcitonin; parathyroid hormone; estrogen therapy; hormone therapy; and recently various biologics.[69] In 2019, a monoclonal antibody romosozumab (Evenity), a drug that promotes bone growth and inhibits bone resorption, was approved by the FDA. Although effective in the prevention of osteoporotic fractures, romosozumab may increase the risk of heart attack, stroke, and cardiovascular death, so careful patient selection is advisable.

Poor compliance is one of the most important treatment problems. Studies show that only 40% of patients take treatment for more than one year. At two years, only 20% of patients are still taking their medication.[70][71][72][73] The use of bone-strengthening drugs has declined after extensive publicity about rare but serious side effects. An estimated one to four of 10,000 patients taking these drugs will sustain an atypical broken thigh bone (femur), and one in 100,000 will suffer from bone death (osteonecrosis) and deterioration of the jawbone with the risk heightened by long-term, high-dose use.

Summary of the essential facts[74]

Support bone health by:

- Engaging in regular high-impact, weight-bearing, and strength-training physical activity.
- Getting enough vitamin D, preferably from food and sunshine.
- Getting enough calcium, preferably from plant-based foods.
- Avoiding smoking.
- Avoiding alcohol or at least limit it to one drink per day .
- Avoiding intake of preformed vitamin A (retinol) of 2000 IU or higher.
- Reducing the risk of falls by balance and strength-training.
- Maintaining a healthy weight.
- Getting a bone mineral density test when recommended.
- Not fearing and taking the treatment for osteopenia and osteoporosis when indicated.

13
Sexual and Reproductive Health

This chapter addresses sexual and reproductive health issues, with a focus on women and men of reproductive ages, 15 to 45. Good sexual and reproductive health is a state of wellbeing relating to reproduction and the body's reproductive system. It includes the ability to have a satisfying and safe sex life, the capability to reproduce and to bear children safely, and the freedom and means to decide if, when, and how often to have children. Sexual and reproductive health plays a prominent role in overall health and is highly dependent on preventive measures that are taken through healthy behaviors. Sexual and reproductive health depends on a good understanding of and appropriate behaviors related to:

- Sexuality
- Contraception, abortion, and infertility
- Sexually transmitted diseases
- Maternal health
- Reproductive cancers
- Urologic and gynecologic disorders

The goal of this chapter is to improve your understanding of sexual and reproductive health, including how to avoid unintended pregnancies and births with contraception and abortion, how to prevent sexually transmitted infections (STIs), and provide information about the safety of childbirth. How to minimize the risk of reproductive system cancers is described in more detail in Chapter 7, "Preventing Cancer." This chapter does not address conditions and diseases involving the urologic and reproductive systems that are not susceptible to prevention through healthy behavioral and lifestyle choices.

Sexuality education

An important basis for sexual and reproductive health is knowledge. Sexuality education enables people to make decisions about their sexuality and sexual health that are informed, responsible, and healthy.[1] In addition to attaining information, sexuality education can facilitate the acquisition of life skills and the formation of values that increase responsible behaviors, respect individual rights, and enhance gender equity.

Sexuality education should contribute to mature, sexually healthy adults who:

- Have accurate information about human sexuality.
- Have developed their values, attitudes, and insights about sexuality.
- Are free to adopt their own gender identities and interact with all genders in respectful and appropriate ways.
- Express love and intimacy in appropriate ways.
- Develop and maintain meaningful relationships.
- Avoid exploitative or manipulative relationships.
- Take responsibility for their behavior.
- Engage in sexual relationships that are consensual, non-exploitative, honest, pleasurable, and healthy.
- Practice health-promoting behaviors, such as regular check-ups.
- Use contraception and abortion effectively to avoid unintended pregnancy and childbearing.
- Avoid contracting or transmitting a sexually transmitted disease, including HIV.

Comprehensive sex education that provides age-appropriate, medically accurate information related to sexuality can effectively delay sexual activity among young people and increase contraceptive use among sexually active youth. Abstinence-only and abstinence-only-until-marriage programs seek to control young people's sexual behavior, usually by instilling fear, shame, and guilt. These programs often rely on negative messages about sexuality and distort information about condoms and STIs. Evaluations have found that these programs have no beneficial impact on young people's sexual behavior."[2,3] Furthermore, to the extent that they ignore contraception and the benefits of safer-sex practices generally, abstinence-only programs do nothing to help prepare young people for when they will become sexually active.

Healthy living requires making informed and healthy choices about reproduction based on an understanding of the benefits and risks relating to contraception, abortion, sexually transmitted infections (STIs), and childbirth. Getting good information about reproductive health sometimes is complicated by the misinformation promulgated by opponents of various forms of contraception and abortion who exaggerate the risk of using contraception or having an abortion.

Family planning

Unintended pregnancies, that is to say, pregnancies that are unplanned or unwanted, are a frequent occurrence and a global problem.[4] In the United States, nearly half (45%) of the 6 million annual pregnancies are unintended. Assuming no change in current contraceptive failure rates, by age 45, more than half of all U.S. women will have had an unintended pregnancy.[5] Teen pregnancy rates in the U.S. are also very high, about twice as high as the rates in Canada or Sweden, with more than 600,000 pregnancies among young women age 15 to 19 each year. More than 80% of U.S. teen pregnancies are unplanned. Teens account for about one-fifth of all unintended pregnancies, and about 10% of all U.S. births are to teenagers.[6]

By providing access to contraceptive information and services, family planning helps people to attain their desired number of children and determine the spacing of pregnancies. This allows for the healthiest pattern of childbearing. Births that occur among women in their teens, especially among women younger than 18, those among women older than age 35, those that are more closely spaced than two years apart, and those of higher birth orders, (i.e., that occur after the second or third birth), are more dangerous for both the mother and her child. A high-risk pattern of childbearing also is more likely to result in preterm or low birth-weight babies who have higher rates of neonatal mortality.[7]

With every birth, even in wealthy countries, there is a risk of illness and death (maternal mortality), and the infants of mothers who die in childbirth have a much greater risk of poor health and death. Some contraceptive methods, especially male and female condoms, provide dual protection, both against undesired pregnancies and against sexually transmitted infections (STIs), including HIV. Family planning also reduces the risk of unintended pregnancies among women living with HIV, resulting in fewer HIV infected babies and fewer orphans.

In addition to the health risk of pregnancy, there are social issues. As Jennifer Frost and her colleagues noted: "Unintended pregnancy can force women and their families to confront difficult abortion decisions or the potentially negative consequences associated with unplanned childbearing—including child health and development issues, relationship instability, and compromises in education and employment that may exacerbate ongoing poverty."[8] Teen childbearing is associated with reduced educational attainment, and higher educational attainment and income are associated with better health. Teen pregnancy has important consequences for future careers and earning potential as fewer than 2% of teens who have a baby before age 18 attain a college degree by age 30.[9]

What to consider in choosing a contraceptive

Many factors that are not related to health, such as convenience and cost, are appropriate to be considered when choosing a contraceptive. Although currently available contraceptive technologies have greatly improved the regulation of fertility, for many women and men, under typical conditions of use, they still have some drawbacks relating to safety, side effects, and effectiveness. Because some commonly used contraceptives are much less effective than others in preventing pregnancy, choosing the best contraceptive for an individual is important.

Contraceptive effectiveness

Studies of unintended pregnancy in the U.S. reveal that many unintended pregnancies occur because contraceptives are not used, because they are discontinued after only a short period of use, and because there are gaps in use. An estimated 52% of the 3.2 million annual unintended pregnancies in the U.S. result from non-use of contraception, 43% from inconsistent or incorrect use, and only 5% because the method itself failed when being used correctly.[10 11]

Reasons for non-use or inconsistent use of contraception include high cost, limited access, infrequent sexual activity, ambivalence about becoming pregnant, and underestimating the risk of becoming pregnant. Other prominent reasons for inconsistent use include dissatisfaction with methods, often after experiencing side effects, but also because of concerns about safety, worries they might cause unpleasant side effects, and inconvenience.[12]

When considering which contraceptive to choose, an important distinction must be made between theoretical effectiveness—when a contraceptive is used perfectly; and use effectiveness—the effectiveness achieved by a typical or average user. The permanent contraceptive methods, male and female sterilization, and the LARC (long-acting reversible contraceptive) methods (IUDs and implants) are highly effective in preventing pregnancy. Their theoretical and use effectiveness is essentially identical. But for commonly used methods, including oral contraceptives (OC), the patch, the ring, injectables (Depo-Provera), and condoms, there is a substantial difference between their effectiveness in typical use compared to the effectiveness measured in carefully controlled clinical trials.

One reason there are so many unintended pregnancies in the U.S. is that almost half of U.S. contraceptive users rely on methods that, in typical use, have both high failure and high discontinuation rates: the pill, the condom, and the 3-month injectable. Among teenagers, condoms and withdrawal are the most commonly used methods. While with perfect use, these methods are highly effective, on average, 9% of pill users, 18% of condom users, and 6% of injectable users will become pregnant during the first year of typical use.[13] In a recent study of high-risk teenagers, pregnancy rates were still higher, with 16% of pill and injectable users becoming pregnant during their first year of use.[14] Figure 13.1 presents the failure rates of various methods of contraception.

Figure 13.1. Risk of pregnancy over one year using different contraceptive methods

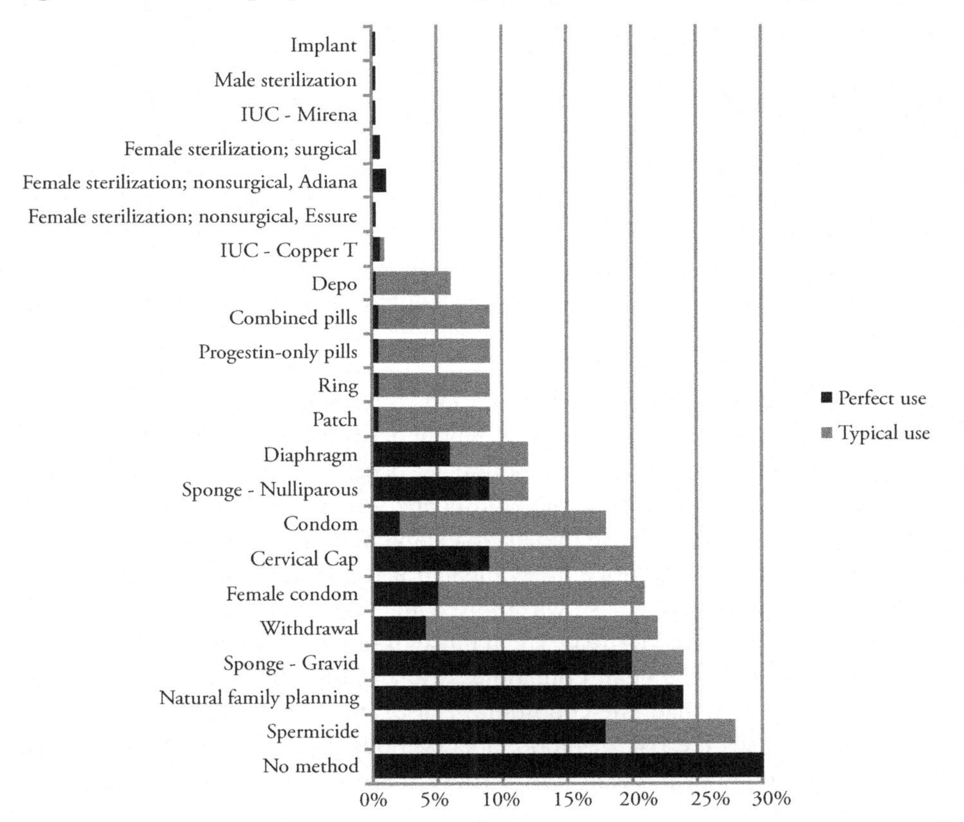

Source: J. Russell, "Contraceptive Failure in the United States. Contraception, 2011, 83:397-404.

Another problem is that the effectiveness of the mix of contraceptives in use in the U.S. is substantially impaired because of high discontinuation rates. About half of condom and injectable contraception users—and almost one-third of pill users—will discontinue use within a year, and they may become non-users of contraception.[15 16] Because they do not require continuing motivation for use, LARCs have the best one-year continuation rates at 78% for the copper T 380A (ParaGard®), 80% for the LNG-IUS (Mirena®), and 84% for the implant (Nexplanon®).[17] Risk of unintended pregnancy in the U.S. is therefore closely related to both non-use of contraception and the frequent choice of contraceptive methods that are likely to be used incorrectly or inconsistently or are likely to be discontinued shortly after they are adopted.

Contraceptive methods: risks and benefits

The risk of serious harm from contraceptives is low for most women, particularly when compared to the risks to health associated with pregnancy.[18 19] Some contraceptives have health benefits beyond preventing pregnancy. But because healthy women and men use them for long periods of time, contraceptives are often held to a higher standard of safety than drugs used to cure diseases.[20] Blood clots among users of the original high-dose combined oral contraceptives (COCs), controversy about hormone replacement therapy, and problems with a flawed intrauterine contraceptive (IUC or IUD), the Dalkon shield, increased the perception that contraceptives are risky. This perception has been reinforced by television advertising campaigns seeking women harmed by various contraceptives to join product liability lawsuits.

The perception of health-related risks of all kinds often does not coincide well with reality. Women end up pregnant because they underestimate the risk of becoming pregnant and decide not to use contraception, or because they discontinue contraception because they overestimate the significance of minor side effects, or they discontinue contraception because they have exaggerated fears about contraceptive safety.[21] For example, a majority of women in a recent pilot study inaccurately believed that oral contraceptive use was more dangerous than pregnancy.[22] In fact, the risks of a pregnancy are far greater than those of oral contraceptive use for most women. The risks of some health outcomes are strongly affected by the simultaneous presence of more than one condition. For example, being both over age 35 and smoking increases the risk of blood clots (venous thromboembolism or VTE) among hormonal contraception users far more than either being over age 35 or smoking alone.

Contraceptive failure or non-use of contraception is common, so the reproductive health risks of an unplanned pregnancy must be considered as a risk inherent to non-use of contraception or choice of a contraceptive with low effectiveness and a high likelihood of early discontinuation. The following section provides a brief summary of the risks and benefits of the most effective and commonly used contraceptive methods. Before adopting any particular contraceptive method, it is highly advisable to thoroughly discuss the method's risks, benefits, and side effects with a health care provider.

Contraceptive implants[23]

The contraceptive implant Nexplanon® is a highly effective long-acting reversible contraceptive (LARC) method. Nexplanon® has FDA approval for three years of use but remains effective for four years. The implant slowly releases a progestin, so it is also free from the side effects and cardiovascular risks of estrogen-containing contraceptives, such as combined oral contraceptives (COCs). The implant also relieves painful menses and endometriosis symptoms, decreases acne, reduces risk of ectopic pregnancy, and is rapidly reversible. The principal disadvantage of Nexplanon® is disrupted menstrual bleeding patterns—either by irregular bleeding or complete cessation of menstrual periods (amenorrhea). Implants may also promote weight gain and may be associated with an increased incidence of ovarian cysts. Improperly performed insertions are also a rare cause of contraceptive failure.

Female and male sterilization[24]

The benefits of sterilization include safety, high effectiveness, lack of significant long-term side effects, no need for continuing motivation or action for use, no need for supplies, and no need for partner compliance. Female sterilization with various techniques and male sterilization by vasectomy are permanent methods. They should be chosen only when no more children are desired. Sterilization is very safe, but like all surgical procedures, it carries some degree of risk, with mortality rates from female surgical sterilization in the U.S. estimated at 1 to 4 deaths per 100,000 procedures, and deaths from vasectomy at 0.5 per 100,000 procedures. When the rare pregnancies after female sterilization occur, about 30% are likely to be outside the uterus (ectopic) and require medical intervention to avoid serious health consequences.

Intrauterine devices (IUDs)[25 26 27]

Intrauterine devices (IUDs), also known as intrauterine contraceptives or IUCs, have a proven record of very high effectiveness, and suitability for a wide variety of women. Women who are childless (nulliparous), are in their teens, immediately post-abortion or postpartum or have had a sexually transmitted infection (STI) are all appropriate candidates for IUDs, as are women with medical conditions that might contraindicate the use of combined hormonal contraceptives.[28 29]

IUDs have important health benefits. The LNG-IUS (Mirena® and Liletta™) that release a small amount of a progestin hormone usually decreases menstrual blood loss, improves iron-deficiency anemia, and helps manage heavy menstrual bleeding (HMB) from various causes. The copper IUD and probably the LNG-IUS provide protection against endometrial cancer, and they protect against infections causing pelvic inflammatory disease (PID). The copper T 380A is the most effective emergency contraceptive method. The long duration of action of each of the IUDs is an advantage.

The most prominent problems caused by IUDs are cramping and pain at the time of insertion disrupted menstrual bleeding patterns and expulsions that occur among 2% to 10% of IUD users. A more serious risk of IUC use is perforation of the uterus that occurs in 0.03% to 0.06% of IUD insertions. The issue of increased risk or greater severity of infection among IUD users has been a prominent concern. However, the pelvic inflammatory disease (PID) rate in IUD users is low, with cases concentrated in the first 20 days after insertion.[30]

Injectable contraceptives[31]

Injectable progestin contraceptives (e.g., Depo-Provera or DMPA), do not contain an estrogen, so they do not increase the risk of the adverse cardiovascular problems experienced by some combined oral contraceptives COCs, patch and ring users. They also decrease the risk of pelvic inflammatory disease (PID), provide privacy since their use cannot be detected, and may cause amenorrhea (the cessation of menses) that some women consider to be desirable. One significant drawback of Depo-Provera is unpredictable vaginal bleeding and spotting, and 40% to 50% of users experience amenorrhea after one year of use and 80% after five years of use. The time for fertility to return to normal is often delayed for 6 to 12 months after the last injection. Other risks include weight gain among some users and bone loss that is reversible on discontinuation of the method. The possibility of increased susceptibility to HIV infection among DMPA users was suspected, but a clinical trial in eastern and southern Africa has found no substantial difference in the risk for acquiring HIV among women using any of three common methods of contraception, DMPA, Copper IUD, and a levonorgestrel implant.[32]

Combined oral contraceptives (COCs)[33 34 35]

Combined oral contraceptives contain synthetic versions of naturally occurring estrogen and progesterone. COC users may experience a variety of minor side effects that are not likely to have important health implications but may result in dissatisfaction with the method and early discontinuation. The estrogens in COCs increase the risk of adverse cardiovascular events, but for women who do not smoke or have other high-risk cardiovascular conditions, the increase is small.

COC Benefits

Health benefits conferred by the use of oral contraceptives include decreases in:

- Irregular and painful menstrual cycles
- Blood loss during menstruation
- Premenstrual symptoms, premenstrual and mood disorders
- Ovarian cysts
- Ectopic pregnancy
- Acne and excessive body hair
- Noncancerous cysts or lumps in the breast
- Acute pelvic inflammatory disease
- Colorectal cancer and cancer of the ovary and endometrium

COC risks

COC use increases the risk of venous blood clots called thrombotic and thrombo-embolic events (VTE), including pulmonary embolism and deep vein thrombosis. The background risk of venous thromboembolism (VTE) in women of childbearing age is approximately 4 to 5/10,000 women over a year. VTE risk is increased by two to three times by using COCs and possibly by as many as four times among users of some types (third generation) of COCs to the range of 9 to 10/10,000 woman-years of use.[36 37] The risk of VTE is greatly increased among women who have certain genetic mutation disorders that increase the risk of blood clots.[38]

Increased risk of an arterial thrombosis such as those causing strokes and heart attacks is primarily among smokers or women with other underlying risk factors for vascular disease such as hypertension, high cholesterol, morbid obesity, and diabetes. There is no measurable increased risk of heart attacks among healthy young women on the lowest dose COC formulations. Most studies have shown no increase in the risk of stroke from the use of low-dose COCs among healthy users who do not smoke or have high blood pressure. Other studies indicate a slight increase in the risk of stroke in non-smokers and about a doubling of risk for stroke among smokers. Women with severe high blood pressure are at risk of stroke, and the use of COCs increases this risk additionally—they should avoid COCs and use a different form of contraception.

Studies of lifetime risk of cancer among COC users are generally reassuring. The Royal College of General Practitioners' Oral Contraception Study found that ever use of oral contraceptives was associated with reduced colorectal (incidence rate ratio, 0.81), endometrial (incidence rate ratio, 0.66), ovarian (incidence rate ratio, 0.67), and lymphatic and hematopoietic cancer (incidence rate ratio, 0.74).[39] An increased risk of lung cancer was seen only among ever users who smoked at recruitment. An increased risk of breast cancer (incidence rate ratio, 1.48) and cervical cancer (incidence rate ratio, 2.32) that was seen in current and recent users appeared to be lost within approximately five years of stopping oral contraception, and long-term hormonal contraceptive use has been found not to be associated with any increase in total cancer risk.[40]

Numerous studies show that the use of hormonal contraceptives is associated with a significantly lower overall risk of death than occurs among non-users.[41] Studies suggest that the net effect of the use of oral contraceptives for five years or longer is a slight reduction in the total risk of cancer.[42] The authors of a Royal College study concluded, "the overall balance of cancer risk among past users of oral contraceptives was neutral with the increased risks counterbalanced by the endometrial, ovarian, and colorectal cancer benefits that persist at least 30 years."[43]

The short-term increase in the risk of dying from the use of COCs, mostly from cardiovascular disease, can be compared to the risk of death from pregnancy and childbirth. In the U.S., about one of every 10,000 births is fatal to the woman giving birth.[44] For healthy women aged 15 to 34 who do not smoke, the risk of death over a year of oral contraceptive use is one out of 1,667,000 (.006/10,000). For smokers aged 15 to 34, the risk of death increases to one out of 33,330 (0.3/10,000). For women aged 35 to 44, the risk of death over a year is one out of 57,803 (0.2/10,000), and for smokers ages 35 to 44, the risk of death increases to one out of 5,155 (1.9/10,000). This data shows why COC use is relatively safe, except for women over age 35 who smoke. They should consider the use of a contraceptive other than the COC.[45]

Contraceptive patch and vaginal contraceptive ring[46]

Because the transdermal contraceptive patch and vaginal contraceptive ring release an estrogen and a progestin, the risk and benefit profile is similar to that of COCs. About half of users will experience skin reactions at the patch site. Side effects among ring users include vaginal symptoms and very rarely, toxic shock syndrome. The advantages of the patch and ring are considered to be similar to those afforded by COCs. However, the one-patch-per-week dosing schedule for the patch and a 21 days-in-place or a longer schedule for some rings may be easier to adhere to than a daily pill.

Abortion

International research shows that women with unintended pregnancies in all countries use abortion to attain their childbearing goals, regardless of its legal status. In the U.S., half of women will experience an unintended pregnancy by age 45, and about three in 10 will have an abortion by age 45.[47 48 49] Unlike the situation in countries where abortion is illegal, abortion in the U.S. is legal and quite safe.[50] Although restrictive state laws make it increasingly difficult to obtain an abortion in some places, the approximately 860,000 abortions performed in the U.S. each year entail very little risk to health. By reducing rates of unintended pregnancies, family planning also reduces the need for abortion, and in settings where abortion is unsafe, family planning also reduces the risks of unsafe abortion.

Almost 90% of abortions are carried out with a pregnancy duration of 13 weeks or less[51] Whether performed with aspiration or medication, abortion is extremely safe, entailing about the same risks as a miscarriage and far fewer risks than continuing a pregnancy.[52] For abortions carried out before 13 weeks, only 1% to 4% of women experience a minor complication, and only 5 in 10,000 experience a major complication. The risk of maternal death is minuscule and increases with higher gestational ages, ranging from 1 per 1,000,000 procedures for abortions carried out at eight weeks or earlier, 4 per 1,000,000 for procedures at 11 to 12 weeks, and 34 per 1,000,000 at 16 to 20 weeks.[53]

Menopausal hormone therapy

Hormone therapy for women after their menopause was once advocated as a way to prevent both menopausal symptoms and cardiovascular disease—this proved to be only partially correct. The use of menopausal hormone therapy does support bone health and relieve hot flashes and other postmenopausal symptoms. Years of research have revealed that hormone therapy with estrogens and progestins taken together or estrogen alone creates a complex pattern of potential risks and benefits.

The Women's Health Initiative (WHI) study found that there were increases in the risk of cardiovascular disease (blood clots and strokes) with 5 to 7 years of use of either estrogen plus progestin or estrogen alone.[54] Combination (estrogen plus progestin) hormone therapy also increased the likelihood of breast cancer, but estrogen alone seemed to have no effect. Instead of the desired reduction in mortality, there was no significant effect on life expectancy among hormone users compared to non-users. A longer-term follow-up of the WHI concluded that hormone therapy decreased overall mortality among the youngest women but after 18 years is not associated with either increased or decreased mortality rates except that the estrogen-only group may have had a slight longevity advantage.[55 56 57]

Research suggests that estrogen plus progestin therapy reduces the risk of diabetes, fractures, and colorectal cancer but increases the risk of invasive breast cancer, coronary heart disease, dementia, stroke, and venous thromboembolism.[58] Estrogen alone decreases the risk of invasive breast cancer, diabetes, and fractures but increases the risk for endometrial cancer, stroke, venous thromboembolism, and gallbladder disease. It would appear that there is cardiovascular benefit from hormone therapy started within 10 years of the onset of menopause but harm if started more than 10 years after onset or in women older than age 60.[59] However, estrogen (with or without progestins) is still, by far, the most effective therapy for menopausal vasomotor symptoms such as hot flashes and vaginal symptoms.[60]

The 2017 hormone therapy position statement of the North American Menopause Society is:

> For women aged younger than 60 years or who are within 10 years of menopause onset and have no contraindications, the benefit-risk ratio is most favorable for treatment of bothersome vasomotor symptoms (VMS) and for those at elevated risk for bone loss or fracture. For women who initiate hormone therapy (HT) more than 10 or 20 years from menopause onset or are aged 60 years or older, the benefit-risk ratio appears less favorable because of the greater absolute risks of coronary heart disease, stroke, venous thromboembolism, and dementia. Longer durations of therapy should be for documented indications such as persistent VMS or bone loss, with shared decision making and periodic reevaluation. For bothersome genitourinary syndrome of menopause (GSM) symptoms not relieved with over-the-counter therapies and without indications for use of systemic HT, low-dose vaginal estrogen therapy or other therapies are recommended.[61]

Discontinuation of hormone therapy is typically recommended after 3 to 5 years or by the age of 60.[62]

The U.S. Preventive Services Task Force recommends against the use of hormone replacement therapy (HRT).[63] They concluded that the magnitude of both the benefits and the harms of hormone therapy in postmenopausal women is small to moderate. The USPSTF concluded with moderate certainty that combined estrogen and progestin has no net benefit for the primary prevention of chronic conditions for most postmenopausal women with an intact uterus and that estrogen alone has no net benefit for the primary prevention of chronic conditions for most postmenopausal women who have had a hysterectomy.

Testosterone–is the Low-T epidemic real?

To get around the stringent rules that apply to prescription drug advertising, the ads on TV offering help for Low-T do not advertise a specific product. Because they can be considered to be "disease awareness" campaigns, they are regulated by the Federal Trade Commission (FTC) and not the FDA.[64] They assert that there are many problems associated with Low-T relating to strength, energy, and libido but don't tell the viewers that abnormally low testosterone, or hypogonadism, is not common, that testosterone treatment has risks, and the benefits are questionable. These TV campaigns have resulted in greatly increased prescribing of testosterone supplement therapy, with sales estimated at $5 billion in 2017.[65]

Fatigue, depression, muscle weakness, loss of erectile function, and interest in sex can be caused by androgen (testosterone) deficiency, but these symptoms can have many other causes. Since the aging process leads to a decline in sex hormone levels, in addition to a cluster of symptoms, a blood test is needed to determine if blood testosterone levels are normal or low for a person's age.[66] One estimate is that perhaps 5% of men have both low testosterone deficiency symptoms and abnormally low blood testosterone.[67] However, a careful study found that only 1.5% of those screened for testosterone treatment eligibility had both low testosterone and symptoms.[68 69]

In the hope of restoring youthful vigor, many men are treated with testosterone for the Low T Syndrome without a blood test. There is substantial, but not fully definitive evidence that testosterone products increase CVD risks. For example, one study found that after three years, an adverse cardiovascular event (e.g., heart attack, stroke, death) was 29% higher among the men on testosterone therapy.[70] Another study with a small number of subjects found a doubling in CVD risk.[71] A study evaluating the risk of a heart attack 90 days after getting a prescription for testosterone therapy found little increase in risk among men younger than 55, no increases in risk for men age under age 65 (unless there was a prior history of heart disease), a doubling of risk among men age 65 to 75, and a tripling of risk for men older than age 75.[72] A study of insurance records of men with venous thromboembolism (VTE) found that having taken testosterone within six months doubled the risk of a VTE, some of which will result in a pulmonary embolism.[73] Other studies of testosterone therapy have not found an increased risk of CVD, at least one study found a decrease, and they found no convincing evidence that higher testosterone levels increase the risk of prostate cancer.[74 75]

A study among older men with an average age of 72, found that testosterone therapy only modestly enhanced strength and sexual function and cannot be considered indicative of the benefits, or lack of benefits, for a younger population of men with higher testosterone levels.[76,77] The data needed to evaluate long-term risks and benefits of testosterone therapy are still inadequate. For most men, rather than opting for testosterone treatment, endocrinologists recommend first trying a healthy diet, cutting back on alcohol, increasing exercise, and losing weight. These actions alone can boost testosterone by up to 15%.

Sexually transmitted infections (STIs)[78]

Because a person can have an STI without having obvious symptoms of a disease, the term sexually transmitted infections (STIs) is the preferred usage, but the term sexually transmitted diseases (STDs) is still in use and considered to be acceptable terminology. More than 1 million people worldwide get a sexually transmitted infection every day. Chlamydia, gonorrhea, syphilis, and trichomoniasis cause about half of these infections, and millions of people are living with herpes simplex virus (HSV) and human papillomavirus (HPV) infections. Genital herpes is one of the most prevalent STIs in the U.S., caused either by herpes simplex virus subtype 2 (HSV-2), a virus that almost exclusively causes genital infections or increasingly by HSV type 1 (HSV-1), a type that causes both oral herpes ("cold sores") and genital herpes. More than 10% to 20% of new genital herpes infections are now caused by HSV-1.[79]

STIs are caused by bacteria, viruses, and parasites and are spread predominantly by sexual contact, including vaginal, anal, and oral sex. Some organisms causing STIs can be spread through non-sexual means such as by blood products and tissue transfer. Of the more than 30 pathogens known to be transmitted through sexual contact, eight cause the greatest incidence of illness. Of these, four are currently curable with antibiotics: syphilis, gonorrhea, chlamydia, and trichomoniasis. The other four are viral infections that are not curable, but their impact on health can be lessened through treatment: hepatitis B, herpes (HSV), HIV, and HPV. Hepatitis B and HPV are preventable by vaccination, but HSV and HIV are not. The impossibility of curing viral STIs and the increasing number of antibiotic-resistant bacterial STIs highlights the importance of prevention by safe sexual practices.

The Center for Communicable Diseases and Prevention (CDC) estimates that there are nearly 20 million new sexually transmitted infections every year in the U.S., with half occurring among young people ages 15 to 24. (See Table 13.2.) HPV (human papillomavirus) and chlamydia are among the most frequently newly diagnosed STI in the U.S.[80,81,82] HSV-2 (herpes simplex virus) is estimated to infect more than 45 million individuals (15.3%) living in the United States ages 14 to 49 years.[83] Both young men and young women are greatly affected by STIs, but young women face the most severe long-term health consequences. The CDC estimates that undiagnosed STIs cause 24,000 U.S. women to become infertile each year.[84]

STIs are estimated to cause nearly $16 billion in U.S. health care costs each year.[85]

Table 13.2. 2017 Incidence of Sexually Transmitted Infections in the U.S.

Sexually Transmitted Infection	Incidence
Chlamydia[86]	1,708,569
Gonorrhea[87]	555,608
HIV[88]	38,739
Syphilis (primary and secondary)[89]	30,644
Hepatitis B (HBV)[90]	20,900
Hepatitis C (HCV)[91]	41,200
Human Papillomavirus (HPV)[92]	14 million

According to the WHO.[93]

- Worldwide, more than 1 million sexually transmitted infections (STIs) occur every day.
- Mother-to-child transmission of STIs can cause stillbirth, neonatal death, low-birth-weight and prematurity, sepsis, pneumonia, neonatal conjunctivitis, and congenital deformities.
- HPV infection worldwide causes 570,000 cases of cervical cancer and 300,000 cervical cancer deaths each year. Most of these cases occur in developing countries that do not have adequate availability of Pap smear cervical cancer screening and care.
- Some STIs can increase the risk of HIV acquisition three-fold or more.
- STIs such as gonorrhea and chlamydia are major causes of pelvic inflammatory disease, ectopic pregnancies, and other adverse pregnancy outcomes and infertility.
- Adolescents, young adults, and marginalized, vulnerable populations, such as sex workers, men who have sex with men, people who inject drugs, prison inmates, and mobile communities have the highest rates of STIs.

Prevention of sexually transmitted infections—STIs

Measures to reduce STIs include comprehensive sexuality education; STI and HIV testing and pre- and post-screening counseling; condom promotion; interventions targeted at vulnerable populations and people who inject drugs; and counseling to improve people's ability to recognize the symptoms of STIs.

Safe and highly effective vaccines are available for two STIs: HPV and hepatitis B (see Chapter 7, "Preventing Cancer"). The vaccine against hepatitis B is included in infant immunization programs in 93% of countries worldwide. Male circumcision reduces the risk of penile cancer, heterosexually acquired HIV infection in men by approximately 60%, and provides some protection against other STIs, such as herpes and HPV.

Many STIs, including chlamydia, gonorrhea, hepatitis B, HIV, HPV, HSV2, and syphilis, can also be transmitted from mother to child during pregnancy and childbirth. All sexually active women age 24 or younger and older women at risk should be screened for gonorrhea and chlamydia infection, according to the U.S. Preventive Services Task Force (USPSTF) Recommendation Statement.[94] When used correctly and consistently, condoms offer one of the most effective methods of protection against STIs, including HIV. There is less evidence about the effectiveness of female condoms, but they too appear to be effective and safe.

In the U.S., the estimated incidence of HIV is slowly declining, and becoming HIV positive is no longer a death sentence thanks to the availability of antiretroviral drug treatment (ART). About 38,739 new HIV infections occurred in 2017.[95] More than 1.1 million people in the United States are living with HIV infection, and about 15% are unaware of their infection.[96] Some groups are much more likely to be affected by HIV than others.[97] Men who have sex with men (MSM) account for two-thirds of new infections, and Blacks continue to be disproportionately affected. The CDC reports that although Blacks represent approximately 14% of the U.S. population, in 2017, they acquired an estimated 43% of new HIV infections with the greatest incidence among men who have sex with men.

Transmission of HIV can be reduced by ART that reduces the viral load of those with infections, by use of condoms and other safe sex practices, and by avoiding the sharing of drug injection paraphernalia among those addicted to opiates and other drugs that are injected.[98] There is good evidence that when the HIV virus is suppressed with ART to the point that it becomes undetectable, it only rarely can be sexually transmitted.[99][100] This may take six months of ART treatment and requires careful adherence to taking ART. Another key element of prevention is the use of ART drugs for preexposure prophylaxis (PrEP) by those at risk of becoming infected.[101] If taken daily, PrEP, which contains two antiretrovirals, has been shown to be 86% effective in preventing new HIV infections.[102]

Those aware of their HIV infection but not in regular care contributed to more than 40% of new cases.[103] Those unaware of infection contributed to more than one-third, and those receiving treatment but not virally suppressed contributed to about 20%. This data is one reason the USPSTF recommends screening for HIV infection in adolescents and adults aged 15 to 65.[104] Younger adolescents and older adults who are at increased risk of infection should also be screened. The USPSTF recommends screening for HIV infection in all pregnant women, including those who present in labor or at delivery whose HIV status is unknown.

Maternal health

The risks associated with pregnancy and childbirth are often underestimated. In a recent study in the U.S., only about half of women were aware that pregnancy entails significant health risks, and only about half of the women surveyed were aware that pregnancy increased the risk of venous thromboembolism (VTE), diabetes and hypertension. The majority of women surveyed (76%) erroneously considered oral contraception to be more dangerous than pregnancy.[105] Even with access to modern medical care, about 1 to 2 of every 10,000 U.S. births results in a maternal death, with hemorrhage, cardiovascular conditions (coronary disease, cardiomyopathy, stroke) infection, embolism, eclampsia and conditions related to mental health such as drug overdose being the leading causes.[106 107 108 109 110] Most of these deaths can be avoided by improving women's access to quality care before, during, and after pregnancy and childbirth from a skilled birth attendant and, if necessary, hospital-based emergency care.

Teen pregnancy and birth increase the risks for both mothers and their newborns.[111] The younger the mother, the greater the risk to her and her baby. In low- and middle-income countries, babies born to mothers under 20 years of age face a 50% higher risk of being stillborn or dying in the first few weeks versus those born to mothers aged 20 to 29. Babies born to adolescent mothers are more likely to have low birth weight, with the risk of long-term detrimental health effects.

The risks of pregnancy and childbirth are amplified for the many women who live with pre-existing medical conditions. Conditions that can be made worse by pregnancy include cardiovascular disease, kidney disease, thyroid disease, asthma, and diabetes. These problems are becoming increasingly common among women of reproductive ages.[112] If the 33% of caesarean births are included, almost half of deliveries in the U.S. involve at least one medical complication.[113] Excluding caesarean births, more than one in four U.S. births is associated with at least one complication, including obstetric trauma and laceration (8%), infection (6%), hemorrhage (4%), gestational diabetes (4%), and severe preeclampsia and eclampsia (1%).[114] Postpartum depression occurs in 11% to 18% of deliveries and at more than twice that rate among adolescent deliveries.[115]

Urological disorders

There are many conditions and diseases involving the urologic and reproductive systems, such as bladder infections that require treatment with antibiotics. They are more common in women and may recur frequently. Another ailment, overactive bladder (OAB) is a very common problem that is at least partially responsive to healthy behavioral and lifestyle choices. It is estimated that at least 50 million American women and men suffer to some degree from overactive bladders that cause sudden, involuntary, and difficult to control urges to urinate and frequent urination, often when the bladder is only partially full. Individuals with OAB often have urinary incontinence that causes wetting accidents because they cannot always prevent urination when an urge occurs. A similar common problem is the involuntary leakage of urine because of the stress incontinence that occurs when int[116]ra-abdominal pressure spikes from a cough, sneeze, laughter, or physical exertion.[116]

Although OAB occurs more frequently among older adults, it is not a universal consequence of aging. Conditions that increase the likelihood of OAB include obesity, neurological disorders such as dementia, various medications (e.g., those taken for hypertension), enlarged prostates, and among women, weak pelvic floor muscles from childbearing or lack of physical fitness. The consumption of some foods and beverages that irritate the bladder can also increase the likelihood of OAB symptoms.

Lifestyle changes for Overactive Bladder (OAB)

The American Urological Association recommends a thorough evaluation before treatment of OAB, and the Urology Care Foundation suggests that the first thing to try to manage overactive bladder is lifestyle changes. In their experience, most patients don't get rid of all their symptoms with lifestyle changes, but many do have fewer symptoms. The following advice is modified from that provided by the Urology Care Foundation.[117]

Limit food and drinks that you find "bladder irritating"

Foods and drinks that increase OAB symptoms among some people include coffee, tea, artificial sweeteners, caffeine, alcohol, soda, and other fizzy drinks, citrus fruit, food made with tomatoes, chocolate, and spicy foods. One strategy is to avoid all "bladder irritating" foods and then add them back one at a time.

Keep a daily "bladder diary"

Write down what you eat and drink, and when and how many trips you make to the bathroom for a few days. This can help you and your health care provider better understand your condition. A diary may help identify foods or other things that make symptoms worse. For example, are they worse when you don't drink enough or drink too much liquid?

Double voiding (emptying your bladder twice)

This may be helpful, especially for men with enlarged prostates who have trouble emptying their bladder completely. After you urinate, wait a few seconds or minutes and then try again to urinate.

Delayed voiding

To retrain your bladder, put off urination, even when you feel an urge. At first, you wait just a few minutes. Gradually you will be able to wait much longer between bathroom visits. The Urology Care Foundation suggests that it is important to try this only if your health care provider tells you to. Some people will have worse symptoms or have urine leaks when they ignore an urge or wait too long to urinate.

Scheduled voiding

Instead of going when you feel the urge, you urinate on a schedule at set times during the day. Depending on how often you urinate now, your health care provider may ask you to urinate every 2 to 4 hours, whether you feel you have to go or not.

Exercises to relax your bladder muscle

These can help decrease urgency. Some call these exercises "quick flicks" because you quickly squeeze and release the muscles in your pelvis several times. When you get the urge to urinate, squeeze, and then relax your pelvic floor muscles as quickly as you can. Do this several times in a row when you feel the urge to go. This sends a message to your nervous system and back to your bladder to stop contracting. As your bladder stops contracting and starts relaxing, your urge to urinate should lessen. When you do this exercise, it helps to be still, relax, and concentrate just on the "quick flick" contractions. Your health care provider can explain this exercise in more detail. Regularly doing these "Kegel" pelvic floor exercises may benefit both women and men by reducing the involuntary contraction of bladder muscles. It can take up to two months for these exercises to be beneficial.

Prescription drugs and injections

When lifestyle changes don't help enough, your health care provider may offer a prescription drug to relax the bladder muscle. Common side effects include dry mouth and eyes, constipation, and blurred vision. If lifestyle changes and prescription drugs don't work, a urologist may recommend injections of botulinum toxin (Botox®) into your bladder muscle to partially paralyze and relax it. The drug may help keep your bladder from contracting too often, but it could cause urinary retention (not emptying your bladder completely) and require temporary use of a catheter to empty your bladder.

Nerve stimulation

When drugs or lifestyle changes don't work, neuromodulation therapy can be used to deliver electrical pulses to nerves to change how they work. There are two types of neuromodulation therapy. Sacral neuromodulation (SNS) entails the placement of a "bladder pacemaker," a device that delivers electrical impulses via the sacral nerves to the bladder to stop the signals that can cause OAB. The other form is percutaneous tibial nerve stimulation (PTNS). This therapy stimulates the tibial nerve, which runs along your knee to the sacral nerves. The electrical pulses help block the nerve signals that aren't working correctly.

Finally, if treatment is not successful in controlling urinary incontinence, a person can manage their bladder problems with one of the many devices and products that collect and hold urine.[118]

Summary of the essential facts

- Young and healthy men and women often face reproductive health risks that they need to address by sexuality education and by the adoption of safe behaviors.
- The use of effective contraceptives, especially the highly effective long-acting reversible contraceptive (LARC) methods, IUDs, and implants, can reliably prevent the detrimental social and health consequences of unintended pregnancies.
- The use of condoms and other safe sexual practices can effectively prevent the acquisition of potentially fatal sexually transmitted infections.
- The safest pattern of childbearing for both a mother and her child is to avoid births at teen ages, older than age 35, more closely spaced than two years apart, and of higher birth orders, i.e., after the second or third birth. Always get prenatal care, and hospital delivery is the safest for mother and child.
- Abortion carried out by well-trained health care providers is very safe and many times safer than childbirth, especially when carried out early in pregnancy.
- Overactive bladder often improves after making healthy behavioral and lifestyle choices.

14
Environmental Pollutants and Toxins

Toxic substances in our environment have important implications for health. Although there are many actions that an individual can take to avoid exposure, some exposures will occur, and increased government regulation of sources of toxic exposure is needed. Environmental toxins include a wide variety of chemicals, minerals, metals, and ionizing radiation that can harm health. Of an estimated 85,000 known chemicals, only a few have been thoroughly tested to assess their impact on health.

Over the past 50 years, the production of industrial chemicals has risen rapidly, and the U.S. generates or imports some 42 billion pounds of them per day. We are exposed to a wide variety of chemicals that are in thousands of household products. We ingest pesticide residues with our food, cover our skin with potentially toxic cosmetics and insect repellents, and breathe air that is polluted from vehicle exhaust, power plant, and industrial emissions. If we understand these challenges, we can take action to protect our health.

Air pollution

A wide array of chronic illnesses and acute health impacts is associated with air pollution exposure. Research has shown that long-term exposure to air pollutants can reduce lung growth and development, and increase the risk of developing many diseases including asthma, reduced lung function, susceptibility to infection, emphysema, chronic obstructive pulmonary disease (COPD), lung cancer, and cardiovascular disease.[1,2] Air pollution increases the risk of preterm birth, impaired brain development and developmental disabilities, and acute pneumonia in children under 5.[3] In 2013, the World Health Organization concluded that outdoor air pollution is a carcinogen.[4,5]

According to the National Institute of Environmental Health Sciences (NIEHS), air pollution is a mixture of natural and human-made substances in the air we breathe.[6] Ozone and particulates are major components of air pollution.[7] Particulates are the microscopic particles released into the air from motor vehicle exhaust, burning, and dust. Particulates are classified according to these sizes, coarse particulates, PM10 (10 to 2.5 microns), fine particulates, PM2.5 (equal or smaller than 2.5 microns), and ultrafine particulates (equal or smaller than 0.1 microns). In general, the smaller particulates, fine and ultrafine, are a greater health risk since they can penetrate deeply into the lungs, and the ultrafines can even reach the bloodstream. A warming climate is increasing levels of the ozone that is formed when sunlight interacts with fossil fuel emissions. Heat, sunlight, and lack of wind are conditions that favor the combination of particulates and ozone into thick smog— a frequent air quality hazard in densely populated cities such as Beijing and Delhi.

Outdoor air pollution involves exposures that take place outside of the built environment. Examples include fine particles produced by the burning of fossil fuels and fires of all kinds (e.g., from wildfires and the coal and petroleum used in energy production and that caused by traffic); noxious gases (sulfur dioxide, nitrogen oxides, carbon monoxide, chemical vapors); ground-level ozone (a reactive form of oxygen and a primary component of urban smog); and tobacco smoke. Outdoor air pollution is difficult to avoid, but we can take action when alerted to the level of pollution.

The U.S. Environmental Protection Agency (EPA) establishes an air quality index (AQI) for five major air pollutants regulated by the Clean Air Act. Each of these pollutants has a national air quality standard set by EPA to protect public health:

- Ground-level ozone
- Particle pollution (also known as particulate matter, including PM2.5 and PM10)
- Carbon monoxide
- Sulfur dioxide
- Nitrogen dioxide

Pollution levels are predicted based on wind and weather forecasts. The AQI scale runs from 0 to 500. The higher the AQI value, the greater the level of air pollution, and the greater the health concern. For example, a red alert would go into effect if there is a prediction that the air quality index will stay above 200 for more than 72 hours.

The color levels, index, and levels of health concern for ozone and particle pollution are:

- Green: Good, 0 to 50, Air quality is satisfactory, and air pollution poses little or no risk.
- Yellow: Moderate, 51 to 100, Air quality is acceptable. However, there may be a risk for some people, particularly those who are unusually sensitive to air pollution.
- Orange: Unhealthy for Sensitive Groups, 101 to 150, Members of sensitive groups may experience health effects. The general public is less likely to be affected.
- Red: Unhealthy, 151 to 200, Some members of the general public may experience health effects; members of sensitive groups may experience more severe health effects.
- Purple: Very Unhealthy, 201 to 300, Health alert: The risk of health effects is increased for everyone.
- Maroon: Hazardous, 301 and higher, Health warning of emergency conditions: everyone is more likely to be affected.

It is not unusual for outdoor air pollution to come indoors by way of open windows, doors, and ventilation. Indoor air pollution involves exposures to particulates, carbon oxides, and other pollutants carried by indoor air or dust. Examples include gases (e.g., carbon monoxide, radon, ozone); household products and chemicals; building materials (e.g., asbestos, formaldehyde, lead); outdoor to indoor allergens (e.g., cockroach and mouse droppings); tobacco smoke; mold; and pollen. When we are aware of the health consequences of exposure, we can take action to avoid exposure to many of these pollutants.

An estimated 85% of deaths from chronic respiratory disease are attributable to chronic obstructive pulmonary disease (COPD), a leading cause of death in the U.S.[8] A study of the causes of chronic respiratory disease mortality among U.S. counties between 1980 and 2014, found that differing incidence and care for asthma, and differing exposure to tobacco, coal dust, asbestos and silica accounted for much of the geographic and occupational variations in rates of death from COPD.[9] A twenty-year study of lung function among children found that decreased smog and other air pollution in the Los Angeles region brought about substantial improvements in lung function.[10]

The NIEHS-supported Harvard Six Cities Study, a large database on the health effects of outdoor and indoor air pollution, found a strong association between exposure to ozone, fine particles, and sulfur dioxide, and an increase in respiratory symptoms, reduced lung capacity, and risk of early death.[11] There is evidence that even short term and low levels of particulate matter and ozone air pollution increase the risk of death. A study among more than 60 million Medicare beneficiaries found that every ten micrograms per cubic meter increase of fine particulates smaller than 2.5 microns (PM2.5) was associated with a 7.3% increase in mortality. Each increase in 10 parts per billion of ozone was associated with a 1.1% increase in mortality.[12 13]

A study that included almost 60 million deaths from 652 cities in 24 countries found that all-cause (nonaccidental), cardiovascular, and respiratory mortality was associated with short-term exposures to both PM10 and PM2.5 particulates.[14] The difference in mortality between the best air quality and the worst observed was estimated to be up to 6%.

People living in some places may find it difficult to avoid the adverse health effects of air pollution. Indoor air pollution from mold, building materials, furniture, paints, varnishes, cleaning supplies, and other chemicals may be easier to avoid.

Environmental toxins and how they are regulated

Until 2016, toxic substances in the U.S. were regulated by the 1976 Toxic Substances Control Act (TSCA), which left the burden of proving that chemicals are dangerous almost entirely up to the government. Industry confidentiality privileges built into the TSCA prevented federal regulators from having access to information about how substances are made and what their health effects might be. In the years since the TSCA became law, the Environmental Protection Agency (EPA) has issued restrictions on only a few chemicals.

Two classes of chemicals have had stricter regulation than that required of most chemicals. Drugs are regulated by the U.S. Food and Drug Administration (FDA). Pesticides are regulated by both the federal Environmental Protection Agency (EPA) and by the states, usually by the state's agriculture office. Manufacturers must register or license pesticides for use before distribution. The EPA receives its authority to register pesticides under the Federal Insecticide, Fungicide, and Rodenticide Act (FIFRA). States are authorized to regulate pesticides under FIFRA and state pesticide laws, and they may place more restrictive requirements on pesticides than the EPA.[15]

For years experts on environmental toxins believed that stricter regulation of other chemicals and other toxic health hazards was a long-overdue safety step. In 2007, the European Union implemented a new regulatory framework for chemicals, Registration, Evaluation, and Authorization of Chemicals (REACH). REACH shifts the burden of proof to industry, requiring chemical companies to prove that their products don't harm human health or the environment and requiring manufacturers to obtain special authorization to manufacture and distribute any chemicals designated to be of very high concern to human and environmental health.

Even though the American chemical industry had reservations about adopting a REACH-style program for the U.S., citing the cost of additional regulations, in 2016, with the safety laws in place in Europe as a model, Congress passed the Frank R. Lautenberg Chemical Safety for the 21st Century Act. The act improves and strengthens TSCA by:[16]

- Subjecting all new and existing chemicals to an EPA safety review.
- Requiring EPA to focus on chemicals that are the highest priorities for full risk-based safety assessments.
- Strengthening transparency and the quality of science used to make EPA decisions.
- Expanding EPA's ability to require additional health and safety testing of chemicals.
- Allowing industry to request that EPA conduct a safety assessment on a specific chemical.
- Providing EPA with a full range of options to address the risks of substances including labeling requirements, use restrictions, phase-outs or other appropriate actions.
- Setting aggressive and attainable timelines for EPA to complete its work.
- Promoting cooperation between state and federal regulators while creating a strong national chemical regulatory system, ensuring interstate commerce is not disadvantaged.
- Strengthening protections for the most vulnerable like infants, children and the elderly.
- Protecting confidential business information.

Although the new chemical safety act has the potential to increase the protection of environmental health, the EPA has not vigorously implemented its new regulatory powers, and many consumer products that are banned for sale in the European Union are still sold in the U.S. Industry critics of stronger regulation point out that humans are exposed not only to human-made toxins but also to a broad array of naturally occurring and potentially dangerous chemicals and substances found in our environment, including in the air and our food. Furthermore, it is undeniable that many of the thousands of chemicals that have been synthesized and introduced into our environment serve beneficial purposes that are important to human welfare.

Are the dangers of environmental toxins well established?[17]

Very few chemicals, minerals, and metals have been thoroughly tested for their impact on human health. Almost all testing that has been done has focused on individual chemicals, so there is very little understanding of how chemicals might act in various combinations. It is probable that many toxic effects are dose-related; that is, they are essentially harmless if we are exposed to them in very small amounts or if they are present in our bodies in very small quantities. The theory is that toxic substances can be safe as long as the amount remains below a certain threshold. Unfortunately for many toxins, the level at which subtle adverse effects begin to occur is not known or is poorly understood. Research strongly suggests that the recommended safe exposure levels of many chemicals are set too high. For example, for metals such as lead and mercury, levels that were once considered safe were found to be too high—the trend is to set lower levels for safe exposure to many environmental toxins.

It is known that we all have hundreds of chemicals in our bodies today, including many that didn't even exist a few decades ago. Many of these chemicals are stored in body fat, so they are eliminated very slowly. Biomonitoring surveys by the Centers for Disease Control and Prevention (CDC) have found traces of 265 environmental chemicals in the bodies of Americans, including toxic metals like arsenic and cadmium, pesticides, flame retardants and even perchlorate, an ingredient of rocket fuel.[18 19]

Writing in the *New York Times* in 2020, Jane Brody presented research that suggests that an observed increase in Parkinson's disease is linked to exposure to toxic chemicals in industrialized countries. The increase in risk is especially prominent after occupational exposures to industrial solvents and degreasing agents such as trichloroethylene (TCE) and exposure to pesticides such as chlorpyrifos, rotenone and paraquat.[20]

Although more research is needed, it has become clear that developing fetuses, infants, children, pre-teens, and teenagers are far more vulnerable to toxins in the environment than adults.[21 22 23] Exposure to even tiny amounts of some toxic substances, at particularly vulnerable stages of development, can lead to significant harm to human health. For example, reports suggest that some children's congenital heart defects may be associated with their mothers' exposure to environmental toxins during pregnancy.

The harmful effects of lead have been well documented and found to be proportional to its concentration in a person's blood. The primary route for lead exposure to children is from oral ingestion via food, water, soil, dust, and flaking paint in older houses that were painted with lead-containing paint. Both pre- and post-birth exposure of children to lead has toxic effects and leads to impaired cognitive development, reduced IQ, and increased non-adaptive classroom behavior. Heavy exposures to lead can cause miscarriage, and even paralysis and blindness. Blood lead limit recommendations have been decreased progressively from 60 μg/dl in the

1960s to the current U.S. and WHO guidelines of a maximum level of 10 μg/dl. The banning of lead additives in paint and gasoline has reduced exposures from those sources, but industrial emissions continue to cause environmental contamination with lead.

Mercury, like lead, is toxic to the brain, especially to the developing brain. Significant sources of mercury are coal-fired power plants and waste incinerators. Methylmercury, the more toxic form of mercury, is produced by microorganisms acting on mercury in deposits in the sea and the soil. Since mercury accumulates through the food chain, the highest levels of methylmercury are found in large predatory fish that are at the top of the food chain. These fish are a major source of human exposure. Mercury exposure, especially during fetal brain development, can impair children's memory, attention, and language abilities and interfere with fine motor and visual-spatial skills. The FDA and EPA advise pregnant women not to eat swordfish, shark, king mackerel, and tilefish and limit consumption of albacore tuna to 6 ounces or less a week. (See Chapter 3, "Optimal Nutrition," for more on fish and health.)

Exposure to tobacco smoke and other forms of air pollution in pregnancy is associated with a wide range of behavioral, neurological, and physical difficulties in babies including stillbirth, placental disruption, prematurity, lower mean birth weight, congenital disabilities, reductions in lung function, and increased risk of infant mortality. Children should not be exposed to secondhand smoke. The effect of exposure to marijuana smoke and vaping is less well established, but it may be similar to the risks of tobacco smoke.

Persistent organic pollutants (POPs) are carbon-containing chemicals that are extremely stable, can be spread over long distances, accumulate in high concentrations in fat tissues, and are concentrated through the food chain. Some 5000 of these stable chemicals are grouped in a class called per- and polyfluoroalkyl substances (PFASs). They are used in a wide range of products including nonstick cookware. The Environmental Protection Agency reports that the two best studied PFASs, PFOA (perfluorooctanoic acid) and PFOS (perfluorooctane sulfonate), can cause tumors and have reproductive, developmental, liver, kidney, and immunological effects in laboratory animals.[24] Limited findings in humans relate to infant birth weights, effects on the immune system, cancer (for PFOA), and thyroid hormone disruption (for PFOS). *Consumer Reports* (*CR*) has observed that there is little monitoring or regulation of contamination of community water supplies and bottled water with PFASs beyond voluntary guidelines of a concentration of 70 parts per trillion.[25] Up to 110 million people in the U.S. may have tap water contaminated with PFASs at a higher level than the one part per trillion recommended by the scientists they have consulted. *CR* suggests that consumers check their municipal supply or well water, filter their water, and choose carpet and furniture brands that do not include stain resistant fabric. Avoiding fast food packaging and microwaveable popcorn bags will also reduce exposure. *CR* has published a list of carbonated and non-carbonated bottled water brands that are low in PFASs.

Some POPs, including DDT, are pesticides that, because of their persistence and accumulation within the food chain, have resulted in widespread human exposures. Exposure to DDT before the age of 14 is associated with an increased risk of breast cancer. Dioxins (polychlorinated-p-dioxins), and polychlorinated-biphenyls (PCBs) that are dioxin-like compounds, are examples of POPs that continue to cause human exposure. Exposure to dioxins in pregnancy has been associated with subtle developmental changes in the fetus. Effects on the child later in life include changes in liver function, thyroid hormone levels, and decreased performance in learning and intelligence tests. PCBs were manufactured in large amounts until the 1970s, and although the widespread use of PCBs is now banned, there is a damaging legacy from the persistence of the chemical. To date, human data do not provide an accurate basis for establishing a tolerable intake of most POPs, either for the general population or for children, probably a more vulnerable subgroup.

Developmental neurotoxicity (DNT)

Some toxins, such as pesticides, affect the nervous system, and there is thought to be a link between exposure to them and increases in learning and developmental disabilities such as autism, attention-deficit/hyperactivity disorder, and other chronic conditions and diseases. It is not clear if there are real increases in learning problems among children in recent years, or just better recognition and diagnosis, but currently, about one in six U.S. children under the age of 18 have some kind of learning, developmental, or behavioral disorder.

The developing fetus and young children are particularly vulnerable to certain environmental toxins because critical neurodevelopmental processes occur in the human central nervous system during fetal development and in the first three years of life. Protection of infants and children from exposure to environmental toxins is very difficult because they may enter a child's body across the placenta during fetal development or by direct ingestion of house dust, soil, breast milk, and other dietary sources during early childhood. Increased knowledge of the toxicity of environmental chemicals, including testing for developmental neurotoxicity and reproductive toxicity, is needed. Animal experiments make it clear that pesticides have the potential to cause serious damage to a developing fetus. For pesticides intended for use on food crops, regulations require only that developmental neurotoxicity testing be evaluated for substances already known or suspected of being toxins. Even though more than 140 registered pesticides are neurotoxic (i.e., specifically designed to act against pests by interfering with neurotransmitters or other processes shared by mammals and insects), the EPA has received developmental neurotoxicity testing results for fewer than a dozen pesticides.

Endocrine disruptors

An endocrine disruptor is a substance or mixture of chemicals that alter functions of the endocrine system and causes adverse health effects in an intact organism, or its progeny. Endocrine disruptors may mimic the biological activity of a hormone, usually, estrogen; prevent or alter the usual effects of a naturally occurring hormone; or affect the synthesis or breakdown rates of natural hormones. Although the hormonal activity of endocrine disrupter chemicals is many times weaker than the body's natural hormones, there is evidence that they cause endocrine changes. These chemicals include some pesticides (e.g., DDT and other chlorinated compounds), chemicals in some consumer and medical products (e.g., some plastic additives), and a number of industrial chemicals (e.g., polychlorinated biphenyls, PCBs), and dioxins.

Suspected effects of endocrine disruptors include male genital organ abnormalities, low sperm counts, precocious female puberty, lowered female fecundity (fertility), polycystic ovary syndrome, endometriosis, uterine fibroids, breast cancer, prostate cancer, testis cancer, thyroid cancer, developmental neurotoxicity, and metabolic syndrome. Endocrine-disrupting chemicals have been implicated in the causation of the metabolic syndrome and obesity by altering fat cell development and increasing energy storage in fat tissue.[26] Endocrine disruptors also affect wildlife including invertebrates, fish, amphibians, reptiles, birds and mammals.

Chemicals of concern as endocrine disruptors include:

- PCBs, PCDFs (Polychlorinated dibenzofurans), PCDDs (polychlorinated dibenzodioxins)
- Polybrominated diphenyl ethers (PBDEs)
- Perfluorinated compounds (PFCs)
- DDT/DDE
- Pesticides
- Heavy metals
- Alkylphenols, bisphenol A (BPA), parabens
- Phthalates
- Pharmaceutical estrogens
- Phytoestrogens (estrogen-like chemicals naturally occurring in plants)

Among the chemicals suspected of being endocrine disruptors, bisphenol A (BPA) and phthalates (key ingredients in plastics) are probably the best studied and the research is indicative that they can disrupt the developing endocrine system.[27] BPA is widely used globally; some 6 billion pounds are produced each year. BPA is used to harden polycarbonate plastics and make the epoxy resin used in the lining of food and beverage containers. Polycarbonates can sometimes be identified in plastics by the resin identification code or recycling number 7.

BPA is a useful and pervasive industrial chemical, but it is also a synthetic estrogen. When heated, worn, or washed, plastics containing BPA can erode or break down, allowing the chemical to leach into food and water and enter the human body. The CDC has found BPA in the urine of 93% of surveyed Americans over the age of 6. Unlike many other chemicals we are exposed to, BPA is readily excreted, so if ingestion of BPA stops, the body eliminates it quickly.

The scientific consensus has been moving away from the idea that BPA is completely safe. Animal studies link low-level fetal BPA exposure to a broad spectrum of developmental and reproductive effects, including breast cancer, early-onset puberty, male genital defects, decreased testosterone levels, reduced sperm counts, and neurobehavioral problems. In 2008, Canada deemed infant exposure to BPA potentially unsafe. It banned the sale of baby bottles that use the chemical—a step later taken by several U.S. states and major retailers, including Wal-Mart. Although European regulators declared BPA safe in a 2008 assessment, Denmark has enacted a ban on BPA in baby bottles. In 2009, the International Endocrine Society released a statement declaring that endocrine disrupters were a significant concern for public health and called for regulation to reduce human exposure.

Although the FDA has reviewed the chemical and ruled it safe, the decision has been criticized for relying almost exclusively on industry-funded studies. The FDA is continuing to study the safety of BPA, and in 2012 and 2013, the FDA amended the food additive regulations to no longer provide for the use of BPA-based epoxy resins as coatings in baby bottles, sippy cups, and infant formula packaging. The FDA stated that the actions were based solely on a determination of abandonment of those uses and was not related to the safety of BPA.[28] In 2018 the FDA continued to support the safety of BPA for "currently authorized uses." However, the Endocrine Society and other scientists who study the health effects of BPA are concerned about the numerous studies linking BPA and adverse health outcomes relating to reproduction, behavior, and metabolic disease.[29] One action anyone can take to minimize BPA exposure is to use BPA free water bottles.

Phthalates are a widely-used class of industrial chemicals that may affect the endocrine system. They are found in polyvinyl chloride plastics and many consumer products, including nail polish, hair spray, deodorant, and shampoo. Imported cosmetics may be particularly suspect in that FDA testing has found that about 15% of those it tests are contaminated or contain dangerous ingredients. There is a trend toward the use of non-phthalate plasticizers in products such as nail polish.[30] Products that are labeled "3-Free" means they do not contain DnBP (an endocrine disrupter), toluene, or formaldehyde. A label that says 5-Free or 10-Free does not guarantee they are safer because the ingredients that are omitted from the polish may be non-toxic. It is not known what level of exposure to nail polish may be a health risk, but many nail polishes still contain triphenyl phosphate (THPH), also a known endocrine disrupter, and choosing products with "free" labeling is a reasonable precaution.

The male children of women who have been exposed to phthalates in pregnancy may suffer from abnormal genital development. In animal studies, phthalates have been shown to disrupt hormones and are linked to reduced sperm counts and other signs of feminization in male rodents. Similar effects are caused by a class of long-lived chemical fire retardants known as polybrominated diphenyl ethers (PBDEs) used in electronics, polyurethane foam and other plastics. These chemicals can leak out of polyurethane cushions in car seats or changing table pads and can be inhaled or absorbed through a baby's skin. Although they are being phased out, unlike BPA and phthalates that are excreted within a few days, PBDEs can remain in the body for years.

Higher levels of phthalates and other endocrine disrupters have been linked to earlier breast development in girls and male genital abnormalities like undescended testicles and smaller penises. However, the science around endocrine disrupters is not settled, and some peer-reviewed studies fail to show a link between endocrine disrupters and health effects. Human exposure to BPA and phthalates is still well below safety levels set by most governments, and most health agencies around the world say the chemicals are safe for humans, but the precautionary principle suggests that choosing products that minimize exposure, especially for pregnant women, infants and children is a good idea.

Pharmaceuticals

Although pharmaceuticals are designed to enhance health, some have the potential to cause problems. When outdated and unused drugs are put into trash or flushed, they may end up in our water system and may not be eliminated by water-treatment techniques. New programs to encourage proper disposal of unused drugs would address just 10% of the source of the problem because 90% of drug contamination comes from pharmaceuticals passing through the body largely unaltered and into the sewage system. There are about 3,000 prescription pharmaceuticals in use in the U.S. and thousands of over-the-counter drugs, as well as the creams and ointments we apply to our skin and then shower off. Pharmaceutical pollutants are worrisome because they are specifically designed to be metabolically active in humans.

In the 1990s, synthetic estrogens, principally from birth control pills, began showing up in the water, leading to male fish with androgynous sex organs. It did not take much estrogen to affect the fish — just 5 or 6 nanograms, or billionths of a gram, per liter of lake water. Even though very tiny amounts of many other classes of drugs are found in many water supplies, most of these drugs are in such low concentrations that they do not appear to have an impact on human health. Among those drugs identified are antidepressants, anticonvulsants, tranquilizers, antibacterials, antipsychotics, ACE inhibitors for hypertension, steroids, analgesics (like ibuprofen), and caffeine. While short-term exposure to these drugs at thousandths of their effective dose levels does not seem to entail a risk, there is essentially no data on long-term low-level exposures and interactions between drugs.

Exposure to pharmaceuticals in water is largely dependent on the source of municipal water. A study by *Consumer Reports* found that bottled water is not guaranteed to be free from pharmaceuticals. Many water systems start with pure water, and their treated wastewater does not come into contact with humans, even if it contains traces of pharmaceuticals. But for other water systems, for example, those that take water from the Mississippi or Colorado rivers, cleaned-up wastewater can end up in the water supply of a city or town.

Many communities have established safe disposal systems for unused drugs. The Food and Drug Administration's advice for old, unused, unwanted, or expired prescription and over-the-counter medicines is to drop them off at a take-back site. If you cannot get to a take-back location or there is none near you, the FDA has a list of medicines that can be flushed and a list of others that should be discarded in the trash. (See https://www.fda.gov/drugs/disposal-unused-medicines-what-you-should-know/drug-disposal-drug-take-back-locations.)

Priority list of environmental toxins

In an effort to reduce exposures to environmental toxins, the U.S. has established a National Priorities List (NPL) of hazardous waste sites eligible for long-term remedial cleanup financed under the federal Superfund program.[31] To assist this program, the Agency for Toxic Substances and Disease Registry (ATSDR) maintains a Substance Priority List (SPL), a list of hazardous substances that will be the candidates for toxicological profiles prepared by the ATSDR.[32] The SPL is not a list based on an evaluation of which are the most toxic substances, but rather a prioritization of substances based on the frequency of occurrence at National Priorities List (NPL) sites, toxicity, and potential for human exposure to the substances found at sites. Many of these chemicals listed in Table 14.1 below can be found on the Substance Priority List, and exposure to them should be minimized because most are already established to harm health.

Avoiding environmental toxins

Given the great uncertainty regarding what exactly is toxic in our environment, the levels that are harmful, and the health effects of environmental toxins, it is best to limit exposure to all potentially toxic substances as much as possible. It should be recognized that it is impossible to avoid all environmental toxins. What can be done is to minimize exposure. There are ways to limit exposures for yourself, your family, at work, and in the community.

The University of California, San Francisco Program on Reproductive Health and the Environment offers the following advice excerpted from their publication: "Toxic Matters Protecting Our Families from Toxic Substances" and available online at www.prhe.ucsf.edu/prhe/toxicmatters.html

Prevent exposure to yourself and at home

Don't smoke

Don't smoke and don't let people smoke around you and stay away from public places where people are smoking.

Become a smart consumer

Use non-toxic personal care products, including cosmetics, hair products, and toothpaste. These products may contain toxic substances.[33] Many of these products have ingredients that can harm reproductive health. Find safer products at www.prhe.ucsf.edu/prhe/tmlinks.html#personalcare and www.prhe.ucsf.edu/prhe/tmlinks.html#consumerguide.

Table 14.1. Substances in the environment known to harm health

Acetone	Chlorine	Mold	Radon
Ammonia	Dioxins	Nitrogen Oxides	Solvents
Artificial Turf	Drinking-Water Contaminants	Ozone	Sulfur Dioxides
Arsenic	Endocrine Disruptors (BPA and Phthalates)	Particulate Matter	Sun Exposure
Asbestos	Ethylene Glycol (antifreeze)	Perchloroethylene	Toluene

Benzene	Flame Retardants (PBDEs or BFRs)	Perfluorooctanoic Acid (PFOA)	Vinyl chloride
Benzo(a)pyrene	Formaldehyde	Pesticides	Volatile Organic Compounds (VOCs)
Bisphenol-a	Gasoline	Phthalates	Tobacco Smoke
Cadmium	Lead	Polychlorinated Biphenyls (PCBs)	
Carbon Monoxide	Mercury	Polycyclic Aromatic Hydrocarbons (PAHs)	

Pick your plastics carefully

Some plastics release toxic chemicals like vinyl chloride, phthalates, and bisphenol-A (BPA).

- Don't buy products made with soft PVC. For example, some shower curtains and toys are made with soft PVC.
- Don't use plastic containers for hot food or drinks. Use glass or stainless steel.
- Use glass instead of plastics in the microwave.
- Learn more about plastics at: www.prhe.ucsf.edu/prhe/tmlinks.html#plastics.

Avoid pesticides and other toxic substances in food and water

Consumer Reports (*CR*) recommends to always buy organic foods to avoid pesticides but notes that eating many conventionally grown foods is low risk and that high consumption of fruits and vegetables is more important to health than limiting fruit and vegetable consumption just to organics. If you can't afford to buy organic produce, buy the fruits and vegetables with the lowest pesticide levels and avoid the most contaminated ones. Because specific foods have a higher risk of pesticide contamination, based on their 2020 analysis, *CR* considers it particularly important to choose organically grown celery, kale, fresh green beans, spinach, apples, blueberries, nectarines, pears, cherries, fresh peaches and potatoes. Higher than desirable levels of pesticide contamination were also found in imported summer squash, lettuce, strawberries and watermelon.[34 35]

Choose fish that are less contaminated with mercury. Find information on healthy and environmentally sustainable fish at www.prhe.ucsf.edu/prhe/tmlinks.html#mercury. Check local fish advisories. Fish advisories are warnings about the safety of eating fish. Don't eat the fish you or others catch before checking these warnings to make sure the fish is safe to eat. See Chapter 3, "Optimal Nutrition," for more on fish.

Limit foods with a lot of animal fat. Many toxic substances build up in animal fat. Avoid canned foods and beverages as much as you can. Eat fresh or frozen fruits and vegetables. This helps you avoid exposure to BPA because BPA is a toxic substance used in the lining of most cans.

To learn how to reduce toxic substances in your drinking water, go to www.prhe.ucsf.edu/prhe/tmlinks.html#foodandwater. Learn more about reducing your exposure to pesticides from food at www.prhe.ucsf.edu/prhe/tmlinks.html#foodandwater. (See Chapter 7, "Preventing Cancer," for more on pesticides.)

Don't use pesticides for pests

Pesticides are toxic chemicals for killing insects, rodents, weeds, bacteria, and mold.

- Keep insects and rodents out of your home. Clean up crumbs and spills. Store food in tightly closed containers. Seal cracks around doors, windowsills, and baseboards. Repair drips and holes. Get rid of standing water.
- Use baits and traps instead of sprays, dusts, and bombs.
- Don't use chemical tick-and-flea collars, flea baths, or flea dips on pets.
- Hire only licensed pest exterminators.
- Find pesticide-free alternatives at: www.prhe.ucsf.edu/prhe/tmlinks.html#pestcontrol.

Use a wet mop

Toxic substances like lead, pesticides, and flame retardants are present in dust.

- Sweeping or dusting with a dry cloth can spread the dust into the air instead of removing it.
- Use a wet mop or wet cloth to clean floors and surfaces.

Take off your shoes at the door

Shoes can carry toxic chemicals into your home. Wipe shoes on a sturdy doormat if you want to keep them on.

Clean your home with non-toxic products

It is easy and cheap to make effective, non-toxic cleaners.

- Use common items like vinegar and baking soda.
- Find out how to shop for non-toxic cleaning products and get recipes to make your own at: www.prhe.ucsf.edu/prhe/tmlinks.html#cleaningproducts

Don't dry-clean your clothes

Most dry-cleaning systems use a chemical called perchloroethylene (PERC). Dry-cleaned clothes release PERC, polluting the air in your home. Use water instead. Most clothes labeled "dry-clean only" can be washed with water. Hand wash these clothes or ask your dry cleaner to "wet clean" them for you.

Choose safer home improvements

Many paints, types of glue, and flooring materials can release toxic chemicals long after you complete a project.

- Ask for "VOC-free" and "water-based" materials.
- If you are pregnant, don't work on or near remodeling projects.
- Stay away from recently remodeled rooms.
- Learn more about safer materials at www.prhe.ucsf.edu/prhe/tmlinks html# remodeling.

Avoid lead exposure

There may be lead in house paint, dust, and garden soil. Any home built before 1978 may have lead paint.

- Call the National Lead Information Center for information about how to prevent exposure to lead at 800-424-LEAD.
- If you have lead paint in your home, cover it with a fresh coat of paint, wallpaper or tiles.
- Never sand or remove lead paint yourself. Hire a contractor who is certified in lead abatement.

Test your home for radon

Radon is a radioactive gas found in many basements and ground floors.

- Purchase a testing kit at your local hardware store. Kits are cheap and easy to use.
- Learn more about radon by calling 1-800-SOS-RADON or at: www.prhe.ucsf.edu/prhe/tmlinks.html#radon. (See Chapter 6, "Preventing Cancer," for more on radon.)

Prevent exposure at work

Many substances used on the job, in office buildings, or in workplace renovation projects are toxic to reproductive health. By law, you have a right to a safe and healthy work environment. Your employer is required by law to provide information and training about workplace hazards, including access to handouts about toxic substances called Material Safety Data Sheets (MSDS).

- Follow guidelines to avoid exposure. Use protective gear. Ask your employer about substitutes for toxic substances and other ways to prevent harmful exposures.

- If you live with anybody who works with toxic chemicals, that person should change and shower after work. The person should also keep work tools and clothing away from other people and living areas in the home. Work clothes should be washed separately.
- Get more information or file a complaint with your regional Occupational Safety and Health Administration (OSHA) office if you believe that your employer is violating OSHA standards or that your workplace poses serious hazards. You can find a directory of regional OSHA offices by calling 800-232-4636 or at www.prhe.ucsf.edu/prhe/tmlinks.html#work.
- If you are a farmworker, you can find information about reducing your exposure to agricultural pesticides at www.prhe.ucsf.edu/prhe/tmlinks.html#work.

Prevent exposure in your community

Help create a better environment for your family and everyone around you. The University of California, San Francisco, has developed community guidelines for avoiding environmental toxins that are excerpted below:

- Drive less. Carpool, take public transportation, ride your bike, or walk.
- Never burn trash, especially furniture, tires, and plastics.
- Don't use pesticides. Use organic or integrated pest management techniques in lawns and gardens.
- Never throw toxic substances down drains or toilets or in the garbage.

Learn more at www.prhe.ucsf.edu/prhe/tmlinks.html#community.

Examples of toxic substances include car oil, gasoline, pesticides, paints, solvents, and medicines. Contact your local health department to find out how to dispose of those substances safely. Check the government section of your phone book or call the U.S. Centers for Disease Control and Prevention (CDC) at 800-232-4636.

Consumer guides and sources of additional information:

1. Healthy Stuff.org is a project of the Ecology Center (a Michigan-based non-profit) and has basic information and rankings on a range of consumer products based on research conducted by environmental health organizations and other researchers around the country. http://www.ecocenter.org/healthy-stuff/

2. Environmental Working Group's Skin Deep Cosmetics Database displays online safety profiles for cosmetics and personal care products; it allows you to search for products and rank them according to their health hazard. http://www.ewg.org/skindeep/splash.php?URI=/index.php

3. United States Department of Health and Human Services' Household Products Database is sponsored by the National Institutes of Health and National Library of Medicine. It contains searchable information on household products, manufacturers, ingredients, and health effects for everyday items. https://householdproducts.nlm.nih.gov

4. The California Department of Public Health's Safe Cosmetics Program. https://www.cdph.ca.gov/Programs/CCDPHP/DEODC/OHB/CSCP/Pages/CSCP.aspx

5. Good Guide provides searchable rankings for companies and products. Products are ranked according to health hazards, environment, and social responsibility. Good Guide also offers a mobile app. https://www.goodguide.com/#/

6. The National Geographic Green Guide website includes buying guides and information on sustainable choices for food, travel, home, and garden. The Green Guide publishes a monthly magazine, weekly newsletter, product reports, and reviews focused on practical every day, environmentally responsible, and health-minded product choices and actions. http://environment.nationalgeographic.com/environment/green-guide/

7. Natural Resources Defense Council (NRDC) publishes a variety of reports and policy papers on environmental health topics such as children's health; health threats and effects; farming and pesticides; chemicals at home, school and work; and science and public policy. https://www.nrdc.org/issues/toxic-chemicals

8. The Environmental Protection Agency (EPA) provides information on how to protect children from toxins, the sun, lead, and other potential environmental health threats at children's health protection and read what you can do to protect children from environmental risks. http://www.epa.gov/epahome/children.htm

9. Centers for Disease Control and Prevention (CDC), National Center for Environmental Health (NCEH). On the basis of research and surveillance results, the NCEH works to protect human health. https://www.cdc.gov/nceh/

10. Environmental Public Health Online Courses (EPHOC) is a comprehensive online/on-demand package of courses for environmental public health practi-

tioners including a module on solid and hazardous materials.

11. TOXNET (National Library of Medicine) is a public database tool to produce information on toxic chemical releases and other waste management activities. https://toxnet.nlm.nih.gov

12. National Institute of Environmental Health Sciences. http://www.niehs.nih.gov/about/od/ocpl/contact/

13. The Agency for Toxic Substances and Disease Registry (ATSDR). http://www.atsdr.cdc.gov/substances/index.asp

14. National Institute of Health Household Products Database. https://household-products.nlm.nih.gov

15. National Institute of Health Tox Town. https://toxtown.nlm.nih.gov

15
More Advice About Healthy Living

This chapter addresses some important health issues that so far have not been discussed. They include preserving your hearing and vision, oral health, the importance of getting enough sleep, and preventing accidents.

Avoiding hearing loss[1]

Hearing loss is common; 23% of Americans aged 12 or older have hearing loss that significantly impairs the quality of their lives. An estimated 25.4 million Americans have mild, 10.7 million moderate, 1.8 million severe, and 0.4 million have profound hearing loss in the better ear. By age 70 or older, more than half of adult Americans suffer from some degree of hearing loss in both ears.[2] Trouble understanding conversations in noisy situations is a common sign of a form of hearing loss.

Hearing loss has important deleterious consequences for academic success, employment, health, and social wellbeing. The hearing-impaired person may feel isolated, angry, embarrassed, depressed, and may suffer a loss of self-esteem. Family members and co-workers are often frustrated by the difficulty in communicating with individuals who avoid seeking help for their hearing problem because they think wearing a hearing aid would be embarrassing or demeaning.

Disease involving the ear and simply aging may contribute to hearing loss, but the commonest preventable cause is exposure to loud sounds for an extended time. Damage to the fragile structures of the ears in childhood or youth may lead to hearing loss decades later. Unfortunately, noise-related hearing loss is usually irreversible. So, avoiding loud noise is essential to keeping hearing intact. Workplace noise used to be the leading cause of hearing loss, but today it is loud recreational noise, for example, from concerts, clubs, MP3 players, and smartphones. Damage to hearing from loud noises depends on how loud the noises are and the length of exposure. Infants and children are more susceptible to hearing damage from loud sounds than adults are.

There are standards for permissible exposure to sound, according to loudness (in decibels) and duration. For example, 8 hours of exposure to 85 decibels (dB), similar to loud traffic, is considered permissible according to the National Institute for Occupational Safety and Health (NIOSH) and the CDC. For every three dBs over 85dB, the permissible exposure time before possible damage can occur is cut in half. For example, the permissible time exposure for 94 dBs, the level of a power lawnmower or hairdryer, is only one hour. Long-term exposure to 85dB can cause hearing loss, so it is not a safe sound level for anyone. The EPA has calculated that the average noise level to prevent hearing loss should be no more than a 70dB time-weighted average over 24 hours.[3] A rock concert could reach levels of 105-115 dBs, and any exposure beyond a few minutes could damage hearing. Lower levels, such as between 80dB and 90dB, can cause permanent hearing damage if you are exposed to them for many hours every day.

Some measures of loudness:

- Normal conversation: 60-65dB
- A busy street: 75-85dB
- Lawn mower/heavy traffic: 85dB
- Forklift truck: 90dB
- Hand drill: 98dB
- Heavy truck 20-25 feet away: 95-100dB
- Motorbikes: 100dB
- Movies: some films regularly top 100dB during big action scenes
- Disco/nightclub/car horn: 110dB
- MP3 player on loud: 112dB
- Chainsaw: 115-120dB
- Rock concert/ambulance siren: 120dB

There are many precautions to take to reduce the risk of noise-induced hearing loss:

- Turn down the volume of your television, radio, or music. You should be able to have a comfortable conversation with someone who is 6-7 feet away from you.
- Use headphones that block out or cancel outside noise, rather than turning up the volume. In-the-ear, ear-bud style headphones are less effective at keeping out background noise.
- Use the volume limiter when listening to MP3 players. Follow a 60:60 rule for listening to an MP3 player safely, listen to music at 60% of the maximum

volume for no more than 60 minutes a day.

- Use ear protection equipment such as earmuffs or earplugs when working in a noisy environment. Don't tolerate loud noise at work.
- Avoid loud concerts or use ear protection at loud concerts and at other events where there are high noise levels.
- Know the symptoms of common causes of hearing loss, such as ear infections, and get prompt treatment for them.
- Visit a health care professional if you or your child are experiencing hearing problems. An audiologist can determine if you need Personal Sound Amplification Products (PSAPs or hearing aids) and help with the choice and adjustment of a PSAP.
- The key to healthy hearing is prevention— know how much loud sound you're exposed to and avoid loud noises.

Avoiding visual impairment and blindness[4 5]

Visual impairment may make normal daily activities such as driving and reading difficult or impossible. Fortunately, 80% of all visual impairment can be prevented or corrected. About two-thirds of visual impairment occurs among people age 50 or older. It is estimated that in 2012, 285 million people worldwide were visually impaired, and, of these, 39 million had no vision and were blind. People with vision that is worse than 20/200 with glasses or contact lenses are considered legally blind in most states in the U.S. An estimated 23.7 million adults and 19 million children in the U.S. are visually impaired or blind. Of the children, 12 million are visually impaired due to focus (refractive) errors, a condition that could be easily corrected, but 1.4 million children are irreversibly blind and need visual rehabilitation interventions to help them attain full psychological and personal development.

Worldwide, uncorrected refractive errors cause an estimated 43% of moderate and severe visual impairment. Refractive errors include myopia (nearsightedness), hyperopia (farsightedness), astigmatism, and presbyopia (difficulty focusing close-up). For reasons that are not entirely clear, the incidence of myopia is soaring—perhaps related to screen time and lack of exposure to the UVB radiation in sunlight.[6] Most refractive errors can be compensated for with glasses or contact lenses. One widely used procedure to correct vision, LASIK surgery, is not foolproof. Some people who have had LASIK surgery are left with permanent problems, including chronic dry eyes, double vision, pain, and light sensitivity.[7 8] More than 95% of people who have had LASIK are satisfied with the results. However, if you are concerned about possible side effects, stick to glasses or contacts.[9]

Cataracts are estimated to cause about one-third and glaucoma about 2% of visual impairment in the middle- and low-income countries. Cataract formation is associated with ultraviolet light exposure, smoking, diabetes, excessive alcohol use, and age. Wearing dark glasses to filter out ultraviolet light can help prevent cataracts and age-related macular degeneration. Wearing photochromic glasses that darken when exposed to UV light and glasses with polarized lenses is a good idea. More than half of Americans over the age of 80 have had cataract surgery. Other disorders that may cause visual problems include age-related macular degeneration,[10] diabetic retinopathy, corneal clouding, injury, detached retina, several infections including onchocerciasis and trachoma, and tumors, such as retinoblastoma and optic glioma. Brain damage from stroke, prematurity, or head trauma can also cause visual impairment.

In the United States, other than refractive errors, the leading causes of visual impairment are:

- Accidents or injuries to the corneal surface of the eye, for example from chemical burns or sports injuries
- Diabetic retinopathy
- Glaucoma
- Macular degeneration
- Cataracts

The following is a modified version of the National Eye Institute's advice for preserving eye health[11]

Have a comprehensive dilated eye exam at least every two years

Many people think that their vision is fine but don't realize that they could see better with glasses or contact lenses. In addition, many common eye diseases such as glaucoma, diabetic eye disease, and age-related macular degeneration often have no warning signs. A dilated eye exam is the only way to detect these diseases in their early stages when they are the most treatable.

Know your family's eye health history

It's important to know if anyone in your family has been diagnosed with an eye disease or condition because some are hereditary.

Healthy eating helps protect sight

A healthy diet rich in fruits and vegetables, particularly dark leafy greens such as spinach, kale, or collard greens, will help keep eyes healthy, as will fish such as salmon, tuna, and halibut that are high in omega-3 fatty acids.[12]

Maintain a healthy weight

Being overweight or obese increases the risk of developing diabetes and other systemic conditions that can lead to vision loss, such as diabetic eye disease or glaucoma.

Wear protective eyewear to prevent injuries

There are an estimated 30,000 sports-related eye injuries in the U.S. each year, with 80% occurring in males. The most frequent cause is the result of playing basketball, baseball, or softball, as well as injuries from paintball and air guns.[13] Wear protective eyewear when playing sports or engaged in activities around the home. Protective eyewear includes safety glasses and goggles, safety shields, and eye guards specially designed to provide the correct protection for a specific activity. Most protective eyewear lenses are made of polycarbonate, which is 10 times stronger than other plastics. Many eye care providers sell protective eyewear, as do some sporting goods stores.

Practice workplace eye safety

Employers are required to provide a safe work environment. When protective eyewear is required as a part of your job, make a habit of wearing the appropriate type at all times, and encourage your co-workers to do the same.

Quit smoking or never start

Smoking is as bad for your eyes as it is for the rest of your body. Research has linked smoking to an increased risk of developing age-related macular degeneration, cataract, and optic nerve damage, all of which can lead to blindness.[14 15]

Wear sunglasses

Sunglasses help to protect your eyes from the sun's ultraviolet rays. When purchasing sunglasses, look for ones that block out 99 to 100% of both UV-A and UV-B radiation. Both adult and children's sunglasses should be labeled "UV absorption up to 400 nm" or "Meets ANSI UV Requirements" and block at least 99% of UV rays. Those labeled "cosmetic" block about 70% of UV rays. Sunglasses without a label may not provide any UV protection. UV protection comes from an invisible chemical in or applied to the lenses, not from the color or darkness of the lenses. However, exposure to the UVB in sunlight in childhood may help prevent the growing epidemic of nearsightedness.[16]

Give your eyes a rest

If you spend a lot of time at the computer or focusing on any one thing, you sometimes forget to blink, and your eyes can get fatigued. Try the 20-20-20 rule: Every 20 minutes, look away about 20 feet in front of you for 20 seconds. This can help reduce eyestrain.

Clean your hands and your contact lenses properly

To avoid the risk of infection, always wash your hands thoroughly before putting in or taking out your contact lenses. Make sure to disinfect contact lenses as instructed and replace them as appropriate.

Oral and Dental Health

According to the CDC, oral health affects our ability to speak, smile, eat, and show emotions. It also affects self-esteem, school performance, and attendance at work and school. Oral health problems include untreated tooth decay, gum disease, tooth loss, and oral cancer. By age 34, more than 80% of people have had at least one cavity. On average, the nation spends more than $113 billion a year on costs related to dental care.[17]

Although fluoridated water, improved toothpaste, and brushes can help to reduce tooth decay, adherence to good habits of flossing and brushing is necessary. Tooth decay, also known as cavities—the scientific term is dental caries—is a common condition afflicting children and adults in the United States, and access to dental care is limited in some places.[18]

Below are some additional Oral and Dental Health facts:

- Tooth decay affects up to two-thirds of adolescents.[19]
- About 1 of 5 (20%) children aged 5 to 11 years have at least one untreated decayed tooth.
- 1 of 7 (13%) adolescents aged 12 to 19 years have at least one untreated decayed tooth.
- The percentage of children and adolescents aged 5 to 19 years with untreated tooth decay is twice as high for those from low-income families (25%) compared with children from higher-income households (11%).

Oral health problems of adults

Untreated tooth decay

More than one in four (27%) adults in the United States have untreated tooth decay.[20] Among those aged 20 to 64 years, more than 90% have had at least one cavity, and 27% had untreated decay.[21]

Gum disease

Nearly half (46%) of all adults aged 30 years or older show signs of gum disease; severe gum disease affects about 9% of adults.[22]

Tooth loss

Complete tooth loss among adults aged 65 to 74 years has steadily declined over time, but disparities exist among some population groups.[23] If left untreated, tooth decay and periodontal (gum) disease lead to tooth loss.

Oral cancer

Oral cancers are most common in older adults, particularly in people older than 55 years who smoke and are heavy drinkers.[24] In 2012, there were nearly 40,000 new cases of cancer of the oral cavity and pharynx diagnosed in the United States and almost 9,000 deaths. The 5-year survival rate for these cancers is about 59%.[25] (See Chapter 7, 'Preventing Cancer.") People who receive cancer chemotherapy may suffer from oral problems such as painful mouth ulcers, impaired taste, and dry mouth.

Chronic diseases

Obesity and chronic diseases, such as arthritis, heart disease, stroke, diabetes, emphysema, hepatitis C, temporomandibular joint (TMJ) disorder and temporomandibular disorder (TMD), autoimmune conditions, and osteoporosis may compromise oral health and functioning and increase the risk of having missing teeth.[26]
Patients with weakened immune systems, such as those infected with HIV and those on drugs that suppress the immune system (e.g., after organ transplants) and on some medications (e.g., steroids), are at higher risk for some oral problems.[27]

The causes of oral health problems

Tooth decay, or cavities, are caused by an erosion of the tooth's enamel by the acids produced by bacteria. Initially, bacteria form a film called plaque that collects on the surface of teeth, especially along the gum line and in the crevices on the chewing surfaces of the teeth. Eating and drinking foods high in sugar and other simple carbohydrates make it easier for bacteria to produce the acids that can demineralize the enamel, or when exposed, cause the root surface to break down. Untreated tooth decay can lead to an abscess in the jaw under the tooth. Like all infections, it can spread to other parts of the body and have serious, and in rare cases, fatal results.

Gum disease, or periodontal disease, is mainly the result of bacterial infections and inflammation (i.e., gingivitis) of the gums. Plaque can lead to hard deposits of calculus that contribute to the periodontal disease process that, in turn, can weaken and destroy the bone that surrounds and supports the teeth. Teeth with little bone support can become loose and may eventually have to be extracted. Chronic conditions that increase the risk for periodontal disease include diabetes, a weakened immune system, poor oral hygiene, and heredity.

The risk of oral cancers can be minimized by avoiding high-risk behaviors, including cigarette, cigar or pipe smoking, use of smokeless tobacco, and excessive use of alcohol. And early detection can increase the survival rate for oral cancers. Oral human papillomavirus (HPV), the most common sexually transmitted disease, can also cause cancers of the mouth, tongue, and throat, called oropharyngeal cancers.

Preventing oral health problems[28 29]

It is only recently that the majority of people will keep most of their natural teeth over their entire lifetime. Public health experts attribute this progress in oral health largely to the benefits of water fluoridation and the use of fluoride toothpaste. However, threats to oral health continue throughout life and may increase with age because of problems with saliva production, receding gums that expose "softer" root surfaces to decay-causing bacteria; or difficulties flossing and brushing because of poor vision, cognitive problems, chronic disease, and physical limitations.

Although some adults may have difficulty accessing regular professional dental care, it is essential.[30] Continuing dental care includes at least once daily brushing and flossing. The American Dental Association recommends, "brushing for two minutes, twice a day with a fluoride toothpaste, cleaning between teeth once a day with an interdental cleaner and regular dental visits advised by your dentist." The ADA also stated that interdental cleaners, including floss, "are an essential part of taking care of your teeth and gums."[31] Professional cleaning by a dental hygienist two or three times a year, periodic dental X-rays, and a dentist's evaluation at regular intervals and restorative dentistry as needed is also essential to maintain good oral health. Minimizing the consumption of high sugar foods, sugar-sweetened beverages, and other refined carbohydrates is also advisable for both children and adults.

One procedure that many authorities consider to be greatly overused is the removal of third molars (wisdom teeth). About 50% of insured individuals in the U.S. will have their third molar removed by the age of 20. Because of little or no benefit and substantial side effects (pain, bleeding, dry socket, nerve damage), the American Public Health Association recommends against the removal of asymptomatic third molars that are not causing any trouble, such as crowding other teeth out of proper alignment.[32 33 34]

Sleep is crucial for good health[35 36]

Even though we know that lack of sleep makes us feel tired, sluggish, and irritable, most Americans don't get enough sleep. We stay up too late watching television, to study, to work, or to party and then struggle to get out of bed when the alarm clock goes off in the morning. Many of us have days when we are sleepy. Lack of sleep impairs attention, judgment, problem-solving, ability to learn, thinking, and mood. Because a lack of sleep impairs attention and thinking, it makes a person prone to accidents and dangerous to ourselves and others. Lack of sleep increases the risk of unintentional injuries. They can happen anywhere and during almost any activity, at home, during sports and other recreation such as in or on the water, as a pedestrian or in a motor vehicle.

In the process of learning something new, there is good evidence for the theory that sleep helps to establish a stable memory and the ability to recall the information. Conversely, with a sleep deficit, memory, and many other aspects of cognitive functioning are impaired, and we may become dangerous—for example, prone to cause medical errors in our hospitals. Investigators believe that slowed thinking and impaired decision making from sleep deprivation was a significant factor in many well-known disasters, including the 1979 nuclear accident at Three Mile Island, the 1986 nuclear meltdown at Chernobyl, the grounding of the Exxon Valdez oil tanker, and the explosion of the space shuttle Challenger.[37 38]

More than a third of American adults are not getting enough sleep on a regular basis, according to a 2016 Centers for Disease Control and Prevention (CDC) study.[39] A National Sleep Foundation survey found that 60% of adult drivers have driven a vehicle when drowsy and more than one-third have fallen asleep at the wheel. The Division of Sleep Medicine at the Harvard Medical School reports that "The Institute of Medicine estimates—based on recent high quality naturalistic and epidemiologic studies—that drowsy driving is responsible for fully 20% of all motor vehicle crashes. That would mean that drowsy driving causes approximately 1 million crashes, 500,000 injuries, and 8,000 deaths each year in the U.S." The National Sleep Foundation convened a panel of experts to consider how to avoid drowsy driving. They agreed upon the following expert consensus statement: "Drivers who have slept for two hours or less in the preceding 24 hours are not fit to operate a motor vehicle." Panelists further agreed that most healthy drivers would likely be impaired with only 3 to 5 hours of sleep during the prior 24 hours.[40]

As was described in Chapter 8, "Preventing Dementia," the brain eliminates waste products such as the beta-amyloid associated with Alzheimer dementia, mainly during sleep.[41] Furthermore, sleep apnea, a cause of disrupted sleep, is associated with mild cognitive impairment and Alzheimer disease 10 years sooner than its occurrence among those without the disorder.[42] So there is a strong association between sleep disturbance and dementia. In one study, researchers found that men who spent less time in slow-wave sleep — the deep, restorative stage of sleep —

tended to show more atrophy in their brain tissue.[43]

Research on the function and benefits of sleep reveals it has an important role in repair and restoration of muscles, the brain, and many vital bodily functions, including maintenance of a healthy balance of hormones, regulating hunger, supporting the immune system, and facilitating memory and learning. One estimate is that inadequate sleep causes more than $400 billion in economic losses and results in 1.23 million lost days of work annually in the U.S. Chronic sleep deprivation is associated with an increased risk of mental distress and major illnesses, obesity, diabetes, high blood pressure and cardiovascular disease including stroke. Epidemiological studies have found that sleeping five hours or less per night is associated with an increased all-cause mortality risk of about 15%.[44,45,46,47,48]

Addressing sleep problems

According to Harvard's Division of Sleep Medicine, an estimated 50 to 70 million Americans suffer from some type of sleep disorder, and on an average night, 30 to 40 million Americans have insomnia.[49] People with insomnia have difficulty falling asleep, staying asleep, or wake up too early and cannot get back to sleep. Many people experience short periods of insomnia due to worry, stress, or from the time zone changes that cause jet lag. Fortunately, for most people, these disruptions in sleep last only a few nights.

Chronic insomnia can result from poor sleep habits, such as irregular bedtimes and wake-up times (including on weekends) and daytime naps. Insomnia can also result from over-stimulation close to bedtime, for example, from exercise late in the evening or consuming too much alcohol or caffeine too late in the day. Because alcohol acts as a sedative, it is commonly used by people with insomnia to help them get to sleep. But its effect is only temporary. Its use frequently leads to awakenings and uneasy sleep later in the night. Other medications, such as antidepressants, steroids, and allergy and cold products, can also disrupt sleep as can a psychiatric disorder or a painful medical condition.[50]

Excessive daytime sleepiness, suddenly falling asleep on the job or while driving is dangerous and not normal. It can be the sign of a medical condition that requires treatment. These conditions include obstructive sleep apnea (OSA), periodic limb movements of sleep (PLMS—the repeated involuntary kicking and jerking movements of the legs and arms that frequently occurs among adults over the age of 60), sleepwalking, and narcolepsy, a brain disorder causing sudden attacks of falling asleep.

Obstructive sleep apnea (OSA) is underdiagnosed but common in the U.S., with

17% of men and 9% of women age 50 to 70 affected.[51] It occurs when a person's airway becomes partially or completely blocked many times during a night of sleep, leading to decreased airflow or short-term cessation of breathing, repetitive awakenings, and severely disrupted sleep. Medical care for individuals with OSA is indicated because it causes episodes of oxygen deprivation that can lead to high blood pressure, insulin resistance, heart and other cardiovascular diseases, and mood and memory problems.[52 53] Obesity is the greatest risk factor for OSA and has been reported to be present in 40% of persons with a BMI greater than 30. Weight loss may ease its severity or eliminate it. However, other treatments may be necessary, including the use of a continuous positive airway pressure (CPAP) machine, optimizing sleep position, sleeping with dental devices that reposition the lower jaw, and surgical procedures that widen the airway. Of these measures, regular use of CPAP is the most effective.

Other treatments that may help sleep disorders include cognitive behavioral therapy, meditation, and biofeedback to ease stress and prescription medications.[54] Over-the-counter sleep medications and remedies, including a low dose of melatonin, may help some people. Melatonin supplements the body's natural production of the sleep-inducing hormone, but it may have side-effects, such as headache, dizziness, and daytime grogginess, and interfere with blood pressure medications. The long-term effects and safety for adults and children are not known. Because melatonin can be sold as a dietary supplement, its quality may be poorly regulated. It is best to obtain melatonin in a pharmaceutical-grade from a reputable source. Herbal sleep remedies have not been proven to be effective. After taking melatonin, drowsiness the following day that may lead to poor work performance and accidents and, possibly, to serious mental and physical problems. Drugs should be a last resort.

The optimal duration of sleep varies according to age and among individuals. The National Sleep Foundation (NSF) recommends that school-age children (ages 6 to 13) get between 9 and 11 hours of sleep per night, teens (ages 14 to 17) should get 8 to 10 hours, and adults 7 to 9 hours. Although some people think they do fine on five or six hours a night, the optimal sleep duration for most people is between seven and eight hours a night.[55 56] For a chart showing NSF recommendations go to https://www.sleepfoundation.org/sites/default/files/2018-10/NSF_sleep_duration_recommendations_chart.png

The most likely reason for the average American's lack of sleep is that we do not set aside enough time for it. We stay up too late and are groggy when the alarm goes off the next morning. In addition to planning for enough time for sleep, the Division of Sleep Medicine at the Harvard Medical School offers this advice for getting the rest you need:[57]

- Create a sleep sanctuary. Reserve your bedroom for sleep and intimacy. Keep it dark and on the cool side. Banish the television, computer, smartphone or tablet, and other diversions from that space.
- Nap only if necessary. Taking a nap at the peak of sleepiness in the afternoon can help to supplement hours missed at night. But naps can also interfere with your ability to sleep at night and throw your sleep schedule into disarray. If you need to nap, limit it to 20 to 30 minutes.
- Avoid caffeine after noon, and go light on alcohol. Caffeine may stay in your body for up to 12 hours. Alcohol can act as a sedative, but it also disturbs sleep.
- Get regular exercise, but not within three hours of bedtime. Exercise acts as a short-term stimulant.
- Avoid backsliding into a sleep debt cycle. Try to go to bed and get up at the same time every day — at the very least, on weekdays. If need be, use weekends to make up for lost sleep but recognize that it will not be fully restorative of the harmful metabolic changes such as increased appetite and reduced insulin sensitivity that are caused by sleep deficit.[58]

Prevention of unintentional injuries

A healthy lifestyle requires attention to avoiding accidents. With about 161,374 deaths in 2016, unintentional injuries were the third leading cause of death. A leading cause of unintentional injury deaths was from falls, with about 25,000 deaths among those aged 75 or older, and there were about 40,000 motor vehicle traffic deaths.[59][60] In 2020, deaths from injuries are being exceeded in number only by diseases of the heart, cancer, and COVID-19.

Avoiding drug overdoses and other poisonings[61]

A wide variety of chemicals and products can cause poisoning. Antifreeze stored in old whiskey bottles has killed children who thought they would try alcohol. In 2016, more than 63,000 persons died from the use of legal or illegal drugs.[62][63] About 42,000 of these deaths were from opioids. To reduce the risk of drug overdoses and other poisonings:

- Keep medicines and toxic products, such as cleaning solutions and detergent pods in their original packaging and where children can't see or get them.
- Know the nationwide poison control center phone number, 1-800-222-1222; they can be reached 24/7. Call 911 if you have a poison emergency, and your child or someone else has collapsed or is not breathing.
- Read the label, warnings, and follow directions carefully.

- Safely dispose of medicines and toxic products if you don't need them. Many localities have take-back programs for medications.
- Carbon monoxide poisoning can occur from running a motor vehicle or a gasoline-powered generator without proper ventilation.

Safety in the home

Among older adults, falls are the leading cause of injuries, both fatal and nonfatal. Some preventive measures to avoid falls include staying active to maintain strength and balance, getting physical checkups that include vision screening and eye care, attention to any medications with side effects like feeling dizzy or sleepy, and safety precautions at home.[64] Among these measures, boosting physical exercise is the most effective way to prevent falls.[65 66 67] A Cochrane Review of 108 studies concluded that exercise could prevent falls by about 23% and the number of people who fall by 15%.[68] Most falls happen at home, and their risk can be diminished by keeping a home well lit; the floors clutter-free by dispensing with small throw rugs or using double-sided tape to secure them to the floor; adding grab bars in the bathroom both beside and inside the tub and next to the toilet. Handrails and lights on all staircases are especially important.

Ways to stay safe from fires[69 70]

In 2018, there were 1,318,500 fires reported in the United States. These fires caused an estimated 3,655 civilian deaths.[71] Here are some ways to prevent fire-related injuries:

- Do not smoke. If you do smoke, never smoke in bed. Avoid smoking while consuming alcoholic beverages.
- Never throw a lighted cigarette or a match anywhere. Extinguish and dispose of them in proper ashtrays.
- Be very cautious around any type of open flames, including backyard grills.
- When around any source of fire, supervise children carefully.
- Follow electrical safety rules. Never put electrical appliances or cords in or near water.
- Do not touch downed power lines.
- Install smoke and carbon monoxide alarms on every floor, test, and maintain them.
- Create and practice a family fire escape plan
- Use safe cooking practices, such as never leaving food unattended heating on the stove.
- Check water heater temperature and to prevent scalding of infants and small

children set water heater thermostats to 120 degrees Fahrenheit or lower.

Water safety[72]

Drowning is the fifth leading cause of unintentional injury death for people of all ages and the second leading cause of injury death for children ages 1 to 14 years. Water safety precautions include the following:

- Learn life-saving skills such as cardiopulmonary resuscitation (CPR).
- Know the basics of swimming.
- Fence in backyard swimming pools.
- Require life jackets in and around water, including in pools for weaker swimmers.
- When around pools or open water, closely supervise children at all times.
- Adults watching kids in or near water should avoid distracting activities like playing cards, reading books, talking on the phone, and using alcohol or drugs.
- Learn and practice the rules for safe boating.

Sports safety[73]

Sports contribute to health but are also a cause of many minor injuries and, unfortunately, more severe injuries that may end a career in a sport, cause disability, or rarely even death. To help prevent sports injuries:

- Use proper safety equipment for the sport, especially helmets.
- Learn and enforce concussion protocols.
- Slowly increase intensity and duration of physical activities to improve physical fitness—being in good condition can protect you from injury.
- Practice sports skills to prevent injuries, e.g., in football and soccer.
- Pay attention to extreme temperatures to prevent heat-related injuries or illness—make sure that players are hydrated, appropriately dressed and not overworked in hot weather.
- Don't risk your health to win a game.

Motor vehicle safety[74]

There were about 37,113 traffic deaths in the U.S. in 2017, an increase since 2014 that is attributed to more driving thanks to low gas prices, an improving economy, and more use of smartphones and other causes of distracted driving.[75] Even hands-free use of phones is a distraction.[76] Driving defensively, staying within legal speed limits, and avoiding distracted driving are critical to driving safely. As described in the preceding section on sleep, lack of sleep impairs attention, judgment, and thinking, making a person more likely to have a crash. Defensive driving means that to reduce the risk of a collision, a driver will both stick to the rules of the road and go beyond them by anticipating and being ready to compensate for errors made by other drivers or other dangerous situations caused by weather or other adverse road conditions.

Per mile driven, teen drivers ages 16 to 19 are nearly three times more likely than drivers aged 20 and older to be in a fatal crash. Speeding is one of the most prevalent factors contributing to traffic crashes. The National Highway Traffic Safety Administration (NHTSA) estimated that the annual economic cost to society of speeding-related crashes in 2012 was $40.4 billion. That year speeding was a contributing factor in 30% of all fatal crashes, with more than 10,000 lives lost. Among males, 37% of 15 to 24-year-old drivers involved in fatal crashes were speeding. Among speeding drivers involved in fatal crashes, 42% had blood alcohol concentrations (BACs) of .08 grams per deciliter (g/dl) or higher, compared to only 16% of non-speeding drivers involved in fatal crashes.[77]

The use of appropriate in-vehicle restraints is important to avoid injury or death when a motor vehicle crash does occur. Seat belts reduce serious and fatal injuries by more than half. All adults and especially parents and caregivers should always wear a seat belt and set a good example for children. Infants and children should be buckled in age- and size-appropriate car seats or booster seats. Buckle all children aged 12 and under in the back seat and seat children in the middle of the back seat when possible, because it is the safest spot in the vehicle. Don't seat children in front of an airbag; they can kill young children riding in the front seat. Never place a rear-facing car seat in front of an airbag.

Distracted driving

The chance of being distracted when driving is increasing with the popularity of smartphone use, eating, texting, using a navigation system, and other interactive dashboard controls and displays. According to the NHTSA, 71% of young people say that they have sent a text while driving. In 2013, nearly one in five crashes (18%) in which someone was injured involved distracted driving. In 2014, 431,000 people were injured in motor vehicle crashes involving distracted drivers, an almost 10% increase since 2011, and more than 3,000 deaths were attributed to distracted driving.[78]

There are three main types of distraction:

1. Visual: taking your eyes off the road;
2. Manual: taking your hands off the wheel; and
3. Cognitive: taking your mind off of driving.

While any of these distractions can endanger the driver and others, texting while driving is especially dangerous because it combines all three types of distraction.

Elderly drivers

Elderly adults are at heightened risk of having an accident because of mild cognitive impairment, cataracts, and other health conditions. They should consider potential alternatives to driving, such as riding with a friend or using public transit. They can also take several steps to stay safe on the road, including:

- Exercising regularly to increase strength and flexibility.
- Asking your doctor or pharmacist to review medicines, both prescription and over-the-counter, to reduce side effects and interactions.
- Having eyes checked by an eye doctor at least every two years. Wear glasses and corrective lenses as required.
- Driving during daylight and in good weather.
- Finding the safest route with well-lit streets, intersections with left-turn arrows, and easy parking.
- Planning your route before you drive.
- Leaving an extra-large following distance behind the car in front of you.
- Avoiding distractions in your car, such as listening to a loud radio, talking on your cell phone, texting, and eating.
- Taking a safe driving course—it might earn you an insurance discount.

Driving under the influence

Avoid driving under the influence of alcohol or drugs (DUI). Buzzed driving is DUI. Experimental studies show a clear and dose-dependent relationship between marijuana use and a number of driving impairment indicators. One estimate is that marijuana users were about 25% more likely to be involved in a crash than drivers with no evidence of marijuana use, but it is possible that age and gender may account for the increased crash risk among marijuana users.[79] A meta-analysis of nine studies published in 2012 in the *British Medical Journal* found that drivers who consume cannabis within three hours of driving are nearly twice as likely to cause a vehicle collision with serious injury or death as those who are not under the influence of drugs or alcohol.[80] Other studies suggest a 1.2 to 2.0 fold increase in crash risk.[81] And various studies have shown that the combined use of cannabis and alcohol is associated with greater crash risk than the use of either alone.[82]

The National Highway Traffic Safety Administration reported that fatal crashes where drugs other than alcohol were involved increased from 2,003 in 1993 to 7,438 in 2015. Some of these deaths seem to have been related to losing consciousness after opioid overdoses. A 2016 report found that 44% of drivers who died and were tested for drugs had positive results, up from 28% in 2006.[83] About 20% of the drug positive drivers were found to have an opioid in their system, and 41% were positive for marijuana. However, data concerning crash fatality rates after marijuana legalization is more reassuring. Surprisingly, a study of some states that enacted medical marijuana laws and legalized dispensaries experienced reductions in traffic fatalities.[84] The trend line in such deaths was not statistically different in Washington and Colorado in the three years after legalization compared to 8 states that did not change their marijuana laws.[85] However, the legalization of marijuana in Colorado has increased cases of marijuana intoxication and the poisoning of both children by accident and adults from poorly standardized edible marijuana products.[86]

Unlike marijuana, alcohol-impaired driving is recognized to be a common cause of collisions, injuries, and deaths. In 2016, 10,497 people died in alcohol-impaired driving crashes, accounting for 28% of all traffic-related deaths in the United States. Every day, 28 people in the United States die in motor vehicle crashes that involve an alcohol-impaired driver. Alcohol involvement for the driver or the pedestrian was reported for 49% of the traffic crashes that resulted in pedestrian death. The annual cost of alcohol-related crashes totals more than $44 billion.[87]

In most jurisdictions, a quantitative measurement such as a blood alcohol content (BAC) above a specific threshold level, such as 0.05% or 0.08%, defines the offense with no other requirement to prove impairment or intoxication. In some jurisdictions, there is an aggravated category of the offense at a higher BAC level, such as 0.12%. In California, where I live, it's illegal to operate a motor vehicle with any of the following blood alcohol concentration (BAC) percentages:

0.08% or higher if 21 years old or older operating a regular passenger vehicle.
0.04% or higher if operating a commercial vehicle.
0.01% or higher if younger than 21 years old.

Table 15.1 shows approximate blood alcohol percentages according to the number of drinks and weight for men and women. The calculators are only an estimate and do not take into account the many other factors that can affect BAC. They include your body fat, muscle, metabolism, intake of liquids and food, and medications. You can't use BAC calculators to determine if you can be a safe driver after con-

Table 15.1. Approximate blood alcohol (%) based on sex, body weight and number of drinks

Women										
Approximate Blood Alcohol Percentage										
Drinks	Body Weight in Pounds									
	90	100	120	140	160	180	200	220	240	
0	.00	.00	.00	.00	.00	.00	.00	.00	.00	Only Safe Driving Limit
1	.05	.05	.04	.03	.03	.03	.02	.02	.02	Driving Skills Significantly Affected
2	.10	.09	.08	.07	.06	.05	.05	.04	.04	
3	.15	.14	.11	.10	.09	.08	.07	.06	.06	
4	.20	.18	.15	.13	.11	.10	.09	.08	.08	Possible Criminal Penalties
5	.25	.23	.19	.16	.14	.13	.11	.10	.09	
6	.30	.27	.23	.19	.17	.15	.14	.12	.11	Legally Intoxicated
7	.35	.32	.27	.23	.20	.18	.16	.14	.13	
8	.40	.36	.30	.26	.23	.20	.18	.17	.15	Criminal Penalties
9	.45	.41	.34	.29	.26	.23	.20	.19	.17	
10	.51	.45	.38	.32	.28	.25	.23	.21	.19	Death Possible

Men									
Approximate Blood Alcohol Percentage									
	Body Weight in Pounds								
	100	120	140	160	180	200	220	240	
0	.00	.00	.00	.00	.00	.00	.00	.00	Only Safe Driving Limit
1	.04	.03	.03	.02	.02	.02	.02	.02	Driving Skills Significantly Affected
2	.08	.06	.05	.05	.04	.04	.03	.03	
3	.11	.09	.08	.07	.06	.06	.05	.05	
4	.15	.12	.11	.09	.08	.08	.07	.06	Possible Criminal Penalties
5	.19	.16	.13	.12	.11	.09	.09	.08	
6	.23	.19	.16	.14	.13	.11	.10	.09	Legally Intoxicated
7	.26	.22	.19	.16	.15	.13	.12	.11	
8	.30	.25	.21	.19	.17	.15	.14	.13	Criminal Penalties
9	.34	.28	.24	.21	.19	.17	.15	.14	
10	.38	.31	.27	.23	.21	.19	.17	.16	Death Possible

Source: This table is from the Virginia Tech Alcohol Abuse Prevention website

suming alcohol. After drinking any amount of alcohol, let someone else do the driving.

Firearm safety

Gun deaths are the third leading cause of death from injuries. The 39,733 deaths from firearms in the United States in 2017 nearly equaled the number of deaths from motor vehicle traffic crashes that year (40,100).[88] In 2012, an estimated 74,000 nonfatal gunshot injuries were treated in emergency departments, of which 72% were classified as being the result of an assault, 18% unintentional, and 5% self-harm. Between 2003 and 2010, hospital costs from firearm injuries were estimated to total $18.9 billion. The U.S. averages about 12,000 homicides committed with a firearm each year, about three-quarters of all U.S. homicides.[89][90] Most deaths from firearms are homicides (37%) or suicides (60%).[91]

Right-to-carry laws are associated with a 24% increase in levels of homicide in the workplace.[92] Household gun ownership levels vary greatly by state, from 60% in Wyoming to 9% in Hawaii. States with higher levels of household gun ownership have higher rates of firearm homicide and overall homicide.[93] States with the highest levels of gun ownership have 114% higher firearm homicide rates and 60% higher homicide rates than states with the lowest gun ownership.[94] This toll could be reduced by reducing access to guns by mandating safe storage of firearms, screening of all purchasers, age limits on gun ownership, safety training requirements, and other measures that have been proven to be effective in reducing firearm misuse.[95][96][97]

The most important ways to reduce injuries

- Wear the proper helmet for your activity.
- Wear a life jacket when on water.
- Have your eyes checked and protect them from injury.
- Remove tripping hazards around your house.
- Learn how to swim.
- Store medicine out of reach of children.
- Take medication only as directed and avoid intoxicating drugs.
- Place children in the proper booster or car seat.
- Wear your seatbelt.
- Walk on a sidewalk when possible.
- If you are a gun owner practice firearm safety.
- Gain or maintain physical fitness.

Concluding thoughts about the Building Blocks of Health

Describing the Building Blocks of Health and how to use a Lifestyle Checklist to put them into place, has taken the reader of this book through many pages. I have focused on the most important things you can do for yourself to enhance and preserve your health. As noted in the first chapter of the book, the principles of healthy living are not complicated or difficult to learn. You should maintain a normal weight; adopt a diet low in added sugar and saturated fat, and high in natural unrefined whole plant-based foods (fruits, vegetables, legumes, soy, and wholegrains); get enough sleep and physical activity; manage stress; avoid high-risk behaviors like misuse of drugs, alcohol, and tobacco; and guard against infectious diseases such as COVID-19 and influenza with vaccinations and other preventive measures.

Your physician or other health care provider should be a partner in your quest for healthier living. Healthy adults can usually follow this book's advice about nutrition and other lifestyle changes without difficulty. But getting the advice and approval of your health care provider before a lifestyle change is a good idea. Especially if you are taking medication or have a health problem such as diabetes, you must obtain medical advice and supervision when changing your lifestyle. Your health care provider will provide individualized advice and care for your specific health needs, including by helping you monitor and control your cholesterol level and blood pressure and by prescribing medications if needed.

With knowledge and discipline, you can meet the goals laid out in the Lifestyle Checklist and enjoy the many rewards of better health. The greater the number of the health enhancing behaviors you can adopt, the healthier you will become. I hope the advice in this book will help you to preserve your health and lengthen your years of living in good health.

16
Understanding Scientific Data

This book is based on medical science, so throughout this book, you will find presentations of the results of scientific studies. I have included the references for many of these studies as would be found in a peer-reviewed scientific publication, but at times they have been omitted. This chapter, "Understanding Scientific Data," aims to help you understand the studies referred to and cited in the book, provides background to how medical research is conducted, and defines key terms used to describe the results of studies.

Thomas Frieden, former director of the Centers for Disease Control and Prevention (CDC), lists eleven different study design types and notes that each type has strengths and weaknesses.[1] He also points out that the highest quality studies, such as cohort and randomized controlled trials (RCTs), are not always feasible. You often can't do RCTs if 1) the exposure isn't something you can randomize people to (e.g., alcohol, smoking), and 2) adherence can be low (e.g., dietary factors). Furthermore, they are not likely or practical to be undertaken for the treatment of rare diseases.

The following descriptions of various research study types, considerations of the validity and accuracy of research findings from each methodology, and definitions of some terms you will find in the book are presented to help the reader. When evaluating the link between a lifestyle or other factors, such as exercise, and a health outcome, such as heart disease, randomized controlled trials, randomized trials, and cohort studies are generally considered to provide the highest level of evidence for causality.[2]

Study Designs

Randomized controlled trials

Randomized controlled trials are considered to be the "gold standard" for validity in medical research. Investigators randomly (by chance) assign participants to two or more groups and follow them. They compare health outcomes in a group or groups that get treatment or other intervention with the health outcomes in an untreated control group. Because group assignment is conducted randomly, there's a good chance that the treatment and intervention groups will be similar to one another in measurable and unmeasurable ways that might also affect the health outcome. The treatment or behavior change may be diet, drugs, devices, or procedures, and control measures may include placebos or no-treatment. To minimize study bias, the best of these studies are single-blinded, so the study subjects or the investigators do not know who is in a treatment or control group. Better yet, some studies are double-blinded, so neither the investigators nor study subjects know to which group each subject has been assigned. These studies are usually among the more difficult and expensive types of studies to conduct and have the weakness that adherence to the intervention may be easy if it is just taking a drug, but difficult if it is a specified diet.

Cohort studies

Cohort studies follow groups of people over time. These studies have the advantage that you do not have to have large numbers of people, nor do you have to follow them for long. The primary difference from a randomized study is that, in cohort studies, people typically self-select to the exposure of interest. That is, investigators might compare people who smoke to those who do not. Researchers then gather information from the cohort members on a wide variety of variables and compare their health outcomes. For example, vegetarians might be found to have a different incidence of cardiovascular disease than individuals who eat meat. Cohort studies are more reliable than case-control studies because the collection of information is ongoing before anyone develops the disease being studied, and less reliant on recall of past events. This book presents data about the link between lifestyle factors and disease derived from two of the largest and longest-running cohort studies of diet, the Harvard-based Nurses' Health Study and the Health Professionals Follow-up Study.

Case-control studies

Case-control studies begin with the health outcomes themselves. Investigators recruit a group of study subjects who already have a certain good or bad health outcome (the cases) and a similar group of subjects who do not have the outcome (the controls). They then look at differences in past experiences (e.g., behavior, toxic exposure, use of a medication, etc.) between those who have and do not have the outcome. The advantage of these studies is that they are relatively easy to conduct. But they have the disadvantage of the potential for inaccurate findings based on recall bias. Some important information may be difficult to recall, and study subjects with an illness often recall past behaviors differently from those without illness. It also may be difficult to identify a control group of people who are similar to those who have the outcome under study.

Observational study

In this type of study, participants are observed, or certain outcomes are measured. No attempt is made to affect the exposure, for example, no treatment is given. A cross-sectional study is a type of observational study that involves data collection from a population, or a representative subset, at one specific point in time. A case-control study is also a type of observational study.

Cross-sectional study

In this type of study, the observation of a defined population is taken at a single point in time or time interval. Both the exposure and the outcome are determined simultaneously.

Systematic review

A systematic review is a critical assessment and evaluation of all research studies that address a particular scientific issue.

Meta-analysis

A meta-analysis is a statistical process that combines data from many different individual research studies and generates a summary estimate of effect. Many studies of this type are presented in this book, but the reader should be aware that experts point out that there are many ways in which meta-analyses can yield misleading information. For example, there may be important differences between the populations being studied or between treatments or interventions. An additional potential problem is that, like all studies, some of the trials included in the meta-analysis may have methodological errors that distort the outcomes of the meta-analysis.[3] Discrepancies between meta-analyses and subsequent large randomized clinical trials have been found.[4]

Other terms

Incidence and prevalence

The incidence of a disease or condition refers to the number of new cases that develop in a certain place during a given period of time, such as a day, week, month or year. The prevalence is the number of people who have a certain disease or condition at a specified point in time. The prevalence of a disease is affected by the incidence (how many people get it), the duration (for how long they have it), and the fatality rate (how many people die of it).

Percent difference

The results of many studies are often reported by the percent differences of one group of participants compared to another. As described below, absolute numbers are usually preferable to percentages.

Relative risk and absolute risk

In medical studies, the probability of seeing a certain event in a group is usually called risk. For comparison of risks between groups, the ratio of risks, or the relative risk (RR), is a measure of effect. If 10/100 exposed people get a disease and 5/100 unexposed people get a disease, the RR of the disease is 2.0, so the exposure doubles the risk. This might be reported as a 100% increase in relative risk. In this example, the absolute risk is 10/100 – 5/100 = 0.05, so 5/100 cases are attributable to the exposure. This might be reported as a 5% increase in absolute risk. Absolute risk is a better measure than the relative risk in understanding how likely and individual will experience a condition. Many studies report relative risk. For example, it might be reported that patients taking a statin had a 25% lower likelihood of a cardiovascular event than the control group that was not on the drug. The duration of a study is important. A study period might be only a few years or less, or it might be 30 years or even a lifetime. Also, keep in mind that a very large percentage increase, or decrease, in the risk of an event with a very low absolute risk, i.e., a very rare event, is not important. Doubling the risk of a rare event is still a rare event.

Odds ratio

An odds ratio (OR) is a measure of association between an exposure and an outcome. The OR represents the odds that an outcome will occur given a particular exposure, compared to the odds of the outcome occurring in the absence of that exposure. Odds are the ratio of the probability of an event occurring in a group, divided by the probability of that event not occurring. If 10/100 exposed people get a disease and 5/100 unexposed people get a disease, the OR of the disease is 10/90 / 5/95, or 2.1.

Hazard ratio

The hazard ratio (HR) is the difference in risk in two experimental groups. It represents an estimate at any given point of time; it is not a cumulative estimate like relative risk and odds ratio. The hazard ratio is a ratio of two hazard functions and is not the same as the relative risk, but it is similar for small time intervals. To put it another way, an HR is the difference in the rate of a disease over a given time period between those with and without the exposure. Unlike the RR and OR, the HR takes into account the time in an interval the disease occurs. If 10/100 exposed people get a disease and 5/100 unexposed people get a disease, and all cases occur at the midpoint, the HR is 10/95 person-years over 5/97.5 person-years = 2.06.

Statistical significance

Statistical significance, as defined by a p-value, is the likelihood that a relationship between two or more variables is caused by something other than random chance. In general, a p-value of 5% or lower is considered to be statistically significant. This means that the probability of the phenomenon being random is, or is less than one out of every 20, which is why the p-value is set at 5%. Another way of stating this is that a p-value of .05 means that the probability a particular outcome occurred by chance is 5 in 100. The lower the p-value is, the less likely that a positive result is false.

Confidence intervals

Study results are often reported with a numerical finding and a confidence interval (CI). The confidence interval is presented with a range of numbers with a statistical likelihood selected by the investigator (often set at 95%) that would bracket the numerical result of the study. If the p-value is set at 5%, and the investigator offers a 95% confidence interval, that means there is a 5% chance that the true value falls outside of the confidence interval brackets. To make it easier to read this book, I have usually omitted the confidence intervals reported in the medical literature, so it is good to keep in mind that there is a certain lack of precision in the numbers presented. For example, I described the findings of a Dutch study that found that when comparing women with least healthy to those with the healthiest lifestyle, the healthiest women lived 15.1 years longer (95% CI: 9.9, 20.2 years).[5] The confidence interval in this instance is very broad: statistically, there is a 95% chance the "true" value could be as low as 9.9 years or as high as 20.2 years and a 5% chance the true value would be even lower or higher.

Confounding variables

When designing an experiment, investigators choose an exposure they want to study and hypothesize that it is related to a health outcome. For example, in a study considering an association between lack of exercise and weight gain, lack of exercise is the exposure, and weight gain is the outcome. Confounding variables are traits, such as age or behaviors that are associated both with the exposure and with the outcome that can either exaggerate or mask the degree to which they appear associated. Confounders are sometimes known but often unknown other variables or factors that also influence dependent variables. Confounding variables can cause two major problems: an increase in the variance of the study result and introduce bias.

Bias

Bias is any deviation of results or inferences from the truth or processes leading to such deviation. Bias can result from several sources: systematic variations in measurement from the true value (systematic error); flaws in study design; deviation of inferences, interpretations, or analyses based on flawed data or data collection. There is no sense of prejudice or subjectivity implied in the assessment of bias under these conditions, but this too can occur. Confounding is a type of bias.

The placebo and nocebo effects

In brief, the placebo effect occurs when the expectation of an improvement in health or symptoms occurs because of a strong belief in the efficacy of a treatment that has no biological basis for being effective, for example, after swallowing a sugar pill with no drugs in it. There are many examples of treatments with sham drugs or procedures that bring about subjective and, at times, even functional improvements in health or symptoms through initiating a self-healing or self-medicating process.[6] Often a supportive relationship with a health practitioner is the key to creating belief in a successful treatment outcome. Exposure to the trappings of a health care environment, for example, nurses, doctors, waiting rooms, etc., often called the theatre of medicine, also seems to be important. The nocebo effect is when a person expects symptoms from a treatment or other intervention, and the usual discomforts of day to day living are interpreted as the result of the treatment or intervention.

Acknowledgments

First, among the many who deserve thanks for supporting my work on this book, is my wife Melissa. Not only did she graciously tolerate the past five years of many closeted hours researching and writing, she helped with editing, expertly carried out all of the cover and interior design, and helped with many of the complicated steps needed to publish a book. High on the list of those to whom I am grateful is my sister Dr. Ann Ferren. Ann is a superstar academic who provided critical review of three versions of the entire book.

Dr. Peter Ferren, my nephew and colleague on the UCSF faculty, helped enormously with Chapter 10, "Stress and Mental Health." Dr. Corinne Rocca, a UCSF colleague in the UCSF Bixby Center for Global Reproductive Health, designed the figure on risk of pregnancy according to various contraceptive methods that appears in Chapter 13, "Sexual and Reproductive Health," and corrected my errors and perfected the information in Chapter 16, "Understanding Scientific Data." Another UCSF colleague and successful author, Dr. Robert Lustig, provided excellent advice and encouragement for the project, and for Chapter 4, "Weight Control," I relied on much of the science in his book, *Fat Chance, Beating the Odds Against Sugar, Processed Food, Obesity and Disease*. A special thanks goes to Dr. John Swartzberg, chair, and all of the members of the Editorial Board of the *University of California, Berkeley Wellness Letter*. My participation on the *UCB Wellness Letter* Board has been a rewarding learning experience.

Some material in this book has been modified from presentations that appeared on the website of Catalyst for Children.

Finally, I want to acknowledge and pay tribute to the thousands of medical researchers whose data and publications have informed this book as has the work and publications of many professional associations including the American Heart

Association and the American Cancer Society. Their work to advance the science of medicine has provided the expert science-based guidance about how to adopt a healthier lifestyle that is the basis of this book. I have tried to accurately interpret the medical evidence that is the basis for this book, and apologize for any errors or omissions. I caution the reader that future research will provide new information that will influence and hopefully improve our efforts to stay healthy.

About the Author

J. Joseph Speidel MD, MPH is a physician, author, scholar and advocate in the field of public health. He is a graduate of Harvard College, Harvard Medical School, and the Harvard School of Public Health and a professor emeritus at the University of California, San Francisco (UCSF) School of Medicine. Previous positions include serving in the U.S. Army Medical Corps Office of the Surgeon General with a rank of Major, directing the U.S. Agency for International Development (USAID) Office of Population, president of Population Action International (PAI), directing the population grants program at the William and Flora Hewlett Foundation, and Co-director of the UCSF Bixby Center for Global Reproductive Health. Dr. Speidel has served on the board of directors of more than 20 non-profit organizations. As director of USAID and Hewlett Foundation programs, Dr. Speidel was responsible for the management of international development assistance and charitable awards totaling more than $1 billion.

Dr. Speidel is board certified in Preventive Medicine and serves on the Editorial Board of the *University of California, Berkeley Wellness Newsletter*. He is the author of more than 300 scientific publications in the field of health and population. In addition, Dr. Speidel has helped prepare more than 50 health-related scientific reports that are posted on the website Catalyst for Children (http://catalystforchildren.org), a resource that provides educational materials to improve the welfare of children and youth.

As president and spokesperson for Population Action International, Dr. Speidel gave more than 750 interviews with print media and made more than 250 radio, TV, and personal appearances including on ABC, NBC, CBS, CNN, BBC, Voice of America, and on talk shows including Good Morning America, The Charlie Rose Show, and Larry King Live.

Dr. Speidel is a recipient of the Arthur S. Flemming Award for outstanding young men in government, the Carl S. Schulz Award of the American Public Health Association, the Family Planning Visionary Award of the National Family Planning and Reproductive Health Association, and the Allan Rosenfield Award for Lifetime Contributions to International Family Planning of the Society of Family Planning.

The goal of Dr. Speidel's new book, *The Building Blocks of Health: How to Optimize Wellness with a Lifestyle Checklist*, is to help Americans adopt a lifestyle that will reverse much of the damage from their unhealthy way of living that leads to illness and premature death.

Each of the book's chapters focuses on an important health-related topic such as nutrition, weight control, heart disease, cancer and dementia. This is a book that all Americans should read, and doctors will want to give to their patients because they do not have enough time to provide good counseling about an optimally healthy lifestyle. The behaviors described in *The Building Blocks of Health* are highly effective in restoring and maintaining health.

Dr. Speidel's website is: jjspeidel.com.

References

Chapter 1 - Introduction

1 Biener AI, Decker SL, Rohde F. Source of Increased Health Care Spending in the United States. JAMA. 2019; 321(12):1147. doi:10.1001/jama.2019.0679

2 Colditz GA, Philpott SE, Hankinson SE. The Impact of the Nurses' Health Study on Population Health: Prevention, Translation, and Control. AJPH. 2016;106(9):1540-1545. DOI: 10.2105/AJPH.2016.303343

3 Merchant RM, Asch DA. Protecting the Value of Medical Science in the Age of Social Media and "Fake News." JAMA. 2018;320(23):2415–2416. doi:10.1001/jama.2018.18416

4 Chou WS, Oh A, Klein WMP. Addressing Health-Related Misinformation on Social Media. JAMA.2018;320(23):2417–2418. doi:10.1001/jama.2018.16865

5 Ioannidis JPA. Neglecting Major Health Problems and Broadcasting Minor, Uncertain Issues in Lifestyle Science. JAMA. 2019;322(21):2069–2070. doi:10.1001/jama.2019.17576

6 Speidel JJ, Weltman A, North TC, Brenton JT, and Melcher GW. Cardiovascular Diseases - Prevention and Treatment. Rocky Mountain Medical Journal, a supplement to Colorado Medicine. 1982;Scientific Section: 49-53.

7 Excerpt From: Michael Greger, MD & Gene Stone. How Not to Die. iBooks. https://itun.es/us/z9E38.l

8 Monte T, Pritikin I. Pritikin: the Man Who Healed America's Heart. Emmaus, PA: Rodale Press; 1988.

9 Excerpt From: Michael Greger, MD & Gene Stone. How Not to Die. iBooks. https://itun.es/us/z9E38.l

10 Antognoli EL, Seeholzer EL, Gullett H, Jackson B, Smith S, FlocS.A SA. Primary care resident training for obesity, nutrition, and physical activity counseling: a mixed-methods study. Health Promot Pract. 2016 July 08 (Epub ahead of print).

11 Miller G, Roehrig C, Hughes-Cromwick P, Lake C. Quantifying national spending on wellness and prevention. Adv Health Econ Health Serv Res 2008;19:1-24.

12 Sensenig AL. Refining estimates of public health spending as measured in national health expenditures accounts: the United States experience. J Public Health Manag Pract. 2007;13(2):103-14.

13 Forsberg V, Fichtenberg C. The Prevention and Public Health Fund: A critical investment in our nation's physical and fiscal health. Center for Public Health Policy, Issue Brief, American Public Health Association, June 2012. https://apha.org/~/media/files/pdf/factsheets/apha_prevfundbrief_june2012.ashx

14 Baicker K, Cutler D, Song Z. Workplace Wellness Programs Can Generate Savings, Health Affairs. 2010;29(2):304-11. doi: 10.1377/hlthaff.2009.0626. Epub 2010 Jan 14.

15 Alonso-Zaldivar R. "$10,345 Per Person U.S. Health Care Spending Reaches New Peak." PBS News

Hour. July 13, 2016. http://Www.Pbs.Org/Newshour/Rundown/New-Peak-Us-Health-Care-Spending-10345-Per-Person/ and National Health Expenditures 2014 Highlights. Centers for Medicare and Medicaid Services

16 Farley TA. When is it Ethical to Withhold Prevention? New Eng J Med. 2016;374(14):1303-1306.

Chapter 2 – Lifestyle Checklist

1 Leading Causes of Death, 1900-1998. U.S. Centers for Disease Control and Prevention. https://www.cdc.gov/nchs/data/dvs/lead1900_98.pdf

2 Kochanek KD, Murphy SL, Xu JQ, Tejada-Vera B. Deaths: Final data for 2014. National vital statistics reports;65(4). Hyattsville, MD: National Center for Health Statistics. 2016.

3 World Health Organization. Global status report on noncommunicable diseases. Geneva:WHO, 2014.

4 World Health Organization. Noncommunicable Diseases Fact Sheet. Geneva:WHO, January 2015.

5 Kochanek KD, Murphy SL, Xu J, Arias E. Division of Vital Statistics: Deaths: Final data for 2017. National Vital Statistics Reports;68(9). Hyattsville, MD: National Center for Health Statistics. June 24, 2019.

6 Overdose Death Rates. National Institute on Drug Abuse. August 2018. https://www.drugabuse.gov/related-topics/trends-statistics/overdose-death-rates.

7 Katz J. U.S. Drug Deaths Climbing Faster Than Ever. New York Times. June 6, 2017.

8 Lee LK, Mannix R. Increasing Fatality Rates From Preventable Deaths in Teenagers and Young Adults. JAMA.2018;320(6):543–544. doi:10.1001/jama.2018.6566.

9 National Center for Injury Prevention and Control, Centers for Disease Control and Prevention. Web-based injury statistics query and reporting system. https://webappa.cdc.gov/sasweb/ncipc/leadcause.html.

10 General Health Status. Office of Disease Prevention and Health Promotion. U. S. Department of Health and Human Services. https://www.healthypeople.gov/2020/about/foundation-health-measures/General-Health-Status.

11 Berry JD, Dyer A, Cai X, Garside DB, Ning H, Thomas A, Greenland P, Van Horn L, Tracy RP, Lloyd-Jones DM. Lifetime risks of cardiovascular disease. N Engl J Med. 2012;366(4):321-9. doi: 10.1056/NEJMoa1012848.

12 Wilkins JT, Ning H. Berry J, Zhao L, Dyer AR, Lloyd-Jones DM. Lifetime risk and years lived free of total cardiovascular disease. JAMA. 2012;308(17):1795-801. doi: 10.1001/jama.2012.14312.

13 Lifetime Risk of Developing or Dying from Cancer. American Cancer Society. https://www.cancer.org/cancer/cancer-basics/lifetime-probability-of-developing-or-dying-from-cancer.html.

14 Seshadri S, Beiser A, Kelly-Hayes M, et al. The Lifetime Risk of Stroke, Estimates from the Framingham Study. Stroke. 2006;37:345-350. https://doi.org/10.1161/01.STR.0000199613.38911.b2.

15 Gershon AS, Warner L, et al. Lifetime risk of developing chronic obstructive pulmonary disease: a longitudinal population study. Lancet. 2011;378(9795):991-6. doi: 10.1016/S0140-6736(11)60990-2.

16 Preston S, Fishman E, Stokes A. "Lifetime Probability of Developing Diabetes in the United States" (2014).

17 Hoerčger TJ, Simpson SA, Yarnoff BO, et al. The Future Burden of CKD in the United States: A Simulation Model for the CDC CKD Initiative. Am J Kidney Dis. 2015;65(3):403-411.

18 Boudette N. U.S. Traffic Deaths Rise for a Second Straight Year. New York Times. February 15, 2017.

19 Murray CJ, Atkinson C, Bhalla K, and US Burden of Disease Collaborators. The State of US Health, 1990-2010: Burden of Diseases, Injuries, and Risk Factors. JAMA. 2013;310(6):591-606. doi:10.1001/jama.2013.13805.

20 Liu Y, Croft JB, Wheaton AG, Kanny D, Cunningham TJ, Lu H, et al. Clustering of Five Health-Related Behaviors for Chronic Disease Prevention Among Adults, United States, 2013. Prev Chronic Dis. 2016;13:160054.

21 Flegal KM, Kruszon-Moran D, Carroll MD, Fryar CD, Ogden CL. Trends in Obesity Among Adults in the United States, 2005 to 2014. JAMA. 2016;315(21):2284-2291. doi:10.1001/jama.2016.6458.

22 Hales CM, Carroll MD, Fryar CD, Ogden CL. Prevalence of obesity among adults and youth: United-States, 2015–2016. NCHS Data Brief. 2017;(288):1-8.

23 Segal LM, Rayburn J, Martin A. Physical Inactivity in the United States, 2015. The State of Obesity: Better Policies for a Healthier America. Trust for America's Health and Robert Wood Johnson Foundation. Washington, D.C. Trust for America's Health, 2016. https://stateofobesity.org/physical-inactivity/

24 Fast facts, smoking and tobacco use. Centers for Disease Control and Prevention (CDC). https://www.cdc.gov/tobacco/data_statistics/fact_sheets/index.htm

25 National Diabetes Statistics Report, 2017. Centers for Disease Control and Prevention (CDC). https://www.cdc.gov/diabetes/pdfs/data/statistics/national-diabetes-statistics-report.pdf

26 Newort F. In U.S., 5% Consider Themselves Vegetarians—Even smaller 2% say they are vegans. Well-Being. July 26, 2012. http://www.gallup.com/poll/156215/consider-themselves-vegetarians.aspx

27 Shay CM, Ning H, Allen NB, et al. Status of cardiovascular health in US adults: prevalence estimatesfrom the National Health and Nutrition Examination Surveys (NHANES) 2003-2008. Circulation.2012;125(1):45-56. doi: 10.1161/Circulation AHA.111.035733. Epub 2011 Nov 17.

28 Substance Abuse and Mental Health Services Administration. (2019). Key substance use and mentalhealth indicators in the United States: Results from the 2018 National Survey on Drug Use and Health (HHS Publication No. PEP19-5068, NSDUH Series H-54). Rockville, MD: Center for Behavioral Health Statistics and Quality, Substance Abuse and Mental Health Services Administration. Retrieved from https://www.samhsa.gov/data/

29 Cullen KA, Gentzke AS, Sawdey MD, et al. e-Cigarette Use Among Youth in the United States, 2019. JAMA. 2019;322(21):2095–2103. doi:https://doi.org/10.1001/jama.2019.18387

30 Health, United States. Table 21. Centers for Disease Control and Prevention (CDC). https://www.cdc.gov/nchs/data/hus/2018/021.pdf

31 Hales CM, Carroll MD, Fryar CD, Ogden CL. Prevalence of obesity among adults and youth: United-States, 2015–2016. NCHS Data Brief. 2017;(288):1-8.

32 Watson KB, Carlson SA, Gunn JP, et al. Physical Inactivity Among Adults Aged 50 Years and Older — United States, 2014. MMWR Morb Mortal Wkly Rep 2016;65:954–958. DOI: http://dx.doi. org/10.15585/mmwr.mm6536a3. http://www.cdc.gov/mmwr/volumes/65/wr/pdfs/mm6536.pdf

33 Physical Activity. Centers for Disease Control and Prevention (CDC). http://www.cdc.gov/physicalactivity/everyone/health/index.html

34 Substance Abuse and Mental Health Services Administration. (2019). Key substance use and mentalhealth indicators in the United States: Results from the 2018 National Survey on Drug Use and Health (HHS Publication No. PEP19-5068, NSDUH Series H-54). Rockville, MD: Center for Behavioral Health Statistics and Quality, Substance Abuse and Mental Health Services Administration. Retrieved from https://www.samhsa.gov/data/

35 Lloyd-Jones DM, Hong Y, Labarthe D, Mozaffarian D, Appel LJ, Van Horn L, Greenlund K, Daniels S, Nichol G, Tomaselli GF, Arnett DK, Fonarow GC, Ho PM, Lauer MS, Masoudi FA, Robertson RM, Roger V, Schwamm LH, Sorlie P, Yancy CW, Rosamond WD. American Heart Association Strategic Planning Task Force and Statistics Committee. Defining and setting national goals for cardiovascular health promotion and disease reduction: the American Heart Association's strategic Impact Goal through 2020 and beyond. Circulation. 2010;121(4):586-613. doi: 10.1161/Circulation AHA.109.192703. Epub 2010 Jan 20.

36 Yancy C W. Is ideal cardiovascular health attainable? Circulation. 2011;123(8):835-7. doi: 10.1161/ Circulation AHA.110.016378. Epub 2011 Feb 14.

37 Shay CM, Ning H, Allen NB, et al. Status of cardiovascular health in US adults: prevalence estimatesfrom the National Health and Nutrition Examination Surveys (NHANES) 2003-2008. Circulation.2012;125(1):45-56. doi: 10.1161/Circulation AHA.111.035733. Epub 2011 Nov 17.

38 Kim JI, Sillah A, Boucher JL, Sidebottom AC, Knickelbine T. Prevalence of the American Heart Association's "ideal cardiovascular health" metrics in a rural, cross-sectional, community-based study: the Heartof New Ulm Project. J Am Heart Assoc. 2013 Apr 25;2(3):e000058. doi: 10.1161/JAHA.113.000058.

39 Yang Q, Cogswell ME, Flanders WD, Hong Y, Zhang Z, Loustalot F, Gillespie C, Merritt R, Hu FB. Trends in cardiovascular health metrics and associations with all-cause and CVD mortality among US-adults. JAMA. 2012 Mar 28;307(12):1273-83. doi: 10.1001/jama.2012.339. Epub 2012 Mar 16. http://www.ncbi.nlm.nih.gov/pubmed/22427615

40 Khaw K-T, Wareham N, Bingham S, Welch A, Luben R, Day N. Combined Impact of Health Behaviours and Mortality in Men and Women: The EPIC-Norfolk Prospective Population Study. PLoS Med. 2008;5(1): e12. doi:10.1371/journal.pmed.0050012

41 Ford ES, Bergmann MM, Boeing H, Li C, Capewell S. Healthy lifestyle behaviors and all-cause mortality among adults in the United States. Prev Med. 2012;55(1):23-7. doi: 10.1016/j.ypmed.2012.04.016. Epub 2012 Apr 29.

42 Loef M, Walach H. The combined effects of healthy lifestyle behaviors on all cause mortality: a systematic review and meta-analysis. Prev Med. 2012;55:163–170. doi: 10.1016/j.ypmed.2012.06.017.

43 Ford ES, Bergmann MM, Kröger J, Schienkiewitz A, Weikert C, Boeing H. Healthy living is the bestrevenge: findings from the European Prospective Investigation Into Cancer and Nutrition-Potsdam study. Arch Intern Med. 2009;169(15):1355-1362. doi: 10.1001/archinternmed.2009.237.

44 Van den Brandt PA. The impact of a Mediterranean diet and healthy lifestyle on premature mortality in men and women Am J Clin Nutr. doi: 10.3945/ajcn.110. 008250.

45 Li Y, Pan A, Wang DD, Liu X, Dhana K, Franco OH, Kaptoge S, Di Angelantonio E, Stampfer M, Willett WC, Hu FB. Impact of Healthy Lifestyle Factors on Life Expectancies in the US Population. Circulation, published online April 30, 2018; doi: 10.1161/CIRCULATIONAHA.117.032047. http://circ.ahajournals. org/content/early/2018/04/25/CIRCULATIONAHA.117.032047

46 Rucker C, Hoffman J. The Seventh-Day Diet. New York: Random House; 1991

47 Kahn HA, Phillips RI, Snowdon DA, Choi W. Association between reported diet and all-cause mortality: twenty-one year follow-up on27,530 adult Seventh-Day Adventists. Am J Epidemiol. 1984;119(5):775-87.

48 Pritikin N, McGrady PM. Pritikin Program for Diet and Exercise. New York, Bantam Books: 1980.

49 Capewell S, O'Flaherty M. Rapid mortality falls after risk-factor changes in populations. Lancet 2011;378:752-753.

50 Healthfinder. Office of Disease Prevention and Health Promotion. U. S. Department of Health and Human Services. http://healthfinder.gov/myhealthfinder/

51 Bortz WM, Next Medicine: The Science and Civics of Health. New York:Oxford University Press 2011.

52 Pizzo PA. A Prescription for Longevity in the 21st Century: Renewing Purpose, Building and Sustaining Social Engagement, and Embracing a Positive Lifestyle. JAMA. 2020;323(5):415–416. doi:10.1001/jama.2019.21087

53 Schroeder SA. We Can Do Better — Improving the Health of the American People. N Engl J Med. 2007;357:1221-8.

54 Fuchs VR. Social Determinants of Health Caveats and Nuances. JAMA. 2017;317(1):25-26. doi:

doi:10.1001/jama.2016.17335.

55 Pantell M, Rehkopf D, Jutte D, et al. Social Isolation: A Predictor of Mortality Comparable to Traditional Clinical Risk Factors. American Journal of Public Health. 2013;103(11):2056-2062.

56 Sapolsky RM. The health-wealth gap. Scientific American. November 2018:63-67.

57 Chetty R, Stepner M, Abraham S, Lin S, Scuderi B, Turner N, Bergeron A, MA; David Cutler D. The-Association Between Income and Life Expectancy in the United States, 2001-2014. JAMA. doi:10.1001/jama.2016.4226. Published online April 10, 2016.

58 McGinnis JM, Foege WH. Actual causes of death in the United States. JAMA. 1993;270(18):2207-2212.

59 Frieden TR, Framework for Public Health Action: The Health Impact Pyramid. AJPH. 2010;100(4):590-595.|

60 Robertson TL, Kato H, Rhoads GG, Kagan A, Marmot M, Syme SL, Gordon T, Worth RM, Belsky JL, Dock DS, Miyanishi M, Kawamoto S. Epidemiologic studies of coronary heart disease and stroke in Japanese men living in Japan, Hawaii, and California. Incidence of myocardial infarction and death from coronary heart disease. Am J Cardiol. 1977;39(2):239-43.

61 Willett WC. Balancing life-style and genomics research for disease prevention. Science. 2002;296(5568):695-8.

62 Tchkonia T, Kirkland JL. Aging, Cell Senescence, and Chronic DiseaseEmerging Therapeutic Strategies. JAMA. 2018;320(13):1319–1320. doi:10.1001/jama.2018.12440

63 Kirkwood T. Why can't we live forever? Scientific American, September 2010.

64 Ornish D, Lin J, Chan JM, et al. Effect of comprehensive lifestyle changes on telomerase activity and-telomere length in men with biopsy-proven low-risk prostate cancer: 5-year follow-up of a descriptive pilot-study. Lancet Oncol. 2013 Oct;14(11):1112-20. doi: 10.1016/S1470-2045(13)70366-8. Epub 2013 Sep 17.

65 Mason C, et al. Independent and Combined Effects of Dietary Weight Loss and Exercise on Leukocyte Telomere Length in Postmenopausal Women. Obesity. 2013;21(12): E549-54

66 Barzilai N, Cuervo AM, Austad S. Aging as a Biological Target for Prevention and Therapy. JAMA.2018;320(13):1321–1322. doi:10.1001/jama.2018.9562.

67 Olshansky SJ. From Lifespan to Healthspan. JAMA. 2018;320(13):1323–1324. doi:10.1001/jama.2018.12621.

68 Zimmer C. What's the Longest Humans Can Live? 115 Years, New Study Says. New York Times, October 6, 2013.

69 Dong X, Milholland B, Vijg J. Evidence for a limit to human lifespan. Nature. 538:257–259 (13 October 2016). doi:10.1038/nature19793.

70 Tchkonia T, Kirkland JL. Aging, Cell Senescence, and Chronic DiseaseEmerging Therapeutic Strategies. JAMA. 2018;320(13):1319–1320. doi:10.1001/jama.2018.12440.

Chapter 3 - Optimal Nutrition

1 Excerpt From: Greger M, Stone G, "How Not to Die." iBooks. p.9 https://itun.es/us/z9E38.l

2 Singh PN, Arthur KN, Orlich MJ1, James W, Purty A, Job JS, Rajaram S, Sabaté J. Global epidemiologyof obesity, vegetarian dietary patterns, and noncommunicable disease in Asian Indians. Am J Clin Nutr. 2014 Jul;100 Suppl 1:359S-64S. DOI: 10.3945/ajcn.113.071571. Epub 2014 May 21.

3 World Health Organization. Global status report on noncommunicable diseases. Geneva, WHO, 2014.

4 association of saturated fat with cardiovascular disease. Am J Clin Nutr. 2010;91(3):535-546.

5 Scientific Report of the 2015 Dietary Guidelines Advisory Committee. Advisory Report to the Secretaryof Health and Human Services and the Secretary of Agriculture. http://www.health.gov/dietaryguidelines/2015-scientific-report/

6 Sifferlin A. Here's What 10 Experts Think of the Government's New Diet Advice. Time Magazine. January 7, 2016. http://time.com/4170928/dietary-guidelines-nutrition-experts/

7 Scientific Report of the 2015 Dietary Guidelines Advisory Committee. Advisory Report to the Secretaryof Health and Human Services and the Secretary of Agriculture. http://www.health.gov/dietaryguidelines/2015-scientific-report/

8 Dietary Guidelines Advisory Committee. 2020. Scientific Report of the 2020 Dietary Guidelines Advisory Committee: Advisory Report to the Secretary of Agriculture and the Secretary of Health and HumanServices. U.S. Department

9 Moss M, Salt Sugar Fat. New York. Random House. 2013.

10 Moss M, Salt Sugar Fat. New York. Random House. 2013.

11 Schnabel L, Kesse-Guyot E, Allès B, et al. Association Between Ultraprocessed Food Consumption-and Risk of Mortality Among Middle-aged Adults in France. JAMA Intern Med. 2019;179(4):490–498. doi:10.1001/jamainternmed.2018.7289

12 Fryar CD, Ervin RB, Caloric Intake From Fast Food Among Adults: United States, 2007–2010 NCSH-Data Brief No. 114, February 2013

13 Hsu T. Bigger, Saltier, Heavier: How Fast Food Changed Over 30 Years. New York Times. March 4,2019.

14 National Center for Health Statistics. Health, United States, 2014: With Special Feature on AdultsAged 55–64. Hyattsville, MD. 2015.

15 Scientific Report of the 2015 Dietary Guidelines Advisory Committee. Advisory Report to the Secretary of Health and Human Services and the Secretary of Agriculture. http://www.health.gov/dietaryguidelines/2015-scientific-report/

16 Ornish D, Brown SE, Scherwitz LW, et al. Can lifestyle changes reverse coronary heart disease? Lancet.1990;336:129-133.

17 Ornish D, Scherwitz LW, Billings JH, Gould LK, Merritt TA, MS, Sparler S, Armstrong WT, Ports TA, Kirkeeide RL, Hogeboom C, Brand RJ. Intensive Lifestyle Changes for Reversal of Coronary Heart Disease. JAMA. 1998;280(23):2001-2007.

18 Esselstyn CB Jr. Updating a 12-year experience with arrest and reversal therapy for coronary heart disease (an overdue requiem for palliative cardiology). Am J Cardiol. 1999;84:339-341.

19 Ervin, RB, Ogden CL. U.S. Department of Health and Human Services, Centers for Disease Control and Prevention. (2013). NCHS Data Brief, No. 122: Consumption of Added Sugars Among U.S. Adults, 2005–2010. Retrieved from http://www.cdc.gov/nchs/data/databriefs/db122.pdf

20 United States Department of Agriculture, Economic Research Service. (2012). USDA Sugar Supply: Tables 51-53: US Consumption of Caloric Sweeteners. Retrieved from http://www.ers.usda.gov/data-products/sugar-and-sweeteners-yearbook-tables.aspx

21 Moss M, Salt Sugar Fat. New York. Random House. 2013.

22 The American Heart Association's Diet and Lifestyle Recommendations, http://www.heart.org/HEARTORG/GettingHealthy/NutritionCenter/HealthyEating/The-American-Heart-Associations-Diet-and-Lifestyle-Recommendations_UCM_305855_Article.jsp

23 Moore LV, Thompson, FE, Adults Meeting Fruit and Vegetable Intake Recommendations — United States, 2013, Morbidity and Mortality Weekly Report (MMWR)July 10, 2015;64(26):709-713. http://www.cdc.gov/mmwr/preview/mmwrhtml/mm6426a1.htm

24 USDA Food Patterns http://www.cnpp.usda.gov/sites/default/files/usda_food_patterns/USDAFoodPternsSummaryTable.pdf

25 Mozaffarian D, Appel LJ, Van Horn L. Components of a Cardioprotective Diet: New Insights. Circulation. 2011;123:2870-2891. DOI: 10.1161/Circulation AHA.110.968735

26 Mozaffarian D. The Great Fat Debate: Taking the focus off of saturated fat. J Am Diet Assoc. 2011;111:665-666.

27 Mozaffarian D, Kumanyika SK, Lemaitre RN, Olson JL, Burke GL, Siscovick DS. Cereal, Fruit, and Vegetable Fiber Intake and the Risk of Cardiovascular Disease in Elderly Individuals. JAMA. 2003;289(13):1659-1666. DOI:10.1001/jama.289.13.1659

28 Reynolds A, Mann J, Cummings J, Winter N, Mete E, Te Morenga L. Carbohydrate quality and humanhealth: a series of systematic reviews and meta-analyses. Lancet. 2019;393(10170):434-445. https://doi.org/10.1016/s0140-6736(18)31809-9

29 Levine, Morgan E. et al. Low Protein Intake Is Associated with a Major Reduction in IGF-1, Cancer, and Overall Mortality in the 65 and Younger but Not Older Population. Cell Metabolism. 2014;19(3):407–417.

30 Ornish D, The Spectrum. New York, NY: Ballantine Books: 2007.

31 Cheski LJ, Roberts C, Margolis S. Nutrition, and Weight Control. Johns Hopkins White Paper, New York. Remedy Media, 2014

32 Mozaffarian D, Katan MB, Ascherio A, Stampfer MJ, Willett WC. Trans-fatty acids and cardiovascular disease. N Engl J Med. 2006;354:1601-1613

33 Lichtenstein AH, Ausman LM, Jalbert SM, Schaefer EJ. effects of different forms of dietary hydrogenated fats on serum lipoprotein cholesterol levels. N Engl J Med. 1999;340:1933-40.

34 Brownell KD, Pomeran JL. The Trans-Fat Ban — Food Regulation and Long-Term Health. N Engl J Med. 2014; 370:1773-1775May 8, 2014DOI: 10.1056/NEJMp1314072

35 Kiage JN, Merrill PD, Robinson CJ, et al. Intake of trans-fat and all-cause mortality in the Reasons forGeographical and Racial Differences in Stroke (REGARDS) cohort. The A J Clin Nutr. 2013;97(5):1121-1128. doi:10.3945/ajcn.112.049064.

36 FDA Cuts Trans-Fat in Processed Foods. FDA Consumer Health Information, U.S. Food and Drug Administration. June 2015. http://www.fda.gov/ForConsumers/ConsumerUpdates/ucm372915.htm

37 Mozaffarian D, Katan MB, Ascherio A, Stampfer MJ, Willett WC. Trans-fatty acids and cardiovascular disease. N Engl J Med. 2006;354:1601–13.

38 U.S. Department of Agriculture, Agricultural Research Service, Nutrition Data Laboratory. USDA National Nutrient Database for Standard Reference. Release 27, 2015. Available at http://ndb.- nal.usda.gov/ (http://ndb.nal.usda.gov/).

39 2015-2020 Dietary Guidelines for Americans. https://health.gov/dietaryguidelines/2015/guidelines/

40 Ganio MS, Armstrong LE, Casa DJ, et al. Mild dehydration impairs cognitive performance and mood of men. British Journal of Nutrition. 2011;106(10):1535-1543.

41 Armstrong, L.E., Ganio, M.S., Casa, D.J. et al. Mild dehydration affects mood in healthy young women. Journal of Nutrition. 2012;142(2):382-388.

42 Dietary Reference Intakes for Water, Potassium, Sodium, Chloride, and Sulfate. Panel on Dietary Reference Intakes for Electrolytes and Water, Standing Committee on the Scientific Evaluation of Dietary Reference Intakes. ISBN: 0-309-53049-0, 640 pp. (2004) http://www.nap.edu/catalog/10925.html

43 Brody J. Dehydration: Risks and Myths. New York Times. May 9, 2016

44 Reynolds G. Intoxicateed by Water. New Yourk Times. September 1, 2015.

45 Lustig R. Sugar, the Bitter Truth. https://www.youtube.com/watch?v=dBnniua6-oM

46 Lustig RH. Fructose: it's "alcohol without the buzz." Adv Nutr. 2013;4(2):226-235.

47 2015-2020 Dietary Guidelines for Americans. https://health.gov/dietaryguidelines/2015/

48 Lustig RH, Schmidt LA, Brindis CD. The toxic truth about sugar. Nature. 2012;482:27-29.

49 Lustig RH. Fructose: it's "alcohol without the buzz." Adv Nutr. 2013;4(2):226-235.

50 Ludwig DS. Examining the Health Effects of Fructose. JAMA. 2013;310(1):33-34. doi:10.1001/jama.2013.6562.

51 Jensen MD. Role of body fat distribution and the metabolic complications of obesity. J Clin Endocrinol-Metab. 2008;93(11)(suppl 1):S57-S63.

52 Mozaffarian D, Appel LJ, Van Horn L. Components of a Cardioprotective Diet: New Insights. Circulation. 2011;123:2870-2891. DOI: 10.1161/Circulation AHA.110.968735

53 Malik VS, Popkin BM, Bray GA, Despres JP, Willett WC, Hu FB. Sugar-sweetened beverages and risk of metabolic syndrome and type 2 diabetes: a meta-analysis. Diabetes Care. 2010;33:2477–2483.

54 Fung TT, Malik V, Rexrode KM, Manson JE, Willett WC, Hu FB. Sweetened beverage consumption and risk of coronary heart disease in women. Am J Clin Nutr. 2009;89:1037–1042.

55 Malik VS, Pan A, Willett WC, and Hu FB. Sugar-sweetened beverages and weight gain in children and adults: a systematic review and meta-analysis. Am J Clin Nutr. 2014 First published ahead of print August 21, 2013 as doi: 10.3945/ajcn.113.058362.

56 Bray GA. Energy and Fructose From Beverages Sweetened With Sugar or High-Fructose Corn Syrup-Pose a Health Risk for Some People. Adv Nutr. 2013;4:220-225; doi:10.3945/an.112.002816

57 Singh GM, Micha R, Khatibzadeh S, Lim S, Ezzati M, Mozaffarian D, on behalf of the Global Burden of Diseases Nutrition and Chronic Diseases Expert Group (NutriCoDE). Estimated Global, Regional, and National Disease Burdens Related to Sugar-Sweetened Beverage Consumption in 2010. Circulation 2015;132(8):639-66.

58 International Diabetes Federation. IDF Diabetes Atlas, 7th edn. Brussels, Belgium: International Diabites Federation, 2015. http://www.diabetesatlas.org

59 Global Report on Diabetes. Geneva. World Health Organization. 2016. ISBN 978 92 4 156525 7 (NLM classification: WK 810) http://www.who.int/diabetes/en/

60 Statistics About Diabetes: American Diabetes Association. March 22, 2018. http://www.diabetes.org/diabetes-basics/statistics/?loc=superfooter

61 Statistics About Diabetes: American Diabetes Association. March 22, 2018. http://www.diabetes.org/

diabetes-basics/statistics/?loc=superfooter

62 American Diabetes Association. Economic costs of diabetes in the US in 2012. Diabetes Care. 2013;36(4):1033-1046.

63 Seaquist ER. Addressing the Burden of Diabetes. JAMA. 2014;311(22):2267-2268. doi:10.1001/jama.2014.6451.

64 Boyle JP, Thompson TJ, Gregg EW, Barker LE, Williamson DF. Projection of the year 2050 burden of diabetes in the US adult population: dynamic modeling of incidence, mortality, and prediabetes prevalence. Popul Health Metr. 2010;8:29

65 CDC Morbidity and Mortality Weekly Report MMWR 2003

66 Basu S, Yoffe P, Hills N, Lustig RH (2013) The Relationship of Sugar to Population-Level Diabetes Prevalence: An Econometric Analysis of Repeated Cross- Sectional Data. PLoS ONE. 8(2): e57873.

doi:10.1371/journal.pone.0057873

67 Pan A, Sun Q, Bernstein AM, Manson JE, Willett WC, Hu FB. Changes in Red Meat Consumption and Subsequent Risk of Type 2 Diabetes Mellitus: Three Cohorts of US Men and Women. JAMA Intern Med. 2013;173(14):1328-1335. doi:10.1001/jamainternmed.2013.6633.

68 Global report on diabetes. World Health Organization 2016 ISBN 978 92 4 156525 7 (NLM classifiction: WK 810)

69 International Diabetes Federation. IDF Diabetes Atlas, 7th edn. Brussels, Belgium: International Diabtes Federation, 2015. http://www.diabetesatlas.org

70 Simple Steps to Preventing Diabetes. The Nutrition Source. https://www.hsph.harvard.edu/nutritiosource/diabetes-prevention/preventing-diabetes-full-story/#references

71 Hu FB, Manson JE, Stampfer MJ, et al. Diet, lifestyle, and the risk of type 2 diabetes mellitus in women. N Engl J Med. 2001; 345:790-7.

72 Tanasescu M, Leitzmann MF, Rimm EB, Hu FB. Physical activity in relation to cardiovascular diseaseand total mortality among men with type 2 diabetes. Circulation. 2003;107:2435 - 2439.

73 de Munter JS, Hu FB, Spiegelman D, Franz M, van Dam RM. Whole grain, bran, and germ intake and risk of type 2 diabetes: a prospective cohort study and systematic review. PLoS Med. 2007; 4:e261.

74 Simple Steps to Preventing Diabetes. The Nutrition Source. https://www.hsph.harvard.edu/nutritiosource/diabetes-prevention/preventing-diabetes-full-story/#references

75 Baliunas DO, Taylor BJ, Irving H, et al. Alcohol as a risk factor for type 2 diabetes: A systematic review and meta-analysis. Diabetes Care. 2009;32:2123-32.

76 Hu FB, Satija A, Manson JE. Curbing the Diabetes Pandemic: The Need for Global Policy Solutions. JAMA. 2015;313(23):2319-2320. doi:10.1001/jama.2015.5287.

77 Gregg EW, Chen H, Wagenknecht LE, et al. Association of an Intensive Lifestyle Intervention With Remission of Type 2 Diabetes. JAMA. 2012;308(23):2489-2496. doi:10.1001/jama.2012.67929.

78 Arterburn DE, O'Connor PJ. A Look Ahead at the Future of Diabetes Prevention and Treatment. JAMA. 2012;308(23):2517-2518. doi:10.1001/jama.2012.144749.

79 Fung TT, Malik V, Rexrode KM, Manson JE, Willett WC, Hu FB. Sweetened beverage consumption and risk of coronary heart disease in women. Am J Clin Nutr. 2009;89:1037–1042

80 Welsh JA, Sharma A, Abramson JL, Vaccarino V, Gillespie C, Vos MB. Caloric Sweetener Consumption and Dyslipidemia Among US Adults. JAMA. 2010;303(15):1490-1497. doi:10.1001/jama.2010.449.

81 Te Morenga LA, Howatson A, Jones RM, Mann J. Dietary sugars and cardiometabolic risk: systematic review and meta-analyses of randomized controlled trials of the effects on blood pressure and lipids. doi: 10.3945/ ajcn.113.081521Am J Clin Nutr. Am J Clin Nutr doi: 10.3945/ajcn.113.081521

82 de Koning L, Malik VS, Kellogg MD, Rimm EB, Willett WC, Hu FB. Sweetened Beverage Consumption, Incident Coronary Heart Disease, and Biomarkers of Risk in Men. Circulation. 2012;125:1735-1741.

83 Yang Q, Zhang Z, Gregg EW, Flanders WD, Merritt R, Hu FB. Added sugar intake and cardiovascular diseases mortality among US adults. JAMA Intern Med. 2014;174(4):516-524.

84 Malik VS, Li Y, Pan A, De Koning L, Schernhammer E, Willett WC, Hu FB. Long-Term Consumptionof Sugar-Sweetened and Artificially Sweetened Beverages and Risk of Mortality in US Adults. Circulation. 2019;139(18):2113–2125. https://doi.org/10.1161/CIRCULATIONAHA.118.03740185

85 Hu Y, Costenbader KH, Gao X, Al-Daabil M, Sparks JA, Solomon DH, Hu FB, Karlson EW, Lu B. Sugar-sweetened soda consumption and risk of developing rheumatoid arthritis in women. Am J Clin Nutr.2014 Sep;100(3):959-67. doi: 10.3945/ajcn.114.086918. Epub 2014 Jul 16.

86 Ervin RB., Ogden CL. U.S. Department of Health and Human Services, Centers for Disease Control and Prevention. (2013). NCHS Data Brief, No. 122: Consumption of Added Sugars Among U.S. Adults,

2005–2010. http://www.cdc.gov/nchs/data/databriefs/db122.pdf

87 United States Department of Agriculture, Economic Research Service. (2012). USDA Sugar Supply: Tables 51-53: US Consumption of Caloric Sweeteners. Retrieved from http://www.ers.usda.gov/data-products/sugar-and-sweeteners-yearbook-tables.aspx

88 Dietary Guidelines Advisory Committee. Scientific Report of the 2020 Dietary Guidelines Advisory-Committee: Advisory Report to the Secretary of Agriculture and the Secretary of Health and Human Services. U.S. Department of Agriculture, Agriculture Research Service, Washington, D.C.

89 Johnson RK, Appel LJ, Brands M, Howard BV, Lefevre M, Lustig RH, Sacks F, Steffen LM, Wylie-Rosett, J. Dietary Sugars Intake and Cardiovascular Health, A Scientific Statement From the American Heart Association. Circulation. 2009;120:1011-1020.

90 Guideline: Sugars intake for adults and children. Geneva: World Health Organization; 2015. http://apps.who.int/iris/bitstream/10665/149782/1/9789241549028_eng.pdf?ua=1

91 Dietary Guidelines Advisory Committee. Scientific Report of the 2020 Dietary Guidelines Advisory-Committee: Advisory Report to the Secretary of Health and Human Services and the Secretary of Agriculture. U.S. Department of Agriculture, Agriculture Research Service, Washington, D.C.

92 Shan Z, Rehm CD, Rogers G, et al. Trends in Dietary Carbohydrate, Protein, and Fat Intake and Diet Quality Among US Adults, 1999-2016. JAMA. 2019;322(12):1178–1187. doi:https://doi.org/10.1001/jama.2019.13771

93 Mozaffarian D, Ludwig DS. The 2015 US Dietary GuidelinesLifting the Ban on Total Dietary Fat. JAMA. 2015;313(24):2421-2422. doi:10.1001/jama.2015.5941

94 Ludwig DS. Lowering the Bar on the Low-Fat Diet. JAMA. Published online September 28, 2016. doi:10.1001/jama.2016.15473

95 Mozaffarian D, Appel LJ, Van Horn L. Components of a Cardioprotective Diet: New Insights. Circulation. 2011;123:2870-2891. DOI: 10.1161/CIRCULATION AHA.110.968735

96 Mozaffarian D, Appel LJ, Van Horn L. Components of a Cardioprotective Diet: New Insights. Circulation. 2011;123:2870-2891. DOI: 10.1161/CIRCULATION AHA.110.968735

97 Zheng Y, Li Y, Satija A, et al. Association of changes in red meat consumption with total and cause specific mortality among US women and men: two prospective cohort studies. BMJ. 2019;365:l2110. doi:10.1136/bmj.l2110.

98 Zheng Y, Li Y, Satija A, et al. Association of changes in red meat consumption with total and cause specific mortality among US women and men: two prospective cohort studies. BMJ. 2019; 365:l2110. doi:10.1136/bmj.l2110.

99 Micha R, Wallace S, Mozaffarian D. Red and processed meat consumption and risk of incident coronary heart disease, stroke, and diabetes:a systematic review and meta-analysis. Circulation. 2010;121:2271–2283.

100 Mozaffarian D, Appel LJ, Van Horn L. Components of a Cardioprotective Diet: New Insights. Circulation. 2011;123:2870-2891. DOI: 10.1161/CIRCULATION AHA.110.968735

101 Bernstein AM, Sun Q, Hu FB, Stampfer MJ, Manson JE, Willett WC. Major dietary protein sources and risk of coronary heart disease in women. Circulation. 2010;122:876–883.

102 Larsson SC, Orsini N. Red meat and processed meat consumption and all-cause mortality: a meta-analysis. Am J Epidemiol. 2014;179: 282-9.

103 Abete I, Romaguera D, Vieira AR et al. Association between total, processed, red and white meat consumption and all-cause, CVD and IHD mortality: a meta-analysis of cohort studies. Br J Nutr. 2014;112, 762–775.

104 Pan A, Sun Q, Bernstein AM, Schulze MB, Manson JE, Stampfer MJ, Willett WC, Hu FB. Red meat

consumption and mortality: results from 2 prospective cohort studies. Arch Intern Med. 2012;172(7):555-63. doi: 10.1001/archinternmed.2011.2287. Epub 2012 Mar 12.

105 Ornish D. Holy Cow! What's Good for You Is Good for Our Planet Comment on "Red Meat Consumption and Mortality". Arch Intern Med. 2012;172(7):563-564. doi:10.1001/archinternmed.2012.174

106 Fung TT, van Dam RM, Hankinson SE, Stampfer M, Willett WC, Hu FB. Low-carbohydrate diets and all-cause and cause-specific mortality: two cohort studies. Ann Intern Med. 2010;153(5):289-98. doi: 10.7326/0003-4819-153-5-201009070-00003.

107 Levine ME, Suarez JA, Brandhorst S, et al. Low Protein Intake is Associated with a Major Reduction in IGF-1, Cancer, and Overall Mortality in the 65 and Younger but Not Older Population. Cell metabolism. 2014;19(3):407-417. doi:10.1016/j.cmet.2014.02.006.

108 Wang X, Lin X, Ouyang YY, Liu J, Zhao G, Pan A, Hu FB. Red and processed meat consumption and mortality: dose-response meta-analysis of prospective cohort studies. Public Health Nutr. 2016 Apr;19(5):893-905. doi: 10.1017/S1368980015002062. Epub 2015 Jul 6.

109 Etemadi A, Sinha R, Ward MH, et al. Mortality from different causes associated with meat, heme iron, nitrates, and nitrites in the NIH-AARP Diet and Health Study: population cohort study. BMJ. 2017;357:j1957.

110 Bullo M, Virgili P, Heller S, Fonarow G. May 8, 2015, presentation, European Congress on Obesity, Prague, Czech Republic

111 Guasch-Ferré M, Satija A, Blondin SA, et al. Meta-analysis of randomized controlled trials of red-meat consumption in comparison with various comparison diets on cardiovascular risk factors. Circulation. 2019;139(15):1828-1845. doi:10.1161/ CIRCULATIONAHA.118.035225.

112 Zheng Y, Li Y, Satija A, et al. Association of changes in red meat consumption with total and cause specific mortality among US women and men: two prospective cohort studies. BMJ. 2019; 365:l2110. doi:10.1136/bmj.l2110.

113 Zhong VW, Van Horn L, Greenland P, et al. Associations of Processed Meat, Unprocessed Red Meat, Poultry, or Fish Intake With Incident Cardiovascular Disease and All-Cause Mortality. JAMA Intern Med. Published online February 03, 2020. doi:10.1001/jamainternmed.2019.6969

114 Johnston BC, Zeraatkar D, Han MA, et al. Unprocessed Red Meat and Processed Meat Consumption: Dietary Guideline Recommendations From the Nutritional Recommendations (NutriRECS) Consortium. Ann Intern Med. 2019;171:756–764. [Epub ahead of print 1 October 2019]. doi: https://doi.org/10.7326/M19-1621

115 Rubin R. Backlash Over Meat Dietary Recommendations Raises Questions About Corporate Ties to-Nutrition Scientists. JAMA. 2020;323(5):401–404. doi:10.1001/jama.2019.21441

116 Ioannidis JPA. The challenge of reforming nutritional epidemiologic research. JAMA. 2018;320:969-970.

117 Hu FB, Otis BO, McCarthy G. Can Plant-Based Meat Alternatives Be Part of a Healthy and Sustainable Diet? JAMA. Published online August 26, 2019. doi:10.1001/jama.2019.13187

118 IPCC. Summary for Policymakers. In: Global Warming of 1.5°C. An IPCC Special Report on the impacts of global warming of 1.5°C above pre-industrial levels and related global greenhouse gas emission pathways, in the context of strengthening the global response to the threat of climate change, sustainable development, and efforts to eradicate poverty [Masson-Delmotte, V., P. Zhai, H.-O. Pörtner, D. Roberts, J. Skea, P.R. Shukla, A. Pirani, W. Moufouma-Okia, C. Péan, R. Pidcock, S. Connors, J.B.R. Matthews, Y. Chen, X. Zhou, M.I. Gomis, E. Lonnoy, T. Maycock, M. Tignor, and T. Waterfield (eds.)]. World Meteorological Organization, Geneva, Switzerland, 2018. 32 pp.

119 Teicholz N, The Government's Bad Diet Advice" New York Times, February 21, 2015.

120 Teicholz N. The Big Fat Surprise: Why Butter, Meat and Cheese Belong in a Healthy Diet. 2014, Simon & Schuster, New York.

121 Mozaffarian D, Ludwig DS. Stop Fearing Fat. New York Times July 9, 2015

122 Mozaffarian D, Appel LJ, Van Horn L. Components of a Cardioprotective Diet: New Insights. Circulation. 2011;123:2870-2891. DOI: 10.1161/CIRCULATION AHA.110.968735.

123 Mozaffarian D, Ludwig DS. The 2015 US Dietary Guidelines Lifting the Ban on Total Dietary Fat. JAMA. 2015;313(24):2421-2422. doi:10.1001/jama.2015.5941

124 Willett WC. The Great Fat Debate: Total fat and health. J Am Diet Assoc. 2011;111:660-662.

125 Willett WC, Yu FB. Optimal diets for prevention of coronary heart disease. JAMA. 2002 Nov 27;288(20):2569-78.

126 Food and Agriculture Organization, World Health Organization. Fats and fatty acids in human nutrition. Ann Nutr Metab. 2009;55: 1-308.

127 Appel LJ, Sacks FM, Carey VJ, et al; OmniHeart Collaborative Research Group. Effects of protein, monounsaturated fat, and carbohydrate intake on blood pressure and serum lipids: results of the OmniHeart-randomized trial. JAMA. 2005;294(19):2455-2464.

128 Estruch R, Ros E, Salas-Salvadó J, et al; PREDIMED Study Investigators. Primary prevention of cadiovascular disease with a Mediterranean diet. N Engl J Med. 2013;368(14):1279-1290.

129 Scientific Report of the 2015 Dietary Guidelines Advisory Committee. Advisory Report to the Secretary of Health and Human Services and the Secretary of Agriculture, p.2; http://www.health.gov/di etaryguidelines/2015-scientific-report/

130 Hu FB. Are refined carbohydrates worse than saturated fat? Am J Clin Nutr. 2010; 91:1541-1542.

131 Ludwig DS. Lowering the Bar on the Low-Fat Diet. JAMA. Published online September 28, 2016. doi:10.1001/jama.2016.15473

132 Mozaffarian D, Micha R, Wallace S. Effects on coronary heart disease of increasing polyunsaturatedfat in place of saturated fat: A systematic review and meta-analysis of randomized controlled trial. PLoS Med. 2010;7; e1000252.

133 Pritikin N, McGrady PM. Pritikin Program for Diet and Exercise. New York, Bantam Books: 1980.

134 Ornish D, Brown SE, Scherwitz LW, et al. Can lifestyle changes reverse coronary heart disease? Lancet. 1990;336:129-133.

135 Esselstyn CB Jr. Resolving the coronary artery disease epidemic through plant-based nutrition. Prev-Cardiol. 2007;4:171-177.

136 Scientific Report of the 2015 Dietary Guidelines Advisory Committee. Advisory Report to the Secretary of Health and Human Services and the Secretary of Agriculture http://www.health.gov/dietaryguidelines/2015-scientific-report/

137 Saturated Fat. American Heart Association. Accessed 8/6/2015 at http://www.heart.org/HEARTORG/GettingHealthy/NutritionCenter/HealthyEating/Saturated-Fats_UCM_301110_Article.jsp

138 Hu FB, Stampfer MJ, Manson JE, Ascherio A, Colditz GA, Speizer FE, Hennekens CH, Willett WC. Dietary saturated fats and their food sources in relation to the risk of coronary heart disease in women. Am JClin Nutr. 1999;70:1001–8.

139 Hooper L, Summerbell CD, Thompson R, Sills D, Roberts FG, Moore HJ, et al. Reduced or modified dietary fat for preventing cardiovascular disease. Cochrane Database Syst Rev. 2012;5:CD002137. PMID: 22592684. http://www.ncbi.nlm.nih.gov/pubmed/22592684.

140 Guasch-Ferr. M, Babio N, Mart.nez-Gonz.lez MA, et al. Dietary fat intake and risk of cardiovascular disease and all-cause mortality in a population at high risk of cardiovascular disease. Am J Clin Nutr. 2015;

102: 1563–73.

141 de Souza RJ, Mente A, Maroleanu A, et al. Intake of saturated and trans unsaturated fatty acids and risk of all cause mortality, cardiovascular disease, and type 2 diabetes: systematic review and meta-analysis of observational studies. BMJ. 2015; 351: h3978.

142 Jakobsen MU, O'Reilly EJ, Heitmann BL, Pereira MA, Bälter K, Fraser GE, et al. Major types of dietary fat and risk of coronary heart disease: a pooled analysis of 11 cohort studies. Am J Clin Nutr. 2009;89(5):1425-32. PMID: 19211817.

143 Farvid MS, Ding M, Pan A, Sun Q, Chiuve SE, Steffen LM, et al. Dietary Linoleic Acid and Risk of Coronary Heart Disease: A Systematic Review and Meta-Analysis of Prospective Cohort Studies. Circulation. 2014. PMID: 25161045. 1284 http://www.ncbi.nlm.nih.gov/pubmed/25161045.

144 Siri-Tarino PW, Sun Q, Hu FB, Krauss RM. Meta-analysis of prospective cohort studies evaluating the association of saturated fat with cardiovascular disease. Am J Clin Nutr. 2010;91:502–509.

145 Mozaffarian D, Micha R, Wallace S (2010) Effects on Coronary Heart Disease of Increasing Polyu saturated Fat in Place of Saturated Fat: A Systematic Review and Meta-Analysis of Randomized Controlled Trials. PLoS Med. 7(3): e1000252. doi:10.1371/journal.pmed.1000252

146 Mozaffarian D, Micha R, Wallace S (2010) Effects on Coronary Heart Disease of Increasing Polyunsaturated Fat in Place of Saturated Fat: A Systematic Review and Meta-Analysis of Randomized Controlled Trials. PLoS Med. 7(3): e1000252. doi:10.1371/journal.pmed.1000252

147 Hooper L, Martin N, Abdelhamid A, Davey Smith G. Reduction in saturated fat intake for cardiovascular disease. Cochrane Database Syst Rev. 2015; 6: CD011737

148 Li Y, Hruby A, Bernstein AM, Ley SH, Wang DD, Chiuve SE, Sampson L, Rexrode KM, Rimm EB, Willett WC, Hu FB. Saturated Fats Compared With Unsaturated Fats and Sources of Carbohydrates in Relation to Risk of Coronary Heart Disease: A Prospective Cohort Study. J Am Coll Cardiol. 2015;66(14):1538-48. doi: 10.1016/j.jacc.2015.07.055.

149 Bell GA, Kantor ED, Lampe JW, Kristal AR, Heckbert SR, White E. Intake of long-chain ω-3 fattyacids from diet and supplements in relation to mortality. Am J Epidemiol. 2014;179(6):710-720.

150 Willett WC, Yu FB. Optimal diets for prevention of coronary heart disease. JAMA. 2002 Nov 27;288(20):2569-78.

151 Avanzini F, Caimi V, Longoni P, Marchioli R, Roncaglioni MC et al. Risk and Prevention Study Collaborative Group. n-3 fatty acids in patients with multiple cardiovascular risk factors. N Engl J Med. 2013 May 9;368(19):1800-8. doi: 10.1056/NEJMoa1205409.

152 Lee JH, O'Keefe JH, Lavie CJ, Marchioli R, Harris WS. Omega-3 fatty acids for cardioprotection. Mayo Clin Proc. 2008;83:324–32.

153 Hooper L, Thompson RL, Harrison RA, et al. Risks and benefits of omega 3 fats for mortality, cardiovascular disease, and cancer: systematic review. BMJ. 2006;332:752–60.

154 von Schacky C, Harris WS. Cardiovascular benefits of omega-3 fatty acids. Cardiovasc Res. 2007;73:310–5.

155 Hu FB, Bronner L, Willett WC, Stampfer MJ, Rexrode KM, Albert CM, Hunter D, Manson JE: Fish and omega-3 fatty acid intake and risk of coronary heart disease in women. JAMA 2002, 287(14):1815–1821.

156 Greene J, Ashburn SM, Razzouk L, Smith DA. Fish Oils, Coronary Heart Disease, and the Environment. AJPH. 2013;103(9):1568-1576. doi: 10.2105/AJPH.2012.300959

157 Aung T, Halsey J, Kromhout D, et al. Associations of Omega-3 Fatty Acid Supplement Use With Cardiovascular Disease RisksMeta-analysis of 10 Trials Involving 77 917 Individuals. JAMA Cardiol. 2018;3(3):225–234. doi:10.1001/jamacardio.2017.5205.

158 Balk EM, Adam GP, Langberg V, Halladay C, Chung M, Lin L, Robertson S, Yip A, Steele D, Smith BT, Lau J, Lichtenstein AH, Trikalinos TA. Omega-3 Fatty Acids and Cardiovascular Disease: An Updated Systematic Review. Evidence Report/Technology Assessment No. 223. (Prepared by the Brown Evidence-based Practice Center under Contract No. 290-2012-00012-I.) AHRQ Publication No. 16-E002-EF. Rockville, MD: Agency for Healthcare Research and Quality; August 2016. www.effectivehealthcare.ahrq.gov/reports/final.cfm. DOI: https://doi.org/10.23970/ AHRQEPCERTA223.

159 Abdelhamid AS, Brown TJ, Brainard JS, et al. Omega-3 fatty acids for the primary and secondary prevention of cardiovascular disease. Cochrane Database of Systematic Reviews 2018, Issue 7. Art. No.: CD003177. DOI: 10.1002/14651858.CD003177.pub3

160 Manson JE, Cook NR, Lee I-M, et al. Marine n–3 fatty acids and prevention of cardiovascular disease and cancer. N Engl J Med. DOI: 10.1056/NEJMoa1811403.

161 Hu Y, Hu FB, Manson JE. Marine Omega–3 Supplementation and Cardiovascular Disease: An Updated Meta–Analysis of 13 Randomized Controlled Trials Involving 127 477 Participants. J Am Heart Assn. 2019;8(19):e013543. https://doi.org/10.1161/JAHA.119.013543

162 Willett WC. The Great Fat Debate: Total fat and health. J Am Diet Assoc. 2011;111:660-662.

163 Skeaff CM, Miller J. Dietary fat and coronary heart disease: summary of evidence from prospective cohort and randomised controlled trials. Ann Nutr Metab. 2009;55(1-3):173-201. PMID: 19752542. http://www.ncbi.nlm.nih.gov/pubmed/19752542.

164 Siri-Tarino PW, Sun Q, Hu FB, Krauss RM. Meta-analysis of prospective cohort studies evaluating the association of saturated fat with cardiovascular disease. Am J Clin Nutr. 2010;91(3):535-46. PMID: 20071648. http://www.ncbi.nlm.nih.gov/pubmed/20071648.

165 de Souza RJ, Mente A, Maroleanu A, et al. Intake of saturated and transunsaturated fatty acids and risk of all cause mortality, cardiovascular disease, and type 2 diabetes: systematic review and meta-analysis of observational studies. BMJ. 2015; 351: h3978.

166 Chowdhury R, Warnakula S, Kunutsor S, Crowe 1277 F, Ward HA, Johnson L, et al. Association of dietary, circulating, and supplement fatty acids with coronary risk: a systematic review and meta-analysis. Ann Intern Med. 2014;160(6):398-406. PMID:24723079. http://www.ncbi.nlm.nih.gov/pubmed/24723079.

167 The end of the debate? Fat chance. The University of California, Berkeley Wellness Letter. 30;13 July 2014.

168 Mann J, Morenga LT, McLean R, Swinburn B, Mhurchu CN, Jackson R, Kennedy J, Beaglehole R. Dietary guidelines on trial: the charges are not evidence based. Lancet. 2016;388:851-852.

169 de Souza RJ, Mente A, Maroleanu A, et al. Intake of saturated and transunsaturated fatty acids and risk of all cause mortality, cardiovascular disease, and type 2 diabetes: systematic review and meta-analysis of observational studies. BMJ. 2015; 351: h3978.

170 Willett W, Skerrett PJ. Eat, Drink, and Be Healthy. New York: Free Press/ Simon & Schuster; 2017 ISBN13: 9781501164774

171 Rimm E. Harvard Public Health. Winter 2019:8-9.

172 Barnard ND, Willett WC, Ding EL. The Misuse of Meta-analysis in Nutrition Research. JAMA. Published online September 18, 2017. doi:10.1001/jama.2017.12083

173 Wallström P, Sonestedt E, Hlebowicz J, et al. Dietary fiber and saturated fat intake associations with cardiovascular disease differ by sex in the Malmö Diet and Cancer cohort: a prospective study. PLoS One. 2012;7(2):e31637.

174 Appleby PN, Thorogood M, Mann JI, Key TJA. The Oxford Vegetarian Study: an overview. Am J Clin Nutr. 1999;70(3)(suppl):525S-531S.

175 Wang DD, Li Y, Chiuve SE, Stampfer MJ, Manson JE, Rimm EB, Willett WC, Hu FB. Association of

Specific Dietary Fats With Total and Cause-Specific Mortality. JAMA Intern Med. 2016;176(8):1134-1145. doi:10.1001/jamainternmed.2016.2417.

176 Saturated Fat. American Heart Association. Accessed at: http://www.heart.org/HEARTORG/Getting-Healthy/NutritionCenter/HealthyEating/Saturated-Fats_UCM_301110_Article.jsp

177 Li Y, Hruby A, Bernstein AM, Ley SH, Wang DD, Chiuve SE, Sampson L, Rexrode KM, Rimm EB, Willett WC, Hu FB. Saturated Fats Compared With Unsaturated Fats and Sources of Carbohydrates in Relation to Risk of Coronary Heart Disease: A Prospective Cohort Study. J Am Coll Cardiol. 2015;66(14):1538-48. doi: 10.1016/j.jacc.2015.07.055.

178 2015-2020 Dietary Guidelines for Americans. https://health.gov/dietaryguidelines/2015/

179 Mozaffarian D. Nutrition and cardiovascular disease and metabolic diseases. In: Mann DL, Zipes DP, Libby P, Bonow RO, eds. Braunwald's Heart Disease: A Textbook of Cardiovascular Medicine. 10th ed. Philadelphia, PA: Elsevier/Saunders; 2014.

180 Levin S, Wells C, Barnard N. Dietary Cholesterol and Blood Cholesterol Concentrations. JAMA.2015;314(19):2083-2084. doi:10.1001/jama.2015.12595

181 Berger S, Raman G, Vishwanathan R, Jacques PF, Johnson EJ. Dietary cholesterol and cardiovascular disease: a systematic review and meta-analysis. Am J Clin Nutr. 2015;102(2):276-294.

182 Fuller NR, Sainsbury A, Caterson ID, Markovic TP. Egg Consumption and Human Cardio-Metabolic Health in People with and without Diabetes. Nutrients. 2015;7(9):7399-420. Epub 2015 Sep 3.

183 Mozaffarian D, Ludwig DS. Dietary Cholesterol and Blood Cholesterol Concentrations—Reply. JAMA.2015;314(19):2084-2085. doi:10.1001/jama.2015.12604

184 Dehghan M, Mente A, Rangarajan S, et al., on behalf of the PURE investigators, Association of egg intake with blood lipids, cardiovascular disease, and mortality in 177,000 people in 50 countries,. A J Clin-Nutrition, , nqz348, https://doi.org/10.1093/ajcn/nqz348

185 Astrup A. Goodbye to the egg-white omelet—welcome back to the whole-egg omelet. A J Clin Nutrtion, 2018;107(6):853–854, https://doi.org/10.1093/ajcn/nqy106

186 Choi Y, Chang Y, Lee JE, et al. Egg consumption and coronary artery calcification in asymptomatic men and women. Atherosclerosis. 2015 Aug;241(2):305-12. doi: 10.1016/j.atherosclerosis.2015.05.036. Epub 2015 Jun 3.

187 Zhong VW, Van Horn L, Cornelis MC, et al. Associations of Dietary Cholesterol or Egg Consumption With Incident Cardiovascular Disease and Mortality. JAMA. 2019;321(11):1081–1095. doi:10.1001/jama.2019.1572

188 Drouin-Chartier J-P, Chen S, Li Y, Schwab AL, et al. Egg consumption and risk of cardiovascular disease: three large prospective US cohort studies, systematic review, and updated meta-analysis BMJ 2020;368:m513. doi: https://doi.org/10.1136/bmj.m513

189 2015-2020 Dietary Guidelines for Americans. https://health.gov/dietaryguidelines/2015/

190 U.S. News, Best Diets Rankings for 2020. https://health.usnews.com/best-diet

191 The best (and worst) diets of 2018. University of California, Berkeley Wellness Letter. April 2018.

192 Pontzer, Wood BM, Raichlen. Hunter-gatherers as models in public health. Obesity Reviews. 2018;19(S1):24-35. https://doi.org/10.1111/obr.12785

193 Scientific Report of the 2015 Dietary Guidelines Advisory Committee. Advisory Report to the Secretary of Health and Human Services and the Secretary of Agriculture. http://www.health.gov/dietaryguidelines/2015-scientific-report/

194 Scientific Report of the 2015 Dietary Guidelines Advisory Committee. Advisory Report to the Secretary of Health and Human Services and the Secretary of Agriculture.

http://www.health.gov/dietaryguidelines/2015-scientific-report/

195 Katz DL, Meller S. Can We Say What Diet Is Best for Health?. Annu. Rev. Public Health. 2014. 35:83-103

196 Katz DL, Meller S. Can We Say What Diet Is Best for Health?. Annu. Rev. Public Health. 2014. 35:83–103

197 Hu FB. Plant-based foods and prevention of cardiovascular disease: an overview. Am J Clin Nutr. 2003;78(suppl):544S–51S.

198 Craig WJ, Mangels AR. Position of the American Dietetic Association: vegetarian diets. J Am Diet Assoc. 2009;109:1266 –1282.

199 Scientific Report of the 2015 Dietary Guidelines Advisory Committee. Advisory Report to the Secretary of Health and Human Services and the Secretary of Agriculture http://www.health.gov/dietaryguidelines/2015-scientific-report/

200 Key TJ, Fraser GE, Thorogood M, et al. Mortality in vegetarians and non-vegetarians: a collaborative analysis of 8300 deaths among 76,000 men and women in five prospective studies. Public Health Nutr. 1998;1:33– 41.

201 Viguiliouk E, et al., Effect of vegetarian dietary patterns on cardiometabolic risk factors in diabetes: A systematic review and meta-analysis of randomized controlled trials, Clinical Nutrition. 2018. https://doi.org/10.1016/j.clnu.2018.05.032

202 Wang F, Zheng J, Yang B, Jiang J, Fu Y, Li D. Effects of vegetarian diets on blood lipids: a systematic review and meta-analysis of randomized controlled trials. J Am Heart Assoc 2015;4(10):e002408.

203 Song M, Fung TT, Hu FB, et al. Association of Animal and Plant Protein Intake With All-Cause and Cause-Specific Mortality. JAMA Intern Med. 2016;176(10):1453–1463. doi:10.1001/jamainternmed.2016.4182

204 Campbell TC, Campbell TM, The China Study. Dallas, Benbella Books: 2006

205 Willcox BJ, Willcox DC, Suzuki M. The Okinawa Diet Plan. New York, Clarkson Potter: 2004.

206 McMurry MP, Cerqueira MT, Connor SL, Connor WE. Changes in Lipid and Lipoprotein Levels and Body Weight in Tarahumara Indians after Consumption of an Affluent Diet. N Engl J Med. 1991; 325:1704-1708December 12, 1991DOI: 10.1056/NEJM199112123252405

207 Fraser GE. Associations between diet and cancer, ischemic heart disease, and all-cause mortality in non-Hispanic white California Seventh-day Adventists. Am J Clin Nutr. 1999;70:532S–538S.

208 Hu FB. Plant-based foods and prevention of cardiovascular disease: an overview. Am J Clin Nutr. 2003;78(suppl):544S–51S.

209 Huang T, Yang B, Zheng J, Li G, Wahlqvist ML, Li D. Cardiovascular disease mortality and cancer incidence in vegetarians: a meta-analysis and systematic review. Ann Nutr Metab. 2012;60(4):233-40. PMID: 22677895.1749 http://www.ncbi.nlm.nih.gov/pubmed/22677895.

210 Appleby PN, Thorogood M, Mann JI, Key TJ. The Oxford Vegetarian Study: an overview. Am J Clin Nutr. 1999;70(3 Suppl):525S-531S.

211 Bellavia A1, Larsson SC, Bottai M, Wolk A, Orsini N. Fruit and vegetable consumption and all-cause mortality: a dose-response analysis. Am J Clin Nutr. 2013;98(2):454-9. doi: 10.3945/ajcn.112.056119. Epub 2013 Jun 26.

212 Swartzberg J, Making the case for fruit, If you eat your veggies can you skip the fruit? University of-California, Berkeley Wellness Letter. October 2014; 31:1,1-2

213 Du H, Li L, Bennett D, et al. Fresh fruit consumption and major cardiovascular disease in China. N Engl J Med. 2016;374:1332-1343.

214 Najjar RS, Moore CE, Montgomery BD. A defined, plant–based diet utilized in an outpatient cardiovascular clinic effectively treats hypercholesterolemia and hypertension and reduces medications. Clin Cardiol. 2018;41:307–313. https://doi.org/10.1002/clc.22863

215 Kahleova, H., Levin, S.M., & Barnard, N.D. Vegetarian Dietary Patterns and Cardiovascular Disease. Progress in cardiovascular diseases. 2018(611): 54-61.

216 Craig WJ, Mangels AR. Position of the American Dietetic Association: vegetarian diets. J Am Diet Assoc. 2009;109:1266 –1282.

217 Wong K. Rise of the Human Predator. Scientific American. April, 2014. p. 46-51.

218 Satija A, Shilpa N. Bhupathiraju SN, Spiegelman D, et al. Healthful and Unhealthful Plant-Based Diets and the Risk of Coronary Heart Disease in U.S. Adults. J Am College Cardiology. 2017;70(4):411-422.

219 Willett WC, Stampfer MJ. Rebuilding the Food Pyramid, Scientific American. January 2003, 64-71.

220 World Health Organization. Healthy diet. Fact sheet N°394 Updated September 2015; http://www.who.int/mediacentre/factsheets/fs394/en/

221 Pritikin N, McGrady PM. Pritikin Program for Diet and Exercise. New York, Bantam Books: 1980

222 Ornish D, Brown SE, Scherwitz LW, et al. Can lifestyle changes reverse coronary heart disease? Lancet. 1990;336:129-133.

223 Esselstyn CB Jr. Resolving the coronary artery disease epidemic through plant-based nutrition. Prev Cardiol. 2007;4:171-177.

224 Connor WE, Connor SL, The Case for a Low-Fat High-Carbohydrate Diet, Should a Low-Fat High-Carbohydrate Diet Be Recommended for Everyone? N Engl J Med 1997;337:562-563

225 McDougall J, Litzau K, Haver E, Saunders V, Spiller GA. Rapid reduction of serum cholesterol and blood pressure by a twelve-day, very low-fat, strictly vegetarian diet. J Am Coll Nutr. 1995;14:491-496.

226 McDougall J. The McDougall Program for a Healthy Heart, Dutton, Boston,1996.

227 Fuhrman J. Eat to Live. New York. Little, Brown and Company. 2011

228 Barnard N. Physician's Committee for Responsible Medicine. Every Meal PowerPlate. http://www.pcrm.org/sites/default/files/images/health/pplate/EveryMealPowerPlate.pdf

229 Barnard N. Physician's Committee for Responsible Medicine. Healthy Eating for Life. http://www.pcrm.org/sites/default/files/pdfs/health/HealthyEatingforLife.pdf

230 Barnard N. Physician's Committee for Responsible Medicine. Cholesterol and Heart Disease. http://www.pcrm.org/sites/default/files/pdfs/health/chol_heartdisease.pdf

231 Campbell TC, Campbell TM, The China Study. Dallas, Benbella Books: 2006

232 Jenkins DJ, Kendall CW, Popovich DG, et al. Effect of a very-high-fiber vegetable, fruit and nut diet on serum lipids and colonic function. Metabolism 2001;(4):494-503.

233 Greger, M, Stone G. How Not to Die. New York, Flatiorn Books, 2015.

234 Shintani TT, Beckham S, Brown AC, O'Connor HK. The Hawaii Diet: ad libitum high carbohydrate, low-fat multi-cultural diet for the reduction of chronic disease risk factors: obesity, hypertension, hypercholesterolemia, and hyperglycemia. Hawaii Med J. 2001;60(3):69-73.

235 Esselstyn CB. Prevent and Reverse Heart Disease. New York, Penguin Group, 2007.

236 Ornish D, The Spectrum. New York, Ballantine Books: 2007.

237 McDougall JA, McDougall MA, The McDougall Plan. Clinton NJ, New Win Publishing, 1983, p. 89

238 Wang DD, Li Y, Chiuve SE, et al. Association of Specific Dietary Fats With Total and Cause-Specific Mortality JAMA Intern Med. 2016;176(8):1134-1145. doi:10.1001/jamainternmed.2016.2417

239 Campbell TC, Campbell TM. The China Study. Dallas, Benbella Books: 2006

240 Buttner D. The Blue Zones, Second Edition. Washington DC, National Geographic, 2012

241 A Recipe For Longevity? Beans, Friends, Purpose And Movement. Here and Now. https://hereandnow.wbur.org/2015/08/26/blue-zones-recipe-for-longevity

242 Fraser GE. Associations between diet and cancer, ischemic heart disease, and all-cause mortality in non-Hispanic white California Seventh-day Adventists. Am J Clin Nutr. 1999;70:532S–538S.

243 McMurry MP, Cerqueira MT, Connor SL, Connor WE. Changes in Lipid and Lipoprotein Levels and Body Weight in Tarahumara Indians after Consumption of an Affluent Diet. N Engl J Med. 1991;325:1704-1708December 12, 1991DOI: 10.1056/NEJM199112123252405.

244 Mortality Trends. Trends in national mortality rates. Mortality Trends. http://www.mortality-trends.org

245 Shimazu T, Kuriyama S, Hozawa A, Ohmori K, Sato Y, Nakaya N, Nishino Y, Tsubono Y, Tsuji I. Dietary patterns and cardiovascular disease mortality in Japan: a prospective cohort study. Int J Epidemiol. m2007;36:600–609.

246 Mozaffarian D, Appel LJ, Van Horn L. Components of a Cardioprotective Diet: New Insights. Circ lation. 2011;123:2870-2891. DOI: 10.1161/CIRCULATION AHA.110.968735

247 Willcox BJ, Willcox DC, Suzuki M. The Okinawa Diet Plan. New York, Clarkson Potter: 2004

248 Willcox DC, Willcox BJ, Todoriki H, Suzuki M. The Okinawan diet: health implications of a low-caloric, nutrient-dense, antioxidant-rich dietary pattern low in glycemic load. J Am Coll Nutr. 2009;28(suppl): 500S–516S.

249 Ornish D. Lifestyle Medicine Cardiobuzz. A MedPage Today Blog July 31, 2014

250 Moss M, Salt Sugar Fat. New York. Random House. 2013.

251 Ornish D, Brown SE, Scherwitz LW, et al. Can lifestyle changes reverse coronary heart disease? Lancet. 1990;336:129-133.

252 Esselstyn CB. Prevent and Reverse Heart Disease. New York, Penguin Group, 2007. p 61-62

253 Ornish D, The Spectrum. New York, Ballantine Books: 2007. p 51-52.

254 Ornish D. Dr. Dean Ornish's Program for Reversing Heart Disease. New York: Ballantine Books, 1990.

255 Ornish D, for the Multicenter Lifestyle Demonstration Project Research Group. Avoiding revascularization with lifestyle changes: the Multicenter Lifestyle Demonstration Project. Am J Cardiol 1998;82:72T–76T.

256 Ornish D. The Spectrum. New York, Ballantine Books: 2007. P. 210

257 Lustig RH, Schmidt LA, Brindis CD. The toxic truth about sugar. Nature. 2012;482:27-29.

258 Ornish D. The Spectrum. New York, Ballantine Books: 2007 and http://ornishspectrum.com/proven-program/nutrition/

259 Ornish D, Brown SE, Scherwitz LW, et al. Can lifestyle changes reverse coronary heart disease? Lancet. 1990;336:129-133.

260 Ornish D, Scherwitz LW, Billings JH, et al. Intensive Lifestyle Changes for Reversal of Coronary Heart Disease. JAMA. December 16, 1998—Vol 280, No. 23 2001-2007

261 Ornish D, Brown SE, Scherwitz LW, et al. Can lifestyle changes reverse coronary heart disease? Lancet. 1990;336:129-133.

262 Gould KL, Ornish D, Scherwitz L, et al. Changes in myocardial perfusion abnormalities by positron emission tomography after long-term, intense risk factor modification. JAMA. 1995; 274:894-901.

263 Ornish D. Avoiding revascularization with lifestyle changes: The Multicenter Lifestyle Demonstration Project. Am J Cardiol. 1998;82(10B):72T-76T. DOI: 10.1016/S0002-9149(98)00744-9.

264 Silberman A1, Banthia R, Estay IS, Kemp C, Studley J, Hareras D, Ornish D. The effectiveness and efficacy of an intensive cardiac rehabilitation program in 24 sites. Am J Health Promot. 2010;24(4):260-6. doi: 10.4278/ajhp.24.4.arb.

265 Moyer MW, Ornish D. Why Almost Everything Dean Ornish Says about Nutrition Is Wrong. UPDATED: With Dean Ornish's Response. June 1, 2015 Scientific American

266 Ornish D, Scherwitz LW, Billings JH, et al. Intensive lifestyle changes for reversal of coronary heart-disease. JAMA. 1998;280: 2001-7 Medline. [Erratum, JAMA 1999;281:1380.]

267 Gould KL, Ornish D, Scherwitz L, et al. Changes in myocardial perfusion abnormalities by positron emission tomography after long-term, intense risk factor modification. JAMA. 1995; 274:894-901.

268 Ornish DM, Brown SE, Scherwitz LW, et al. Can lifestyle changes reverse coronary heart disease? The Lifestyle Heart Trial. Lancet. 1990;336:129-33.

269 Daubenmier JJ, Weidner G, Sumner MD, Mendell N, Merritt-Worden T, Studley J, Ornish D.The contribution of changes in diet, exercise, and stress management to changes in coronary risk in women and men in the multisite cardiac lifestyle intervention program. Ann Behav Med. 2007;33(1):57-68.

270 Moyer MW, Ornish D. Why Almost Everything Dean Ornish Says about Nutrition Is Wrong. UPDATED: With Dean Ornish's Response. June 1, 2015 Scientific American.

271 Esselstyn CB. Prevent and Reverse Heart Disease. New York, Penguin Group, 2007.

272 Esselstyn, CB. Resolving the Coronary Artery Disease Epidemic Through Plant-Based Nutrition. Preventive Cardiology. 2001;4, 171-177.

273 Esselstyn CB. Updating a 12-year experience with arrest and reversal therapy for coronary heart disease (an overdue requiem for palliative cardiology). Am J Cardiol. 1999;84:339-341.

274 Shintani TT, Beckham S, Brown AC, O'Connor HK. The Hawaii Diet: ad libitum high carbohydrate, low-fat multi-cultural diet for the reduction of chronic disease risk factors: obesity, hypertension, hyperch lesterolemia, and hyperglycemia. Hawaii Med J. 2001;60(3):69-73.

275 Speidel JJ, Weltman A, North TC, Brenton JT, and Melcher GW. Cardiovascular Diseases - Prevention and Treatment. Rocky Mountain Medical Journal, a supplement to Colorado Medicine. 1982;Scientific Section: 49-53.

276 Advocating for avocados. University of California, Berkeley Wellness Letter. July 2015;31(12):1-2.

277 Mayhew AJ, de Souza RJ, Meyre D, et al. A systematic review and meta-analysis of nut consumption and incident risk of CVD and all-cause mortality. Br J Nutr. 2016;115:212–25.

278 Grosso G, Yang J, Marventano S, et al. Nut consumption on all-cause, cardiovascular, and cancer mortality risk: a systematic review and meta-analysis of epidemiologic studies. Am J Clin Nutr. 2015;101:783–93.

279 van den Brandt PA, Schouten LJ. Relationship of tree nut, peanut and peanut butter intake with total and cause-specific mortality: a cohort study and meta-analysis, International Journal of Epidemiology. 2015;44(3):1038–1049. https://doi.org/10.1093/ije/dyv039

280 Aune D, Keum N, Giovannucci E, et al. Nut consumption and risk of cardiovascular disease, totalcancer, all-cause and cause-specific mortality: a systematic review and dose-response meta-analysis of prospective studies. BMC Med. 2016;14:207.

281 Larsson SC, Drca N, Björck M, et al. Nut consumption and incidence of seven cardiovascular diseases. Heart. Published Online First: 16 April 2018. doi: 10.1136/heartjnl-2017-312819

282 A Recipe For Longevity? Beans, Friends, Purpose And Movement. Here and Now. https://hereandnow.

wbur.org/2015/08/26/blue-zones-recipe-for-longevity

283 Katz DL, Meller S. Can We Say What Diet Is Best for Health? Annu. Rev. Public Health. 2014;35:83-103.

284 I'll have what Olaf is having. University of California, Berkeley Wellness Letter. June 2014.

285 Serra-Majem L, Roman B, Estruch R. Scientific evidence of interventions using the Mediterranean diet: a systematic review. Nutr. Rev. 2006:64:S27–47

286 Sofi F, Abbate R, Gensini GF, Casini A. Accruing evidence about benefits of adherence to the Mediterranean diet on health: an updated systematic review and meta-analysis. Am J Clin Nutr. 2010;92:1189–1196.

287 Estruch R, Ros E, Salas-Salvado′ J, Covas MI, Corella D, Aro′ s F, et al. PREDIMED Study Investigators. Primary prevention of cardiovascular disease with a Mediterranean diet. N Engl J Med. 2013;368:1279-90. [PMID: 23432189] doi:10.1056/NEJMoa1200303

288 Serra-Majem L, Roman B, Estruch R. 2006. Scientific evidence of interventions using the Mediterranean diet: a systematic review. Nutr. Rev. 64:S27–47

289 de Lorgeril M, Salen P. Mediterranean diet in secondary prevention of coronary heart disease. Clin Invest Med. 2006;29(3):154-158

290 de Lorgeril M, Salen P, Martin JL, Monjaud I, Delaye J, Mamelle N. 1999. Mediterranean diet, traditional risk factors, and the rate of cardiovascular complications after myocardial infarction: final report of the Lyon Diet Heart Study. Circulation. 99:779–85

291 Wengreen H, Munger RG, Cutler A, et al. Prospective study of Dietary Approaches to Stop Hypertension–and Mediterranean-style dietary patterns and age-related cognitive change: the Cache County Study on Memory, Health and Aging. Am J Clin Nutr. 2013;98:1263–71.

292 Samieri C, Sun Q, MD, Townsend MK, et al. The Association Between Dietary Patterns at Midlife and Health in Aging: An Observational Study. Ann Intern Med. 2013;159(9):584-591. doi:10.7326/0003- 4819-159-9-201311050-00004

293 Chiuve SE, Fung TT, Rexrode KM, Spiegelman D, Manson JE, Stampfer MJ, Albert CM. Adherence to a Low-Risk, Healthy Lifestyle and Risk of Sudden Cardiac Death Among Women. JAMA. 2011;306(1):62-69. doi:10.1001/jama.2011.907

294 Mitrou PN, Kipnis V, Thiebaut AC, Reedy J, Subar AF, Wirfalt E, Flood A, Mouw T, Hollenbeck AR, Leitzmann MF, et al. Mediterranean dietary pattern and prediction of all-cause mortality in a US population: results from the NIH-AARP Diet and Health Study. Arch Intern Med. 2007;167:2461–8.

295 van den Brandt PA. The impact of a Mediterranean diet and healthy lifestyle on premature mortality in men and women. Am J Clin Nutr. doi: 2011, 10.3945/ajcn.110. 008250.

296 Estruch R, Ros E, Salas-Salvado J, et al. Primary prevention of cardiovascular disease with a Mediterranean diet. N Engl J Med. 2013;368:1279-90.

297 Ornish D, Mediterranean Diet for Primary Prevention of Cardiovascular Disease, Correspondence. N Engl J Med. 2013; 369;7. 675-676. DOI: 10.1056/NEJMc1306659

298 Ruiz-Canela M, Estruch R, Corella D, Salas-Salvadó J, Martínez-González MA. Association of Mediterranean Diet With Peripheral Artery Disease The PREDIMED Randomized Trial. JAMA. 2014;311(4):415-417. doi:10.1001/jama.2013.280618.

299 Li Y, Hruby A, Bernstein AM, Ley SH, Wang DD, Chiuve SE, Sampson L, Rexrode KM, Rimm EB, Willett WC, Hu FB. Saturated Fats Compared With Unsaturated Fats and Sources of Carbohydrates in Relation to Risk of Coronary Heart Disease. J Am Coll Cardiol. 2015;66(14):1538-1548. doi:10.1016/j.jacc.2015.07.055

300 Bloomfield HE, Koeller E, Greer N, MacDonald R, Kane R, Wilt TJ. Effects on health outcomes of

a Mediterranean Diet with no restriction on fat intake: a systematic review and meta-analysis. Ann Intern Med. 2016; published online 2016 July 19. DOI:10.7326/M16-0361.

301 Esselstyn CB. Prevent and Reverse Heart Disease. New York, Penguin Group, 2007.

302 Katz DL, Meller S. Can We Say What Diet Is Best for Health?. Annu. Rev. Public Health 2014. 35:83-103.

303 Natl. Heart Lung Blood Inst. 2012. What is the DASH eating plan? Updated July 2. NHLBI, Bethesda, Md. http://www.nhlbi.nih.gov/health/health-topics/topics/dash/

304 Blumenthal JA, Babyak MA, Hinderliter A, Watkins LL, Craighead L, et al. Effects of the DASH diet alone and in combination with exercise and weight loss on blood pressure and cardiovascular biomarkers in men and women with high blood pressure: the ENCORE study. Arch. Intern. Med. 2010;170:126–35.

305 Miller ER 3rd, Erlinger TP, Appel LJ. The effects of macronutrients on blood pressure and lipids: an overview of the DASH and OmniHeart trials. Curr Atheroscler Rep. 2006;8:460–465.

306 OmniHeart Diets Provide More Options for Heart Health http://www.health.harvard.edu/PDFs/Omni-Diets.pdf

307 Natl. Heart Lung Blood Inst. 2012. What is the DASH eating plan? Updated July 2. NHLBI, Bethesda, Md. http://www.nhlbi.nih.gov/health/health-topics/topics/dash/

308 Blumenthal JA, Babyak MA, Hinderliter A, Watkins LL, Craighead L, et al. 2010. Effects of the DASH diet alone and in combination with exercise and weight loss on blood pressure and cardiovas-cularbiomarkers in men and women with high blood pressure: the ENCORE study. Arch. Intern. Med. 2010;170:126–35.

309 Miller ER 3rd, Erlinger TP, Appel LJ. The effects of macronutrients on blood pressure and lipids: an overview of the DASH and OmniHeart trials. Curr Atheroscler Rep. 2006;8:460–465.

310 Swain JF, McCarron PB, Hamilton EF, Sacks FM, Appel LJ. Characteristics of the diet patterns tested in the Optimal Macronutrient Intake Trial to Prevent Heart Disease (OmniHeart): options for a hearthealthy diet. J Am Diet Assoc. 2008;108:257–265.

311 Two more reasons to DASH. University of California, Berkeley Wellness Letter. December 2016.

312 Knowler WC, Barrett-Connor E, Fowler SE, Hamman RF, Lachin JM, et al. 2002. Reduction in the incidence of type 2 diabetes with lifestyle intervention or metformin. N. Engl. J. Med. 346:393–403.

313 Ludwig DS. The Glycemic Index: Physiological Mechanisms Relating to Obesity, Diabetes, and Car-diovascular Disease. JAMA. 2002;287(18):2414-2423. doi:10.1001/jama.287.18.2414.

314 http://nutritiondata.self.com/topics/glycemic-index

315 Ma XY, Liu JP, Song ZY. Glycemic load, glycemic index and risk of cardiovascular diseases: meta-analyses of prospective studies. Atherosclerosis. 2012;223:491–96

316 Goff LM, Cowland DE, Hooper L, Frost GS. Low glycaemic index diets and blood lipids: a systemat-ic review and meta-analysis of randomised controlled trials. Nutr Metab Cardiovasc Dis. 2013;23(1):1-10.

317 Ludwig DS. The Glycemic Index: Physiological Mechanisms Relating to Obesity, Diabetes, and Car-diovascular Disease. JAMA. 2002;287(18):2414-2423. doi:10.1001/jama.287.18.2414.

318 Katz DL, Meller S. Can We Say What Diet Is Best for Health?. Annu. Rev. Public Health 2014. 35:83-103.

319 Katz DL, Meller S. Can We Say What Diet Is Best for Health?. Annu. Rev. Public Health 2014. 35:83-103.

320 Mansoor, N., Vinknes, K.J., Veierød, M.B. and Retterstøl, K. Effects of low-carbohydrate diets v. low-fat diets on body weight and cardiovascular risk factors: a meta-analysis of randomised controlled trials. British Journal of Nutrition. 2016;115(3):466–479. doi:10.1017/S0007114515004699.

321 Smith SR. A Look at the Low-Carbohydrate Diet. N Engl J Med. 2009;361:2286-2288. DOI: 10.1056/NEJMcibr0908756.

322 Banach M. Low carbohydrate diets are unsafe and should be avoided. European Society of Cardiology. Https://www.eurekalert.org/pub_releases/2018-08/esoc-lcd082318.php

323 Jenkins DJ, Wong JM, Kendall CW, Esfahani A, Ng VW, et al. The effect of a plant-based low-carbohydrate ("Eco-Atkins") diet on body weight and blood lipid concentrations in hyperlipidemic subjects. Arch. Intern. Med. 2009;169:1046–54

324 Chiavaroli L, Nishi SK, Khan TA et al. Portfolio Dietary Pattern and Cardiovascular Disease: A Systematic Review and Meta-Analysis of Controlled Trials. Progress in Cardiovascular Diseases. 2018;61(1):43-53. doi: 10.1016/j.pcad.2018.05.004. Epub 2018 May 26.

325 Katz DL, Meller S. Can We Say What Diet Is Best for Health?. Annu. Rev. Public Health 2014. 35:83-103.

326 Whalen KA, Judd S, McCullough ML, Flanders WD, Hartman TJ, Bostick RM. Paleolithic and Mediterranean Diet Pattern Scores Are Inversely Associated with All-Cause and Cause-Specific Mortality in Adults. J Nutr. 2017;147(4):612–620. doi:10.3945/jn.116.241919

327 U.S. News, Best Diets Rankings for 2019. https://health.usnews.com/best-diet

328 Smith MM, Trexler ET, Sommer AJ, Starkoff BE, Devor ST. Unrestricted Paleolithic Diet is Associated with Unfavorable Changes to Blood Lipids in Healthy Subjects. Int J Exercise Sci. 2014; 7(2):128-139.

329 https://www. eurekalert.org/pub_releases/2018-08/esoc-lcd082318.php

330 Manheimer EW, van Zuuren EJ, Fedorowicz Z, Pijl H. Paleolithic nutrition for metabolic syndrome: systematic review and meta-analysis. Am J Clin Nutr. 2015;102(4):922–932. doi:10.3945/ajcn.115.113613

331 de Menezes EVA, Sampaio HAC, Carioca AAF, et al. Influence of Paleolithic diet on anthropometric markers in chronic diseases: systematic review and meta-analysis. Nutr J. 2019;18(1):41. Published 2019 Jul 23. doi:10.1186/s12937-019-0457-z

332 Whalen KA, Judd S, McCullough ML, Flanders WD, Hartman TJ, Bostick RM. Paleolithic and Mediterranean Diet Pattern Scores Are Inversely Associated with All-Cause and Cause-Specific Mortality in Adults. J Nutr. 2017;147(4):612–620. doi:10.3945/jn.116.241919

333 Katz DL, Meller S. Can We Say What Diet Is Best for Health? Annu. Rev. Public Health. 2014. 35:83-103.

334 Ketogenic diets: beyond the hype. University of Californa, Berkeley Wellness Letter. November 2018.

335 The best (and worst) diets of 2018. University of California, Berkeley Wellness Letter. April 2018.

336 Ornish D, Brown SE, Scherwitz LW, et al. Can lifestyle changes reverse coronary heart disease? Lancet. 1990;336:129-133.

337 Esselstyn CB Jr. Resolving the coronary artery disease epidemic through plant-based nutrition. Prev Cardiol. 2007;4:171-177.

338 Connor WE, Connor SL, The Case for a Low-Fat High-Carbohydrate Diet, Should a Low-Fat High-Carbohydrate Diet Be Recommended for Everyone? N Engl J Med. 1997;337:562-563 339 McDougall J, Litzau K, Haver E, Saunders V, Spiller GA. Rapid reduction of serum cholesterol and blood pressure by a twelve-day, very low-fat, strictly vegetarian diet. J Am Coll Nutr. 1995;14:491-496.

340 Fuhrman J, Eat to Live. New York, Little. Brown and Company: 2011

341 Ornish D, The Spectrum. New York, Ballantine Books: 2007 and http://ornishspectrum.com/proven-program/nutrition/

342 Daubenmier JJ, Weidner G, Sumner MD, Mendell N, Merritt-Worden T, Studley J, Ornish D. The contribution of changes in diet, exercise, and stress management to changes in coronary risk in women and

men in the multisite cardiac lifestyle intervention program. Ann Behav Med. 2007 Feb;33(1):57-68.

343 Dansinger ML, Gleason JA, Griffith JL, Selker HP, Schaefer EJ. Comparison of the Atkins, Ornish, Weight Watchers, and Zone Diets for Weight Loss and Heart Disease Risk ReductionA Randomized Trial. JAMA. 2005;293(1):43-53. doi:10.1001/jama.293.1.43.

344 Ornish D, The Spectrum. New York, Ballantine Books: 2007 and http://ornishspectrum.com/proven-program/nutrition/

345 Ornish D, The Spectrum. New York, Ballantine Books: 2007 and http://ornishspectrum.com/proven-program/nutrition/

346 Esselstyn CB. Prevent and Reverse Heart Disease. New York, Penguin Group, 2007. p 69

347 Esselstyn CB. Prevent and Reverse Heart Disease. New York, Penguin Group, 2007. p 69

348 Guideline: Sugars intake for adults and children. Geneva: World Health Organization; 2015. http://apps.who.int/iris/bitstream/10665/149782/1/9789241549028_eng.pdf?ua=1

349 Moss M, Salt Sugar Fat. New York. Random House. 2013.

350 Healthy eating for life: food choices for cancer prevention and survival. Physician's Committee for Responsible Medicine, Washington, DC, 2013. www.PCRM.org.

351 Katan MB, Grundy SM, Willett WC. Beyond Low-Fat Diets, Should a Low-Fat High-Carbohydrate-Diet Be Recommended for Everyone? N Engl J Med. 1997;337:563-566

352 Stampfer MJ, Hu FB, Manson JE, Rimm EB, Willett WC. Primary Prevention of Coronary Heart Disease in Women Through Diet and Lifestyle. N Engl J Med. 2000;343:16-22.

353 Hu FB, Willett WC. Optimal Diets for Prevention of Coronary Heart Disease. JAMA. 2002;288:2569-2578.

354 Hu FB. Plant-based foods and prevention of cardiovascular disease: an overview Am J Clin Nutr 2003;78(suppl):544S–51S.

355 Hu FB, Willett WC. Optimal Diets for Prevention of Coronary Heart Disease. JAMA. 2002;288:2569-2578.

356 Mozaffarian D, Appel LJ, Van Horn L. Components of a cardioprotective diet: new insights. Circulation. 2011;123:2870-91.

357 Ludwig DS. Lowering the Bar on the Low-Fat Diet. JAMA. Published online September 28, 2016. doi:10.1001/jama.2016.15473.

358 New thinking on daily food goals. Harvard Health Letter. July 2019:5

359 Willett W, Rockström J, Loken B, et al. Food in the Anthropocene: the EAT-Lancet Commission on healthy diets from sustainable food systems. Lancet. 2019;393(10170):447-492. doi: 10.1016/S0140-6736(18)31788-4

360 Aune, D, Navarro Rosenblatt D.A, Chan D.S, et al. Dairy products, calcium, and prostate cancer risk:A systematic review and meta-analysis of cohort studies. Am. J. Clin. Nutr. 2015, 101, 87–117.

361 Li X, Zhao J, Li P, Gao Y. Dairy Products Intake and Endometrial Cancer Risk: A Meta-Analysis of Observational Studies. Nutrients. 2017;10(1). pii: E25. doi: 10.3390/nu10010025.

362 Cho E, Smith-Warner SA, Spiegelman D, et al. Dairy foods, calcium, and colorectal cancer: A pooled analysis of 10 cohort studies. J. Natl. Cancer Inst. 2004;96:1015–1022.

363 Patterson E, Larsson SC, Wolk A, Akesson A. Association between dairy food consumption and risk of myocardial infarction in women differs by type of dairy food. J. Nutr. 2013;143:74–79.

364 Hu D, Huang J, Wang Y, Zhang D, Qu Y. Dairy foods and risk of stroke: A meta-analysis of prospective cohort studies. Nutr. Metab. Cardiovasc. Dis. 2014;24:460–469.

365 Huth PJ, Park KM. Influence of dairy product and milk fat consumption on cardiovascular disease risk: A review of the evidence. Adv. Nutr. 2012;3:266–285.

366 Aune D, Norat T, Romundstad P, Vatten LJ. Dairy products and the risk of type 2 diabetes: A systematic review and dose-response meta-analysis of cohort studies. Am. J. Clin. Nutr. 2013;98:1066–1083.

367 Chen M, Sun Q, Giovannucci E, Mozaffarian D, Manson JE, Willett WC, Hu FB. Dairy consumption-and risk of type 2 diabetes: 3 cohorts of US adults and an updated meta-analysis. BMC Med. 2014;12:215.

368 Bischoff-Ferrari HA, Dawson-Hughes B, Baron JA, et al. Milk intake and risk of hip fracture in men and women: A meta-analysis of prospective cohort studies. J. Bone Miner. Res. 2011;26:833–839.

369 Benatar JR, Sidhu K, Stewart RA. Effects of high and low-fat dairy food on cardio-metabolic risk factors: a meta-analysis of randomized studies. PLoS One. 2013;8:e76480.

370 Larsson SC, Crippa A, Orsini N, et al. Non-fermented milk consumption and mortality from all causes, cardiovascular disease, and cancer: a systematic review and meta-analysis. Nutrients. 2015;7(9):7749–7763.

371 Lu W, Chen H, Niu Y, Wu H, Xia D, Wu Y. Dairy products intake and cancer mortality risk: a meta-analysis of 11 population-based cohort studies. Nutr J. 2016;15(1):91.

372 Guo J, Astrup A, Lovegrove JA, Gijsbers L, Givens DI, Soedamah-Muthu SS. Milk and dairy consumption and risk of cardiovascular diseases and all-cause mortality: dose-response meta-analysis of prospective cohort studies. Eur J Epidemiol. 2017;32(4):269-287. Epub 2017 Apr 3.

373 Michaëlsson K, Wolk A, Melhus H, Byberg L. Milk, Fruit and Vegetable, and Total Antioxidant Intakes in Relation to Mortality Rates: Cohort Studies in Women and Men. American Journal of Epidemiology. 2017;185(5):345-361. doi:10.1093/aje/kww124.

374 Chen M, Li Y, Sun Q, et al. Dairy fat and risk of cardiovascular disease in 3 cohorts of US adults. Am J Clin Nutr. 2016;104:1209–1217.

375 Dehghan M, Mente A, Rangarajan S, et al. Association of dairy intake with cardiovascular disease and mortality in 21 countries from five continents (PURE): a prospective cohort study. Lancet. Published Online September 11, 2018. http://dx.doi.org/10.1016/S0140-6736(18)31812-9

376 Barnard ND, Henner M. The Cheese Trap: How Breaking a Surprising Addiction Will Help You Lose Weight, Gain Energy and Get Healthy. Hachette Book Group. New York, 2017.

377 Say Cheese. University of California, Berkeley Wellness Letter. Vol 31, Issue 14, September 2015.

378 Praagman J, Dalmeijer GW, van der Schouw YT, Soedamah-Muthu SS, Monique Verschuren WM, Bas Bueno-de-Mesquita H, Geleijnse JM, Beulens JW. The relationship between fermented food intake and-mortality risk in the European Prospective Investigation into Cancer and Nutrition-Netherlands cohort. Br J Nutr. 2015 Feb 14;113(3):498-506.

379 Tong X, Chen G-C, Zhang Z, Wei Y-L, Xu J-Y, Qin L-Q. Cheese Consumption and Risk of All-Cause Mortality: A Meta-Analysis of Prospective Studies. Nutrients. 2017;9(1):63. doi:10.3390/nu9010063.

380 Mozaffarian D, Appel LJ, Van Horn L. Components of a Cardioprotective Diet: New Insights. Circulation. 2011;123:2870-2891. DOI: 10.1161/CIRCULATION AHA.110.968735.

381 Lee JH, O'Keefe JH, Lavie CJ, Marchioli R, Harris WS. Omega-3 fatty acids for cardioprotection. Mayo Clin Proc. 2008;83:324–32.

382 Hooper L, Thompson RL, Harrison RA, et al. Risks and benefits of omega 3 fats for mortality, cardiovascular disease, and cancer: systematic review. BMJ. 2006;332:752–60.

383 Hu FB, Bronner L, Willett WC, Stampfer MJ, Rexrode KM, Albert CM, Hunter D, Manson JE. Fish and omega-3 fatty acid intake and risk of coronary heart disease in women. JAMA. 2002; 287(14):1815–1821.

384 Bell GA, Kantor ED, Lampe JW, Kristal AR, Heckbert SR, White E. Intake of long-chain ω-3 fatty acids from diet and supplements in relation to mortality. Am J Epidemiol. 2014;179(6):710-720.

385 Avanzini F, Caimi V, Longoni P, Marchioli R, Roncaglioni MC et al. Risk and Prevention Study Collaborative Group. n-3 fatty acids in patients with multiple cardiovascular risk factors. N Engl J Med. 2013;368(19):1800-8. doi: 10.1056/NEJMoa1205409.

386 Greene J, Ashburn SM, Razzouk L, Smith DA. Fish Oils, Coronary Heart Disease, and the Environment. AJPH. 2013;103(9):1568-1576. doi: 10.2105/AJPH.2012.300959.

387 Chew EY. Dietary Intake of Omega-3 Fatty Acids From Fish and Risk of Diabetic Retinopathy. JAMA. 2017;317(21):2226-2227. doi:10.1001/jama.2017.1926

388 Leung SSL, Yinko, RD, Stark KD, Thanassoulis G, Pilote L. Fish Consumption and Acute Coronary Syndrome: A Meta-Analysis. Am J Med. 2014;127:848-857.

389 The Risk and Prevention Study Collaborative Group. n−3 Fatty Acids in Patients with Multiple Cardiovascular Risk Factors. N Engl J Med. 2013;368:1800-1808.

390 Budtz-Jorgensen E, Grandjean P, Weihe P: Separation of risks and benefits of seafood intake. Environ-Health Perspect. 2007;115(3):323–327.

391 The American Heart Association Diet and Lifestyle Recommendations. American Heart Association. http://www.heart.org/HEARTORG/HealthyLiving/HealthyEating/Nutrition/The-American-Heart-Associations-Diet-and-Lifestyle-Recommendations_UCM_305855_Article.jsp#.WFWzo7GtpaM

392 EPA-FDA Advisory on Mercury in Fish and Shellfishhttps://www.epa.gov/fish-tech/epa-fda-advisory-mercury-fish-and-shellfish.

393 Parker-Pope T, The Tuna Debate Still Swirls. New York Times, March 3, 2015.

394 Report of the Joint United Nations Food and Agriculture Organization/World Health Organization Expert Consultation on the Risks and Benefits of Fish Consumption. Rome, 25–29 January 2010. FAO Fisheries and Aquaculture Report No. 978.27

395 Report of the Joint Food and Agriculture Organization of the United Nations (FAO) and the World-Health Organization (WHO) Expert Consultation on the Risks and Benefits of Fish Consumption, 2011. Rome. 2011. http://www.fao.org/docrep/014/ba0136e/ba0136e00.pdf

396 Report of the 1970 Joint FAO/WHO Expert Consultation on the Risks and Benefits of Fish Consumption. Food and Agriculture Organization of the United Nations; Geneva WHO. 1971

397 A tilapia tell-all. University of California Berkeley Wellness Letter. Vol 31, Issue 8, April 2015.

398 Greene J, Ashburn SM, Razzouk L, Smith DA. Fish Oils, Coronary Heart Disease, and the Environment. AJPH. 2013;103(9):1568-1576. doi: 10.2105/AJPH.2012.300959.

399 What is the meaning of 'natural' on the label of food? USFDA http://www.fda.gov/AboutFDA/Transparency/Basics/ucm214868.htm. http://www.fda.gov/Food/GuidanceRegulation/GuidanceDocumentsRegulatoryInformation/LabelingNutrition/ucm456090.htm

400 Smith-Spangler C, Brandeau ML, Hunter GE, et al. Are Organic Foods Safer or Healthier Than Conventional Alternatives?: A Systematic Review. Annals of Internal Medicine. 2012;157(5):348–366. doi:10.7326/0003-4819-157-5-201209040-00007. PMID 22944875.

401 Smith-Spangler C, Brandeau ML, Hunter GE, et al. Are Organic Foods Safer or Healthier Than Conventional Alternatives?: A Systematic Review. Annals of Internal Medicine. 2012;157(5):348–366. doi:10.7326/0003-4819-157-5-201209040-00007. PMID 22944875.

402 Bradbury KE, Balkwill A, Spencer EA, et al; Million Women Study Collaborators. Organic food consumption and the incidence of cancer in a large prospective study of women in the United Kingdom. Br J Cancer. 2014;110(9):2321-2326. doi:10.1038/bjc.2014.148

403 Baudry J, Assmann KE, Touvier M, et al. Association of Frequency of Organic Food ConsumptionWith Cancer Risk: Findings From the NutriNet-Santé Prospective Cohort Study. JAMA Intern Med. 2018;178(12):1597–1606. doi:10.1001/jamainternmed.2018.4357

404 A. Dangour, S.K. Dodhia, A. Hayter, E. Allen, K. Lock, R. Uauy, Nutritional quality of organic foods: a systematic review. Am. J. Clin. Nutr. 2009;90:680–685.

405 Smith-Spangler C, et al. Are organic foods safer or healthier than conventional alternatives? A systematic review. Ann Intern Med. 157(5):348–366 (2012); http://www.ncbi.nlm.nih.gov/pubmed/22944875.

406 Brandt M. Little evidence of health benefits from organic foods, Stanford study finds. Inside Stanford Medicine (3 Sep 2012). Stanford, CA: School of Medicine, Stanford University. Available: http://med.stanford.edu/ism/2012/september/organic.html [accessed 14 Nov 2012].

407 Holzman, David C. PESTICIDES. Organic Food Conclusions Don't Tell the Whole Story. Environmental Health Perspectives. 2017:120(12):A458.

408 Huber M, Rembiałkowska E, Srednicka D, Bügel S, van de Vijver LPL. Organic food and impact on human health: Assessing the status quo and prospects of research. NJAS - Wageningen Journal of Life-Sciences. 2011;58:103-109.

409 Bouchard MF, Chevrier J, Harley KG, et al. Prenatal exposure to organophosphate pesticides and IQ in 7-year-old children. Environ Health Perspect. 2011;119(8):1189–1195. http://dx.doi.org/10.1289/ehp.1003185.

410 Engel SM, et al. Prenatal exposure to organophosphates, paraoxonase 1, and cognitive development in childhood. Environ Health Perspect. 2011:119(8):1182–1188. http://dx.doi.org/10.1289/ehp.1003183.

411 Rauh V, et al. Seven-year neurodevelopmental scores and prenatal exposure to chlorpyrifos, a common agricultural pesticide. Environ Health Perspect. 2011;119(8):1196–1201. http://dx.doi.org/10.1289/ehp.1003160.

412 Bellinger DC. A strategy for comparing the contributions of environmental chemicals and other risk-factors to neurodevelopment of children. Environ Health Perspect. 2012;120(4):501–507. http://dx.doi.org/10.1289/ehp.1104170.

413 Vandenberg LN, et al. Hormones and endocrine-disrupting chemicals: low-dose effects and nonmonotonic dose responses. Endocr Rev. 33(3):378–455 (2012); http://dx.doi.org/10.1210/er.2011-1050.

414 Guerrero-Bosagna C, et al. Epigenetic transgenerational inheritance of vinclozolin induced mouse adult onset disease and associated sperm epigenome biomarkers. Reprod Toxicol; http://dx.doi.org/10.1016/j.reprotox.2012.09.005 [online 2 Oct 2012].

415 Hemler EC, Chavarro JE, Hu FB. Organic Foods for Cancer Prevention—Worth the Investment? JAMA Intern Med. 2018;178(12):1606–1607. doi:10.1001/jamainternmed.2018.4363

416 Forman J, et al. Organic foods: health and environmental advantages and disadvantages. Pediatrics. 2012;130(5):e1406–e1415. http://dx.doi.org/10.1542/peds.2012-2579.

417 Artificial sweeteners and cancer. National Cancer Institute. https://www.cancer.gov/about-cancer/causes-prevention/risk/diet/artificial-sweeteners-fact-sheet

418 High intensity sweeteners FDA. http://www.fda.gov/food/ingredientspackaginglabeling/foodadditives-ingredients/ucm397716.htm

419 Is Stevia an 'FDA approved' sweetener? http://www.fda.gov/AboutFDA/Transparency/Basics/ucm214864.htm

420 High intensity sweeteners FDA. http://www.fda.gov/food/ingredientspackaginglabeling/foodadditives-ingredients/ucm397716.htm.

421 Artificial sweeteners and cancer. National Cancer Institute. https://www.cancer.gov/about-cancer/

causes-prevention/risk/diet/artificial-sweeteners-fact-sheet

422 Food, Nutrition, Physical Activity, and the Prevention of Cancer: a Global Perspective.Washington DC: World Cancer Research Fund / American Institute for Cancer Research;2007.

423 Bosetti C, Gallus S, Talamini R, et al. Artificial sweeteners and the risk of gastric, pancreatic, and endometrial cancers in Italy. Cancer Epidemiol Biomarkers Prev. 2009;18(8):2235-8. PMID: 19661082. http://www.ncbi.nlm.nih.gov/pubmed/19661082

424 Lim U, Subar AF, Mouw T, et al. Consumption of aspartame-containing beverages and incidence of hematopoietic and brain malignancies. Cancer Epidemiol Biomarkers Prev. 2006;15(9):1654–1659.

425 Wolraich ML, Lindgren SD, Stumbo PJ, Stegink LD, Appelbaum MI, Kiritsy MC. Effects of diets high in sucrose or aspartame on the behavior and cognitive performance of children. N Engl J Med. 1994;330(5):301-7. PMID: 8277950. http://www.ncbi.nlm.nih.gov/pubmed/8277950.

426 Shaywitz BA, Anderson GM, Novotny EJ, et al. Aspartame has no effect on seizures or epileptiform discharges in epileptic children. Ann Neurol. 1994;35(1):98-103. PMID: 7506878. http://www.ncbi.nlm.nih.gov/pubmed/7506878.

427 Kruesi MJ, Rapoport JL, Cummings EM, et al. Effects of sugar and aspartame on aggression and activity in children. Am J Psychiatry. 2367 1987;144(11):1487-90. PMID: 3674234. http://www.ncbi.nlm.nih.gov/pubmed/3674234.

428 Ryan-Harshman M, Leiter LA, Anderson GH. Phenylalanine and aspartame fail to alter feeding behavior, mood and arousal in men. Physiol Behav. 1987;39(2):247-53. PMID:3575461. http://www.ncbi.nlm.nih.gov/pubmed/3575461.

429 Spiers PA, Sabounjian L, Reiner A, Myers DK, Wurtman J, Schomer DL. Aspartame: neuropsychologic and neurophysiologic evaluation of acute and chronic effects. Am J Clin Nutr. 1998;68(3):531-7. PMID: 9734727. http://www.ncbi.nlm.nih.gov/pubmed/9734727.

430 Stokes AF, Belger A, Banich MT, Bernadine E. Effects of alcohol and chronic aspartame ingestion upon performance in aviation relevant cognitive tasks. Aviat Space Environ Med. 1994;65(1):7-15. PMID: 8117231. http://www.ncbi.nlm.nih.gov/pubmed/8117231.

431 Pivonka EE, Grunewald KK. Aspartame- or sugar-sweetened beverages: effects on mood in young women. J Am Diet Assoc. 1990;90(2):250-4. PMID: 2303661. http://www.ncbi.nlm.nih.gov/pubmed/2303661.

432 Stokes AF, Belger A, Banich MT, Taylor H. Effects of acute aspartame and acute alcohol ingestion upon the cognitive performance of pilots. Aviat Space Environ Med. 1991;62(7):648-53. PMID: 1898300. http://www.ncbi.nlm.nih.gov/pubmed/1898300.

433 European Food Safety Authority (EFSA). Food Additives and Nutrient Sources Added to food Panel. Scientific Opinion on the re-evaluation of aspartame (E 951) as a food additive. Parma, Italy,2013. Available from: http://www.efsa.europa.eu/en/efsajournal/doc/3496.pdf.

434 Gougeon R, Spidel M, Lee K, Field CJ. Canadian Diabetes Association National Nutrition Committee Technical Review: Non-nutritive Intense Sweeteners in Diabetes Management. Canadian Journal Of Diabetes. 2004;28(4):385-399.

435 Weighing in on sugar substitutes. University of California, Berkeley, Wellness Letter. August 2017.

436 Bernstein AM, de Koning L, Flint AJ, Rexrode KM, Willett WC. Soda consumption and the risk of stroke in men and women. Am J Clin Nutr. 2012;95(5):1190–1199. doi:10.3945/ajcn.111.030205

437 Pase MP, Himali JJ, Beiser AS, et al. Sugar- and Artificially Sweetened Beverages and the Risks of Incident Stroke and Dementia, A Prospective Cohort Study. Stroke. 2017;48(5):1139-1146. doi: 10.1161/STROKEAHA.116.016027.

438 Toews I, Lohner S, de Gaudry DK, Sommer H, Meerpohl JJ. Association between intake of non-sugar

sweeteners and health outcomes: systematic review and meta-analyses of randomised and non-randomised-controlled trials and observational studies. BMJ. 2019;364:k4718. doi: https://doi.org/10.1136/bmj. k4718.

439 Schernhammer ES, Bertrand KA, Birmann BM, Sampson L, Willett WC, Feskanich D. Consumptionof artificial sweetener- and sugar-containing soda and risk of lymphoma and leukemia in men and women. Am J Clin Nutr. 2012;96(6):1419-28. PMID:2345 23097267. http://www.ncbi.nlm.nih.gov/pubmed/23097267

440 Scientific Report of the 2015 Dietary Guidelines Advisory Committee. Advisory Report to the Secretary of Health and Human Services and the Secretary of Agriculture.http://www.health.gov/dietaryguidelines/2015-scientific-report/

441 Scientific Report of the 2015 Dietary Guidelines Advisory Committee. Advisory Report to the Secretary of Health and Human Services and the Secretary of Agriculture.http://www.health.gov/dietaryguidelines/2015-scientific-report/

442 The Truth About Gluten. Consumer Reports. January 2015.

443 Fasano A. Surprises from Celiac Disease. Scientific American. August 2009.

444 The Truth About Gluten. Consumer Reports. January 2015.

445 Arsenic in Your Rice: The Latest. Consumer Reports. January 2015.

446 Dagfinn A, NaNa K, Giovannucci E, Fadnes LT, Boffetta P, Greenwood DC, et al. Whole grain consumption and risk of cardiovascular disease, cancer, and all cause and cause specific mortality: systematic review and dose-response meta-analysis of prospective studies. BMJ. 2016;353:i2716.

447 Zong G, Gao A, Hu FB, Sun Q. Whole Grain Intake and Mortality From All Causes, Cardiovascular Disease, and Cancer A Meta-Analysis of Prospective Cohort Studies. Circulation. 2016;133:2370-2380 https://doi.org/10.1161/CIRCULATION.AHA.115.021101

448 Brody JE. Fear, Not Fact, Behind G.M.O. Labeling. New York Times. June 9, 2015.

449 Harmon A. How Square Watermelons Get Their Shape, and Other G.M.O. Misconceptions. New York Times. Updated August 2, 2016

450 United States Department of Agriculture, Economic Research Service. Adoption of Genetically Engineered Crops in the U.S. Updated July 9, 2015, http://www.ers.usda.gov/data-products/adoption-of-genetically-engineered-crops-in-the-us/recent-trends-in-ge-adoption.aspx

451 Landrigan PJ, Benbrook C. GMOs, Herbicides and Public Health. New Engl J Med. 2015;373(8):693-695.

452 Hakim D. Doubts About the Promised Bounty of Genetically Modified Crops. New York Times. October 29, 2016

453 National Academies of Sciences, Engineering, and Medicine. 2016. Genetically Engineered Crops: Experiences and Prospects. Washington, DC: The National Academies Press. doi: 10.17226/23395.

454 Ley RE. Obesity and the human microbiome. Curr Opin Gastroenterol. 2010 Jan;26(1):5-11. doi: 10.1097/MOG.0b013e328333d751.

455 Ursell LK, Metcalf JL, Parfrey LW, Knight R. Defining the Human Microbiome. Nutrition reviews. 2012;70(Suppl 1):S38-S44. doi:10.1111/j.1753-4887.2012.00493.x.

456 Shen J, Obin MS, Zhao L. The gut microbiota, obesity and insulin resistance. Mol Aspects Med. 2013;34(1):39-58. doi: 10.1016/j.mam.2012.11.001. Epub 2012 Nov 16.

457 Molinaro F, Paschetta E, Cassader M, Gambino R, Musso G. Probiotics, prebiotics, energy balance, and obesity: mechanistic insights and therapeutic implications. Gastroenterol Clin North Am. 2012;41(4):843-54.

458 Ackerman J. The Ultimate Social Network. Scientific American. June 2012.

459 Lynch SV, Pedersen O. The Human Intestinal Microbiome in Health and Disease. New Eng. J Med. 2016;375(24):2369-2377.

460 LaMont JT. Probiotics for children with gastroenteritis. New Eng. J Med. 2018;329(21):2076-2077.

461 O'Connor A. For Coffee Drinkers, the Buzz May Be in Your Genes. New York Times. July 19, 2016, p. D4.

462 Salazar-Martinez E, Willett WC, Ascherio A, Manson JE, Leitzmann MF, Stampfer MJ, Hu FB. Coffee Consumption and Risk for Type 2 Diabetes Mellitus. Annals of Internal Medicine. 2004;140:1-8.

463 Guallar E, Blasco-Colmenares E, Arking DE, Zhao D. Moderate Coffee Intake Can Be Part of a Healthy Diet. Ann Intern Med. [Epub ahead of print 11 July 2017] doi: 10.7326/M17-1503

464 Coffee: Love it or leave it? Harvard Health Letter. May 2016.

465 Coffee: grounds for optimism. University of California Berkeley Wellness Letter. vol. 29, Issue 13, August 2013.

466 Van Dam RM, Hu FB, Willett WC. Coffee, Caffeine and Health. N Engl J Med. 2020;383:369-378.

467 Blumberg JB. Introduction to the proceedings of the Fifth International Scientific Symposium on Tea and Human Health. Am J Clin Nutr. 2013;98(suppl):1607S–10S.

468 Arab L, Khan F, Lam H. Tea consumption and cardiovascular disease risk. Am J Clin Nutr. 2013;98(suppl):1651S–9S.

469 Proceedings of the Fifth International Scientific Symposium on Tea and Human Health. Am J Clin Nutr. 2013;98(suppl):1607S–.

470 Reading the tea leaves. University of California, Berkeley Wellness Letter. vol. 30, Issue 7, February 2014.

Chapter 4 – Weight Control

1 Heymsfield SB, Wadden TA. Mechanisms, Pathophysiology, and Management of Obesity. N Engl J Med 2017; 376:254-266 January 19, 2017DOI: 10.1056/NEJMra1514009

2 Drexler M. Obesity. Can we stop the epidemic. Harvard Public Health Spring 2017, pp. 12-35.

3 Greger M. How Not to Diet. New York: Flatiron Books. 2019. p35.

4 Roberto CA, Swinburn B, Hawkes C, et al. Patchy progress on obesity prevention: emerging examples, entrenched barriers, and new thinking. Lancet. 2015;385(9985):2400–9.

5 FAO, IFAD and WPF, 2015. The State of Food Insecurity in the World 2015. International hunger targets: taking stock of uneven progress. Rome, Italy: FAO.

6 Flegal KM, Kruszon-Moran D, Carroll MD, Fryar CD, Ogden CL. Trends in Obesity Among Adults in-the United States, 2005 to 2014. JAMA. 2016;315(21):2284-2291. doi:10.1001/jama.2016.6458

7 Cheskin LJ, Roberts C, Margolis S. Nutrition and Weight Control. Johns Hopkins White Paper, New York. Remedy Media, 2014.

8 Hales CM, Carroll MD, Fryar CD, Ogden CL. Prevalence of obesity and severe obesity among adults: United States, 2017–2018. NCHS Data Brief, no 360. Hyattsville, MD: National Center for Health Statistics, 2020

9 Hales CM, Fryar CD, Carroll MD, Freedman DS, Ogden CL. Trends in Obesity and Severe Obesity Prevalence in US Youth and Adults by Sex and Age, 2007-2008 to 2015-2016. JAMA. 2018;319(16):1723–1725. doi:10.1001/jama.2018.3060

10 National Center for Health Statistics. Health, United States, 2014: With Special Feature on Adults Aged 55–64. Hyattsville, MD. 2015. Table 59

11 Ogden CL, Carroll MD, Fryar CD, Flegal KM. Prevalence of Obesity Among Adults and Youth: United States, 2011–2014 National Center for Health Statistics Data Brief, No. 219, November 2015. http://www.cdc.gov/nchs/data/databriefs/db219.pdf

12 Ward JZ, Bleich SN, Cradock AL, et al. Projected U.S state-level prevalence of adult obesity and severe obesity. N Engl J Med. 2019; 381(25):2440-2450.

13 Cheskin LJ, Roberts C, Margolis S. Nutrition and Weight Control. Johns Hopkins White Paper, New York. Remedy Media, 2014

14 Facts: With a Very Heavy Heart, obesity and cardiovascular disease (CVD) https://www.heart.org/idc/groups/heart-public/@wcm/@adv/documents/downloadable/ucm_305059.pdf

15 Finkelstein EA, Trogdon JG, Cohen JW, Dietz W. Annual medical spending attributable to obesity: payer-and service-specific estimates. Health Aff (Millwood). 2009 Sep-Oct;28(5):w822-31. doi: 10.1377/hlthaff.28.5.w822.

16 Campaign to End Obesity. http://www.obesitycampaign.org.

17 Wang Y, Beydoun WY, Liang L, Caballero B, Kumanyika SK. Will All Americans Become Overweight or Obese? Estimating the Progression and Cost of the US Obesity Epidemic. Obesity. 2008;(16):2323–2330. doi:10.1038/oby.2008.351

18 National Heart, Lung, and Blood Institute https://www.nhlbi.nih.gov/health/educational/lose_wt/BMI/bmi_tbl.pdf

19 Michelle G. Swainson, Alan M. Batterham, Costas Tsakirides, Zoe H. Rutherford, Karen Hind. Prediction of whole-body fat percentage and visceral adipose tissue mass from five anthropometric variables. PLOS ONE, 2017; 12 (5): e0177175 DOI: 10.1371/journal.pone.0177175

20 Maffetone PB, Rivera-Dominguez I, Laursen PB. Overfat Adults and Children in Developed Countries: The Public Health Importance of Identifying Excess Body Fat. Front. Public Health. 2017;5:190. doi: 10.3389/fpubh.2017.00190

21 Shah NR, Braverman ER, Measuring Adiposity in Patients: the Utility of Body Mass Index (BMI), Percent Body Fat, and Leptin. PLoS ONE. 2012;7:4, e33308

22 WHO. Physical status: the use and interpretation of anthropometry. Report of a WHO Expert Committee.WHO Technical Report Series 854. Geneva: World Health Organization, 1995.

23 Shah NR, Braverman ER, Measuring Adiposity in Patients: the Utility of Body Mass Index (BMI), Percent Body Fat, and Leptin. PLoS ONE. 2012;7:4, e33308

24 Exercise AC. ACE Lifestyle & Weight Management Consultant Manual, The Ultimate Resource for Fitness Professionals. American Council on Exercise; 2009.

25 Overweight and Obesity Statistics, U.S. Department of Health and Human Services, National Institute of Diabetes and Digestive and Kidney diseases, Weight Control Information Network. http://www.niddk.nih.gov/health-information/health-statistics/Documents/stat904z.pdf

26 The GBD 2015 Obesity Collaborators. Health Effects of Overweight and Obesity in 195 Countries over 25 Years. N Engl J Med. 2017; 377:13-27, July 6, 2017DOI: 10.1056/NEJMoa1614362

27 Cheskin LJ, Roberts C, Margolis S. Nutrition and Weight Control. Johns Hopkins White Paper, New York. Remedy Media, 2014.

28 Fontaine KR, Redden DT, Wang C, Westfall AO, Allison DB. Years of Life Lost Due to Obesity. JAMA.2003;289(2):187-193. doi:10.1001/jama.289.2.187

29 Reis JP, Loria CM, Lewis CE, et al. Association Between Duration of Overall and Abdominal Obesity Beginning in Young Adulthood and Coronary Artery Calcification in Middle Age. JAMA. 2013;310(3):280-288. doi:10.1001/jama.2013.7833.

30 Kuk JL, Katzmarzyk PT, Nichaman MZ, Church TS, Blair SN, Ross R. Visceral fat is an independent predictor of all-cause mortality in men. Obesity (Silver Spring). 2006;14(2):336–41.

31 Koster A, Murphy RA, Eiriksdottir G, Aspelund T, Sigurdsson S, Lang TF, et al. Fat distribution and-mortality: the AGES-Reykjavik Study. Obesity (Silver Spring). 2015;23(4):893–7.

32 Borrell LN, Samuel L. Body Mass Index Categories and Mortality Risk in US Adults: The Effect of Overweight and Obesity on Advancing Death. Am J Publ Hlth. 2014;104(3):512-519. doi: 10.2105/AJPH.2013.301597

33 Zheng Y, Manson JE, Yuan C, Liang MH, Grodstein F, Stampfer MJ, Willett WC, Hu FB. Associations of Weight Gain From Early to Middle Adulthood With Major Health Outcomes Later in Life. JAMA. 2017;318(3):255-269. doi:10.1001/jama.2017.7092

34 Zheng Y, Manson JE, Yuan C, Liang MH, Grodstein F, Stampfer MJ, Willett WC, Hu FB. Associations of Weight Gain From Early to Middle Adulthood With Major Health Outcomes Later in Life. JAMA. 2017;318(3):255-269. doi:10.1001/jama.2017.7092

35 Pischon T, Boeing H, et al. General and Abdominal Adiposity and Risk of Death in Europe. New England Journal of Medicine, November 13, 2008; 359:2105-20

36 Jensen MD. Role of body fat distribution and the metabolic complications of obesity. J Clin Endocrinol Metab. 2008;93(11)(suppl 1):S57-S63.

37 Yusuf S, Hawken S, Ounpuu S, et al. INTERHEART Study Investigators. Obesity and the risk of myocardial infarction in 27,000 participants from 52 countries: a case-control study. Lancet. 2005;366(9497):1640-1649.

38 Emdin CA, Khera AV, Natarajan P, Klarin D, Zekavat SM, Hsiao AJ, Kathiresan S. Genetic Association of Waist-to-Hip Ratio With Cardiometabolic Traits, Type 2 Diabetes, and Coronary Heart Disease. JAMA.2017;317(6):626-634. doi:10.1001/jama.2016.21042

39 Wildman RP, Muntner P, Reynolds K, et al. The Obese Without Cardiometabolic Risk Factor Clustering and the Normal Weight With Cardiometabolic Risk Factor ClusteringPrevalence and Correlates of 2 Phenotypes Among the US Population (NHANES 1999-2004). Arch Intern Med. 2008;168(15):1617–1624. doi:10.1001/archinte.168.15.1617

40 Rubin R. What's the Best Way to Treat Normal-Weight People With Metabolic Abnormalities?. JAMA.2018;320(3):223–225. doi:10.1001/jama.2018.8188

41 Chooi YC, Ding C, Chan Z, et al. Moderate Weight Loss Improves Body Composition and Metabolic Function in Metabolically Unhealthy Lean Subjects. Obesity. 2018;26(6):943-1103. doi:10.1002/oby.22185

42 Lustig RH. Fat Chance, Beating the Odds Against Sugar, Processed Food, Obesity and Disease. New York. Plume. 2012.

43 Ortega FB, Lee D, Katzmarzyk PT, et al. The intriguing metabolically healthy but obese phenotype: cardiovascular prognosis and role of fitness. European Heart Journal, 2012; DOI: 10.1093/eurheartj/ehs174

44 Caleyachetty R, et al. European Association for the Study of Obesity. Healthy' obese people still at higher risk of cardiovascular disease events than general population. ScienceDaily.16 May 2017. www.sciencedaily.com/releases/2017/05/170516190739.htm

45 Caleyachetty R, et al. European Association for the Study of Obesity. Healthy' obese people still at higher risk of cardiovascular disease events than general population. ScienceDaily.16 May 2017. www.sciencedaily.com/releases/2017/05/170516190739.htm

46 Kennedy AB, Lavie CJ, Blair SN. Fitness or Fatness Which Is More Important? JAMA. 2018;319(3):231–232. doi:10.1001/jama.2017.21649.

47 Angerås O, Albertsson P, Karason K, et al.. Evidence for obesity paradox in patients with acute coronary syndromes: A report from the Swedish Coronary Angiography and Angioplasty Registry. European

Heart Journal, 2012; DOI: 10.1093/eurheartj/ehs217

48 Flegal KM, Kit BK, Orpana H, Graubard BI. Association of All-Cause Mortality With Overweight and Obesity Using Standard Body Mass Index Categories, A Systematic Review and Meta-analysis. JAMA. 2013;309(1):71-82. doi:10.1001/jama.2012.113905.

49 Heymsfield SB, Cefalu WT. Does Body Mass Index Adequately Convey a Patient's Mortality Risk? JAMA, January 2, 2013—Vol 309, No. 1 87-88

50 Cheskin LJ, Roberts C, Margolis S. Nutrition and Weight Control. Johns Hopkins White Paper, New York. Remedy Media, 2014. P48.

51 Willett WC, Dietz WH, Colditz GA. Guidelines for Healthy Weight. N Engl J Med. 1999; 341:427-434August 5, 1999DOI: 10.1056/NEJM199908053410607

52 Manson JE, Willett WC, Stampfer MJ, et al. Body weight and mortality among women. N Engl J Med. 1995;333:677-85.

53 Stevens J, Jianwen C, Pamuk ER, Williamson DF, Thun MJ, Wood JL. The effect of age on the association between body-mass index and mortal- ity. N Engl J Med. 1998;338:1-7.

54 Veronese N, Li Y, Manson JE, Willett WC, Fontana L, Hu F. Combined associations of body weight and lifestyle factors with all cause and cause specific mortality in men and women: prospective cohort study. BMJ. 2016;355:i5855 http://dx.doi.org/10.1136/bmj.i5855

55 Kennedy AB, Lavie CJ, Blair SN. Fitness or Fatness Which Is More Important? JAMA. 2018;319(3):231–232. doi:10.1001/jama.2017.21649.

56 Kennedy AB, Lavie CJ, Blair SN. Fitness or Fatness Which Is More Important?. JAMA. 2018;319(3):231–232. doi:10.1001/jama.2017.21649.

57 Tobias DK, Hu FB. Does being overweight really reduce mortality? Obesity (Silver Spring) 2013;21:1746-9. doi:10.1002/oby.20602.

58 Global BMI Mortality Collaboration. Body-mass index and all-cause mortality: individual-participant-data meta-analysis of 239 prospective studies in four continents. Lancet. 2016;388:776-86. doi:10.1016/S0140-6736(16)30175-1.

59 Dagfinn A, Abhijit S, Prasad M, Norat T, Imre J, Tonstad S, et al. BMI and all cause mortality: systematic review and non-linear dose-response meta-analysis of 230 cohort studies with 3.74 million deaths among 30.3 million participants BMJ. 2016;353:i2156

60 Lustig R. Sugar, the Bitter Truth. https://www.youtube.com/watch?v=dBnniua6-oM

61 Super Size Me. https://en.wikipedia.org/wiki/Super Size Me

62 Kechagias S, Ernersson Å, Dahlqvist O, Lundberg P, Lindström T, Nystrom FH. Fast-food-based hyper-alimentation can induce rapid and profound elevation of serum alanine aminotransferase in healthy subjects. Gut. (2008). doi:10.1136/gut.2007.131797

63 Hagström H, Tynelius P, Rasmussen F. High BMI in late adolescence predicts future severe liver disease and hepatocellular carcinoma: a national, population-based cohort study in 1.2 million men. Gut. Published online March 20 2017. 10.1136/gutjnl-2016-313622

64 Diehl AM, Day C. Cause, Pathogenesis, and Treatment of Nonalcoholic Steatohepatitis. N Engl J Med. 2017;377:2063-72. DOI: 10.1056/NEJMra1503519

65 Koutoukidis DA, Astbury NM, Tudor KE, et al. Association of Weight Loss Interventions With Changes in Biomarkers of Nonalcoholic Fatty Liver Disease: A Systematic Review and Meta-analysis. JAMA Intern Med. Published online July 01, 2019. doi:10.1001/jamainternmed.2019

66 Paul S, Davis AM. Diagnosis and Management of Nonalcoholic Fatty Liver Disease. JAMA.2018;320(23):2474–2475. doi:10.1001/jama.2018.17365.

67 Emdin CA, Khera AV, Natarajan P, Klarin D, Zekavat SM, Hsiao AJ, Kathiresan S. Genetic Association of Waist-to-Hip Ratio With Cardiometabolic Traits, Type 2 Diabetes, and Coronary Heart Disease. JAMA.2017;317(6):626-634. doi:10.1001/jama.2016.21042.

68 Canoy D, Boekholdt SM, Wareham N, et al. Body fat distribution and risk of coronary heart disease in men and women in the European Prospective Investigation Into Cancer and Nutrition in Norfolk cohort: a population-based prospective study. Circulation. 2007;116(25):2933-2943.

69 Yusuf S, Hawken S, Ounpuu S, et al; INTERHEART Study Investigators. Obesity and the risk of my cardial infarction in 27,000 participants from 52 countries: a case-control study. Lancet. 2005;366(9497):1640-1649.

70 Shook R. Obesity and energy balance: what is the role of physical activity? Expert Rev Endocrinol Metab. 2016;11(6):511–20.

71 Plachta-Danielzik S, Landsberg B, Bosy-Westphal A, Johannsen M, Lange D, Muller JM. Energy gain and energy gap in normal-weight children: longitudinal data of the KOPS. Obesity (Silver Spring). 2008;16:777–783.

72 Hill JO. Can a small-changes approach help address the obesity epidemic? A report of the Joint Task Force of the American Society for Nutrition, Institute of Food Technologists, and International Food Information Council. Am J Clin Nutr. 2009;89:477– 484.

73 Mozaffarian D, Appel LJ, Van Horn L. Components of a Cardioprotective Diet: New Insights. Circul tion. 2011;123:2870-2891. DOI: 10.1161/CIRCULATIONAHA.110.968735

74 Mozaffarian D, Hao T, Rimm EB, Willett WC, Hu FB. Changes in diet and lifestyle and long-term weight gain in women and men. N Engl J Med 2011; 364:2392-2404June 23, 2011DOI: 10.1056/NEJMoa1014296

75 Roberts SB, Das SK, The Messy Truth about Weight Loss. Scientific American. June 2017, pp.36-41.

76 Lustig RH. Fat Chance, Beating the Odds Against Sugar, Processed Food, Obesity and Disease. New York. Plume. 2012. p. 35.

77 Lustig RH. Fat Chance, Beating the Odds Against Sugar, Processed Food, Obesity and Disease. New York. Plume. 2012. p. 20

78 Lustig RH. Fat Chance, Beating the Odds Against Sugar, Processed Food, Obesity and Disease. New York. Plume. 2012. p. 20

79 Ludwig DS. Lowering the Bar on the Low-Fat Diet. JAMA. 2016;316(20):2087-2088. doi:10.1001/jama.2016.15473

80 Moss M, Salt Sugar Fat. New York. Random House. 2013.

81 Kolata G. The Lost Weight? The Body Finds It. Even for the 'Biggest Loser.' New York Times January 1, 2017 p.16-17.

82 Fothergill E, Guo J, Howard L, et al. Persistent metabolic adaptation 6 years after "The Biggest Loser" competition. Obesity. 2016;24(8):1612–1619. DOI: 10.1002/oby.21538

83 Cheskin LJ, Roberts C, Margolis S. Nutrition and Weight Control. Johns Hopkins White Paper, New York. Remedy Media, 2014.

84 Lustig RH. Fat Chance, Beating the Odds Against Sugar, Processed Food, Obesity and Disease. New York. Plume. 2012. p. 46.

85 Lustig RH. Fat Chance, Beating the Odds Against Sugar, Processed Food, Obesity and Disease. New York. Plume. 2012. p. 52.

86 Lustig RH. Fat Chance, Beating the Odds Against Sugar, Processed Food, Obesity and Disease. New York. Plume. 2012. p. 41.

87 Cheskin LJ, Roberts C, Margolis S. Nutrition and Weight Control. Johns Hopkins White Paper, New York. Remedy Media, 2014.

88 Lustig RH. Fat Chance, Beating the Odds Against Sugar, Processed Food, Obesity and Disease. New York. Plume. 2012. p. 68.

89 Friedman RA. What Cookies and Meth Have in Common. New York Times July 2, 2017

90 Tappy L, Lê, K. Health Effects of Fructose and Fructose-Containing Caloric Sweeteners: Where Do We Stand 10 Years After the Initial Whistle Blowings? Curr Diab Rep. 2015;15:54. doi:10.1007/s11892- 015-0627-0

91 Jew S, Abumweis SS, Jones PJ. Evolution of the human diet: linking our ancestral diet to modern functional foods as a means of chronic disease prevention. J Med Food. 2009;12(5):925–34.

92 Leach JD, Sobolik KD. High dietary intake of prebiotic inulin-type fructans in the prehistoric Chihuahuan Desert. Br J Nutr. 2010;103(11):1558–61.

93 Institute of Medicine. Dietary Reference Intakes for Energy, Carbohydrate, Fiber, Fat, Fatty Acids, Cholesterol, Protein and Amino Acids. Washington, D.C.: National Academies Press; 2005.

94 Clemens R, Kranz S, Mobley AR, et al. Filling America's fiber intake gap: summary of a roundtable to probe realistic solutions with a focus on grain-based foods. J Nutr. 2012;142(7):1390S–401S.

95 Berthoud HR. The vagus nerve, food intake and obesity. Regul Pept. 2008;149(1–3):15–25.

96 Al-Lahham SH, Roelofsen H, Priebe M, et al. Regulation of adipokine production in human adipose tissue by propionic acid. Eur J Clin Invest. 2010;40(5):401–7.

97 Lustig RH. Fat Chance, Beating the Odds Against Sugar, Processed Food, Obesity and Disease. New York. Plume. 2012. pp. 130-138.

98 Roberts SB, Das SK, The Messy Truth about Weight Loss. Scientific American. June 2017, pp.36-41.

99 Heaton KW. Food fibre as an obstacle to energy intake. Lancet. 1973;2(7843):1418–21.

100 Southgate DA, Durnin JV. Calorie conversion factors. An experimental reassessment of the factors used in the calculation of the energy value of human diets. Br J Nutr. 1970;24(2):517–35.

101 Levine AS, Silvis SE. Absorption of whole peanuts, peanut oil, and peanut butter. N Engl J Med. 1980;303(16):917–8.

102 Roberts SB, Das SK, The Messy Truth about Weight Loss. Scientific American. June 2017, pp.36-41.

103 Karl JP, Meydani M, Barnett JB. Substituting whole grains for refined grains in a 6-wk randomized trial favorably affects energy-balance metrics in healthy men and postmenopausal women Am J Clin Nutr ajcn139683; First published online February 8, 2017.

104 Get more zzz's to prevent weight gain? University of California, Berkeley Wellness Letter. 33(9) April 2017, pSR1.

105 Komaroff AL. The Microbiome and Risk for Obesity and Diabetes. JAMA. 2017;317(4):355-356. doi:10.1001/jama.2016.20099

106 Wu GD, Chen J, Hoffmann C, et al. Linking long-term dietary patterns with gut microbial enterotypes. Science. 2011;334(6052):105–8.

107 Shook R. Obesity and energy balance: what is the role of physical activity? Expert Rev Endocrinol Metab. 2016;11(6):511–20.

108 Villablanca PA, Alegria JR, Mookadam F, Holmes DR, Wright RS, Levine JA. Nonexercise activity thermogenesis in obesity management. Mayo Clin Proc. 2015;90(4):509–19.

109 Lustig RH. Fat Chance, Beating the Odds Against Sugar, Processed Food, Obesity and Disease. New York. Plume. 2012. pp.139-149.

110 National Weight Control Registry. http://www.nwcr.ws/Research/default.htm. accessed April 22, 2017.

111 Bailey C. Fit or Fat? Boston, Houghton Mifflin: 1977.

112 Field AE, Haines J, Rosner B, Willett WC. Weight-control behaviors and subsequent weight change among adolescents and young adult females. Am J Clin Nutr. 2010;91(1):147-53. doi: 10.3945/ajcn.2009.28321. Epub 2009 Nov 4.

113 Moyer MW. Can Brown Fat Defeat Obesity? Scientific American. August 2014, p 30-32.

114 Villareal DT, Aguirre L, Gurney AB, et al. Aerobic or Resistance Exercise, or Both, in Dieting Obese Older Adults. N Engl J Med 2017; 376:1943-1955. May 18, 2017 DOI: 10.1056/NEJMoa1616338

115 Church TS. The Underappreciated Synergy of Strength Training. Obesity. 2020;28(2):24-24. https://doi.org/10.1002/oby.22702

116 Bennie JA, De Cocker K, Pavey T, Stamatakis E, et al. Muscle Strengthening, Aerobic Exercise, and Obesity: A Pooled Analysis of 1.7 Million US Adults. Obesity. 2020;28(2):371-378. https://doi.org/10.1002/oby.22673

117 Carroll AE. Diet, Not Exercise Is Crucial to Weight Loss. New York Times June 18, 2015.

118 Pontzer H, et al. Constrained Total Energy Expenditure and Metabolic Adaptation to Physical Activity in Adult Humans. Current Biology 2016; 26(3): 410-417 February 8, 2016.

119 Pontzer H. The Exercise Paradox. Scientific American. February 2017, p26-31.

120 Catenacci VA, Wyatt HR. The role of physical activity in producing and maintaining weight loss. Nat Clin Pract Endocrinol Metab. 2007;3(7):518-29.

121 Miller WC, et al. A meta-analysis of the past 25 years of weight loss research using diet, exercise or diet plus exercise intervention. Int J Obes Relat Metab Disord. 1997; 21:941–947. [PubMed: 9347414]

122 Flack KD, Ufholz K, Johnson L, Fitzgerald JS, Roemmich JN. Energy compensation in response to aerobic exercise training in overweight adults. American Journal of Physiology-Regulatory, Integrative and Comparative Physiology. 2018;315(4):R619-R626 https://doi.org/10.1152/ajpregu.00071.2018

123 Reynolds G. Exercise Alone May Slim After All. New York Times. July 10, 2018 pD6.

124 Schoeller DA, et al. How much physical activity is needed to minimize weight gain in previously obese women? Am J Clin Nutr. 1997;66:551–556.

125 Weinsier RL, et al. Free-living activity energy expenditure in women successful and unsuccessful at maintaining a normal body weight. Am J Clin Nutr. 2002;75:499–504.

126 Astrup A, Grunwald GK, Melanson EL, Saris WH, Hill JO. The role of low-fat diets in body weight control: a meta-analysis of ad libitum dietary intervention studies. Int J Obes Relat Metab Disord. 2000;24: 1545–1552.

127 Howard BV, Manson JE, Stefanick ML, Beresford SA, Frank G, Jones B, Rodabough RJ, Snetselaar L, Thomson C, Tinker L, Vitolins M, Prentice R. Low-fat dietary pattern and weight change over 7 years: the Women's Health Initiative Dietary Modification Trial. JAMA. 2006;295:39–49.

128 Mozaffarian D, Appel LJ, Van Horn L. Components of a Cardioprotective Diet: New Insights. Circulation. 2011;123:2870-2891. DOI: 10.1161/CIRCULATIONAHA.110.968735.

129 Shai I, Schwarzfuchs D, Henkin Y, Shahar DR, Witkow S, Greenberg I, R, Sarusi B, Brickner D, Schwartz Z, Sheiner E, Marko R, Katorza E, Thiery J, Fiedler GM, Bluher M, Stumvoll M, Stampfer MJ. Weight loss with a low-carbohydrate, Mediterranean, or low-fat diet. N Engl J Med. 2008;359:229 –241.

130 Sacks FM, Bray GA, Carey VJ, Smith SR, Ryan DH, Anton SD, McManus K, Champagne CM, Bishop LM, Laranjo N, Leboff MS, Rood JC, de Jonge L, Greenway FL, Loria CM, Obarzanek E, Williamson DA. Comparison of weight-loss diets with different compositions of fat, protein, and carbohydrates. N Engl J Med. 2009;360:859–873.

131 Mozaffarian D, Appel LJ, Van Horn L. Components of a Cardioprotective Diet: New Insights. Circulation. 2011;123:2870-2891. DOI: 10.1161/CIRCULATIONAHA.110.968735

132 Ello-Martin JA, Ledikwe JH, Rolls BJ. The influence of food portion size and energy density on energy intake: implications for weight management.Am J Clin Nutr. 2005;82:236S–241S.

133 Rosenheck R. Fast food consumption and increased caloric intake: a systematic review of a trajectory towards weight gain and obesity risk. Obes Rev. 2008;9:535–547.

134 Shintani TT, Hughes CK, Beckham S, O'Connor HK. Obesity and cardiovascular risk intervention through the ad libitum feeding of traditional Hawaiian diet. Am J Clin Nutr. 1991;53(6 Suppl):1647S–51.

135 Greger M. How Not to Diet. New York: Flatiron Books. 2019. P188.

136 Lustig RH, Schmidt LA, Brindis CD. The toxic truth about sugar. Nature. 2012;482: 27-29

137 Bray GA. Low-Carbohydrate Diets and Realities of Weight Loss. JAMA. 2003;289(14):1853-1855. doi:10.1001/jama.289.14.1853

138 Johnston BC, Kanters S, Bandayrel K, Wu P, Naji F, Siemieniuk RA, Ball GDC, Busse JW, Thorlund K, Guyatt G, Jansen JP, Mills EJ. Comparison of Weight Loss Among Named Diet Programs in Overweight and Obese Adults A Meta-analysis. JAMA. 2014;312(9):923-933. doi:10.1001/jama.2014.10397

139 Jensen MD, Ryan DH, Apovian CM, et al. 2013 AHA/ACC/TOS guideline for the management of overweight and obesity in adults: a report of the American College of Cardiology/American Heart Association Task Force on Practice Guidelines and the Obesity Society. J Am Coll Cardiol. 2014;63(25 pt B):2985-3023. https://www.lipid.org/sites/default/files/ManagementOverweightObesity.pdf

140 Slomski A. Weight Gain Not an Issue With Mediterranean Diet. JAMA. 2016;316(4):385. doi:10.1001/jama.2016.9068

141 Johnston BC, Kanters S, Bandayrel K, et al. Comparison of weight loss among named diet programs in overweight and obese adults: a meta-analysis. JAMA. doi:10.1001/jama.2014.10397

142 Van Horn L. A Diet by Any Other Name Is Still About Energy. JAMA. 2014;312(9):900-901. doi:10.1001/jama.2014.10837

143 Van Horn L. A Diet by Any Other Name Is Still About Energy. JAMA. 2014;312(9):900-901. doi:10.1001/jama.2014.10837

144 de Souza RJ, Bray GA, Carey VJ, et al. Effects of 4 weight-loss diets differing in fat, protein, and carbohydrate on fat mass, lean mass, visceral adipose tissue, and hepatic fat: results from the POUNDS LOST trial. Am J Clin Nutr. 2012;95(3):614-625.

145 Sacks FM, Bray GA, Carey VJ, et al. Comparison of weight-loss diets with different compositions of fat, protein, and carbohydrates. N Engl J Med. 2009;360(9):859-873.

146 Anton SD, Gallagher J, Carey VJ, et al. Diet type and changes in food cravings following weight loss: findings from the POUNDS LOST Trial. Eat Weight Disord. 2012;17(2):e101-e108.

147 Gardner CD, Trepanowski JF, Del Gobbo LC, et al. Effect of Low-Fat vs Low-Carbohydrate Diet on 12-Month Weight Loss in Overweight Adults and the Association With Genotype Pattern or Insulin SecretionThe DIETFITS Randomized Clinical Trial. JAMA. 2018;319(7):667–679. doi:10.1001/jama.2018.0245

148 Sofi F, Dinu M, Pagliai G, Cesari F, Gori AM, Sereni A, Becatti M, Fiorillo C, Marcucci R, Casini A. Low-Calorie Vegetarian Versus Mediterranean Diets for Reducing Body Weight and Improving Cardiovascular Risk Profile: CARDIVEG Study (Cardiovascular Prevention With Vegetarian Diet). Circulation. 2018 Mar 13;137(11):1103-1113. doi: 10.1161/CIRCULATIONAHA.117.030088. Epub 2018 Feb 26.PMID: 29483085

149 Tobias DK, Chen M, Manson J, Ludwig DS, Willett W, Hu FB. Effect of low-fat diet interventions versus other diet interventions on long-term weight change in adults: a systematic review and meta-analysis. The Lancet Diabetes & Endocrinology. 2015;3(12):968-79. doi: 10.1016/S2213-8587(15)00367-8.

150 Abbasi J. Interest in the Ketogenic Diet Grows for Weight Loss and Type 2 Diabetes. JAMA. 2018;319(3):215–217. doi:10.1001/jama.2017.20639

151 Bueno, N., De Melo, I., De Oliveira, S., & Da Rocha Ataide, T. (2013). Very-low-carbohydrate ketogenic diet v. low-fat diet for long-term weight loss: A meta-analysis of randomised controlled trials. British Journal of Nutrition. 2013;110(7):1178-1187. doi:10.1017/S0007114513000548

152 Mansoor N, Vinknes KJ, Veierød MB, Retterstøl K, Effects of low-carbohydrate diets v. low-fat diets on body weight and cardiovascular risk factors: a meta-analysis of randomised controlled trials. British Journal of Nutrition. 2016;115:466–479

153 Noto H, Goto A, Tsujimoto T, Noda M. Low-carbohydrate diets and all-cause mortality: a systematic review and meta-analysis of observational studies. PLoS ONE. 2013;8(1):e55030.

154 Seidelmann SB, Claggett B, Cheng S, et al. Dietary carbohydrate intake and mortality: a prospective cohort study and meta-analysis. Lancet Public Health 2018; published online Aug 16. http://dx.doi.org/10.1016/S2468-2667(18)30135-X.

155 Fleming RM. The effect of high-protein diets on coronary blood flow. Angiology. 2000;51(10):817–26.

156 Schwingshackl L, Hoffmann G. Low-carbohydrate diets impair flow-mediated dilatation: evidence from a systematic review and meta-analysis. Br J Nutr. 2013;110(5):969–70.

157 Bueno, N., De Melo, I., De Oliveira, S., & Da Rocha Ataide, T. (2013). Very-low-carbohydrate ket genic diet v. low-fat diet for long-term weight loss: A meta-analysis of randomised controlled trials. British Journal of Nutrition. 2013;110(7):1178-1187. doi:10.1017/S0007114513000548

158 Bray GA. Low-carbohydrate diets and realities of weight loss. JAMA. 2003;289(14):1853–5.

159 U.S. News, Best Diets Rankings for 2020. https://health.usnews.com/best-diet

160 Hall KD, Bemis T, Brychta R, Chen KY, et al. Calorie for Calorie, Dietary Fat Restriction Results in More Body Fat Loss than Carbohydrate Restriction in People with Obesity. Cell Metabolism, 2015; DOI: 10.1016/j.cmet.2015.07.021

161 Hall KD, Guo J. Obesity energetics: body weight regulation and the effects of diet composition. Ga troenterology. 2017;152(7):1718–27.e3.

162 Hooper L, Abdelhamid A, Moore HJ, Douthwaite W, Skeaff CM, Summerbell CD. Effect of reducing total fat intake on body weight: systematic review and meta-analysis of randomised controlled trials and cohort studies. BMJ 2012; 345: e7666

163 Ornish D, Scherwitz LW, Billings JH, Gould KL, Merritt TA, Sparler S, Armstrong WT, Ports TA, Kirkeeide RL, Hogeboom C, Brand RJ. Intensive Lifestyle Changes for Reversal of Coronary Heart Disease. JAMA, 1998;280(23):2001-2007

164 Silberman A, Banthia R, Estay IS, Kemp C, Studley J, Hareras D, Ornish D. The effectiveness and efficacy of an intensive cardiac rehabilitation program in 24 sites. Am J Health Promot. 2010 Mar-Apr;24(4):260-6. doi: 10.4278/ajhp.24.4.arb.

165 Wright N, Wilson L, Smith M, Duncan B, McHugh P. The BROAD study: a randomised controlled trial using a whole food plant-based diet in the community for obesity, ischaemic heart disease or diabetes. Nutr Diabetes. 2017;7(3):e256.

166 Shintani TT, Hughes CK, Beckham S, O'Connor HK. Obesity and cardiovascular risk intervention through the ad libitum feeding of traditional Hawaiian diet. Am J Clin Nutr. 1991;53(6 Suppl):1647S–51.

167 Huang RY, Huang CC, Hu FB, Chavarro JE. Vegetarian Diets and Weight Reduction: a Meta-Analysis of Randomized Controlled Trials. J Gen Intern Med. 2016;31(1):109-16. doi: 10.1007/s11606-015-3390-7.

168 Turner-McGrievy GM, Davidson CR, Wingard EE, Wilcox S, Frongillo EA. Comparative effectiveness

of plant-based diets for weight loss: a randomized controlled trial of five different diets. Nutrition. 2015;31(2):350-8. Epub 2014 Oct 18.

169 Fernández de la Puebla RA, Fuentes F, Pérez-Martinez P, et al. A reduction in dietary saturated fat decreases body fat content in overweight, hypercholesterolemic males. Nutr Metab Cardiovasc Dis. 2003;13(5):273–7.

170 Piers LS, Walker KZ, Stoney RM, Soares MJ, O'Dea K. The influence of the type of dietary fat on postprandial fat oxidation rates: monounsaturated (olive oil) vs saturated fat (cream). Int J Obes Relat Metab Disord. 2002;26(6):814–21.

171 Anderson JW, Konz EC, Jenkins DJ. Health advantages and disadvantages of weight-reducing diets: a computer analysis and critical review. J Am Coll Nutr. 2000;19(5):578–90.

172 Kim H, Caulfield LE, Rebholz CM. Healthy plant-based diets are associated with lower risk of all-cause mortality in us adults. J Nutr. 2018;148(4):624–31.

173 Cava E, Yeat NC, Mittendorfer B. Preserving healthy muscle during weight loss. Adv Nutr. 2017;8(3):511–9.

174 Backx EM, Tieland M, Borgonjen-van den Berg KJ, Claessen PR, van Loon LJ, de Groot LC. Protein intake and lean body mass preservation during energy intake restriction in overweight older adults. Int J Obes (Lond). 2016;40(2):299–304.

175 Kim JE, O'Connor LE, Sands LP, Slebodnik MB, Campbell WW. Effects of dietary protein intake on body composition changes after weight loss in older adults: a systematic review and meta-analysis. Nutr Rev. 2016;74(3):210–24.

176 Liao CD, Tsauo JY, Wu YT, et al. Effects of protein supplementation combined with resistance exercise on body composition and physical function in older adults: a systematic review and meta-analysis, The American Journal of Clinical Nutrition. 2017;106(4):1078–1091, https://doi.org/10.3945/ajcn.116.143594

177 Sardeli AV, Komatsu TR, Mori MA, Gáspari AF, Chacon-Mikahil MPT. Resistance training prevents muscle loss induced by caloric restriction in obese elderly individuals: a systematic review and meta-analysis. Nutrients. 2018;10(4):423.

178 Morton RW, Murphy KT, McKellar SR. A systematic review, meta-analysis, and meta-regression of the effect of protein supplementation on resistance training-induced gains in muscle mass and strength in healthy adults. Br J Sports Med 2018;52:376–384. doi:10.1136/bjsports-2017-097608

179 Naude CE, Schoonees A, Senekal M, Young T, Garner P, Volmink J. Low carbohydrate versus isoc ergetic balanced diets for reducing weight and cardiovascular risk: a systematic review and meta-analysis. PLoS One. 2014; 9(7):e100652. Epub 2014 Jul 9.

180 Mueller C, Masri B, Hogg J, Mastrogiacomo M, Chiu YL. Carbohydrate- vs fat-controlled diet effect on weight loss and coronary artery disease risk: a pilot feeding study. Nutr Clin Pract. 2010;25(5):542-7.

181 Kones R. Low-fat versus low-carbohydrate diets, weight loss, vascular health, and prevention of coronary artery disease: the evidence, the reality, the challenge, and the hope. Nutr Clin Pract. 2010;25(5):528-41. doi: 10.1177/0884533610380614.

182 Atkins JL, Whincup PH, Morris RW, Lennon LT, Papacosta O,Wannamethee SG. High diet quality is associated with a lower risk of cardiovascular disease and all-cause mortality in older men. J Nutr. 2014;144(5):673-680.

183 U.S. Department of Agriculture, Center for Nutrition Policy and Promotion, September 2011.

184 Guth E. Counting Calories as an Approach to Achieve Weight Control. JAMA. 2018;319(3):225–226. doi:10.1001/jama.2017.21355.

185 Brody J. To Cut Weight: Lose the Diet, Find a Lifestyle. New York Times. March 6, 2018.

186 Wolff E, Dansinger ML. Soft drinks and weight gain: how strong is the link? Medscape J Med.

2008;10:189.

187 Lustig RH, Mulligan K, Noworolski SM. Isocaloric Fructose Restriction and Metabolic Improvement in Children with Obesity and Metabolic Syndrome. Obesity. 2016;24:453–460. doi:10.1002/oby.21371

188 Keller KL, Kirzner J, Pietrobelli A, St-Onge MP, Faith MS. Increased sweetened beverage intake is associated with reduced milk and calcium intake in 3- to 7-year-old children at multi-item laboratory lunches. J Am Diet Assoc. 2009;109:497–501.

189 Te Morenga L, Mallard S, Mann J. Dietary sugars and body weight: systematic review and meta- analyses of randomised controlled trials and cohort studies BMJ 2013; 346:e7492

190 Moss M, Salt Sugar Fat. Random House, New York. 2013.

191 Cheskin LJ, Roberts C, Margolis S. Nutrition and Weight Control. Johns Hopkins White Paper, New York. Remedy Media, 2014.

192 US Preventive Services Task Force. Behavioral Weight Loss Interventions to Prevent Obesity-Related Morbidity and Mortality in Adults US Preventive Services Task Force Recommendation Statement. JAMA.2018;320(11):1163–1171. doi:10.1001/jama.2018.13022

193 American College of Cardiology/American Heart Association Task Force on Practice Guidelines, Obesity Expert Panel, 2013. Expert Panel Report: guidelines (2013) for the management of overweight and obesity in adults. Obesity (Silver Spring) 2014; 22: Suppl 2: S41-410.

194 Heymsfield SB, Wadden TA. Mechanisms, Pathophysiology, and Management of Obesity. N Engl J Med. 2017;376:254-266 January 19, 2017DOI: 10.1056/NEJMra1514009.

195 De Cabo R, Mattson MP. Effects of intermittent fasting on health, aging, and disease. N Engl J Med. 2019;381(26):2541-2551.

196 Abbasi J. Can a Diet That Mimics Fasting Turn Back the Clock?. JAMA. 2017;318(3):227–229. doi:10.1001/jama.2017.6648.

197 Wei M, Brandhorst S, Shelehchi M, et al. Fasting-mimicking diet and markers/risk factors for aging, diabetes, cancer, and cardiovascular disease. Science Translational Medicine. 2017;9(377):eaai8700. DOI: 10.1126/scitranslmed.aai8700

198 Klempel MC, Kroeger CM, Bhutani S, Trepanowski JF, Varady KA. Intermittent fasting combined with calorie restriction is effective for weight loss and cardio-protection in obese women. Nutrition Journal201211: 98 DOI: 10.1186/1475-2891-11-98

199 Mattson MP, Wan R: Beneficial effects of intermittent fasting and caloric restriction on the cardiovascular and cerebrovascular systems. J Nutr Biochem. 2005; 16 (3): 129-137. 10.1016/j.jnutbio.2004.12.007.

200 Harvie MN, Pegington M, Mattson MP, Frystyk J, Dillon B, Evans G, et al: The effects of intermittent or continuous energy restriction on weight loss and metabolic disease risk markers: a randomized trial in young overweight women. Int J Obes (Lond). 2011;35 (5): 714-727. 10.1038/ijo.2010.171.

201 De Cabo R, Mattson MP. Effects of intermittent fasting on health, aging, and disease. N Engl J Med. 2019;381(26):2541-2551.

202 Das SK, Roberts SB, Bhapkar MV, et al. Body-composition changes in the Comprehensive Assessment of Long-term Effects of Reducing Intake of Energy (CALERIE)-2 study: a 2-y randomized controlled trial of calorie restriction in nonobese humans. Am J Clin Nutr. 2017;105(4):913–27.

203 Owen OE, Smalley KJ, D'Alessio DA, Mozzoli MA, Dawson EK. Protein, fat, and carbohydrate requirements during starvation: anaplerosis and cataplerosis. Am J Clin Nutr. 1998;68(1):12–34.

204 Longo VD, Mattson MP. Fasting: molecular mechanisms and clinical applications. Cell Metab. 2014;19(2):181–92.

205 Greger M. How Not to Diet. New York: Flatiron Books. 2019. P464.

206 Horne BD, Grajower MM, Anderson JL. Limited Evidence for the Health Effects and Safety of Intermittent Fasting Among Patients With Type 2 Diabetes. JAMA. 2020;324(4):341–342. doi:10.1001/jama.2020.3908

207 Austad SN. Ageing: Mixed results for dieting monkeys. Nature, 2012;489:210–211(13 September 2012) doi:10.1038/nature11484

208 Greger M. How Not to Diet. New York: Flatiron Books. 2019.

209 Cheskin LJ, Roberts C, Margolis S. Nutrition and Weight Control. Johns Hopkins White Paper, New York. Remedy Media, 2014

210 18 keys to healthy weight loss. The girth of a nation. UC Berkeley Wellness Letter. 31(15) Fall 2015.

211 American College of Cardiology/ American Heart Association Task Force on Practice Guidelines, Obesity Expert Panel, 2013. Expert Panel Report: guidelines (2013) for the management of overweight and obesity in adults. Obesity (Silver Spring) 2014;22:Suppl2:S41-410.

212 Drexler M. Obesity. Can we stop the epidemic. Harvard Public Health Spring 2017, pp. 12-35.

213 Popkin BM, Hawkes C. Sweetening of the global diet, particularly beverages: patterns, trends, and policy responses. Lancet Diabetes Endocrinol. 2016;4:174-86.

214 Ebbeling CB, Feldman HA, Steltz SK, Quinn NL, Robinson LM, Ludwig DS. Effects of Sugar-Sweetened, Artificially Sweetened, and Unsweetened Beverages on Cardiometabolic Risk Factors, Body Composition, and Sweet Taste Preference: A Randomized Controlled Trial. J Am Heart Assoc. 2020 Aug 4;9(15):e015668. doi: 10.1161/JAHA.119.015668. Epub 2020 Jul 22. PMID: 32696704.

215 O'Connor A. Can Artificial Sweeteners Keep Us From Gaining Weight? New York Times. August 20, 2020.

216 Ornish D, The Spectrum. New York, Ballantine Books: 2007

217 Buttner D. The Blue Zones, Second Edition. Washington DC, National Geographic, 2012

218 Church TS, Thomas DM, Tudor-Locke C, et al. Trends over 5 decades in U.S. occupation-related physical activity and their associations with obesity. PLoS One 2011; 6(5): e19657.

219 Heymsfield SB, Wadden TA. Mechanisms, Pathophysiology, and Management of Obesity. N Engl J Med. 2017; 376:254-266 January 19, 2017DOI: 10.1056/NEJMra1514009 220 Heymsfield SB, Wadden TA. Mechanisms, Pathophysiology, and Management of Obesity. N Engl J Med. 2017; 376:254-266 January 19, 2017 DOI: 10.1056/NEJMra1514009

221 Fisher DP, Johnson E, Haneuse S, et al. Association Between Bariatric Surgery and Macrovascular Disease Outcomes in Patients With Type 2 Diabetes and Severe Obesity. JAMA. 2018;320(15):1570–1582. doi:10.1001/jama.2018.14619.

222 Sjöström L, Peltonen M, Jacobson P, et al. Association of bariatric surgery with long-term remission of type 2 diabetes and with microvascular and macrovascular complications. JAMA.

2014;311(22):2297-2304. doi:10.1001/jama.2014.5988

223 Schauer PR, Bhatt DL, Kashyap SR. Bariatric surgery or intensive medical therapy for diabetes after 5 years. N Engl J Med. 2017;376(20):1997.

224 Arterburn DE, Telem DA, Kushner RF, Courcoulas AP. Benefits and Risks of Bariatric Surgery in Adults: A Review. JAMA. 2020;324(9):879–887. doi:10.1001/jama.2020.12567

225 Rosen CJ, Ingelfinger JR. Bariatric Surgery and Restoration of Insulin Sensitivity — It's Weight Loss. N Engl J Med 2020; 383:777-778. DOI: 10.1056/NEJMe2024212

Chapter 5 – Vitamins and Other Supplements

1 Bellows L, Moore R, Gross A. Dietary Supplements: Vitamins and Minerals. Colorado State University Extension Publication no. 9.338 (9/13) http://www.ext.colostate.edu/pubs/foodnut/09338.html

2 Bellows L, Moore R, Gross A. Dietary Supplements: Herbals and Botanicals. Colorado State University Extension Publication no. 9.370 (10/13) http://www.ext.colostate.edu/pubs/foodnut/09370.html

3 Office of Dietary Supplements, National Institutes of Health: Dietary Supplements: What You Need To Know.http://ods.od.nih.gov/HealthInformation/DS_WhatYouNeedToKnow.aspx

4 Office of Dietary Supplements, National Institutes of Health: Frequently Asked Questions. http://ods.od.nih.gov/Health_Information/ODS_Frequently_Asked_Questions.aspx

5 RN 2016 Annual Survey on Dietary Supplements.Council for Responsible Nutrition (CRN). 2016. https://www.crnusa.org/resources/crn-2016-annual-survey-dietary-supplements.

6 Cohen PA. The Supplement Paradox: Negligible Benefits, Robust Consumption. JAMA. 2016;316(14):1453-1454. doi:10.1001/jama.2016.14252

7 Kuehn BM. Dietary Supplement Linked to Cases of Acute Hepatitis. JAMA. 2013;310(17):1784. doi:10.1001/jama.2013.281868

8 Or F, Kim Y, Simms J, Austin SB. Taking Stock of Dietary Supplements' Harmful Effects on Children, Adolescents, and Young Adults. Journal of Adolescent Health. 2019; DOI: https://doi.org/10.1016/j.jadohealth.2019.03.005

9 Interlandi J. Supplements, a complete guide to safety. Consumer Reports. September 2016.

10 Geller AI, Shehab N, Weidle NJ, Lovegrove MC, Wolpert BJ, Timbo BB, Mozersky RP, Budnitz DS. Emergency department visits for adverse events related to dietary supplements. N Engl J Med. 015;373:1531–40.

11 Bakalar N. Take a number $30.2 billion. New York Times. June 28, 2016.

12 Offit P A, Do You Believe in Magic. New York: Harper Collins; 2013.

13 Kaptchuk TJ, Miller FG. Placebo Effects in Medicine. N Engl J Med. 2015; 373:8-9July 2, 2015DOI: 10.1056/NEJMp1504023

14 Colloca L, Barsky AJ. Placebo and nocebo effects. N Engl J Med. 2015; 382(6):554-561.

15 Kaptchuk TJ, Miller FG. Placebo Effects in Medicine. N Engl J Med. 2015; 373:8-9. DOI: 10.1056/NEJMp1504023

16 Food and Drug Administration: Overview of Dietary Supplements, http://www.fda.gov/Food/DietarySupplements/default.htm

17 Bellows L, Moore R, Gross A. Dietary Supplements: Vitamins and Minerals. Colorado State University Extension Publication no. 9.338 (9/13) http://www.ext.colostate.edu/pubs/foodnut/09338.html

18 Cohen PA, Bass S. Injecting safety into supplements—modernizing the dietary supplement law. N Engl J Med. 2019;381(25):2387-2389.

19 Cohen PA. The Supplement Paradox: Negligible Benefits, Robust Consumption. JAMA. 016;316(14):1453-1454. doi:10.1001/jama.2016.14252.

20 Manson JE, Bassuk SS. Vitamin and Mineral SupplementsWhat Clinicians Need to Know. JAMA.2018;319(9):859–860. doi:10.1001/jama.2017.21012

21 Offit P A, Do You Believe in Magic. New York: Harper Collins; 2013.

22 Dietary supplements: we can do better. University of California, Berkeley Wellness Letter. Summer 2019.

23 Shop Smarter for Supplements. Consumer Reports. December 2018.

24 Felton R. A Tattered Safety Net. Consumer Reports. September 2020:30-37.

25 Carroll AE. Given Their Potential for Harm, It's Time to Focus on the Safety of Supplements. JAMA.2018;320(13):1306–1307. doi:10.1001/jama.2018.13147

26 Bellows L, Moore R, Gross A. Dietary Supplements: Vitamins and Minerals. Colorado State University Extension Publication no. 9.338 (9/13) http://www.ext.colostate.edu/pubs/foodnut/09338.html

27 Office of Dietary Supplements, National Institutes of Health: Frequently Asked Questions. http://ods.od.nih.gov/Health_Information/ODS_Frequently_Asked_Questions.aspx

28 Food and Drug Administration: Overview of Dietary Supplements, http://www.fda.gov/Food/Dietary-Supplements/default.htm

29 Abbasi J. Amid Reports of Infant Deaths, FTC Cracks Down on Homeopathy While FDA Investigates. JAMA. 2017;317(8):793-795. doi:10.1001/jama.2016.19090

30 Podolsky SH, Kesselheim AS. Regulating Homeopathic Products — A Century of Dilute Interest. N Engl J Med. 2016; 374:201-203January 21, 2016DOI: 10.1056/NEJMp1513393

31 Dilutions of grandeur U.C. Berkeley Wellness Letter Vol. 32, Issue 1, October 2015.

32 Bellows L, Moore R, Gross A. Dietary Supplements: Vitamins and Minerals. Colorado State University Extension Publication no. 9.338 (9/13) http://www.ext.colostate.edu/pubs/foodnut/09338.html

33 Office of Dietary Supplements, National Institutes of Health: Frequently Asked Questions. http://ods.od.nih.gov/Health_Information/ODS_Frequently_Asked_Questions.aspx

34 Food and Drug Administration: Overview of Dietary Supplements, http://www.fda.gov/Food/Dietary-Supplements/default.htm

35 Dietary supplements: we can do better. University of California, Berkeley Wellness Letter. Summer 2019.

36 Offit P A, Do You Believe in Magic. New York: Harper Collins; 2013.

37 Cohen PA. The Supplement Paradox: Negligible Benefits, Robust Consumption. JAMA. 2016;316(14):1453-1454. doi:10.1001/jama.2016.14252.

38 Cooper L. Your dietary supplement might contain banned drugs. Some manufacturers are flouting the FDA and continuing to sell illegal concoctions, study finds. Consumer Reports October 21, 2014 http://www.consumerreports.org/cro/news/2014/10/your-dietary-supplement-might-contain-banned-drugs/index.htm

39 What's behind our dietary supplements coverage. Consumer Reports. January 2011.http://www.co sum-erreports.org/cro/2012/04/what-s-behind-our-dietary-supplements-coverage/index.htm

40 Interlandi J. Supplements, a complete guide to safety. Consumer Reports. September 2016.

41 Tucker J, Fischer T, Upjohn L, Mazzera D, Kumar M. Unapproved Pharmaceutical Ingredients Included in Dietary Supplements Associated With US Food and Drug Administration Warnings. JAMA Netw Open.2018;1(6):e183337. doi:10.1001/jamanetworkopen.2018.3337

42 Cohen PA. The FDA and Adulterated Supplements—Dereliction of Duty. JAMA Netw Open.2018;1(6):e183329. doi:10.1001/jamanetworkopen.2018.3329

43 Offit P A, Do You Believe in Magic. New York: Harper Collins; 2013.

44 Offit PA, Erush, S. Skip the Supplements. New York Times. December 14, 2013; http://www.nytimes.com/2013/12/15/opinion/sunday/skip-the-supplements.html?_r=0

45 Dietary Reference Intakes: The Essential Guide to Nutrient Requirements http://www.nap.edu/catalog/11537.html; http://www.nal.usda.gov/fnic/DRI/Essential_Guide/DRIEssentialGuideNutReq.pdf

46 Dietary Reference Intakes Tables and Application, Institute of Medicine Last Updated 10/2/2014 http://

www.iom.edu/Activities/Nutrition/SummaryDRIs/DRI-Tables.aspx

47 Guidance for Industry: A Food Labeling Guide (14. Appendix F: Calculate the% Daily Value for the Appropriate Nutrients) January 2013. U. S. Food and Drug Administration http://www.fda.gov/Food/GuidanceRegulation/GuidanceDocumentsRegulatoryInformation/LabelingNutrition/ucm064928.htm

48 Bellows L, Moore R, Gross A. Dietary Supplements: Vitamins and Minerals. Colorado State University Extension Publication no. 9.338 (9/13) http://www.ext.colostate.edu/pubs/foodnut/09338.html

49 Bellows L, Moore R. Fat-Soluble Vitamins: A, D, E, and K. Colorado State University Extension Publication no. 9.315 (11/12) http://www.ext.colostate.edu/pubs/foodnut/09315.html

50 Bellows L, Moore R. Water-Soluble Vitamins: B-Complex and Vitamin C. Colorado State University Extension Publication no. 9.312 (11/12) http://www.ext.colostate.edu/pubs/foodnut/09370.html

51 Meyer HE, Willett WC, Fung TT, Holvik K, Feskanich D. Association of High Intakes of Vitamins B6 and B12 From Food and Supplements With Risk of Hip Fracture Among Postmenopausal Women in the Nurses' Health Study. JAMA Netw Open. Published online May 10, 20192(5):e193591. doi:10.1001/jamanetworkopen. 2019.3591.

52 Bellows L, Moore R. Water-Soluble Vitamins: B-Complex and Vitamin C. Colorado State University Extension Publication no. 9.312 (11/12) http://www.ext.colostate.edu/pubs/foodnut/09370.html

53 Morris MC, Schneider JA, Tangney CC. Thoughts on B-vitamins and dementia. Journal of Alzheimer's disease : JAD. 2006;9(4):429-433.

54 Cobalamin CR. The stomach, and aging. Am J Clin Nutr. 1997;66:750–759.

55 Brody JE, A Vitamin to Protect the Aging Brain. New York Times, September 6, 2016.

56 Should you take a vitamin B12 supplement? Harvard Health Letter. April 2020.

57 Allen LH. How common is vitamin B-12 deficiency? Am J Clin Nutr. 2009;89(2):693S–696S, https://doi.org/10.3945/ajcn.2008.26947A

58 Baik HW, Russell RM. Vitamin B12 deficiency in the elderly. Annu Rev Nutr. 1999;19:357-77.

59 Should you take a vitamin B12 supplement?. Harvard Health Letter. April 2020.

60 Offit P A, Do You Believe in Magic. New York: Harper Collins; 2013

61 Bellows L, Moore R. Fat-Soluble Vitamins: A, D, E, and K. Colorado State University Extension Publication no. 9.315 (11/12) http://www.ext.colostate.edu/pubs/foodnut/09315.html

62 Institute of Medicine (US) Panel on Micronutrients. Dietary Reference Intakes for Vitamin A, Vitamin K, Arsenic, Boron, Chromium, Copper, Iodine, Iron, Manganese, Molybdenum, Nickel, Silicon, Vanadium, and Zinc. Washington (DC): National Academies Press (US); 2001. 4, Vitamin A. Available from http://www.ncbi.nlm.nih.gov/books/NBK222318/

63 Bellows L, Moore R. Fat-Soluble Vitamins: A, D, E, and K. Colorado State University Extension Publication no. 9.315 (11/12) http://www.ext.colostate.edu/pubs/foodnut/09315.html

64 Bellows L, Moore R. Fat-Soluble Vitamins: A, D, E, and K. Colorado State University Extension Publication no. 9.315 (11/12) http://www.ext.colostate.edu/pubs/foodnut/09315.html

65 Wang H, O'Reilly EJ, Weisskopf MG, Logro G. Vitamin E Intake and Risk of Amyotrophic Lateral Sclerosis: A Pooled Analysis of Data From 5 Prospective Cohort Studies. American Journal of Epidemiology. 2011;173:595-602.

66 Miller ER, Pastor-Barriuso R, Dalal D, Riemersma RA, Appel LJ, Guallar E. Meta-Analysis: High-Dosage Vitamin E Supplementation May Increase All-Cause Mortality. Ann Intern Med. 2005;142:37–46. doi: 10.7326/0003-4819-142-1-200501040-00110

67 Bellows L, Moore R. Fat-Soluble Vitamins: A, D, E, and K. Colorado State University Extension

Publication no. 9.315 (11/12) http://www.ext.colostate.edu/pubs/foodnut/09315.html

68 Bellows L, Moore R. Fat-Soluble Vitamins: A, D, E, and K. Colorado State University Extension Publication no. 9.315 (11/12) http://www.ext.colostate.edu/pubs/foodnut/09315.html

69 Huang HY, Caballero B, Chang S, Alberg AJ, Semba RD, Schneyer CR, et al. The efficacy and safety of multivitamin and mineral supplement use to prevent cancer and chronic disease in adults: a systematic review for a National Institutes of Health state-of-the-science conference. Ann Intern Med. 2006;145:372-385.

70 Beste LA, Moseley RH, Saint S, Cornia PB. Too Much of a Good Thing. N Engl J Med. 2016;374:873-878March 3, 2016DOI: 10.1056/NEJMcps1405984

71 Navarro VJ, Barnhart H, Bonkovsky HL, et al. Liver injury from herbals and dietary supplements in the U.S. Drug-Induced Liver Injury Network. Hepatology. 2014;60:1399-1408

72 Bellows L, Moore R. Fat-Soluble Vitamins: A, D, E, and K. Colorado State University Extension Publication no. 9.315 (11/12) http://www.ext.colostate.edu/pubs/foodnut/09315.html

73 Vitamin D. Medline Plus, A service of the U.S. National Library of Medicine National Institutes of Health; http://www.nlm.nih.gov/medlineplus/druginfo/natural/929.html

74 Holick MF. Vitamin D Deficiency. N Engl J Med. 2007; 357:266-281July 19, 2007DOI: 10.1056/ NEJMra070553

75 Szabo L. Shadows on a Sunny Fad. New York Times. August 19, 2018.

76 Kolata G. Why Are So Many People Popping Vitamin D? New York Times. April 10, 2017.

77 Kolata G. D Is for Dilemma. New York Times. April 11, 2017.

78 The vitamin D bandwagon rolls on. U.C. Berkeley Wellness Letter. vol 31 No. 5, Winter 2014-15, p.4

79 Ross AC1, Manson JE, Abrams SA, Aloia JF, Brannon PM, Clinton SK, Durazo-Arvizu RA, Gallagher JC, Gallo RL, Jones G, Kovacs CS, Mayne ST, Rosen CJ, Shapses SA. The 2011 report on dietary reference intakes for calcium and vitamin D from the Institute of Medicine: what clinicians need to know. J Clin Endocrinol Metab. 2011;96(1):53-8. doi: 10.1210/jc.2010-2704. Epub 2010 Nov 29.

80 Dietary Reference Intakes for Calcium and Vitamin D, Report Brief, Washington DC: The Institute of Medicine of the National Academies. November 2010. http://www.nal.usda.gov/fnic/DRI/DRI_Calcium_Vitamin_D/FullReport.pdf

81 Ross AC1, Manson JE, Abrams SA, Aloia JF, Brannon PM, Clinton SK, Durazo-Arvizu RA, Gallagher JC, Gallo RL, Jones G, Kovacs CS, Mayne ST, Rosen CJ, Shapses SA. The 2011 report on dietary reference intakes for calcium and vitamin D from the Institute of Medicine: what clinicians need to know. J Clin Endocrinol Metab. 2011;96(1):53-8. doi: 10.1210/jc.2010-2704. Epub 2010 Nov 29.

82 Dietary Reference Intakes for Calcium and Vitamin D, Report Brief, Washington DC: The Institute of Medicine of the National Academies. November 2010. http://www.nal.usda.gov/fnic/DRI/DRI_Calcium_Vitamin_D/FullReport.pdf

83 Dietary Reference Intakes for Calcium and Vitamin D, Report Brief, Washington DC: The Institute ofMedicine of the National Academies. November 2010. http://www.nal.usda.gov/fnic/DRI/DRI_Calcium_Vitamin_D/FullReport.pdf

84 Hansen KE, Johnson RE, Chambers KR, Johnson MG, Lemon CC, Vo TNT, Marvdashti S. Treatment of Vitamin D Insufficiency in Postmenopausal WomenA Randomized Clinical Trial. JAMA Intern Med. 2015;175(10):1612-1621. doi:10.1001/jamainternmed.2015.3874

85 Theodoratou E, Tzoulaki I, Zgaga L, Ioannidis JPA. Vitamin D and multiple health outcomes: umbrella review of systematic reviews and meta-analyses of observational studies and randomised trials. BMJ. 2014;348:g2035. doi:10.1136/bmj.g2035.

86 Bolland MJ, Avenell A, Grey A. Should adults take vitamin D supplements to prevent disease?

BMJ. 2016;355:i6201.

87 Manson JE, Cook NR, Lee I-M, et al. Vitamin D supplements and prevention of cancer and cardiovascular disease. N Engl J Med. November 10, 2018. DOI: 10.1056/NEJMoa1809944.

88 Rooney MR, Harnack L, Michos ED, Ogilvie RP, Sempos CT, Lutsey PL. Trends in Use of High-Dose Vitamin D Supplements Exceeding 1000 or 4000 International Units Daily, 1999- 2014. JAMA. 2017;317(23):2448–2450. doi:10.1001/jama.2017.4392

89 Ross CR, Taylor CL, Yaktine AL, et al. Dietary Reference Intakes for Calcium and Vitamin D. Washington, DC: National Academies Press; 2011.

90 Lucas A, Wolf M. Vitamin D and Health Outcomes: Then Came the Randomized Clinical Trials. JAMA. 2019;322(19):1866–1868. doi:https://doi.org/10.1001/jama.2019.17302

91 Bellows L, Moore R. Fat-Soluble Vitamins: A, D, E, and K. Colorado State University Extension Publication no. 9.315 (11/12) http://www.ext.colostate.edu/pubs/foodnut/09315.html

92 Vitamin D. Medline Plus, A service of the U.S. National Library of Medicine National Institutes of Health; http://www.nlm.nih.gov/medlineplus/druginfo/natural/929.html

93 Ross AC1, Manson JE, Abrams SA, Aloia JF, Brannon PM, Clinton SK, Durazo-Arvizu RA, Gallagher JC, Gallo RL, Jones G, Kovacs CS, Mayne ST, Rosen CJ, Shapses SA. The 2011 report on dietary reference intakes for calcium and vitamin D from the Institute of Medicine: what clinicians need to know. J Clin Endocrinol Metab. 2011;96(1):53-8. doi: 10.1210/jc.2010-2704. Epub 2010 Nov 29.

94 Manson JE, Brannon PM, Rosen CJ, Taylor CL. Vitamin D Deficiency — Is There Really a Pandemic? N Engl J Med. 2016;375(19):1817-1820

95 Institute of Medicine. Dietary reference intakes: calcium and vitamin D. Washing- ton, DC: National Academies Press, 2011.

96 Offit P A, Do You Believe in Magic. New York: Harper Collins; 2013.

97 Goodman GE, Thornquist MD, Balmes J, Cullen MR, Meyskens FL, Omenn GS, Valanis B, Williams JH. The Beta-Carotene and Retinol Efficacy Trial: Incidence of Lung Cancer and Cardiovascular Disease Mortality During 6-Year Follow-up After Stopping Beta-Carotene and Retinol Supplements J Natl Cancer Inst. 2004;96(23):1743-1750

98 Bjelakovic G, Nikolova D, Simonetti RG, Gluud C. Antioxidant supplements for preventing gastrointestinal cancers. Cochrane Database of Systematic Reviews. 2008;3. Art. No.: CD004183. DOI: 10.1002/14651858.CD004183.pub3.

99 Lonn E, Bosch J, Yusuf S, Sheridan P, Pogue J, Arnold JM, Ross C, Arnold A, Sleight P, Probstfield J, Dagenais GR, HOPE and HOPE-TOO Trial Investigators Effects of long-term vitamin E supplementation on cardiovascular events and cancer: a randomized controlled trial. JAMA. 2005;293(11):1338-1347.

100 Lawson KA, Wright ME, Subar A, Mouw T, Hollenbeck A, Schatzkin A, Leitzmann MF. Multivitamin Use and Risk of Prostate Cancer in the National Institutes of Health–AARP Diet and Health Study. J Natl Cancer Inst. 2007;99(10):754-764 doi:10.1093/jnci/djk177

101 Bjelakovic G, Nikolova D, Gluud L, Simonetti RG, Gluud C. Mortality in Randomized Trials of Antioxidant Supplements for Primary and Secondary Prevention: Systematic Review and Meta-analysis. JAMA. 2007;297(8):842-857. doi:10.1001/jama.297.8.842. http://jama.jamanetwork.com/article.aspx?articleid=205797

102 Bjelakovic G, Nikolova D, Gluud LL, Simonetti RG, Gluud C. Antioxidant supplements for prevention of mortality in healthy participants and patients with various diseases. Cochrane Database Syst Rev. 2008;16(2):CD007176. doi: 10.1002/14651858.CD007176.

103 Offit P A, Do You Believe in Magic. New York: Harper Collins; 2013.

104 Demetrius A. Vitamin Supplements and Cancer Prevention: Where Do Randomized Controlled Trials

Stand? J Natl Cancer Inst. 2009;101 (1): 2-4 doi:10.1093/jnci/djn453 first published online December 30, 2008.

105 Offit P A, Do You Believe in Magic. New York: Harper Collins; 2013.

106 Klein EA, Thompson IM Jr, Tangen CM, Crowley JJ, Lucia MS, Goodman PJ, Minasian LM, Ford-LG, Parnes HL, Gaziano JM, et al. Vitamin E and the risk of prostate cancer: the Selenium and Vitamin E Cancer Prevention Trial (SELECT). JAMA. 2011;306(14):1549-56.

107 National Cancer Institute. Selenium and Vitamin E Cancer Prevention Trial (SELECT) 2/21/14 http://www.cancer.gov/newscenter/qa/2008/selectqa

108 Mursu J, Robien K, Harnack LJ, Harnack LJ, Park K, Jacobs DR Jr. Dietary Supplements and Mortality Rate in Older Women The Iowa Women's Health Study. Arch Intern Med. 2011;171(18):1625-1633

109 Mursu J, Robien K, Harnack LJ, Harnack LJ, Park K, Jacobs DR Jr. Dietary Supplements and Mortality Rate in Older Women The Iowa Women's Health Study. Arch Intern Med. 2011;171(18):1625-1633

110 Fortmann SP, Burda BU, Senger CA, Lin JS, Whitlock EP. Vitamin and mineral supplements in the primary prevention of cardiovascular disease and cancer: an updated systematic evidence review for the U.S. Preventive Services Task Force. Ann Intern Med. 2013;159:824-34.

111 Moyer VA, U.S. Preventive Services Task Force. Vitamin D and calcium supplementation to prevent fractures in adults: U.S. Preventive Services Task Force recommendation statement. Ann Intern Med. 2013; 158:691-6.

112 Grodstein F, O'Brien J, Kang JH, Dushkes R, Cook NR, Okereke O, et al. Long-term multivitamin supplementation and cognitive function in men. A randomized trial. Ann Intern Med. 2013; 159:806-14.

113 Sesso HD, Buring JE, Christen WG, Kurth T, Belanger C, MacFadyen J, Bubes V, Manson JE, Glynn RJ, Gaziano JM. Vitamins E and C in the prevention of cardiovascular disease in men: the Physicians' Health Study II randomized controlled trial. JAMA. 2008 Nov 12;300(18):2123-33. doi: 10.1001/jama.2008.600. Epub 2008 Nov 9.

114 Gaziano JM, Glynn RJ, Christen WG, Kurth T, Belanger C, MacFadyen J, Bubes V, Manson JE, Sesso HD, Buring JE. Vitamins E and C in the Prevention of Prostate and Total Cancer in Men: The Physicians' Health Study II, a Randomized Controlled Trial. JAMA. Jan 7, 2009; 301(1): 52–62.

115 Huang HY, Caballero B, Chang S, Alberg AJ, Semba RD, Schneyer CR, et al. The efficacy and safety of multivitamin and mineral supplement use to prevent cancer and chronic disease in adults: a systematic review for a National Institutes of Health state-of-the-science conference. Ann Intern Med. 2006;145:372-85.

116 Bjelakovic G, Nikolova D, Gluud C. Antioxidant supplements to prevent mortality. JAMA. 2013; 310:1178-9.

117 Guallar E, Stranges S, Mulrow C, Appel LJ, Miller ER. Enough Is Enough: Stop Wasting Money on Vitamin and Mineral Supplements. Ann Intern Med. 2013;159:850-851. doi:10.7326/0003-4819-159-12-201312170-00011

118 Mursu J, Robien K, Harnack LJ, Harnack LJ, Park K, Jacobs DR Jr. Dietary Supplements and Mortality Rate in Older Women The Iowa Women's Health Study. Arch Intern Med. 2011;171(18):1625-1633

119 Gaziano JM, Sesso HD, Christen WG, Bubes V, Smith JP, MacFadyen J, Schvartz M, Manson JE, Glynn RJ, Buring JE. Multivitamins in the Prevention of Cancer in Men, The Physicians' Health Study II Randomized Controlled Trial. JAMA. 2012;308(18):1871–1880. doi:10.1001/jama.2012.14641

120 Bach PB, Lewis RJ. Multiplicities in the Assessment of Multiple Vitamins. Is It Too Soon to Tell Men That Vitamins Prevent Cancer?. JAMA. 2012;308(18):1916–1917. doi:10.1001/jama.2012.53273

121 Omenn GS, Goodman GE, Thornquist MD, et al. Effects of a combination of beta carotene and vitamin A on lung cancer and cardiovascular disease. N Engl J Med. 1996;334(18):1150-1155.

122 Klein EA, Thompson IM Jr, Tangen CM, et al. Vitamin E and the risk of prostate cancer: the Selenium

and Vitamin E Cancer Prevention Trial (SELECT). JAMA. 2011;306(14):1549-1556

123 Willett W, Skerrett PJ. Eat, Drink, and Be Healthy. New York: Free Press/Simon & Schuster; 2017. ISBN13: 9781501164774

124 Manson JE, Cook NR, Lee I-M, et al. Vitamin D supplements and prevention of cancer and cardiovascular disease. N Engl J Med. November 10, 2018. DOI: 10.1056/NEJMoa1809944.

125 Dietary Supplements: What you need to know. NIH Clinical Center. 2011. http://ods.od.nih.gov/HealthInformation/DS_WhatYouNeedToKnow.aspx

126 Bellows L, Moore R, Gross A. Dietary Supplements: Herbals and Botanicals. Colorado State University Extension Publication no. 9.370 (10/13) http://www.ext.colostate.edu/pubs/foodnut/09370.html

127 Abbasi J. Another Nail in the Coffin for Fish Oil Supplements. JAMA. 2018;319(18):1851–1852. doi:10.1001/jama.2018.2498

128 Aung T, Halsey J, Kromhout D, et al. Associations of Omega-3 Fatty Acid Supplement Use With Cardiovascular Disease Risks: Meta-analysis of 10 Trials Involving 77 917 Individuals. JAMA Cardiol. 2018;3(3):225–233. doi:10.1001/jamacardio.2017.5205

129 Hu Y, Hu FB, Manson JE. Marine Omega–3 Supplementation and Cardiovascular Disease: An Updated Meta–Analysis of 13 Randomized Controlled Trials Involving 127 477 Participants. J Am Heart Assn. 2019;8(19):e013543. https://doi.org/10.1161/JAHA.119.013543.

130 Bellows L. Vegetarian Diets. Colorado State University Extension Publication no. 9.324; http://www.ext.colostate.edu/pubs/foodnut/09324.html

131 Gliemann L1, Schmidt JF, Olesen J, Biensø RS, Peronard SL, Grandjean SU, Mortensen SP, Nyberg M, Bangsbo J, Pilegaard H, Hellsten Y. Resveratrol blunts the positive effects of exercise training on cardiovascular health in aged men. J Physiol. 2013;591(20):5047-59. doi: 10.1113/jphysiol.2013.258061. Epub 2013 Jul 22.

132 Reynolds G. Rebranding the Free Radicals. New York Times February 18, 2014. p. D4.

133 Bellows L, Moore R, Gross A. Dietary Supplements: Herbals and Botanicals. Colorado State University Extension Publication no. 9.370 (10/13) http://www.ext.colostate.edu/pubs/foodnut/09370.html

134 Shop Smarter for Supplements. Consumer Reports. December 2018.

135 Safety Alerts & Advisories. U.S. Food and Drug Administration; http://www.fda.gov/Food/RecallsOutbreaksEmergencies/SafetyAlertsAdvisories/default.htm

136 Dangerous supplements: what you don't know about these 12 ingredients could hurt you. Consumer Reports. Last updated: September 2010 http://www.consumerreports.org/cro/2012/05/dangerous-supplements/index.htm

137 Dangerous supplements: what you don't know about these 12 ingredients could hurt you. Consumer Reports. Last updated: September 2010 http://www.consumerreports.org/cro/2012/05/dangerous-supplements/index.htm

138 Sepkowitz KA. Energy Drinks and Caffeine-Related Adverse Effects. JAMA. 2013;309(3):243-244. doi:10.1001/jama.2012.173526.

139 Howland J, Rohsenow DJ. Risks of Energy Drinks Mixed With Alcohol. JAMA. 2013;309(3):245-246. doi:10.1001/jama.2012.187978.

140 Svatikova A, Covassin N, Somers KR, Somers KV, Soucek F, Kara T, Bukartyk J. A Randomized Trial of Cardiovascular Responses to Energy Drink Consumption in Healthy Adults. JAMA. 2015;314(19):2079-2082. doi:10.1001/jama.2015.13744.

141 Torpy JM, Livingston EH. Energy Drinks. JAMA. 2013;309(3):297. doi:10.1001/jama.2012.170614.

142 Torpy JM, Livingston EH. Energy Drinks. JAMA. 2013;309(3):297. doi:10.1001/jama.2012.170614.

143 Sepkowitz KA. Energy Drinks and Caffeine-Related Adverse Effects. JAMA. 2013;309(3):243-244. doi:10.1001/jama.2012.173526.

144 Howland J, Rohsenow DJ. Risks of Energy Drinks Mixed With Alcohol. JAMA. 2013;309(3):245-246. doi:10.1001/jama.2012.187978.

145 O'Brien MC, McCoy TP, Rhodes SD, Wagoner A, Wolfson M. Caffeinated cocktails: energy drink consumption, high-risk drinking, and alcohol-related consequences among college students. Acad Emerg Med. 2008;15(5):453-460.

146 Bachman R. Teen Sports Diet Debate. Wall St. Journal. January 12, 2016.

147 Do Kids Need Supplements? Consumer Reports http://consumerreports.org/cro/2012/03/do-kidsneed-vitamins-and-supplements/index.htm?loginMethod=auto

148 Do Kids Need Supplements? Consumer Reports http://consumerreports.org/cro/2012/03/do-kidsneed-vitamins-and-supplements/index.htm?loginMethod=auto

149 Where we stand: Vitamins-HealthyChildren.org; http://www.healthychildren.org/English/healthy-living/nutrition/Pages/Where-We-Stand-Vitamins.aspx

150 Where we stand: Vitamins-HealthyChildren.org, Caring for Your Baby and Young Child: Birth to Age 5, 6th Edition (Copyright © 2015 American Academy of Pediatrics); http://www.healthychildren.org/English/ages-stages/gradeschool/nutrition/Pages/Vitamin-Supplements-and-Children.aspx

151 Where we stand: Vitamins-HealthyChildren.org, Vitamin supplementation http://www.healthychildren.org/English/ages-stages/gradeschool/nutrition/Pages/Vitamin-Supplements-and-Children.aspx

152 Hoeckler JL Should I give multivitamins to my preschooler? http://www.mayoclinic.org/healthy-living/nutrition-and-healthy-eating/expert-answers/multivitamins/faq-20058310

153 Do Kids Need Supplements? Consumer Reports http://consumerreports.org/cro/2012/03/do-kids-need-vitamins-and-supplements/index.htm?loginMethod=auto

154 Where we stand: Vitamins-HealthyChildren.org; http://www.healthychildren.org/English/healthy-living/nutrition/Pages/Where-We-Stand-Vitamins.aspx

155 Where we stand: Vitamins-HealthyChildren.org, Caring for Your Baby and Young Child: Birth to Age 5, 6th Edition (Copyright © 2015 American Academy of Pediatrics); http://www.healthychildren.org/English/ages-stages/gradeschool/nutrition/Pages/Vitamin-Supplements-and-Children.aspx

156 Where we stand: Vitamins-HealthyChildren.org, Vitamin supplementation http://www.healthychildren.org/English/ages-stages/gradeschool/nutrition/Pages/Vitamin-Supplements-and-Children.aspx

157 Bellows L, Moore R, Gross A. Dietary Supplements: Vitamins and Minerals. Colorado State UniversityExtension Publication no. 9.338 (9/13) http://www.ext.colostate.edu/pubs/foodnut/09338.html

Chapter 6 – Preventing Cardiovascular Disease (CVD)

1 Roth GA, Mohammad H. Forouzanfar MH, Moran AE, et al. Demographic and Epidemiologic Drivers of Global Cardiovascular Mortality. N Engl J Med 2015; 372:1333-1341April 2, 2015DOI: 10.1056/NEJMoa1406656.

2 Heart Disease and Stroke Statistics 2017 At-a-Glance. American Heart Association. https://www.heart.org/idc/groups/ahamah-public/@wcm/@sop/@smd/documents/downloadable/ucm_491265.pdf

3 Appel L, Llinas RH, 2014 Hypertension and Stroke White Paper. Johns Hopkins Medicine. 2014, 81pp.

4 Lloyd-Jones D, Adams RJ, Brown TM, et al. Heart disease and stroke statistics—2010 update: A report from the American Heart Association statistics committee and stroke statistics subcommittee. Circulation. 2010;121:e1-e170.

5 Heart Attack Statistics. AllHeartAttack. http://www.allheartattack.com/statistics.php.

6 Wei J, Cheng S, Bairey Merz CN. Coronary Microvascular Dysfunction Causing Cardiac Ischemia in Women. JAMA. 2019;322(23):2334–2335. doi:https://doi.org/10.1001/jama.2019.15736

7 Kullo IK, Rooke TW. Peripheral Artery Disease. N Engl J Med. 2016; 374:861-871. DOI: 10.1056/NEJMcp1507631

8 Skelly CL, Cifu AS. Screening, Evaluation, and Treatment of Peripheral Arterial Disease. JAMA.2016;316(14):1486-1487. doi:10.1001/jama.2016.11103

9 Berenson GS ed. Bogalusa Heart Study: Evolution of Cardio-metabolic Risk from Childhood to Middle Age. Springer, 2011.

10 Berenson GS, Srinivasan S, Bao W, Newman WP, Tracy RE, Wattigney WA. Association between cardiovascular multiple risk factors and atherosclerosis in children and young adults. N Engl J Med.1998;338:1650-6.

11 Enos WF, Holmes RH, Beyer J. Coronary disease among United States soldiers killed in action in Korea: preliminary report. JAMA. 1953;152(12):1090-1093.

12 McNamara JJ, Molot MA, Stremple JF, Cutting RT. Coronary artery disease in combat casualties in Vietnam. JAMA. 1971;216(7):1185-1187.

13 Webber BJ, Seguin PG, Burnett DG, Clark LL, Otto JL. Prevalence of and risk factors for autopsy-determined atherosclerosis among US service members, 2001-2011. JAMA. 2012;308(24):2577-2583.

14 Mozaffarian D, Benjamin EJ, Go AS, Arnett DK, Blaha MJ, Cushman M, Das SR, de Ferranti S, Despr.s J-P, Fullerton HJ, Howard VJ, Huffman MD, Isasi CR, Jim.nez MC, Judd SE, Kissela BM, Lichtman JH, Lisabeth LD, Liu S, Mackey RH, Magid DJ, McGuire DK, Mohler ER III, Moy CS, Muntner P, Mussolino ME, Nasir K, Neumar RW, Nichol G, Palaniappan L, Pandey DK, Reeves MJ, Rodriguez CJ, Rosamond W, Sorlie PD, Stein J, Towfighi A, Turan TN, Virani SS, Woo D, Yeh RW, Turner MB; on behalf of the American Heart Association Statistics Committee and Stroke Statistics Subcommittee. Heart disease and stroke statistics—2016 update: a report from the American Heart Association. Circulation. 2016;133:e38-e360.

15 Menotti A, Lanti M, Kromhout D, Blackburn H, Jacobs D, Nissinen A, Dontas A, Kafatos A, Nedeljkovic S, Adachi H. Homogeneity in the relationship of serum cholesterol to coronary deaths across different cultures: 40-year follow-up of the Seven Countries Study. Eur J Cardiovasc Prev Rehabil. 2008 Dec;15(6):719-25.

16 Jaquish CE. The Framingham Heart Study, on its way to becoming the gold standard for Cardiovascular Genetic Epidemiology? BMC Med Genet. 2007 Oct 4;8:63.

17 O'Donnell CJ, Elosua R. Cardiovascular risk factors. Insights from Framingham Heart Study. Rev Esp Cardiol. 2008 Mar;61(3):299-310.

18 Appel L, Llinas RH, 2014 Hypertension and Stroke White Paper. Johns Hopkins Medicine. 2014, 81pp.

19 Keaney JF. CHIP-ping Away at Atherosclerosis. N Engl J Med 2017; 377:184-185. DOI: 10.1056/NEJMe1706173

20 Jaiswal S, Natarajan P, Silver AJ, et al. Clonal hematopoiesis and risk of atherosclerotic cardiovascular disease. N Engl J Med 2017;377:111-21.

21 Fenelon A, Preston SH. Estimating smoking-attributable mortality in the United States. Demography. 2012;49(3):797-818. doi:10.1007/s13524-012-0108-x

22 Bakalar N. Risks From E-Cigarettes. New York Times. August 23, 2018.

23 Alzahrani, Talal et al. Association Between Electronic Cigarette Use and Myocardial Infarction. American Journal of Preventive Medicine. 2018;55(4):455 - 461

24 Duncan MS, Freiberg MS, Greevy RA, Kundu S, Vasan RS, Tindle HA. Association of Smoking Cessation With Subsequent Risk of Cardiovascular Disease. JAMA. 2019;322(7):642–650. doi:https://doi.org/10.1001/jama.2019.10298

25 Appel L, Llinas RH, 2014 Hypertension and Stroke White Paper. Johns Hopkins Medicine. 2014, 81pp.

26 Appel L, Llinas RH, 2014 Hypertension and Stroke White Paper. Johns Hopkins Medicine. 2014, 81pp.

27 Dockery DW, Stone PH. Cardiovascular risks from fine particulate air pollution. N Engl J Med 2007;356:511–513.

28 Appel L, Llinas RH, 2014 Hypertension and Stroke White Paper. Johns Hopkins Medicine. 2014, 81pp.

29 Tsimikas S. A test in context: lipoprotein(a)—diagnosis, prognosis, controversies, and emerging therapies. J Am Coll Cardiol 2017; 69: 692–711.

30 Van Buuren F, Horstkotte D, Knabbe C, Hinse D, Mellwig KP. Incidence of elevated lipoprotein (a) levels in a large cohort of patients with cardiovascular disease. Clinical Research in Cardiology Supplements. 2017;12(Suppl 1):55-59. doi:10.1007/s11789-017-0087-y.

31 O'Connor A. A Little-Known Heart Danger. New York Times. January 9, 2018.

32 Watts GF, Boffa MB. Lipoprotein(a): lodestar for future clinical trials. Lancet 2018; Published Online October 4, 2018 http://dx.doi.org/10.1016/S0140-6736(18)31922-6.

33 Tsimikas S, Karwatowska-Prokopczuk E, Gouni-Berthold I, et al. Lipoprotein(a) Reduction in Persons with Cardiovascular Disease. N Engl J Med. 2020; 382:244-255. DOI: 10.1056/NEJMoa1905239

34 Appel L, Llinas RH, 2014 Hypertension and Stroke White Paper. Johns Hopkins Medicine. 2014, 81pp.

35 Moore JX, Chaudhary N, Akinyemiju T. Metabolic Syndrome Prevalence by Race/Ethnicity and Sex in the United States, National Health and Nutrition Examination Survey, 1988–2012. Prev Chronic Dis 2017;14:160287. DOI: http://dx.doi.org/10.5888/pcd14.160287.

36 Stone NJ, Robinson JG, Lichtenstein AH, et al. 2013 ACC/AHA guideline on the treatment of blood cholesterol to reduce atherosclerotic cardiovascular risk in adults: a report of the American College of Cardiology/American Heart Association Task Force on Practice Guidelines. Circulation. 2014;129:S1-45.

37 Eckel RH, Jakicic JM, Ard JD, et al. 2013 AHA/ACC guideline on life-style management to reduce cardiovascular risk: a report of the American College of Cardiology/American Heart Association Task Force on Practice Guidelines. Circulation. 2014;129(suppl 2):S76–S99.

38 Lloyd-Jones DM, Hong Y, Labarthe D, Mozaffarian D, Appel LJ, Van Horn L, Greenlund K, Daniels S, Nichol G, Tomaselli GF, Arnett DK, Fonarow GC, Ho PM, Lauer MS, Masoudi FA, Robertson RM, Roger V, Schwamm LH, Sorlie P, Yancy CW, Rosamond WD; on behalf of the American Heart Association Strategic Planning Task Force and Statistics Committee. Defining and setting national goals for cardiovascular health promotion and disease reduction: the American Heart Association's Strategic Impact Goal through 2020 and beyond. Circulation. 2010;121:586–613.

39 Berry JD, Dyer A, Cai X, et al. Lifetime risks of cardiovascular disease. N Engl J Med. 2012;366(4):321-329.

40 Younus AY, Aneni EC, Spatz ES, et al. A Systematic Review of the Prevalence and Outcomes of Ideal Cardiovascular Health in US and Non-US Populations. Mayo Clin Proc. 2016;91(5):649-670. https://doi.org/10.1016/j.mayocp.2016.01.019

41 Yusuf S, Hawken S, Ounpuu S, on behalf of the INTERHEART Study Investigators. Effect of potentially modifiable risk factors associated with myocardial infarction in 52 countries (the INTERHEART study): case-control study. Lancet. 2004;364:937-952.

42 Ornish D, The Spectrum. New York, Ballantine Books: 2007.

43 Åkesson A, Larsson SC, Discacciati D, Wolk A. Low-Risk Diet and Lifestyle Habits in the Primary Pre-

vention of Myocardial Infarction in Men. J Am Coll Cardiol. 2014;64(13):1299-1306. doi:10.1016/j.jacc.2014.06.1190

44 Khera AV, Emdin CA, Drake I, et al.Genetic Risk, Adherence to a Healthy Lifestyle, and Coronary Disease. n engl j med 375;24:2349-2358.

45 Mozaffarian D. The Promise of Lifestyle for Cardiovascular Health: Time for Implementation. J Am Coll Cardiol. 2014;64(13):1307-1309. doi:10.1016/j.jacc.2014.06.1191.

46 Campbell TC, Campbell TM, The China Study. Dallas, Benbella Books: 2006

47 Fuhrman J. Eat to Live. New York. Little, Brown and Company. 2011

48 O'Keefe JH, et al., "Optimal low-density lipoprotein is 50 to 70 mg/dL: Lower is better and physiologically normal," Journal of the American College of Cardiology, Vol. 43pgs. 2142-2146, 2004, with permssion from the American College of Cardiology Foundation.

49 Virani SS, Alonso A, Benjamin EJ, et al.; on behalf of the American Heart Association Council on Epidemiology and Prevention Statistics Committee and Stroke Statistics Subcommittee. Heart disease and stroke statistics— 2020 update: a report from the American Heart Association. Circulation. 2020;141:e139–e596. doi: 10.1161/CIR.0000000000000757.

50 Go AS, Mozaffarian D, Roger VL, et al. American Heart Association Statistics Committee and Stroke Statistics Subcommittee.Heart disease and stroke statistics—2013 update: a report from the American Heart Association. Circulation. 2013 Jan 1;127(1):e6-e245. doi: 10.1161/CIR.0b013e31828124ad. Epub 2012 Dec 12.

51 Grundy SM, Cleeman JI, et al. for the Coordinating Committee of the National Cholesterol Education Program. Implications of Recent Clinical Trials for the National Cholesterol Education Program Adult Treatment Panel III Guidelines. Endorsed by the National Heart, Lung, and Blood Institute, American College of Cardiology Foundation, and American Heart Association Circulation. 2004;110:227-239

52 Jarcho JA, Keaney JF. Proof That Lower Is Better — LDL Cholesterol and IMPROVE-IT. N Engl J Med 2015; 372:2448-2450June 18, 2015DOI: 10.1056/NEJMe1507041

53 Cannon C. The IDEAL Cholesterol. Lower Is Better. JAMA. 2005;294(19):2492-2494. doi:10.1001/JAMA.294.19.2492

54 Making Sense of Cholesterol Tests. Harvard Health Letter http://www.health.harvard.edu/heart-health/making-sense-of-cholesterol-tests

55 Carroll KK, Giovannetti PM, Huff MW, Moase O, Roberts DC, Wolfe BM. Hypocholesterolemic effect of substituting soybean protein for animal protein in the diet of healthy young women. Am J Clin Nutr.

56 Cholesterol and Heart Disease, the Physicians Committee for Responsible Medicine.

57 Voight BF, Peloso GM, Orho-Melander M, et al. Plasma HDL cholesterol and risk of myocardial infarction: a mendelian randomisation study Lancet 2012; 380: 572–80 Published Online May 17, 2012 http://dx.doi.org/10.1016/ S0140-6736(12)60312-2

58 Kolata G. Dashing Hopes, Study Shows a Cholesterol Drug Had No Effect on Heart Health. New York Times April 4, 2016.

59 Appel L, Llinas RH, 2014 Hypertension and Stroke White Paper. Johns Hopkins Medicine. 2014, 81pp.

60 Navar AM. The Evolving Story of Triglycerides and Coronary Heart Disease Risk. JAMA. 2019;321(4):347–349. doi:10.1001/jama.2018.20044

61 Stone NJ, et al. 2013 Report on the Treatment of Blood Cholesterol to Reduce Atherosclerotic Cardiovascular Disease in Adults: Full Panel Report Supplement. Based on a Systematic Review from the National Heart, Lung and Blood Institute2014? 397pp

62 Stone NJ, et al. 2013 ACC/AHA Guideline on the Treatment of Blood Cholesterol to Reduce Atherosclerotic Cardiovascular Risk in Adults, A Report of the American College of Cardiology/American Heart Association Task Force on Practice Guidelines. Circulation 2014; 129: S1-S45. Published online before print November 12, 2013, doi: 10.1161/01.cir.0000437738.63853.7a

63 Cannon CP. The IDEAL CholesterolLower Is Better. JAMA. 2005;294(19):2492-2494. doi:10.1001/JAMA.294.19.2492.

64 Jarcho JA, Keaney JF. Proof That Lower Is Better — LDL Cholesterol and IMPROVE-IT. N Engl J Med 2015; 372:2448-2450June 18, 2015DOI: 10.1056/NEJMe1507041.

65 Silverman MG, Ference BA, Im K, et al. Association between lowering LDL-C and cardiovascular risk reduction among different therapeutic interventions: a systematic review and meta-analysis. JAMA. 2016;316(12):1289-1297.

66 Rodriguez F, Harrington RA. Cholesterol, Cardiovascular Risk, Statins, PCSK9 Inhibitors, and the Future of LDL-C Lowering. JAMA. 2016;316(19):1967-1968. doi:10.1001/JAMA.2016.16575.

67 American Heart Association (2013) website http://www.heart.org/HEARTORG/Conditions/Cholesterol/AboutCholesterol/What-Your-Cholesterol-Levels-Mean_UCM_305562_Article.jsp)

68 Virani SS, Alonso A, Benjamin EJ, et al.; on behalf of the American Heart Association Council on Epidemiology and Prevention Statistics Committee and Stroke Statistics Subcommittee. Heart disease and stroke statistics— 2020 update: a report from the American Heart Association. Circulation. 2020;141:e139–e596. doi: 10.1161/CIR.0000000000000757.

69 American Heart Association (2013) website http://www.heart.org/HEARTORG/Conditions/Cholesterol/AboutCholesterol/What-Your-Cholesterol-Levels-Mean_UCM_305562_Article.jsp)

70 Glueck CJ. Optimal LDL Cholesterol < 70 Mg/Dl, Scientific Update 3/30/09, Alliance Cholesterol Center. http://www.jewishhospitalcincinnati.com/cholesterol/Research/OPTIMAL_LDL_CHOLESTEROL_3-27-09.pdf

71 Appel L, Llinas RH, 2014 Hypertension and Stroke White Paper. Johns Hopkins Medicine. 2014, 81pp.

72 Sachdeva A, Cannon CP, Deedwania PC, Labresh KA, Smith SC Jr, Dai D, Hernandez A, Fonarow GC. Lipid levels in patients hospitalized with coronary artery disease: an analysis of 136,905 hospitalizations in Get With The Guidelines. Am Heart J. 2009 Jan;157(1):111-117.e2. doi: 10.1016/j.ahj.2008.08.010. Epub 2008 Oct 22.

73 American Heart Association (2013) website http://www.heart.org/HEARTORG/Conditions/Cholesterol/AboutCholesterol/What-Your-Cholesterol-Levels-Mean_UCM_305562_Article.jsp)

74 American Heart Association (2013) website http://www.heart.org/HEARTORG/Conditions/Cholesterol/AboutCholesterol/What-Your-Cholesterol-Levels-Mean_UCM_305562_Article.jsp)

75 Virani SS, Alonso A, Benjamin EJ, et al.; on behalf of the American Heart Association Council on Epidemiology and Prevention Statistics Committee and Stroke Statistics Subcommittee. Heart disease and stroke statistics— 2020 update: a report from the American Heart Association. Circulation. 2020;141:e139–e596. doi: 10.1161/CIR.0000000000000757.

76 Aung T, Halsey J, Kromhout D, et al. Associations of omega-3 fatty acid supplement use with cardiovascular disease risks: meta-analysis of 10 trials involving 77 917 individuals. JAMA Cardiol 2018;3:225-234.

77 The ASCEND Study Collaborative Group. Effects of n−3 fatty acid supplements in diabetes mellitus. N Engl J Med 2018;379:1540-1550.

78 Manson JE, Cook NR, Lee I-M, et al. Marine n−3 fatty acids and prevention of cardiovascular disease and cancer. N Engl J Med. DOI: 10.1056/NEJMoa1811403.

79 Hu Y, Hu FB, Manson JE. Marine Omega-3 Supplementation and Cardiovascular Disease: An Updat-

ed Meta-Analysis of 13 Randomized Controlled Trials Involving 127 477 Participants. J Am Heart Assn. 2019;8(19):e013543. https://doi.org/10.1161/JAHA.119.013543

80 Esselstyn CB. Updating a 12-year experience with arrest and reversal therapy for coronary heart disease (an overdue requiem for palliative cardiology). Am J Cardiol 1999;84:339-341.

81 Connor WE, Connor SL, The Case for a Low-Fat High-Carbohydrate Diet, Should a Low-Fat High-Carbohydrate Diet Be Recommended for Everyone? N Engl J Med. 1997;337:562-563

82 McDougall J, Litzau K, Haver E, Saunders V, Spiller GA. Rapid reduction of serum cholesterol and blood pressure by a twelve-day, very low fat, strictly vegetarian diet. J Am Coll Nutr. 1995;14:491-496.

83 McDougall J. The McDougall Program for a Healthy Heart, Dutton, Boston,1996.

84 Fuhrman J. Eat to Live. New York. Little, Brown and Company. 2011

85 Barnard N. Physician's Committee for Responsible Medicine. Every Meal PowerPlate. http://www.pcrm.org/sites/default/files/images/health/pplate/EveryMealPowerPlate.pdf

86 Barnard N. Physician's Committee for Responsible Medicine. Healthy Eating for Life. http://www.pcrm.org/sites/default/files/pdfs/health/HealthyEatingforLife.pdf

87 Barnard N. Physician's Committee for Responsible Medicine. Cholesterol and Heart Disease. http://www.pcrm.org/sites/default/files/pdfs/health/chol_heartdisease.pdf

88 Campbell TC, Campbell TM, The China Study. Dallas, Benbella Books: 2006

89 Jenkins DJ, Kendall CW, Popovich DG, et al. Effect of a very-high-fiber vegetable, fruit and nut diet on serum lipids and colonic function. Metabolism 2001;(4):494-503.

90 Greger, M, Stone G. How Not to Die. New York, Flatiorn Books, 2015.

91 Shintani TT, Beckham S, Brown AC, O'Connor HK. The Hawaii Diet: ad libitum high carbohydrate, low fat multi-cultural diet for the reduction of chronic disease risk factors: obesity, hypertension, hypercholesterolemia, and hyperglycemia. Hawaii Med J. 2001 Mar;60(3):69-73.

92 Moss M, Salt Sugar Fat. Random House, New York. 2013

93 Esselstyn CB. Prevent and Reverse Heart Disease. New York, Penguin Group, 2007. p 69

94 Hu FB. Plant-based foods and prevention of cardiovascular disease: an overview. Am J Clin Nutr 2003;78(suppl):544S–51S.

95 Ornish D, Scherwitz LW, Billings JH, Gould KL, Merritt TA, Sparler S, Armstrong WT, Ports TA, Kirkeeide RL, Hogeboom C, Brand RJ. Intensive Lifestyle Changes for Reversal of Coronary Heart Disease. JAMA, December 16, 1998, Vol 280, No. 23 2001-2007

96 Ornish D, Brown SE, Scherwitz LW, et al. Can lifestyle changes reverse coronary heart disease? Lancet. 1990;336:129-133.

97 Esselstyn, CB. (2001). Resolving the Coronary Artery Disease Epidemic Through Plant-Based Nutrition. Preventive Cardiology, 4, 171-177.

98 Esselstyn CB. Updating a 12-year experience with arrest and reversal therapy for coronary heart disease (an overdue requiem for palliative cardiology). Am J Cardiol 1999;84:339-341.

99 Liu S, Manson JE, Lee I-M, Cole SR, Hennekens CH, Willett WC, Buring JE. Fruit and vegetable intake and risk of cardiovascular disease: the Women's Health Study. Am J Clin Nutr. 2000;72:922-8.

100 Fraser GE. Associations between diet and cancer, ischemic heart disease, and all-cause mortality in non-Hispanic white California Seventh-day Adventists. Am J Clin Nutr. 1999;70:532S–538S.

101 Tharrey M, Mariotti F, Mashchak A, Barbillon P, Delattre M, Fraser GE. Patterns of plant and animal protein intake are strongly associated with cardiovascular mortality: the Adventist Health Study-2 cohort, International Journal of Epidemiology, April 2, 2018:dyy030. https://doi.org/10.1093/ije/dyy030

102 Kim H, Caulfield LE, Garcia-Larsen V, et al. Plant-Based Diets Are Associated With a Lower Risk of Incident Cardiovascular Disease, Cardiovascular Disease Mortality, and All-Cause Mortality in a General Population of Middle-Aged Adults. J Am Heart Assoc. 2019;8:e012865

103 Willett WC. Eat, Drink, and Be Healthy: The Harvard Medical School Guide to Healthy Eating. Free Press. 2005. ISBN 0-7432-6642-0

104 Willett WC. The Mediterranean diet: science and practice. Public Health Nutr. 2006 Feb;9(1A):105-10.

105 Serra-Majem L, Roman B, Estruch R. 2006. Scientific evidence of interventions using the Mediterranean diet: a systematic review. Nutr. Rev. 64:S27–47

106 Katz DL, Meller S. Can We Say What Diet Is Best for Health?. Annu. Rev. Public Health 2014. 35:85

107 Hu FB, Stampfer MJ, Manson JE, et al. Dietary fat intake and the risk of coronary heart disease in women. N Engl J Med. 1997;337:1491–9.

108 Hu FB, Stampfer MJ, Manson JE, et al. Dietary saturated fats and their food sources in relation to the risk of coronary heart disease in women. Am J Clin Nutr December 1999 vol. 70 no. 6 1001-1008.

109 Oh K, Hu FB, Manson JE, Stampfer MJ, Willett WC (2005) Dietary fat intake and risk of coronary heart disease in women: 20 years of follow-up of the nurses' health study. Am J Epidemiol 161: 672–679.

110 Mozaffarian D, Micha R, Wallace S. Effects on Coronary Heart Disease of Increasing Polyunsaturated Fat in Place of Saturated Fat: A Systematic Review and Meta-Analysis of Randomized Controlled Trials. PLoS Med. 2010;7(3): e1000252. doi:10.1371/journal.pmed.1000252

111 Ahmad S, Moorthy MV, Demler OV, et al. Assessment of Risk Factors and Biomarkers Associated With Risk of Cardiovascular Disease Among Women Consuming a Mediterranean Diet. JAMA Netw Open.2018;1(8):e185708. doi:10.1001/jamanetworkopen.2018.5708

112 de Lorgeril M, Salen P, Martin JL, Monjaud I, Delaye J, Mamelle N. Mediterranean diet, traditional risk factors and the rate of cardiovascular complications after myocardial infarction: final report of the Lyon Diet Heart Study. Circulation. 1999;99:779-785.

113 de Lorgeril M, Renaud S, Mamelle N, et al. Mediterranean alpha-linolenic acid-rich diet in secondary prevention of coronary heart disease [published correction appears in Lancet. 1995;345:738]. Lancet. 1994;343:1454-1459.

114 Ornish D, Scherwitz LW, Billings JH, et al. Intensive lifestyle changes for reversal of coronary heart disease. JAMA. 1998;280:2001-2007.

115 Ekelund LG, Haskell WL, Johnson JL, Wholey FS, Criqui MH, Sheps DS. Physical fitness as a prevention of cardiovascular mortality in asymptomatic North American men. N Engl J Med. 1988; 319:1379-1384.

116 Katz DL, Meller S. Can We Say What Diet Is Best for Health?. Annu. Rev. Public Health 2014. 35:85

117 Moore, LV; Frances E. Thompson, FE, Adults Meeting Fruit and Vegetable Intake Recommendations — United States, 2013, Morbidity and Mortality Weekly Report (MMWR)July 10, 2015 / 64(26);709-713 http://www.cdc.gov/mmwr/preview/mmwrhtml/mm6426a1.htm

118 USDA Food Patterns http://www.cnpp.usda.gov/sites/default/files/usda_food_patterns/USDAFoodPatternsSummaryTable.pdf

119 Mozaffarian D, Appel LJ, Van Horn L. Components of a Cardioprotective Diet: New Insights. Circulation. 2011;123:2870-2891. DOI: 10.1161/Circulation AHA.110.968735.

120 Klatsky A, Friedman GD, Siegelaub AB. Alcohol and mortality: A ten year Kaiser-Permanente experiment. Ann Intern Med. 1981;95:139–145.

121 Marmot MG, Rose G, Shipley MJ, Thomas BJ. Alcohol and mortality: A U-shaped curve. Lancet.

1981;14:580–583.

122 Rehm J, Greenfield TK, Rogers JD. Average volume of alcohol consumption, patterns of drinking, and all-cause mortality: results from the US National Alcohol Survey. Am J Epidemiol. 2001;153:64–71.

123 Klatsky AL, Udaltsova N. Alcohol Drinking and Total Mortality Risk. Ann Epidemiol. 2007;17:S63–S67.

124 Shaper AG, Wannamethee G, Walker M. Alcohol and mortality in British men: Explaining the U-shaped curve. Lancet. 1988;2:1267–1273.

125 Fillmore KM, Stockwell T, Chikritzhs T, et al. Moderate alcohol use and reduced mortality risk: Systematic error in prospective studies and new hypotheses. Ann Epidemiol. 2007;17(suppl):S16-S23.

126 Harriss LR, English DR, Hopper JL, et al. Alcohol consumption and cardiovascular mortality accounting for possible misclassification of intake: 11-year follow-up of the Melbourne Collaborative Cohort Study. Addiction. 2007;102:1574-1585.

127 Stockwell T, Zhao J, Panwar S, et al. Do "Moderate" Drinkers Have Reduced Mortality Risk? A Systematic Review and Meta-Analysis of Alcohol Consumption and All-Cause Mortality. Journal of Studies on Alcohol and Drugs. 2016;77(2):185-198

128 Corrao G, Bagnardi V, Zambon A, La Vecchia C. A meta-analysis of alcohol consumption and the risk of 15 diseases. Prev Med. 2004;38:613–619.

129 Gillis AM. A sober reality? Alcohol, abstinence and atrial fibrillation. N Engl J Med. 2020;382(1):83-84.

130 Voskobo A, Kalman JM, De Silva A, et al. Alcohol Abstinence in Drinkers with Atrial Fibrillation. N Engl J Med. 2020; 382:20-28. DOI: 10.1056/NEJMoa1817591

131 Centers for Disease Control and Prevention (CDC). Alcohol and public health: alcohol-related disease impact (ARDI): average for United States 2006-2010: alcohol-attributable deaths due to excessive alcohol use. https://nccd.cdc.gov/DPH _ARDI/Default/Report.aspx?T=AAM&P=f6d7eda7 -036e-4553-9968-9b17ffad620e&R=d7a9b303 -48e9-4440-bf47-070a4827e1fd&M=8E1C5233 -5640-4EE8-9247-1ECA7DA325B9&F=&D. Accessed April 19, 2018.

132 Centers for Disease Control and Prevention. Excessive drinking is draining the US economy. https://www.cdc.gov/features/costsofdrinking /index.html. Accessed April 19, 2018.

133 Kranzler HR, Soyka M. Diagnosis and Pharmacotherapy of Alcohol Use Disorder A Review. JAMA.2018;320(8):815–824. doi:10.1001/jama.2018.11406

134 Danaei G, Ding EL, Mozaffarian D, Taylor B, Rehm J, Murray CJ, Ezzati M. The preventable causes of death in the United States: comparative risk assessment of dietary, lifestyle, and metabolic risk factors. PLoS Med. 2009;6:e1000058.

135 Mozaffarian D, Appel LJ, Van Horn L. Components of a Cardioprotective Diet: New Insights. Circulation. 2011;123:2870-2891. DOI: 10.1161/Circulation AHA.110.968735.

136 Does alcohol deserve its healthy buzz? University of California, Berkeley Wellness Letter. November 2017:1-2.

137 UK Department of Health. UK Chief Medical Officers' Low Risk Drinking Guidelines. August, 2016. https://www.gov.uk/government/uploads/system/uploads/attachment_data/file/545937/UK_CMOs__ report.pdf (accessed March 16, 2018).

138 Burton R, Sheron N.No level of alcohol consumption improves health. The Lancet. August 23, 2018 http://dx.doi.org/10.1016/S0140-6736(18)31571-X

139 Yang Q, Zhang Z, Gregg EW, Flanders WD, Merritt R, Hu FB. Added Sugar Intake and Cardiovascular Diseases Mortality Among US Adults JAMA Intern Med. 2014;174(4):516-524. doi:10.1001/ JAMAint-

ernmed.2013.13563.

140 Singh GM, Micha R, Khatibzadeh S, Lim S, Ezzati M, Mozaffarian D, on behalf of the Global

Burden of Diseases Nutrition and Chronic Diseases Expert Group (NutriCoDE) Estimated Global, Regional, and National Disease Burdens Related to Sugar-Sweetened Beverage Consumption in 2010 Circulation. 2015;132:639-666 published online before print June 29 2015, doi:10.1161/CIRCULATIONAHA. 114.010636

141 Lustig RH, Schmidt LA, Brindis CD. The toxic truth about sugar. Nature. 2012;482:27-29.

142 Lustig, RH, Mulligan K, Noworolski SM, Tai VW, Wen MJ, Erkin-Cakmak A, Gugliucci A, Schwarz JM. Isocaloric fructose restriction and metabolic improvement in children with obesity and metabolic syndrome. Obesity, 2016;24:453–460. doi:10.1002/oby.21371

143 Basu S, Yoffe P, Hills N, Lustig RH (2013) The Relationship of Sugar to Population-Level Diabetes Prevalence: An Econometric Analysis of Repeated Cross- Sectional Data. PLoS ONE 8(2): e57873. doi:10.1371/journal.pone.0057873

144 Malik VS, Popkin BM, Bray GA, Despres JP, Willett WC, Hu FB. Sugar-sweetened beverages and risk of metabolic syndrome and type 2 diabetes: a meta-analysis. Diabetes Care. 2010;33:2477–2483.

145 de Koning L, Malik VS, Kellogg MD, Rimm EB, Willett WC, Hu FB. Sweetened Beverage Consumption, Incident Coronary Heart Disease, and Biomarkers of Risk in Men Circulation. 2012;125:1735-1741.

146 Ekelund LG, Haskell WL, Johnson JL, Wholey FS, Criqui MH, Sheps DS. Physical fitness as a prevention of cardiovascular mortality in asymptomatic North American men. N Engl J Med. 1988; 319:1379-1384.

147 Centers for Disease Control and Prevention. Public health focus: physical activity and the prevention of coronary heart disease. MMWR Morb Mortal Wkly Rep. 1993;42:669-672.

148 Lee IM, Paffenbarger RS Jr, Hennekens CH. Physical activity, physical fitness and longevity. Aging (Milano). 1997;9:2–11.

149 Blair SN, Jackson AS. Physical fitness and activity as separate heart disease risk factors: a meta-analysis. Med Sci Sports Exerc. 2001;33:762–764.

150 Thompson PD, Buchner D., Piña, IL, Balady G J, Williams MA, Marcus, BH, Wenger, NK. Exercise and physical activity in the prevention and treatment of atherosclerotic cardiovascular disease: A statement from the Council on Clinical Cardiology (Subcommittee on Exercise, Rehabilitation, and Prevention) and the Council on Nutrition, Physical Activity, and Metabolism (Subcommittee on Physical Activity). Circulation, 2003;107(24):3106-3116.DOI: 10.1161/01.CIR.0000075572.40158.77

151 Mandsager K, Harb S, Cremer P, Phelan D, Nissen SE, Jaber W. Association of Cardiorespiratory Fitness With Long-term Mortality Among Adults Undergoing Exercise Treadmill Testing. JAMA Network Open. 2018;1(6):e183605. doi:10.1001/jamanetworkopen.2018.3605

152 Gebel K, Ding D, Chey T, Stamatakis E, Brown WJ, Bauman AE. Effect of Moderate to Vigorous Physical Activity on All-Cause Mortality in Middle-aged and Older Australians. JAMA Intern Med. 2015;175(6):970-977. doi:10.1001/JAMAinternmed.2015.0541

153 Rankin AJ, Rankin AC, MacIntyre P, Hillis WS. Walk or run? Is high-intensity exercise more effective than moderate-intensity exercise at reducing cardiovascular risk? Scott Med J. 2012;57(2):99-102.

154 Sabia S, Dugravot A, Kivimaki M, Brunner E, Shipley MJ, Singh-Manoux A. Effect of intensity and type of physical activity on mortality: results from the Whitehall II cohort study. Am J Public Health. 2012;102(4):698-704.

155 Wen CP, Wai JP, Tsai MK, Chen CH. Minimal amount of exercise to prolong life: to walk, to run, or just mix it up? J AmColl Cardiol. 2014;64(5):482-484.

156 Lee IM, Paffenbarger RS Jr. Associations of light, moderate, and vigorous intensity physical activity

with longevity: the Harvard Alumni Health Study. Am J Epidemiol. 2000;151(3):293-299.

157 Arem H, Moore SC, Patel A, Hartge P, Berrington de Gonzalez A, Visvanathan K, Campbell PT,

Freedman M, Weiderpass E, Adami HO, Linet MS, Lee IM, Matthews CE. Leisure Time Physical Activity and Mortality A Detailed Pooled Analysis of the Dose-Response Relationship. JAMA Intern Med. 2015;175(6):959-967. doi:10.1001/JAMAinternmed.2015.0533

158 Bellettiere J, LaMonte MJ, Evenson KR. et al. Sedentary Behavior and Cardiovascular Disease in Older Women. Circulation. 2019;139:1036–1046.

159 Reynolds G. Exercise and the Aging Heart. New York Times. July 31, 2018.

160 Stefanick ML, Mackey S, Sheehan M, et al. Effects of diet and exercise in men and postmenopausal women with low levels of HDL cholesterol and high levels of LDL cholesterol. N Engl J Med. 1998 Jul 2;339:12-20.

161 Appel L, Llinas RH, 2014 Hypertension and Stroke White Paper. Johns Hopkins Medicine. 2014, 81pp.

162 Wall HK, Hannan JA, Wright JS. Patients With Undiagnosed Hypertension: Hiding in Plain Sight. JAMA. 2014;312(19):1973-1974. doi:10.1001/JAMA.2014.15388.

163 Appel L, Llinas RH, 2014 Hypertension and Stroke White Paper. Johns Hopkins Medicine. 2014, 81pp.

164 Go AS, Mozaffarian D, Roger VL, et al. American Heart Association Statistics Committee and Stroke Statistics Subcommittee. Heart disease and stroke statistics—2013 update: a report from the American Heart Association. Circulation. 2013;127(1):e6-e245.

165 Vasan RS, Beiser A, Seshadri S, et al. Residual lifetime risk for developing hypertension in middle-aged women and men: the Framingham Heart Study. JAMA. 2002;287(8):1003-1010.

166 Chobanian AV, Bakris GL, Black HR, et al. National Heart, Lung, and Blood Institute Joint National Committee on Prevention, Detection, Evaluation, and Treatment of High Blood Pressure; National High Blood Pressure Education Program Coordinating Committee. The Seventh Report of the Joint National Committee on Prevention, Detection, Evaluation, and Treatment of High Blood Pressure: the JNC 7 report. JAMA. 2003;289(19):2560-2572.

167 Yang Q, Cogswell ME, Flanders WD, et al; Trends in cardiovascular health metrics and associations with all-cause and CVD mortality among US adults. JAMA. 2012;307:1273-1283.

168 Go AS, Mozaffarian D, Roger VL., et al; for the AHA Statistics Committee and Stroke Statistics Subcommittee Executive summary: heart disease and stroke statistics–2014 update: a report from the American Heart Association. Circulation. 2014;129:399-410.

169 Olives C, Myerson R, Mokdad AH, Murray CJ, Lim SS; Prevalence, awareness, treatment, and control of hypertension in United States counties, 2001-2009. PloS One. 2013;8:e60308

170 Olives C, Myerson R, Mokdad AH, Murray CJ, Lim SS; Prevalence, awareness, treatment, and control of hypertension in United States counties, 2001-2009. PloS One. 2013;8:e60308

171 Nwankwo T, Yoon SS, Burt V, Gu Q. Hypertension among adults in the United States: National Health and Nutrition Examination Survey, 2011-2012. http://www.cdc.gov/nchs/data/databriefs/db133.pdf. Accessed October 24, 2014.

172 Appel L, Llinas RH, 2014 Hypertension and Stroke White Paper. Johns Hopkins Medicine. 2014, 81pp.

173 U.S. Department of Health and Human Services. The Health Consequences of Smoking—50 Years of Progress: A Report of the Surgeon General. Atlanta: U.S. Department of Health and Human Services, Centers for Disease Control and Prevention, National Center for Chronic Disease Prevention and Health Promotion, Office on Smoking and Health, 2014

174 Smoking doubles stroke risk among African-Americans. Medical Express. March 8, 2019. https://medicalxpress.com/news/2019-03-african-americans.html

175 Jousilahti P. Headache and the risk of stroke. Curr Atheroscler Rep. 2004 Jul;6(4):320-5.

176 Laino C. News From The International Stroke Conference: Does Marijuana Increase The Risk Of Stroke? Neurology Today: 4 April 2013 - Volume 13 - Issue 7 - pp 1,11–12doi: 10.1097/01.NT.0000429368.31764.3c

177 Appel L, Llinas RH, 2014 Hypertension and Stroke White Paper. Johns Hopkins Medicine. 2014, 81pp.

178 Centers for Disease Control and Prevention. http://www.cdc.gov/nchs/fastats/leading-causes-ofdeath.htm

179 Stroke Facts, Centers for Disease Control and Prevention. http://www.cdc.gov/stroke/facts.htm

180 Circulation: Heart Disease and Stroke Statistics—2013 Update. http://circ.ahajournals.org/content/127/1/e6.long

181 The GD 2016 Lifetime Risk of Stroke Collaborators. Global, Regional, and Country-Specific Lifetime Risks of Stroke, 1990 and 2016. New England Journal of Medicine. 2018;379(25):2429-2437. Doi.10.1056/NEJMoa1804492

182 http://www.ninds.nih.gov/disorders/stroke/poststrokerehab.html

183 Maillard P, Seshadri S, Beiser A, et al. Effects of systolic blood pressure on white-matter integrity in young adults in the Framingham Heart Study: a cross-sectional study. Lancet neurology. 2012;11(12):1039-1047. doi:10.1016/S1474-4422(12)70241-7.

184 Sarafidis PA, Bakris GL. Early Patterns of Blood Pressure Change and Future Coronary Atherosclerosis. JAMA. 2014;311(5):471-472. doi:10.1001/JAMA.2013.285123.

185 Allen N, Berry JD, Ning H, Van Horn L, Dyer A, Lloyd-Jones DM. Impact of blood pressure and blood pressure change during middle age on the remaining lifetime risk for cardiovascular disease: the cardiovascular lifetime risk pooling project. Circulation. 2012;125(1):37-44.

186 Allen NB, Siddique J, Wilkins J, et al. Blood pressure trajectories in early adulthood and subclinical atherosclerosis in middle age. JAMA. doi:10.1001/JAMA.2013.285122.

187 Launer LJ, Masaki K, Petrovitch H, Foley D, Havlik RJ. The association between midlife blood pressure levels and late-life cognitive function: the Honolulu-Asia Aging Study. JAMA. 1995;274(23):1846-1851.

188 Stewart R, Xue QL, Masaki K, et al. Change in blood pressure and incident dementia: a 32-year prospective study. Hypertension. 2009;54(2):233-240.

189 DeCarli C. Blood Pressure Control and Cognitive Performance: Something to Think About With Aging. JAMA. 2015;313(19):1963-1964. doi:10.1001/JAMA.2015.3113.

190 Gorelick PB. Blood Pressure and the Prevention of Cognitive Impairment. JAMA Neurol. 2014;71(10):1211-1213. doi:10.1001/JAMAneurol.2014.2014.

191 Gottesman RF, Schneider AL, Albert M, et al. Midlife hypertension and 20-year cognitive change: the Atherosclerosis Risk in Communities Neurocognitive Study. JAMA Neurol. 2014;71(10):1218-1227.

192 Gottesman RF, Schneider AL, Albert M, et al. Midlife hypertension and 20-year cognitive change: the Atherosclerosis Risk in Communities Neurocognitive Study. JAMA Neurol. 2014;71(10):1218-1227.

193 Appel L, Llinas RH, 2014 Hypertension and Stroke White Paper. Johns Hopkins Medicine. 2014, 81pp.

194 Menotti A, Jacobs DR Jr, Blackburn H, Kromhout D, Nissinen A, Nedeljkovic S, Buzina R, Mohacek I, Seccareccia F, Giampaoli S, Dontas A, Aravanis C, Toshima H. Twenty-five-year prediction of stroke

deaths in the seven countries study: the role of blood pressure and its changes. Stroke. 1996 Mar;27(3):381-7.

195 Go AS, Mozaffarian D, Roger VL, et.al. Heart disease and stroke statistics—2014 update: a report from the American Heart Association. Circulation.2013;01.cir.0000441139.02102.80published online before print December 18, 2013, doi:10.1161/01.cir.0000441139.02102.80 http://circ.ahajournals.org/content/early/2013/12/18/01.cir.0000441139.02102.80.full.pdf

196 Cook NR, Appel LJ, Whelton PK. Lower levels of sodium intake and reduced cardiovascular risk. Circulation 2014; 129: 981-9.

197 The American Heart Association's Diet and Lifestyle Recommendations, http://www.heart.org/HEARTORG/GettingHealthy/NutritionCenter/HealthyEating/The-American-Heart-Associations-Diet-and-Lifestyle-Recommendations_UCM_305855_Article.jsp

198 Elijovich, F, et al. Salt Sensitivity of Blood Pressure: A Scientific Statement From the American Heart Association. Hypertension. 2016;68:e7-e46. https://www.ahajournals.org/doi/full/10.1161/HYP.0000000000000047?url_ver=Z39.88-2003&rfr_id=ori:rid:crossref.org&rfr_dat=cr_pub%3dpubmed

199 O'Donnell M, Mente M, Rangarajan S, et al. for the PURE Investigators Urinary Sodium and Potassium Excretion, Mortality, and Cardiovascular Events. N Engl J Med 2014; 371:612-623August 14, 2014DOI: 10.1056/NEJMoa1311889

200 Graudal N, Jurgens G, Baslund B, Alderman MH. Compared with usual sodium intake, lowand excessive-sodium diets are associated with increased mortality: a meta-analysis. Am J Hypertens 2014;27:1129-1137

201 Bibbins-Domingo K, Chertow GM, Coxson PG, et al. Projected effect of dietary salt reductions on future cardiovascular disease. N Engl J Med 2010;362:590-599

202 Mozaffarian D, Fahimi S, Singh GM, et al. Global sodium consumption and death from cardiovascular causes. N Engl J Med 2014;371:624-34.

203 Cogswell ME, Mugavero K, Bowman BA, Frieden TR. Dietary Sodium and Cardiovascular Disease Risk — Measurement Matters. N Engl J Med 2016; 375:580-586August 11, 2016DOI: 10.1056/NEJMsb1607161

204 Strom BL, Yaktine AL, Oria M, eds. Sodium Intake in Populations: Assessment of Evidence.Washington, DC: National Academies Press; 2013.

205 Strom BL, Yaktine AL, Oria M, eds. Sodium Intake in Populations: Assessment of Evidence.Washington, DC: National Academies Press; 2013.

206 Mills KT, Chen J, Yang W, et al. Sodium Excretion and the Risk of Cardiovascular Disease in Patients With Chronic Kidney Disease. JAMA. 2016;315(20):2200-2210. doi:10.1001/JAMA.2016.4447.

207 Powe NR, Bibbins-Domingo K. Dietary Salt, Kidney Disease, and Cardiovascular Health. JAMA. 2016;315(20):2173-2174. doi:10.1001/JAMA.2016.5985.

208 Oparil S. Low Sodium Intake — Cardiovascular Health Benefit or Risk? N Engl J Med 2014; 371:677-679August 14, 2014DOI: 10.1056/NEJMe1407695

209 Strom BL, Yaktine AL, Oria M, eds. Sodium Intake in Populations: Assessment of Evidence.Washington, DC: National Academies Press; 2013.

210 Jin J, Sugerman D. Salt in the Diet. JAMA. 2014;311(12):1265. doi:10.1001/JAMA.2014.90.

211 Cogswell ME, Mugavero K, Bowman BA, Frieden TR. Dietary Sodium and Cardiovascular Disease Risk — Measurement Matters. N Engl J Med 2016; 375:580-586August 11, 2016DOI: 10.1056/NEJMsb1607161

212 Cogswell ME, Zhang Z, Carriquiry AL, et al. Sodium and potassium intakes among US adults. Am J Clin Nutr. 2012;96(3):647-657.

213 Mente A, O'Donnell MJ, Rangarajan S, et al. Association of urinary sodium and potassium excretion with blood pressure. N Engl J Med 2014;371:601-11.

214 Ekelund LG, Haskell WL, Johnson JL, Wholey FS, Criqui MH, Sheps DS. Physical fitness as a prevention of cardiovascular mortality in asymptomatic North American men. N Engl J Med. 1988; 319:1379-1384.

215 Sacks FM, Svetkey LP, Vollmer WM, et al. For The Dash–Sodium Collaborative Research Group. Effects On Blood Pressure Of Reduced Dietary Sodium And The Dietary Approaches To Stop Hypertension (Dash) Diet. N Engl J Med. 2001;344:3-10.

216 James PA, Oparil S, Carter BL, et al. 2014 Evidence-Based Guideline for the Management of High Blood Pressure in Adults: Report From the Panel Members Appointed to the Eighth Joint National Committee (JNC 8). JAMA. 2014;311(5):507-520. doi:10.1001/JAMA.2013.284427.

217 Peterson ED, Gaziano J, Greenland P. Recommendations for Treating Hypertension: What Are the Right Goals and Purposes?. JAMA. 2014;311(5):474-476. doi:10.1001/JAMA.2013.284430.

218 SHEP Cooperative Research Group. Prevention of stroke by antihypertensive drug treatment in older persons with isolated systolic hypertension: final results of the Systolic Hypertension in the Elderly Program (SHEP). JAMA. 1991;265(24):3255-3264.

219 Law MR, Morris JK, Wald NJ. Use of blood pressure lowering drugs in the prevention of cardiovascular disease: meta-analysis of 147 randomised trials in the context of expectations from prospective epidemiological studies. BMJ. 2009;338:b1665.

220 Ventura HO, Lavie CJ. Antihypertensive Therapy for Prehypertension: Relationship With Cardiovascular Outcomes. JAMA. 2011;305(9):940-941. doi:10.1001/JAMA.2011.256.

221 Thompson AM, Hu T, Eshelbrenner CL, Reynolds K, He J, Bazzano LA. Antihypertensive treatment and secondary prevention of cardiovascular disease events among persons with hypertension: a meta-analysis. JAMA. 2011;305(9):913-922

222 Wright, JT, Williamson JD, M.D., M.H.S., Whelton PK, et al. A Randomized Trial of Intensive versus Standard Blood-Pressure Control. N Engl J Med. 2015;373:2103-16. DOI: 10.1056/NEJMoa1511939

223 Williamson JD, Supiano MA, Applegate WB, et al. Intensive vs Standard Blood Pressure Control and Cardiovascular Disease Outcomes in Adults Aged ≥75 Years: A Randomized Clinical Trial. JAMA. 2016;315(24):2673-2682. doi:10.1001/JAMA.2016.7050.

224 Wright JT Jr, Williamson JD, Whelton PK, et al. A randomized trial of intensive vs standard

blood-pressure control. N Engl J Med. 2015;373(22):2103-2116.

225 Chobanian AV. Time to Reassess Blood-Pressure Goals N Engl J Med 2015; 373:2093-2095November 26, 2015DOI: 10.1056/NEJMp1513290

226 Chobanian AV. SPRINT Results in Older Patients: How Low to Go?. JAMA. 2016;315(24):2669-2670. doi:10.1001/JAMA.2016.7070.

227 Perkovic V, Rodgers A. Redefining Blood-Pressure Targets — SPRINT Starts the Marathon N Engl J Med 2015; 373:2175-2178November 26, 2015DOI: 10.1056/NEJMe1513301

228 Beckett NS, Peters R, Fletcher AE, Staessen JA, Liu L, Dumitrascu D, Stoyanovsky V, Antikainen RL, Nikitin Y, Anderson C, Belhani A, Forette F, Rajkumar C, Thijs L, Banya W, Bulpitt C J. for the HYVET Study Group. Treatment of Hypertension in Patients 80 Years of Age or Older. N Engl J Med. 2008;358:1887-98. 10.1056/NEJMoa0801369 [doi]

229 Greenland P, Peterson E. The New 2017 ACC/AHA Guidelines "Up the Pressure" on Diagnosis and Treatment of Hypertension. JAMA. 2017;318(21):2083–2084. doi:10.1001/jama.2017.18605

230 Whelton PK, Carey RM, AronowWS, et al. 2017 ACC/AHA/AAPA/ABC/ACPM/AGS/APhA/ ASH/ ASPC/NMA/PCNA guideline for the prevention, detection, evaluation, and management of high blood pres-

sure in adults: a report of the American College of Cardiology/American Heart Association Task Force on Clinical Practice Guidelines [published online November 13, 2017]. Hypertension. doi:10.1161/

HYP.0000000000000065 also [published online November 13, 2017]. J AmColl Cardiol. doi:10.1016/j.jacc.2017.11.006

231 Cifu AS, Davis AM. Prevention, Detection, Evaluation, and Management of High Blood Pressure in Adults. JAMA. 2017;318(21):2132–2134. doi:10.1001/jama.2017.18706

232 Whelton PK, Carey RM. The 2017 Clinical Practice Guideline for High Blood Pressure. JAMA.2017;318(21):2073–2074. doi:10.1001/jama.2017.18209

233 Blood Pressure: the numbers game. The University of California, Berkeley Wellness Letter. February 2018.

234 Chobanian AV. Hypertension in 2017—What Is the Right Target? JAMA. 2017;317(6):579-580. doi:10.1001/JAMA.2017.0105

235 Blood Pressure Lowering Treatment Trialists' Collaboration. Blood pressure loweringtreatment based on cardiovascular risk: a meta-analysis of individual patient data. Lancet 2014; 384: 591-8.

236 Lonn EM, Bosch J. Blood-Pressure Lowering in Intermediate-Risk Persons without Cardiovascular Disease. N Engl J Med 2016;374:2009-20. DOI: 10.1056/NEJMoa1600175

237 Cushman WC, Evans GW, Byington RP, et al. Effects of intensive blood-pressure control in type 2 diabetes mellitus. N Engl J Med. 2010;362(17):1575-1585.

238 Cushman WC, Evans GW, Byington RP, et al. Effects of intensive blood-pressure control in type 2 diabetes mellitus. N Engl J Med. 2010;362(17):1575-1585.

239 Sim JJ, Shi J, Kovesdy CP, Kalantar-Zadeh K, Jacobsen SJ. Impact of Achieved Blood Pressures on Mortality Risk and End-Stage Renal Disease Among a Large, Diverse Hypertension Population. J Am Coll Cardiol. 2014;64(6):588-597. doi:10.1016/j.jacc.2014.04.065.

240 Andersson C, Vasan RS. Lower Is Not Always Better? Blood Pressure Treatment Targets Revisited. J Am Coll Cardiol. 2014;64(6):598-600. doi:10.1016/j.jacc.2014.04.066.

241 Brunstrom M, Carlberg B. Association of blood pressure lowering with mortality and cardiovascular disease across blood pressure levels: a systematic review and meta-analysis. JAMA Intern Med. 2018;178(1):28-36.

242 de Boer IH, Bakris G, Cannon CP. Individualizing Blood Pressure Targets for People With Diabetes and HypertensionComparing the ADA and the ACC/AHA Recommendations. JAMA. 2018;319(13):1319–1320. doi:10.1001/jama.2018.0642

243 Bakris G, Sorrentino, M. Redefining Hypertension — Assessing the New Blood-Pressure Guidelines. N Engl J Med 2018; 378:497-499. DOI: 10.1056/NEJMp1716193

244 McEvoy JW, Daya N, Rahman F, et al. Association of Isolated Diastolic Hypertension as Defined by the 2017 ACC/AHA Blood Pressure Guideline With Incident Cardiovascular Outcomes. JAMA. 2020;323(4):329–338. doi:10.1001/jama.2019.21402

245 Flint AC, Conell C, Ren X, et al. Effect of Systolic and Diastolic Blood Pressure on Cardiovascular Outcomes. N Engl J Med. 2019; 381:243-251. DOI: 10.1056/NEJMoa1803180

246 Lacey B, Lewington S, Clarke R, Kong XL, et al. Age-specific association between blood pressure and vascular and non-vascular diseases in 0.5 million adults in China: a prospective cohort study. The Lancet Global Health. 2018;6:e640-e649.

247 Pfeffer MA, McMurray JJV, Lessons in Uncertainty and Humility — Clinical Trials Involving Hypertension. N Engl J Med. 2016; 375:1756-1766. November 3, 2016. DOI: 10.1056/NEJMra1510067.

248 A major change for daily aspirin therapy. Harvard Health Letter. November 2019.

249 Bibbins-Domingo K, US Preventive Services Task Force. Aspirin use for the primary prevention of cardiovascular disease and colorectal cancer: US Preventive Services Task Force recommendation statement.

Ann Intern Med. 2016; 164: 836.

250 Guirguis-Blake JM, Evans C V, Senger CA, O'Connor EA, Whitlock EP. Aspirin for the primary prevention of cardiovascular events: a systematic evidence review for the US Preventive Services Task Force. Ann Intern Med 2016;164:804–13.

251 Whitlock EP, Burda BU, Williams SB, Guirguis-Blake JM, Evans C V. Bleeding risks with aspirin use for primary prevention in adults: a systematic review for the US Preventive Services Task Force. Ann Intern Med 2016;164:826.

252 Zheng SL, Roddick AJ. Association of Aspirin Use for Primary Prevention With Cardiovascular Events and Bleeding Events: A Systematic Review and Meta-analysis. JAMA. 2019;321(3):277–287. doi:10.1001/jama.2018.20578

253 Gaziano JM, Brotons C, Coppolecchia R, et al. Use of aspirin to reduce risk of initial vascular events in patients at moderate risk of cardiovascular disease (ARRIVE): a randomised, double-blind, placebo-controlled trial. Lancet 2018; published online Aug 26. http://dx.doi.org/10.1016/S0140-6736(18)31924-X.

254 The ASCEND Study Collaborative Group. (2018) Effects of Aspirin for Primary Prevention in Persons with Diabetes Mellitus. N Engl J Med DOI: 10.1056/NEJMoa1804988.

255 McNeil JJ, Nelson MR, Woods RL, et al. Effect of Aspirin on All-Cause Mortality in the Healthy Elderly. N Engl J Med. September 16, 2018. DOI: 10.1056/NEJMoa1803955

256 McNeil JJ, Woods RL, Nelson MR, et al. Effect of Aspirin on Disability-free Survival in the Healthy Elderly. N Engl J Med. 2018. DOI: 10.1056/NEJMoa1800722.

257 McNeil JJ, Wolfe R, Woods RL, et al. Effect of aspirin on cardiovascular events and bleeding in the healthy elderly. N Engl J Med. 2018. DOI: 10.1056/NEJMoa1805819.

258 Ridker PM. Should aspirin be used for primary prevention in the post-statin era? N Engl J Med. 2018;379(16):1572-1574.

259 Blumenthal RS, Llinas RH. 2020 Hypertension and Stroke. White Paper. University of California, Berkeley. 2020, 85pp.

260 Heart Protection Study Collaborative Group. Effects on 11-year mortality and morbidity of lowering LDL cholesterol with simvastatin for about 5 years in 20 536 high-risk individuals: a randomised controlled trial. The Lancet , Volume 378 , Issue 9808 , 2013 – 2020.

261 Appel L, Llinas RH, 2014 Hypertension and Stroke White Paper. Johns Hopkins Medicine. 2014, p.54.

262 Shepherd J, Cobbe SM, Ford I, et al; West of Scotland Coronary Prevention Study Group. Prevention of coronary heart disease with pravastatin in men with hypercholesterolemia. N Engl J Med. 1995;333(20):1301-1307

263 Mihaylova B, Emberson J, Blackwell L, et al; Cholesterol Treatment Trialists' (CTT) Collaborators. The effects of lowering LDL cholesterol with statin therapy in people at low risk of vascular disease: meta-analysis of individual data from 27 randomised trials. Lancet. 2012;380(9841):581-590.

264 Elley CR. ACP Journal Club. Review: Statins reduce mortality and major vascular events in patients with no history of CV disease. Ann Intern Med. 2013 Jul 16;159(2):JC2. doi: 10.7326/0003-4819-159-2-201307160-02002.

265 Downs JR, Clearfield M, Weis S, et al. Primary prevention of acute coronary events with lovastatin in men and women with average cholesterol levels: results of AFCAPS/TexCAPS: Air Force/Texas Coronary Atherosclerosis Prevention Study. JAMA. 1998;279(20):1615-1622.

266 Ridker PM, Danielson E, Fonseca FA, et al; JUPITER Study Group. Rosuvastatin to prevent vascular events in men and women with elevated C-reactive protein. N Engl J Med. 2008;359(21):2195-2207.

267 Blaha MJ, Nasir K, Blumenthal RS. Statin Therapy for Healthy Men Identified as "Increased Risk" JAMA. 2012;307(14):1489-1490. doi:10.1001/JAMA.2012.425

268 Chou R. Error in USPSTF Report on Statin Use. JAMA. 2020;323(7):669. doi:10.1001/jama.2020.0298

269 Mammen AL. Statin-Associated Autoimmune Myopathy. N Engl J Med. 2016;374:664-669 February 18, 2016 DOI: 10.1056/NEJMra1515161

270 Samaras K, Makkar SR, Crawford JD, et al. Effects of Statins on Memory, Cognition, and Brain Volume in the Elderly. J Am Coll Cardiol. 2019;74(21):2554-2568.

271 Swiger KJ, Manalac RJ, Blumenthal RS, Blaha MJ, Martin SS. Statins and Cognition: A Systematic Review and Meta-analysis of Short- and Long-term Cognitive Effects. Mayo Clinic Proceedings. 2013;88(11):1213-1221. https://doi.org/10.1016/j.mayocp.2013.07.013

272 Kokkinos, PF, et al. Interactive effects of fitness and statin treatment on mortality risk in veterans with dyslipidaemia: a cohort study. Lancet. 2013:381(9864):394-399.

273 Psaty BM, Weiss NS. 2013 ACC/AHA Guideline on the Treatment of Blood Cholesterol: A Fresh Interpretation of Old Evidence. JAMA. 2014;311(5):461-462. doi:10.1001/JAMA.2013.284203.

274 Stone NJ, Robinson J, Lichtenstein AH, et al. ACC/AHA Guideline on the Treatment of Blood Cholesterol to Reduce Atherosclerotic Cardiovascular Risk in Adults: a report of the American College of Cardiology/American Heart Association Task Force on Practice Guidelines [published online November 12, 2013]. Circulation. doi:10.1161/01.cir.0000437738.63853.7a. http://circ.ahajournals.org/content/early/2013/11/11/01.cir.0000437741.48606.98.full.pdf

275 Goff DC, Lloyd-Jones DM, Bennett G, et al; American College of Cardiology/American Heart Association Task Force on Practice Guidelines. 2013 ACC/AHA guideline on the assessment of cardiovascular risk: a report of the American College of Cardiology/American Heart Association Task Force on Practice Guidelines. J Am Coll Cardiol. 2014;63(25, pt B):2935-2959.

276 Stone NJ, Robinson JG, Lichtenstein AH, et al; American College of Cardiology/American Heart Association Task Force on Practice Guidelines. 2013ACC/AHA guideline on the treatment of blood cholesterol to reduce atherosclerotic cardiovascular risk in adults. J AmColl Cardiol. 2014;63(25 pt B):2889-2934

277 Collins R, Reith C, Emberson J, et al. Interpretation of the evidence for the efficacy and safety of statin therapy. Lancet. 2016;388(10059):2532-2561.

278 Krumholz HM. Treatment of Cholesterol in 2017. JAMA. 2017;318(5):417–418. doi:10.1001/jama.2017.6753.

279 Pencina MJ, Navar-Boggan AM, D'Agostino RB, et al. Application of New Cholesterol Guidelines to a Population-Based Sample. N Engl J Med. 2014;370:1422-1431April 10, 2014DOI: 10.1056/NEJMoa1315665.

280 Mozaffarian D, Benjamin EJ, Go AS, et al; American Heart Association Statistics Committee and Stroke Statistics Subcommittee. Heart disease and stroke statistics—2015 update. Circulation. 2015;131(4):e29-e322.

281 Ebrahim S, Juan P Casas JP. Statins for all by the age of 50 years? Lancet. 2012;380(9841):545-547, 11 August 2012. DOI: http://dx.doi.org/10.1016/S0140-6736(12)60694-1

282 Greenland P, Lauer MS. Cholesterol Lowering in 2015: Still Answering Questions About How and in Whom. JAMA. 2015;314(2):127-128. doi:10.1001/JAMA.2015.7434.

283 Ioannidis JPA. More Than a Billion People Taking Statins? Potential Implications of the New Cardiovascular Guidelines JAMA. 2014;311(5):463-464. doi:10.1001/JAMA.2013.284657.

284 Redberg RF, Katz MH. Healthy Men Should Not Take Statins. JAMA, April 11, 2012—Vol 307, No. 14 1491-2.

285 Mammen AL. Statin-Associated Autoimmune Myopathy. N Engl J Med. 2016; 374:664-669 February 18, 2016 DOI: 10.1056/NEJMra1515161.

286 Krumholz HM. Treatment of Cholesterol in 2017. JAMA. 2017;318(5):417–418. doi:10.1001/jama.2017.6753.

287 Nasir K, Bittencourt MS, Blaha MJ, et al. Implications of coronary artery calcium testing among statin candidates according to American College of Cardiology/American Heart Association Cholesterol Management Guidelines. J AmColl Cardiol. 2015;66(15):1657-1668.

288 Leening MG, Berry JD, Allen NB. Lifetime Perspectives on Primary Prevention of Atherosclerotic Cardiovascular Disease. JAMA. 2016;315(14):1449-1450. doi:10.1001/JAMA.2016.1654.

289 Shrank WH, Barlow JF, Brennan TA. New Therapies in the Treatment of High Cholesterol: An Argument to Return to Goal-Based Lipid Guidelines. JAMA. 2015;314(14):1443-1444. doi:10.1001/JAMA.2015.10017.

290 Sullivan D, Olsson AG, Scott R, et al. Effect of a Monoclonal Antibody to PCSK9 on Low-Density Lipoprotein Cholesterol Levels in Statin-Intolerant Patients: The GAUSS Randomized Trial. JAMA. 2012;308(23):2497-2506. doi:10.1001/JAMA.2012.25790.

291 The University of California, Berkeley Wellness Letter. Vol 30 issue 8, March 2014.

292 Chou R, Dana T, Blazina I, Daeges M, Jeanne TL. Statins for Prevention of Cardiovascular Disease in Adults Evidence Report and Systematic Review for the US Preventive Services Task Force. JAMA. 2016;316(19):2008-2024. doi:10.1001/JAMA.2015.15629.

293 US Preventive Services Task Force. Statin use for the primary prevention of cardiovascular disease in adults: US Preventive Services Task Force recommendation statement. JAMA. doi:10.1001/JAMA.2016.15450.

294 Greenland P, Bonow RO. Interpretation and Use of Another Statin Guideline. JAMA. 2016;316(19):1977-1979. doi:10.1001/JAMA.2016.15087.

295 Greenland P, Bonow RO. Interpretation and Use of Another Statin Guideline. JAMA. 2016;316(19):1977-1979. doi:10.1001/JAMA.2016.15087.

296 Gurwitz JH, Go AS, Fortmann SP. Statins for Primary Prevention in Older AdultsUncertainty and the Need for More Evidence. JAMA. 2016;316(19):1971-1972. doi:10.1001/JAMA.2016.15212.

297 Shepherd J, Blauw GJ, Murphy MB, et al; PROSPER Study Group. Pravastatin in elderly individuals at risk of vascular disease (PROSPER): a randomised controlled trial. Lancet. 2002;360 (9346):1623-1630.

298 Gotto A, Kjekshus J, Yusuf S, Collins R, Simes J, Baigent C, Keech A, on behalf of the Cholesterol Treatment Trialists' Collaboration. Efficacy and safety of statin therapy in older people: a meta-analysis of individual participant data from 28 randomised controlled trials. Lancet. 2019; 393: 407–15.

299 Orkaby AR, Driver JA, Ho Y, et al. Association of Statin Use With All-Cause and Cardiovascular Mortality in US Veterans 75 Years and Older. JAMA. 2020;324(1):68–78. doi:10.1001/jama.2020.7848

300 Nicholls SJ, Nelson AJ. Statins for Primary Prevention in the Elderly: The Importance of Rigorous Evidence. JAMA. 2020;324(1):45–46. doi:10.1001/jama.2020.8390

301 Redberg RF, Katz MH. Statins for Primary PreventionThe Debate Is Intense, but the Data Are Weak. JAMA. 2016;316(19):1979-1981. doi:10.1001/JAMA.2016.15085.

302 Fernandez G, Spatz ES, Jablecki C, Phillips PS. Statinmyopathy: a common dilemma not reflected in clinical trials. Cleve Clin J Med. 2011;78(6):393-403.

303 Sugiyama T, Tsugawa Y, Tseng C-H, Kobayashi Y, Shapiro MF. Different time trends of caloric and fat intake between statin users and nonusers among US adults: gluttony in the time of statins? JAMA Intern Med. 2014;174(7):1038-1045.

304 Redberg RF, Katz MH. Statins for Primary PreventionThe Debate Is Intense, but the Data Are Weak. JAMA. 2016;316(19):1979-1981. doi:10.1001/JAMA.2016.15085.

305 Navar AM, Peterson ED. Evolving Approaches for Statins in Primary PreventionProgress, but Questions Remain. JAMA. 2016;316(19):1981-1983. doi:10.1001/JAMA.2016.15094.

306 Berry JD, Dyer A, Cai X, et al. Lifetime risks of cardiovascular disease. N Engl J Med. 2012;366(4):321-329.

307 Ford I, Murray H, McCowan C, Packard CJ. Long-term safety and efficacy of lowering low-density lipoprotein cholesterol with statin therapy: 20-year follow-up of West of Scotland Coronary Prevention Study. Circulation. 2016;133(11):1073-1080.

308 Mihaylova B, Emberson J, Blackwell L, et al; Cholesterol Treatment Trialists' (CTT) Collaborators. The effects of lowering LDL cholesterol with statin therapy in people at low risk of vascular disease: meta-analysis of individual data from 27 randomised trials. Lancet. 2012;380(9841):581-590.

309 Silverman MG, Ference BA, Im K, et al. Association between lowering LDL-C and cardiovascular risk reduction among different therapeutic interventions: a systematic review and meta-analysis. JAMA. 2016;316(12):1289-1297.

310 Rist PM, Buring JE, Ridker PM, et al. Lipid levels and the risk of hemorrhagic stroke among women, Neurology. 2019;92(19) e2286-e2294; DOI: 10.1212/WNL.0000000000007454

311 Wechsler LR. Statins and Stroke—Its Complicated. N Engl J Med. 2019; 382(1):81-82

312 Reeskamp LF, Hoogeveen RM. Reader response: Lipid levels and the risk of hemorrhagic stroke among women. Neurology. 2019;92(19) Published July 01, 2019.

313 Gani A. Reader response: Lipid levels and the risk of hemorrhagic stroke among women. Neurology. 2019;92(19) Published April 17, 2019

314 Cholesterol Treatment Trialists' (CTT) Collaboration, Baigent C, Blackwell L, et al. Efficacy and safety of more intensive lowering of LDL cholesterol: A meta-analysis of data from 170,000 participants in 26 randomised trials. Lancet. 2010;376:1670–1681.

315 Grundy SM, Stone NJ, Bailey AL, et al. 2018 AHA/ACC/AACVPR/AAPA/ABC/ACPM/ADA/AGS/APhA/ASPC/NLA/PCNA Guideline on the Management of Blood Cholesterol. A Report of the American College of Cardiology/American Heart Association Task Force on Clinical Practice Guidelines. Circulation. 10 Nov 2018 Circulation. 2018;0:CIR.0000000000000625.

316 Michos ED, McEvoy JW, Blumenthal RS. Lipid management for the prevention of cardiovascular disease. N Engl J Med. 2019;381:1557-1567.

317 Stone NJ, Robinson JG, Lichtenstein AH, et al. 2013 ACC/AHA guideline on the treatment of blood cholesterol to reduce atherosclerotic cardiovascular risk in adults. J AmColl Cardiol. 2014;63(25)(pt B):2889-2934.

318 Ioannidis JPA. Inconsistent Guideline Recommendations for Cardiovascular Prevention and the Debate About Zeroing in on and Zeroing LDL-C Levels With PCSK9 Inhibitors. JAMA. 2017;318(5):419–420. doi:10.1001/jama.2017.6765

319 Collins R, Reith C, Emberson J, et al. Interpretation of the evidence for the efficacy and safety of statin therapy [published online September 8, 2016]. Lancet. doi:10.1016/S0140 -6736(16)31357-5

320 Mihaylova B, Emberson J, Blackwell L, et al; Cholesterol Treatment Trialists' (CTT) Collaborators. The effects of lowering LDL cholesterol with statin therapy in people at low risk of vascular disease: meta-analysis of individual data from 27 randomised trials. Lancet. 2012;380(9841):581-590.

321 Silverman MG, Ference BA, Im K, et al. Association between lowering LDL-C and cardiovascular risk reduction among different therapeutic interventions: a systematic review and meta-analysis. JAMA. 2016;316(12):1289-1297.

322 Taylor F, Huffman MD, Macedo AF, et al. Statins for the primary prevention of cardiovascular disease. Cochrane Database Syst Rev. 2013;1(1):CD004816. doi:10.1002/14651858.CD14004816. pub14651855.

323 Taylor FC, Huffman M, Ebrahim S. Statin therapy for primary prevention of cardiovascular disease, published online November 25, 2013. JAMA. doi:10.1001/JAMA.2013.281348.

324 Robinson JG. Accumulating Evidence for Statins in Primary Prevention. JAMA. 2013;310(22):2405-2406. doi:10.1001/JAMA.2013.281355.

325 Chou R, Dana T, Blazina I, et al. Statins for prevention of cardiovascular disease in adults. JAMA. 2016;316(19):2008-2024.

326 Should you be taking a statin? The University of California, Berkeley Wellness Letter. Vol 32 Issue 8, March 2017.

327 Krumholz HM, An End to Heart Disease? Not Quite. New York Times. March 20, 2017

328 Blumenthal RS. 2020 Heart Attack Prevention. White Paper. University of California, Berkeley. 2020, 78pp.

329 Cannon CP, BlazingMA, Giugliano RP, et al; IMPROVE-IT Investigators. Ezetimibe added to statin therapy after acute coronary syndromes. N Engl J Med. 2015;372(25):2387-2397.

330 Krumholz HM. Treatment of Cholesterol in 2017. JAMA. 2017;318(5):417–418. doi:10.1001/jama.2017.6753

331 Blumenthal RS. 2020 Heart Attack Prevention. White Paper. University of California, Berkeley. 2020, 78pp.

332 Dullaart RPF. PCSK9 Inhibition to Reduce Cardiovascular Events. N Engl J Med. 2017;376:1790-1791. May 4, 2017. DOI: 10.1056/NEJMe1703138

333 Sabatine MS, Giugliano RP, Wiviott SD, et al. Efficacy and safety of evolocumab in reducing lipids and cardiovascular events. N Engl J Med. 2015;372:1500-1509.

334 Robinson JG, Farnier M, Krempf M, et al. Efficacy and safety of alirocumab in reducing lipids and cardiovascular events. N Engl J Med. 2015;372:1489-1499.

335 Sabatine MS, Giugliano RP, Keech AC, et al. Evolocumab and clinical outcomes in patients with cardiovascular disease. N Engl J Med. 2017;376:1713-1722.

336 Ioannidis JPA. Inconsistent Guideline Recommendations for Cardiovascular Prevention and the Debate About Zeroing in on and Zeroing LDL-C Levels With PCSK9 Inhibitors. JAMA. 2017;318(5):419–420. doi:10.1001/jama.2017.6765.

337 Waters DD, Hsue PY, Bangalore S. PCSK9 Inhibitors for Statin Intolerance? JAMA. 2016;315(15):1571-1572. doi:10.1001/jama.2016.3670

338 Honigberg MC, Natarajan P. Bempedoic Acid for Lowering LDL Cholesterol. JAMA. 2019;322(18):1769–1771. doi:10.1001/jama.2019.16598

339 Blumenthal RS. 2020 Heart Attack Prevention. White Paper. University of California, Berkeley. 2020, 78pp.

340 Blumenthal RS. 2020 Heart Attack Prevention. White Paper. University of California, Berkeley. 2020, 78pp.

341 Bhatt DL, Steg PG, Miller M, et al. Cardiovascular risk reduction with icosapent ethyl for hypertriglyceridemia. N Engl J Med 2019;380:11-22.

342 Michos ED, McEvoy JW, Blumenthal RS. Lipid management for the prevention of cardiovascular disease. N Engl J Med. 2019; 381: 1557-1567.

343 Ornish D, The Spectrum. New York, Ballantine Books: 2007.

344 Appel L, Llinas RH, 2014 Hypertension and Stroke White Paper. Johns Hopkins Medicine. 2014, 81pp.

Chapter 7- Preventing Cancer

1 Swartzberg JE, Wolf JL, Preventing Cancer: Strategies to Reduce Your Risk. New York: The Wellness Reports, University of California, Berkeley School of Public Health. Remedy Health Media;2011.

2 Swartzberg JE, Wolf JL, Preventing Cancer: Strategies to Reduce Your Risk. New York: The Wellness Reports, University of California, Berkeley School of Public Health. Remedy Health Media;2011.

3 Doll R, Peto R. The causes of cancer: quantitative estimates of avoidable risks of cancer in the United States today. J Natl Cancer Inst. 1981;66:1191-1308.

4 Song M, Giovannucci E. Preventable Incidence and Mortality of Carcinoma Associated With Lifestyle Factors Among White Adults in the United States. JAMA Oncol. 2016;2(9):1154-1161. doi:10.1001/jamaoncol. 2016.0843

5 Parkin DM, Boyd L, Darby SC, Mesher D, Sasieni P, Walker LC. The Fraction of Cancer Attributable to Lifestyle and Environmental Factors in the UK in 2010. Br J Cancer 2011;105(S2):Si-S81.

6 Emmons KM, Colditz GA. Realizing the Potential of Cancer Prevention— The Role of Implementation Science. N Engl J Med 376;10:986-990.

7 Goodarz Danaei, Stephen Vander Hoorn, Alan D Lopez, Christopher J L Murray, Majid Ezzati, and the Comparative Risk Assessment collaborating group (Cancers) Causes of cancer in the world: comparative risk assessment of nine behavioural and environmental risk factors. Lancet 2005;366:1784–93

8 Emmons KM, Colditz GA. Realizing the Potential of Cancer Prevention— The Role of Implementation Science. N Engl J Med. 376;10:986-990.

9 Rebbeck TR, Kauff ND, Domchek SM. Meta-analysis of risk reduction estimates associated with risk-reducing salpingo-oophorectomy in BRCA1 or BRCA2 mutation carriers. J Natl Cancer Inst. 2009;101:80-7.

10 Calle EE, Rodriguez C, Walker-Thurmond K, Thun MJ. Overweight, obesity, and mortality from cancer in a prospectively studied cohort of US adults. N Engl J Med. 2003;348:1625–38.

11 Chang S, Lacey JV, Brinton LA, et al. Lifetime weight history and endometrial cancer risk by type of menopausal hormone use in the NIH-AARP diet and health study. Cancer Epidemiol Biomarkers Prev. 2007;16:723–30.

12 Luzzatto L, Pandolfi PP. Causality and chance in the development of cancer. N Engl J Med 2005; 373(1): 84–88.

13 Tomasetti C, Bert Vogelstein B. Variation in cancer risk among tissues can be explained by the number of stem cell divisions. Science. 2015;347(6217):78-81. [DOI:10.1126/science.1260825] http://www.sciencemag.org/citmgr?type=refworks&gca=sci%3B347%2F6217%2F78

14 Song Wu, Scott Powers, Wei Zhu & Yusuf A. Hannun. Substantial contribution of extrinsic risk factors to cancer development. Nature 529:43–47. doi:10.1038/nature16166

15 Wild C, Brennan P, Plummer M, Bray F, Straif K, Zavadil J. Cancer risk: Role of chance overstated. Science. 2015:347(6223):728. DOI: 10.1126/science.aaa6799

16 Rozhok AI, Wahl GM, DeGregori J. A critical examination of the "bad luck" explanation of cancer risk. Cancer Prev Res (Phila). 2015;8(9):762-764. 2015;108(3):djv343.

17 Giovannucci EL. Are most cancers caused by specific risk factors acting on tissues with high underlying stem cell divisions? J Natl Cancer Inst. 2015;108(3):djv343.

18 Lefall LD, Kripke ML. Reducing Environmental Cancer Risk: What We Can Do Now. Bethesda MD:

National Institutes of Health, Annual report of the President's Cancer Panel. 2010.

19 Ropeik D, Gray G. Risk. Boston and New York: Houghton Mifflin; 2002.

20 Current Investment by Areas of Research. American Cancer Society. https://www.cancer.org/research/currently-funded-cancer-research/investment-by-research-areas.html

21 NIH Categorical Spending, Research Portfolio Online Reporting Tools (RePORT) https://report.nih.gov/categorical_spending.aspx

22 American Cancer Society. Cancer Facts & Figures 2014. Atlanta, Ga. 2014.

23 U.S. Complete Prevalence Counts, Invasive Cancers Only, January 1, 2016 By Age at Prevalence. SEER Cancer Statistics Review. https://seer.cancer.gov/csr/1975_2016/browse_csr.php?sectionSEL=1&pageSEL=sect_01_table.22

24 Davis MM, Dayoub EJ. A Strategic Approach to Therapeutic Cancer Vaccines in the 21st Century. JAMA. 2011;305(22):2343-2344. doi:10.1001/jama.2011.814.

25 U.S. Department of Health and Human Services. The Health Consequences of Smoking—50 Years of Progress. A Report of the Surgeon General. Atlanta: U.S. Department of Health and Human Services, Centers for Disease Control and Prevention, National Center for Chronic Disease Prevention and Health Promotion, Office on Smoking and Health, 2014.

26 U.S. Department of Health and Human Services. The Health Consequences of Smoking: A Report of the Surgeon General. Atlanta: U.S. Department of Health and Human Services, Centers for Disease Control and Prevention, National Center for Chronic Disease Prevention and Health Promotion, Office on Smoking and Health, 2004.

27 U.S. Department of Health and Human Services. How Tobacco Smoke Causes Disease: What It Means to You. Atlanta: U.S. Department of Health and Human Services, Centers for Disease Control and Prevention, National Center for Chronic Disease Prevention and Health Promotion, Office on Smoking and Health, 2010.

28 U.S. Department of Health and Human Services. How Tobacco Smoke Causes Disease: The Biology and Behavioral Basis for Smoking-Attributable Disease: A Report of the Surgeon General. Atlanta, GA: U.S. Department of Health and Human Services, Centers for Disease Control and Prevention, National Center for Chronic Disease Prevention and Health Promotion, Office on Smoking and Health, 2010. http://www.ncbi.nlm.nih.gov/books/NBK53017/pdf/TOC.pdf

29 Centers for Disease Control and Prevention. Current Cigarette Smoking Among Adults—United States, 2016. Morbidity and Mortality Weekly Report 2018;67(2):53-9 and Current Smoking Among Adults, 2016, in the United States. Centers for Disease Control and Prevention (CDC). https://www.cdc.gov/tobacco/data_statistics/fact_sheets/adult_data/cig_smoking/index.htm

30 Ravenholt RT. Tobacco's global death march. Population and Development Review 16(2) June 1990.

31 Jha P, Ramasundarahettige C, Landsman V, Rostrom B, Thun M, Anderson RN, McAfee T, Peto R. 21st Century Hazards of Smoking and Benefits of Cessation in the United States. [PDF–782 KB]. N. Engl. J. Med. 2013;368(4):341–50.

32 CDC Fact Sheet, Tobacco-Related Mortality, Smoking and Tobacco Use, CDC.gov

33 Hajek P, Phillips-Waller A, Przulj D, et al. A randomized trial of e-cigarettes versus nicotine-replacement therapy. N Engl J Med 2019;380:629-637.

34 Drazen JM, Morrissy S, Campion EW. The dangerous flavors of e-cigarettes. N Engl J Med. 2019;380:679-680. DOI: 10.1056/NEJMe1900484

35 Vaping+smoking=bad news. University of California, Berkeley Wellness Letter. April 2019.

36 Cullen KA, Ambrose BK, Gentzke AS, Apelberg BJ, Jamal A, King BA. Notes from the Field: Use of Electronic Cigarettes and Any Tobacco Product Among Middle and High School Students — United States,

2011–2018. MMWR Morb Mortal Wkly Rep 2018;67:1276–1277. DOI: http://dx.doi.org/10.15585/mmwr.mm6745a5external icon

37 Singh, T., Arrazola, R. A., Corey, C. G., et al. (2016) Tobacco Use Among Middle and High School Students — United States, 2011–2015. Morbidity and Mortality Weekly Report, 65(14), 361–367. Retrieved June 10, 2016, from http://www.cdc.gov/mmwr/volumes/65/wr/mm6514a1.htm.

38 Johnston, L. D., Miech, R. A., O'Malley, P. M., Bachman, J. G., Schulenberg, J. E. & Patrick, M.E. (2018). Monitoring the Future national survey results on drug use, 1975-2017: Overview, key findings on adolescent drug use. Ann Arbor: Institute for Social Research, The University of Michigan. Retrieved March 12, 2018, from http://www.monitoringthefuture.org/pubs/monographs/mtf-overview2017.pdf - PDF

39 Cullen KA, Gentzke AS, Sawdey MD, et al. e-Cigarette Use Among Youth in the United States, 2019 JAMA. 2019;322(21):2095–2103. doi:https://doi.org/10.1001/jama.2019.18387

40 Brownson EG, Thompson CM, Gibran NS. Explosion injuries from e-cigarettes. N Engl J Med. 2016;375:1400-1402.

41 Dinakar C, O'Connor GT. The health effects of electronic cigarettes. N Engl J Med. 2016;375:1372-1381

42 Alzahrani T, Pena I, Temesgen N, Glantz SA. Association Between Electronic Cigarette Use and My cardial Infarction. Am J Preventive Medicine. 2018;55(4):455–461

43 Outbreak of Lung Injury Associated with the Use of E-Cigarette, or Vaping, Products. Centers for Disease Control and Prevention. December 19, 2019. https://www.cdc.gov/tobacco/basic_information/e-cigarettes/severe-lung-disease.html#latest-outbreak-information

44 World Cancer Report 2014. Geneva: WHO, International Agency for Research on Cancer

45 Harms of Cigarette Smoking and Health Benefits of Quitting. National Cancer Institute. http://www.cancer.gov/about-cancer/causes-prevention/risk/tobacco/cessation-fact-sheet#q1

46 Volkow ND, Baler RD, Compton WM, Weiss S. Adverse health effects of marijuana use. N. Engl. J. Med. 2014;370:2219–2227.

47 Ammerman S, Ryan S, Adelman WP. The impact of marijuana policies on youth: clinical, research, and legal update. Pediatrics. 2015;135:e769–e785.

48 WebMD http://www.emedicinehealth.com/lung_cancer/page2_em.htm

49 Secondhand Smoke and Cancer. National Cancer Institute. http://www.cancer.gov/about-cancer/causes-prevention/risk/tobacco/second-hand-smoke-fact-sheet

50 http://www.cdc.gov/tobacco/data_statistics/fact_sheets/health_effects/effects_cig_smoking/#cancer,

51 CDC Fact Sheet-Health Effects of Cigarette Smoking-Smoking and Tobacco Use. https://www.cdc.gov/tobacco/data_statistics/fact_sheets/health_effects/effects_cig_smoking/

52 Carter BD, Abnet CC, Feskanich D, et al. Smoking and Mortality — Beyond Established Causes. N Engl J Med. 2015; 372:631-640February 12, 2015DOI: 10.1056/NEJMsa1407211

53 Smith AL, Chapman S. Quitting Smoking Unassisted, The 50-Year Research Neglect of a Major Public Health Phenomenon. JAMA. 2014;311(2):137-138. doi:10.1001/jama.2013.282618.

54 Godtfredsen NS, Prescott E, Osler M. Effect of Smoking Reduction on Lung Cancer Risk. JAMA. 2005;294(12):1505-1510. doi:10.1001/jama.294.12.1505.

55 U.S. Department of Health and Human Services. How Tobacco Smoke Causes Disease: What It Means to You. Atlanta: U.S. Department of Health and Human Services, Centers for Disease Control and Prevention, National Center for Chronic Disease Prevention and Health Promotion, Office on Smoking and Health, 2010.

56 CDC Fact Sheet - Alcohol Use and Your Health http://www.cdc.gov/alcohol/fact-sheets/alcohol-use.htm

57 Centers for Disease Control and Prevention (CDC). Alcohol-Related Disease Impact (ARDI). Atlanta, GA: CDC.

58 Stahre M, Roeber J, Kanny D, Brewer RD, Zhang X. Contribution of excessive alcohol consumption to deaths and years of potential life lost in the United States. Prev Chronic Dis. 2014;11:130293.

59 Sacks JJ, Gonzales KR, Bouchery EE, Tomedi LE, Brewer RD. 2010 National and State Costs of Excessive Alcohol Consumption. Am J Prev Med. 2015; 49(5):e73–e79.

60 Alcohol and Cancer Risk Fact Sheet. National Cancer Institute http://www.cancer.gov/about-cancer/causes-prevention/risk/alcohol/alcohol-fact-sheet

61 Nelson DE, Jarman DW, Rehm J, et al. Alcohol-Attributable Cancer Deaths and Years of Potential Life Lost in the United States. Am J Public Health. 2013;103: 641–648. doi:10.2105/AJPH.2012.301199.

62 CDC:Fact Sheets - Alcohol Use and Your Health http://www.cdc.gov/alcohol/fact-sheets/alcohol-use.htm

63 National Institute of Alcohol Abuse and Alcoholism. Tenth special report to the U.S. Congress on alcohol and health [PDF - 2.8MB]. Bethesda, MD: National Institute of Health; 2000.

64 CDC:Fact Sheets - Alcohol Use and Your Health http://www.cdc.gov/alcohol/fact-sheets/alcohol-use.htm

65 National Institute of Alcohol Abuse and Alcoholism. Tenth special report to the U.S. Congress on alcohol and health [PDF - 2.8MB]. Bethesda, MD: National Institute of Health; 2000.

66 Klein WMP, Jacobsen PB, Helzlsouer KJ. Alcohol and Cancer Risk: Clinical and Research Implications. JAMA. 2020;323(1):23–24. doi:10.1001/jama.2019.19133

67 World Cancer Report 2014. Geneva: WHO, International Agency for Research on Cancer; 2014:97-100.

68 WHO Cancer Prevention. http://www.who.int/cancer/prevention/en/

69 Does Alcohol deserve its healthy buzz? University of California, Berkeley Wellness Letter. November, 2017.

70 Calle EE, Rodriguez C, Walker-Thurmond K, Thun MJ. Overweight, Obesity, and Mortality from Cancer in a Prospectively Studied Cohort of U.S. Adults. N Engl J Med. 2003; 348:1625-1638April 24, 2003DOI: 10.1056/NEJMoa021423

71 Massetti GM, Dietz WH, Richardson LC. Excessive Weight Gain, Obesity, and Cancer Opportunities or Clinical Intervention. JAMA. 2017;318(20):1975–1976. doi:10.1001/jama.2017.15519

72 Steele CB, Thomas CC, Henley SJ, et al. Vital Signs: Trends in Incidence of Cancers Related to Overweight and Obesity—United States, 2005-2014. October 3, 2017. https://www.cdc.gov/mmwr/volumes/ 66/wr/mm6639e1.htm?s_cid=mm6639e1_w.

73 Byers T, Sadjo RL. Does intentional weight loss reduce cancer risk? Diabetes Obes Metab. 2011 Dec;13(12):1063-72. doi: 10.1111/j.1463-1326.2011.01464.x.

74 Willett WC, Key T, Romieu I, Diet, obesity and physical activity. World Cancer Report 2014. Geneva: WHO, International Agency for Research on Cancer;2014: Chapter 2.6.

75 Lauby-Secretan B, Scocciant C, Loomis D, et al. for the International Agency for Research on Cancer Handbook Working Group. Body Fatness and Cancer — Viewpoint of the IARC Working Group. N Engl J Med. 2016; 375:794-798August 25, 2016DOI: 10.1056/NEJMsr1606602

76 Lauby-Secretan B, Scocciant C, Loomis D, et al. for the International Agency for Research on Cancer Handbook Working Group. Body Fatness and Cancer — Viewpoint of the IARC Working Group. N Engl J Med. 2016; 375:794-798August 25, 2016DOI: 10.1056/NEJMsr1606602

77 Liu P, Wu K, Ng K, et al. Association of Obesity With Risk of Early-Onset Colorectal Cancer Among Women. JAMA Oncol. Published online October 11, 2018. doi:10.1001/jamaoncol.2018.4280

78 Pearson-Stuttard J, Zhou B, et al. Worldwide burden of cancer attributable to diabetes and high body-mass index: a comparative risk assessment. The Lancet Diabetes & Endocrinology. 2018;6(1):95-104.

79 Lakoski SG, Willis BL, Barlow CE, et al. Midlife Cardiorespiratory Fitness, Incident Cancer, and Survival After Cancer in Men: The Cooper Center Longitudinal Study. JAMA Oncol. 2015;1(2):231–237. doi:10.1001/jamaoncol.2015.0226

80 Peel JB, Sui X, Adams SA, Hébert JR, Hardin JW, Blair SN. A prospective study of cardiorespiratory fitness and breast cancer mortality. Med Sci Sports Exerc. 2009;41(4):742–748. doi:10.1249/MSS.0b013e31818edac7

81 Marshall CH, Al-Mallah MH, Dardari Z, Brawner CA, et al. Cardiorespiratory Fitness and Incident Lung and Colorectal Cancer in Men and Women: Results from the Henry Ford Exercise Testing (FIT) Cohort. Cancer. 2019;125(15):2594-2601.

82 Moore SC, Lee I-M,Weiderpass E, et al. Association of leisure-time physical activity with risk of 26 types of cancer in 1.44 million adults [published online May 16, 2016]. JAMA Intern Med. doi:10.1001/jamainternmed.2016.1548.

83 2018 Physical Activity Guidelines Advisory Committee. 2018 Physical Activity Guidelines Advisory Committee Scientific Report. Washington, DC: U.S. Department of Health and Human Services, 2018.

84 Willett WC, Key T, Romieu I, Diet, obesity and physical activity. World Cancer Report 2014. Geneva: WHO, International Agency for Research on Cancer;2014: Chapter 2.6.

85 Schabath MB, Hernandez LM, Wu X, Pillow PC, Spitz MR. Dietary Phytoestrogens and Lung Cancer Risk. JAMA. 2005;294(12):1493-1504. doi:10.1001/jama.294.12.1493.

86 Willett WC. Diet and Cancer: An Evolving Picture. JAMA. 2005;293(2):233-234. doi:10.1001/jama.293.2.233.

87 Willett WC, Key T, Romieu I, Diet, obesity and physical activity. World Cancer Report 2014. Geneva: WHO, International Agency for Research on Cancer;2014: Chapter 2.6.

88 Lavalette C, Adjibade M, Srour B, et al. Cancer-Specific and General Nutritional Scores and Cancer Risk: Results from the Prospective NutriNet-Santé Cohort. Cancer Res July 26,2018 DOI: 10.1158/0008-5472.CAN-18-0155.

89 Farvid S, Chen WY, Rosner BA, Rulla MT, Willett WC, Eliassen AH. Fruit and vegetable consumption and breast cancer incidence: Repeated measures over 30 years of follow-up. Int. J. Cancer. 2019;144:1496–1510

90 WHO. Q&A on the carcinogenicity of the consumption of red meat and processed meat. October 2015. http://www.who.int/features/qa/cancer-red-meat/en/

91 WHO, International Agency for Research on Cancer. Press Release No. 240. October 26, 2015. https://www.iarc.fr/en/media-centre/pr/2015/pdfs/pr240_E.pdf

92 Manson JE, Cook NR, Lee I-M, et al. Marine n−3 fatty acids and prevention of cardiovascular disease and cancer. N Engl J Med. DOI: 10.1056/NEJMoa1811403.

93 World Cancer Report 2014. Geneva: WHO, International Agency for Research on Cancer;2014:129

94 Aune D, Keum NN, Giovannucci E, et al. Nut consumption and risk of cardiovascular disease, total cancer, all-cause and cause- specific mortality: a systematic review and dose-response meta-analysis of prospective studies. BMC Medicine. 2016;14:207. DOI 10.1186/s12916-016-0730-3

95 Er A, Lane JA, Martin RM, et al. Adherence to dietary and lifestyle recommendations and prostate cancer risk in the Prostate Testing for Cancer and Treatment (ProtecT) Trial. Cancer Epidemiol Biomarkers & Prevention 2014;23:2066-2077.

96 Monge A, Lajous M. Ultra-processed foods and cancer BMJ.2018;360:k599. doi: https://doi.org/10.1136/bmj.k599

97 Dietary Reference Intakes for Calcium and Vitamin D, Report Brief November 2010, The Institute of Medicine of the National Academies http://www.nal.usda.gov/fnic/DRI/DRI_Calcium_Vitamin_D/FullReport.pdf

98 Manson JE, Cook NR, Lee IM, et al.; VITAL Research Group. Vitamin D supplements and prevention of cancer and cardiovascular disease. N Engl J Med. 2019;380(1):33-44. doi:10.1056/NEJMoa1809944

99 Barry EL, Passarelli MN, Baron JA. Vitamin D as Cancer Therapy? Insights From 2 New Trials. JAMA.2019;321(14):1354–1355. doi:10.1001/jama.2019.2589

100 World Cancer Report 2014. Geneva: WHO, International Agency for Research on Cancer;2014:105

101 American Cancer Society. Viruses that can lead to cancer. http://www.cancer.org/cancer/cancercauses/othercarcinogens/infectiousagents/infectiousagentsandcancer/infectious-agents-and-cancer-viruses

102 American Cancer Society. Viruses that can lead to cancer. http://www.cancer.org/cancer/cancercauses/othercarcinogens/infectiousagents/infectiousagentsandcancer/infectious-agents-and-cancer-viruses

103 Joura EA, Giuliano AR, Iversen O, et al. for the Broad Spectrum HPV Vaccine Study. A 9-Valent HPV Vaccine against Infection and Intraepithelial Neoplasia in Women. N Engl J Med. 2015; 372:711-723February 19, 2015DOI: 10.1056/NEJMoa1405044

104 Iversen O, Miranda MJ, Ulied A, et al. Luxembourg A. Immunogenicity of the 9-Valent HPV Vaccine Using 2-Dose Regimens in Girls and Boys vs a 3-Dose Regimen in Women. JAMA. 2016;316(22):2411-2421. doi:10.1001/jama.2016.17615.

105 Swartzberg JE, Wolf JL, Preventing Cancer: Strategies to Reduce Your Risk. New York: The Wellness Reports, University of California, Berkeley School of Public Health. Remedy Health Media;2011.

106 World Cancer Report 2014. Geneva: WHO, International Agency for Research on Cancer; 2014:109

107 American Cancer Society. Viruses that can lead to cancer. http://www.cancer.org/cancer/cancercauses/othercarcinogens/infectiousagents/infectiousagentsandcancer/infe tious-agents-and-cancer-viruses

108 American Cancer Society. Viruses that can lead to cancer. http://www.cancer.org/cancer/cancercauses/othercarcinogens/infectiousagents/infectiousagentsandcancer/infectious-agents-and-cancer-viruses

109 American Cancer Society. Viruses that can lead to cancer. http://www.cancer.org/cancer/cancercauses/othercarcinogens/infectiousagents/infectiousagentsandcancer/infectious-agents-and-cancer-viruses

110 American Cancer Society. Bacteria that can lead to cancer. http://www.cancer.org/cancer/cancercauses/othercarcinogens/infectiousagents/infectiousagentsandcancer/infectious-agents-and-cancer-bacteria

111 Herrero R, Parsonnet J, Greenberg E. Prevention of Gastric Cancer. JAMA. 2014;312(12):1197-1198. doi:10.1001/jama.2014.10498.

112 American Cancer Society. Bacteria that can lead to cancer. http://www.cancer.org/cancer/cancercauses/othercarcinogens/infectiousagents/infectiousagentsandcancer/infectious-agents-and-cancer-bacteria

113 American Cancer Society, Parasites and Cancer. https://www.cancer.org/cancer/cancer-causes/infectious-agents/infections-that-can-lead-to-cancer/parasites.html

114 US Department of Health and Human Services. Public Health Service, National Toxicology Program. Report on Carcinogens, Twelfth Edition: Ionizing radiation. 2011. http://ntp.niehs.nih.gov/ntp/roc/twelfth/profiles/IonizingRadiation.pdf.

115 American Cancer Society. Do X-rays and gamma rays cause cancer?http://www.cancer.org/cancer/cancercauses/radiationexposureandcancer/xraysgammaraysandcancerrisk/x-rays-gamma-rays-and-cancer-risk-do-xrays-and-gamma-rays-cause-cancer

116 World Cancer Report 2014. Geneva: WHO, International Agency for Research on Cancer;2014:144

117 Patient Safety-Radiation Dose in X-Ray and CT Exams. http://www.radiologyinfo.org/en/info.cfm?pg=safety-xray

118 Environmental Protection Agency. A Citizen's Guide to Radon. 1/10/2013. Accessed at http://www.epa.gov/radon/pubs/citguide.html on June 28, 2013.

119 Environmental Protection Agency. Consumer's Guide to Radon Reduction. 5/13/2013. Accessed at http://www.epa.gov/radon/pubs/consguid.html on June 28, 2013.

120 National Cancer Institute. Radon and Cancer: Questions and Answers. 12/6/2011. Accessed at www.cancer.gov/cancertopics/factsheet/Risk/radon on June 28, 2013.

121 Lubin JH, Boice JD Jr. Lung cancer risk from residential radon: Meta-analysis of eight epidemiologic studies. J Natl Cancer Inst. 1997;89:49–57.

122 Alberg AJ, Samet JM. Epidemiology of lung cancer. Chest. 2003;123:21S-49S.

123 American Cancer Society. Skin cancer. http://www.cancer.org/cancer/skincancer/

124 Gershenwald JE, Halpern AC, Sondak VK. Melanoma Prevention—Avoiding Indoor Tanning and Minimizing Overexposure to the Sun. JAMA. 2016;316(18):1913-1914. doi:10.1001/jama.2016.16430

125 Matta MK, Zusterzeel R, Pilli NR, et al. Effect of Sunscreen Application Under Maximal Use Conditions on Plasma Concentration of Sunscreen Active Ingredients: A Randomized Clinical Trial. JAMA. Published online May 06, 2019321(21):2082–2091. doi:10.1001/jama.2019.5586

126 Califf RM, Shinkai K. Filling in the Evidence About Sunscreen. JAMA. Published online May 06,

019321(21):2077–2079. doi:10.1001/jama.2019.5528

127 American Cancer Society. Do X-rays and gamma rays cause cancer? http://www.cancer.org/cancer/cancercauses/radiationexposureandcancer/xraysgammaraysandcancerrisk/x-rays-gamma-rays-and-cancer-risk-do-xrays-and-gamma-rays-cause-cancer

128 Storrs C. Do CT scans cause cancer? Scientific American. July 2013. p. 30-32.

129 Redberg RF, Smith-Bindman R. We are Giving Ourselves Cancer. New York Times, January 31, 2014.

130 Patient Safety-Radiation Dose in X-Ray and CT Exams. http://www.radiologyinfo.org/en/info.cfm?pg=safety-xray

131 American Cancer Society. Known and Probable Human Carcinogens. http://www.cancer.org/cancer/cancercauses/othercarcinogens/generalinformationaboutcarcinogens/known-and-probable-human-carcinogens

132 http://monographs.iarc.fr/ENG/Classification/.

133 Alavanja MCR., Ross MK. and Bonner MR. Increased cancer burden among pesticide applicators and others due to pesticide exposure. CA: A Cancer Journal for Clinicians, 2013;63: 120–142. doi:10.3322/caac.21170.

134 Swartzberg JE, Wolf JL, Preventing Cancer: Strategies to Reduce Your Risk. New York: The Wellness Reports, University of California, Berkeley School of Public Health. Remedy Health Media;2011.

135 American Cancer Society. Family cancer syndromes. http://www.cancer.org/cancer/cancercauses/geneticsandcancer/heredity-and-cancer

136 Antoniou, A., Pharoah, P.D.P., Narod, S. et al. Average risks of breast and ovarian cancer associated with BRCA1 or BRCA2 mutations detected in case series unselected for family history: a combined analysis of 22 studies. Am J Hum Genet. 2003; 72: 1117–1130.

137 Ring K L, Garcia C, Thomas MH, et al. Current and future role of genetic screening in gynecologic malignancies. Am J Obstetrics & Gynecology. 2017; 217(5):512-515

138 Antoniou AC, Casadei S, et. al. Breast-Cancer Risk in Families with Mutations in PALB2. N Engl J Med. 2014;371(6):497-506. 10.1056/NEJMoa1400382 [doi]http://www.nejm.org/doi/full/10.1056/NEJMoa1400382

139 Evans MK, Longo DL. PALB2 Mutations and Breast-Cancer Risk. N Engl J Med. 2014;371:566- 568. DOI: 10.1056/NEJMe1405784.

140 Pace LE, Keating NL. Medications to Reduce Breast Cancer Risk: Promise and Limitations. JAMA. 2019;322(9):821–823. doi:https://doi.org/10.1001/jama.2019.9689

141 US Preventive Services Task Force. Medication use to reduce risk of breast cancer: US Preventive Services Task Force recommendation statement [published September 3, 2019]. JAMA. doi:10.1001/jama.2019.11885

142 Shieh Y, Tice JA. Medications for Primary Prevention of Breast Cancer. JAMA. 2020;324(3):291–292. doi:10.1001/jama.2020.9246

143 Breast Cancer Surveillance Consortium Risk Calculator. https://tools.bcsc-scc.org/BC5yearRisk/ calculator.htm

144 Platz EA, Willett WC, Colditz GA, Rimm EB, Spiegelman D, Giovannucci E. Proportion of colon cancer risk that might be preventable in a cohort of middle-aged US men. Cancer Causes Control. 2000;11:579-588

145 Cao Y, Nishihara R, Wu K, Wang M, Ogino S, Willett WC, Spiegelman D, Fuchs CS, Giovannucci EL, Chan AT. Population-wide Impact of Long-term Use of Aspirin and the Risk for Cancer. JAMA Oncol. 2016;2(6):762-9. doi: 10.1001/jamaoncol.2015.6396.

146 Vilar E, Maresso K, Hawk ET. Aspirin for Cancer Prevention: One Step Closer. JAMA Oncol. 2016;2(6):770-771. doi:10.1001/jamaoncol.2015.6395.

147 Cuzick J, Thorat MA, Bosetti C, et al. Estimates of benefits and harms of prophylactic use of aspirin in the general population. Ann Oncol. 2014. doi: 10.1093/annonc/mdu225

148 Sutcliffe P, Connock M, Gurung T, Freeman K, Johnson S, Kandala NB, Grove A, Gurung B, Morrow S, Clarke A. Aspirin for prophylactic use in the primary prevention of cardiovascular disease and cancer: a systematic review and overview of reviews. Health Technol Assess. 2013 Sep; 17(43):1-253.

149 Collaborative Group on Epidemiological Studies of Ovarian Cancer. Menopausal hormone use and ovarian cancer risk: individual participant meta-analysis of 52 epidemiological studies. Lancet. 2015;385: 1835–42.

150 Onwude J. Hormone therapy and ovarian cancer. Lancet. 2015;386:1037–1038

151 Naftolin F, Friedenthal J, Blakemore J, Nachtigall L. Hormone therapy and ovarian cancer. Lancet. 386;9998:1037-1038

152 Ornish D, Weidner G, Fair WR, Marlin R, Pettengill EB, Raisin CJ, Dunn-Emke S, Crutchfield L, Jacobs FN, Barnard RJ, Aronson WJ, McCormac P, McKnight DJ, Fein JD, Dnistrian AM, Weinstein J, Ngo TH, Mendell NR, Carroll PR. Intensive lifestyle changes may affect the progression of prostate cancer. J Urol. 2005 Sep;174(3):1065-9; discussion 1069-70.

153 Still hung up on cell phones. University of California, Berkeley Wellness Letter June 2017; 1-2.

154 Shermer M. Can you hear me now? Scientific American, October 2010. p. 98.

155 Li D-K, Chen H, Ferber JR, et al. Exposure to Magnetic Field Non-Ionizing Radiation and the Risk of Miscarriage: A Prospective Cohort Study. Scientific Reports, 2017; 7 (1) DOI: 10.1038/s41598-017-16623-8

156 Still hung up on cell phones. University of California, Berkeley Wellness Letter. June 2017; 1-2.

157 Environmental Protection Agency. Radiation: Ionizing and Non-Ionizing. 5/17/2013. www.epa.gov/radiation/understand/index.html.

158 International Agency for Research on Cancer. IARC Monographs on the Evaluation of Carcinogenic Risks to Humans. Volume 80: Non-Ionizing Radiation, Part 1: Static and Extremely Low-Frequency (ELF) Electric and Magnetic Fields. 2002. http://monographs.iarc.fr/ENG/Monographs/vol80/index.php.

159 Kheifets L, Ahlbom A, Crespi CM, Draper G, Hagihara J, Lowenthal RM, Mezei G, Oksuzyan S, Schüz J, Swanson J, Tittarelli A, Vinceti M, Wunsch Filho V. Pooled analysis of recent studies on magnetic fields and childhood leukaemia. Br J Cancer. 2010 Sep 28;103(7):1128-35. Erratum in: Br J Cancer. 2011 Jan 4;104(1):228.

160 National Institute of Environmental Health Sciences. Health Effects from Exposure to Power-Line Frequency Electric and Magnetic Fields.1999. www.niehs.nih.gov/health/assets/docs_f_o/niehs-report.pdf.

161 National Institute of Environmental Health Sciences. Electric and Magnetic Fields Associated with the Use of Electric Power. 2002. http://www.niehs.nih.gov/health/materials/electric_and_magnetic_fields_ associated_with_the_use_of_electric_power_questions_and_answers_english_508.pdf

162 Schüz J. Exposure to extremely low-frequency magnetic fields and the risk of childhood cancer: update of the epidemiological evidence. Prog Biophys Mol Biol. 2011 Dec;107(3):339-42. Epub 2011 Sep 19.

163 World Cancer Report 2014. Geneva: WHO, International Agency for Research on Cancer. p148

164 American Cancer Society. Imaging (radiology) tests for cancer cancer.http://www.cancer.org/treatment/understandingyourdiagnosis/examsandtestdescriptions/imaging-radiology-tests-for-cancer

165 Saslow D, Boetes C, Burke W, et al. for the American Cancer Society Breast Cancer Advisory Group. American Cancer Society guidelines for breast screening with MRI as an adjunct to mammography. Cancer J Clin. 2007;57:75-89.

166 Mammograms: still a good idea? University of California, Berkeley Wellness Letter 2010;26(5) 1-3.

167 Longo DL. Detecting breast cancer in women with dense breasts. N Engl J Med. 2019;381(22):2169-2170.

168 Orenstein P. Our-Feel-Good War on Breast Cancer. New York Times Magazine, April 28, 2013.

169 Yi M, Hunt KK. Optimizing Mammography Screening Intervals. JAMA. 2015;314(15):1635-1636. doi:10.1001/jama.2015.13149.

170 Keating NL, Pace LE. New Guidelines for Breast Cancer Screening in US Women. JAMA. 2015;314(15):1569–1571. doi:10.1001/jama.2015.13086

171 Rosenbaum L. Invisible Risks, Emotional Choices — Mammography and Medical Decision Making. N Engl J Med. 2014; 371:1549-1552October 16, 2014DOI: 10.1056/NEJMms1409003

172 American Cancer Society recommendations for early breast cancer detection in women without breast symptoms. https://www.cancer.org/healthy/find-cancer-early/cancer-screening-guidelines/american- cancer-society-guidelines-for-the-early-detection-of-cancer.html; http://www.cancer.org/cancer/breastcancer/moreinformation/breastcancerearlydetection/breast-cancer-early-detection-acs-recs

173 Breast Cancer Risk Assessment and Screening in Average-Risk Women. ACOG Practice Bulletin. Number 179, July 2017.

174 Breast Cancer: Early Detection and the Final Recommendation Statement, Breast Cancer: Screening of the U. S. Preventative Services Task Force. 2016. http://www.uspreventiveservicestaskforce.org/Page/Document/RecommendationStatementFinal/breast-cancer-screening1

175 Nelson HD, Pappas M, Cantor A, Haney E, Holmes R. Risk Assessment, Genetic Counseling, and Genetic Testing for BRCA-Related Cancer in Women: Updated Evidence Report and Systematic Review for the US Preventive Services Task Force. JAMA. 2019;322(7):666–685. doi:10.1001/jama.2019.8430

176 Domchek S, Robson M. Broadening Criteria for BRCA1/2 Evaluation: Placing the USPSTF Recommendation in Context. JAMA. 2019;322(7):619–621. doi:10.1001/jama.2019.9688

177 Lauby-Secretan B, Scoccianti C, Loomis D, et al. Breast-cancer screening — viewpoint of the IARC Working Group. N Engl J Med. 2015;372:2353-8.

178 Jørgensen KJ, Bewley S. Breast-cancer screening — viewpoint of the IARC Working Group. N Engl

J Med. 2015;373:15. http://www.nejm.org/doi/pdf/10.1056/NEJMc1508733

179 Jatoi I. Breast-cancer screening — viewpoint of the IARC Working Group. N Engl J Med 2015;373:15. http://www.nejm.org/doi/pdf/10.1056/NEJMc1508733

180 Welch HG, Passow HJ. Quantifying the benefits and harms of screening mammography. JAMA Intern Med. 2014;174:448-54.

181 Biller-Andorno N, Jüni P. Abolishing Mammography Screening Programs? A View from the Swiss Medical Board. N Engl J Med. 2014; 370:1965-1967May 22, 2014DOI: 10.1056/NEJMp1401875

182 Duffy SW, Tabár L, Ming-Fang Yen A, et al. Mammography screening reduces rates of advanced and fatal breast cancers: Results in 549,091 women. Cancer. 2020;126(13):2971-2979. DOI: 10.1002/cncr.32859

183 Philippe A, Magali B, Alice K, Cécile P, Mathieu B. Effectiveness of and overdiagnosis from mammography screening in the Netherlands: population based study. BMJ. 2017; 359 :j5224.

184 Nelson R. Mammography cuts risk for fatal breast cancers: New data. Ob Gyn News. June 2020.

185 O'Donoghue C, Eklund M, Ozanne EM, Esserman LJ. Aggregate Cost of Mammography Screening in the United States: Comparison of Current Practice and Advocated Guidelines. Ann Intern Med. 2014;160(3):145-153. doi:10.7326/M13-1217

186 Jin J. JAMA Patient Page | October 20, 2015. Breast Cancer Screening Guidelines in the United States. JAMA. 2015;314(15):1658. doi:10.1001/jama.2015.11766. http://jama.jamanetwork.com/article. aspx?articleid=2463258

187 Levin B, Lieberman DA, McFarland, et al. Screening and Surveillance for the Early Detection of Colorectal Cancer and Adenomatous Polyps, 2008: A Joint Guideline from the American Cancer Society, the US Multi-Society Task Force on Colorectal Cancer, and the American College of Radiology. CA Cancer J Clin. 2008;58.

188 Strum WB. Colorectal adenomas. N Engl J Med 2016;374:1065-75. DOI:10.1056/NEJMra1513581

189 Saslow D, Solomon D, Lawson H, et al. American Cancer Society, American Society for Colposcopy and Cervical Pathology, and American Society for Clinical Pathology Screening Guidelines for the Prevention and Early Detection of Cervical Cancer. CA Cancer J Clin. 2012 May-Jun;62(3):147-72. Epub 2012 Mar 14.

190 Smith RA, Brooks D, Cokkinides V, Salsow D, Brawley OW. Cancer screening in the United States, 2013: A review of current American Cancer Society guidelines, current issues in cancer screening, and new guidance on cervical cancer screening and lung cancer screening. CA Cancer J Clin 2013, Mar- Apr;63:87-105. Accessed at http://onlinelibrary.wiley.com/doi/10.3322/caac.21174/full on April 23, 2013.

191 Volerman A, Cifu AS. Cervical Cancer Screening. JAMA. 2014;312(21):2279-2280. doi:10.1001/jama.2014.14992.

192 US Preventive Services Task Force. Screening for Cervical CancerUS Preventive Services Task Force Recommendation Statement. JAMA. 2018;320(7):674–686. doi:10.1001/jama.2018.10897

193 Sawaya GF, Sanstead E, Alarid-Escudero F, et al. Estimated Quality of Life and Economic Outcomes Associated With 12 Cervical Cancer Screening Strategies: A Cost-effectiveness Analysis. JAMA Intern Med. Published online May 13, 2019179(7):867–878. doi:10.1001/jamainternmed.2019.0299

194 Lu KH. Screening for Ovarian Cancer in Asymptomatic Women. JAMA. 2018;319(6):557–558. doi:10.1001/jama.2017.21894

195 US Preventive Services Task Force. Screening for ovarian cancer: US Preventive Services Task Force recommendation statement [published online February 13, 2018]. JAMA. doi:10.1001/ jama.2017.21926

196 Henderson JT, Webber EM, Sawaya GF. Screening for ovarian cancer: updated evidence report and systematic review for the US Preventive Services Task Force [published online February 13, 2018]. JAMA. doi:10.1001/jama.2017.21421

197 Smith RA, Brooks D, Cokkinides V, Salsow D, Brawley OW. Cancer screening in the United States, 2013: A review of current American Cancer Society guidelines, current issues in cancer screening, and new guidance on cervical cancer screening and lung cancer screening. CA Cancer J Clin 2013, Mar- Apr;63:87-105. Accessed at http://onlinelibrary.wiley.com/doi/10.3322/caac.21174/full on April 23, 2013.

198 Wender R, Fontham E, Barrera E, et al. American Cancer Society lung cancer screening guidelines: CA Cancer Journal for Clinicians. 2013 Jan 11 [Epub ahead of print].

199 Davis AM, Cifu AS. Lung Cancer Screening. JAMA. 2014;312(12):1248-1249. doi:10.1001/jama.2014.12272.

200 Garnick MB. The great prostate cancer debate. Scientific Amierican. February 2012:39-43.

201 Etzioni R, Tsodikov A, Mariotto A, et al. Quantifying the role of PSA screening in the US prostate cancer mortality decline. Cancer Causes Control. 2008;19(2):175-181.

202 Lang RS. Changing times for prostate cancer screening. Cleveland Clinic Men's Health Advisor. 2013. Vol 14G

203 Penson DF. The Pendulum of Prostate Cancer Screening. JAMA. 2015;314(19):2031-2033. doi:10.1001/jama.2015.13775.

204 Hayes JH, Barry MJ. Screening for Prostate Cancer With the Prostate-Specific Antigen Test: A Review of Current Evidence. JAMA. 2014;311(11):1143-1149. doi:10.1001/jama.2014.2085.

205 Hayes JH, Barry MJ. Screening for Prostate Cancer With the Prostate-Specific Antigen Test: A Review of Current Evidence. JAMA. 2014;311(11):1143-1149. doi:10.1001/jama.2014.2085.

206 New advice (again) about PSA testing. University of California, Berkeley Wellness Letter. July 2017: 1-2.

207 Schröder FH, Hugosson J, Roobol MJ, et al.; ERSPC Investigators. Screening and prostate cancer mortality: results of the European Randomised Study of Screening for Prostate Cancer (ERSPC) at 13 years of follow-up. Lancet. 2014;384(9959):2027-2035.

208 Schröder FH, Hugosson J, Carlsson S, et al. Screening for prostate cancer decreases the risk of developing metastatic disease: findings from the European Randomized Study of Screening for Prostate Cancer (ERSPC). Eur Urol. 2012;62(5):745-752.

209 Pinsky PF, Prorok PC, Kramer BS. Prostate Cancer Screening — A Perspective on the Current State of the Evidence. N Engl J Med. 2017;376(13):1285-1289.

210 https://www.cancer.org/healthy/find-cancer-early/cancer-screening-guidelines/american-cancer-society- guidelines-for-the-early-detection-of-cancer.html

211 US Preventive Services Task Force. Screening for Prostate Cancer. US Preventive Services Task Force Recommendation Statement. JAMA. 2018;319(18):1901–1913. doi:10.1001/jama.2018.3710

212 Carter HB, Albertsen PC, Barry MJ, et al. Early detection of prostate cancer: AUA guideline. J Urol. 2013;190(2):419-426.

213 Eggener SE, Cifu AS, Nabhan C. Prostate Cancer Screening. JAMA. 2015;314(8):825-826. doi:10.1001/jama.2015.8033.

214 http://auanet.mediaroom.com/2018-05-08-AUA-Responds-to-USPSTF-Final-Recommendations-on-Screening-for-Prostate-Cancer

215 Barry MJ. Screening for Prostate cancer is the Third Trial the Charm?. JAMA. 2018;319(9):868–869. doi:10.1001/jama.2018.0153

216 Martin RM, Donovan JL, Turner EL, et al.; CAP Trial Group. Effect of a low-intensity PSA-based screening intervention on prostate cancer mortality: the CAP randomized clinical trial. JAMA. 2018;319(9):883-895. doi:10.1001/jama .2018.0154

217 Carter HB. Prostate-Specific Antigen (PSA) Screening for Prostate CancerRevisiting the Evidence. JAMA.2018;319(18):1866–1868. doi:10.1001/jama.2018.4914

218 Welch GH, Albertsen PC. Reconsidering prostate cancer mortality—the future of PSA screening. N Engl J Med. 2020;382(16):1557-1563.

219 Shoag JE, Nyame YA, Gulati R, Etzioni R, Hu JC. Reconsidering the Trade-offs of Prostate Cancer Screening. N Engl J Med. 2020; 382:2465-2468 DOI: 10.1056/NEJMsb2000250

220 Brody, JE. Prostate Surgery or 'Active Surveillance'? New York Times. March 3, 2020.

221 Gershenwald JE, Halpern AC, Sondak VK. Melanoma Prevention—Avoiding Indoor Tanning and Minimizing Overexposure to the Sun. JAMA. 2016;316(18):1913-1914. doi:10.1001/jama.2016.16430

222 American Cancer Society. Signs and symptoms of melanoma skin cancer. http://www.cancer.org/cancer/skincancer-melanoma/detailedguide/melanoma-skin-cancer-signs-and-symptoms

223 US Preventive Services Task Force. Screening for Skin CancerUS Preventive Services Task Force Recommendation Statement. JAMA. 2016;316(4):429-435. doi:10.1001/jama.2016.8465

224 Tsao H, Weinstock MA. Visual Inspection and the US Preventive Services Task Force Recommendation on Skin Cancer Screening. JAMA. 2016;316(4):398-400. doi:10.1001/jama.2016.9850

225 Lyon J. Farewell to a Cancer That Never Was. JAMA. 2017;317(18):1824-1825. doi:10.1001/jama.2017.3969

226 US Preventive Services Task Force. Screening for Thyroid Cancer US Preventive Services Task Force Recommendation Statement. JAMA. 2017;317(18):1882-1887. doi:10.1001/jama.2017.4011

227 Lin JS, Bowles EJA, Williams SB, Morrison CC. Screening for Thyroid Cancer Updated Evidence Report and Systematic Review for the US Preventive Services Task Force. JAMA. 2017;317(18):1888-1903. doi:10.1001/jama.2017.0562

228 American cancer Society. Genetics and cancer. http://www.cancer.org/cancer/cancercauses/geneticsandcancer/index

Chapter 8 – Preventing Dementia

1 Roeder A. Light in the Shadows. Harvard Public Health. Fall 2017.

2 Is it normal forgetfulness…or MCI? University of California, Berkeley Wellness Letter. May 2017.

3 Langa KM, Levine DA. The Diagnosis and Management of Mild Cognitive ImpairmentA Clinical Review. JAMA. 2014;312(23):2551–2561. doi:10.1001/jama.2014.13806

4 Alzheimer Association http://alz.org/documents_custom/cms_release_110316.pdf

5 Plassman BL, Langa KM, Fisher GG, et al. Prevalence of dementia in the United States: the aging, demographics, and memory study. Neuroepidemiology. 2007;29(1–2):125–132.

6 Alzheimer Association http://alz.org/documents_custom/cms_release_110316.pdf

7 James BD, Leurgans SE, Hebert LE, Scherr PA, Yaffe K, Bennett DA. Contribution of Alzheimer disease to mortality in the United States. Neurology. 2014;82(12):1045-1050. doi:10.1212/WNL.0000000000000240.

8 Alzheimer Association http://alz.org/documents_custom/cms_release_110316.pdf.

9 Bredesen DE, The End of Alzheimer. New York: Avery, Penguin Random House 2017.

10 Blonz ER. Alzheimer Disease as the Product of a Progressive Energy Deficiency Syndrome in the Central Nervous System: The Neuroenergetic Hypothesis. Journal of Alzheimer Disease. 2017;60:1223–1229 DOI 10.3233/JAD-170549.

11 Blazer DG, Yaffe K, Liverman CT, eds. Cognitive Aging: Progress in Understanding and Opportunities

for Action. Washington, DC: National Academies Press; 2015. http://www.iom.edu/cognitiveaging.

12 Norton, S, Matthews FE, Barnes DE et al. Potential for primary prevention of Alzheimer disease: an analysis of population-based data. The Lancet Neurology. 2014;13(8):788–794.

13 Kivipelto M, Hakansson K. A Rare Success Against Alzheimer. Scientific American April 2017:33-37.

14 Elwood P, Galante J, Pickering J, Palmer S, Bayer A, Ben-Shlomo Y, et al. (2013) Healthy Lifestyles Reduce the Incidence of Chronic Diseases and Dementia: Evidence from the Caerphilly Cohort Study. PLoS ONE. 8(12): e81877. doi:10.1371/journal.pone.0081877

15 Elwood P, Galante J, Pickering J, Palmer S, Bayer A, Ben-Shlomo Y, et al. (2013) Healthy Lifestyles Reduce the Incidence of Chronic Diseases and Dementia: Evidence from the Caerphilly Cohort Study. PLoS ONE. 8(12): e81877. doi:10.1371/journal.pone.0081877

16 http://medicine.cf.ac.uk/media/filer_public/47/61/47612976-a974-44e6-b260-8a1624b65110/peter_elwood_-_the_success_of_the_caerphilly_cohort_study.pdf.

17 Kivipelto M, Hakansson K. A Rare Success Against Alzheimer. Scientific American April 2017: 33-37.

18 Ngandu T, Lehtisalo J, Solomon A, et al. A 2 year multidomain intervention of diet, exercise, cognitive training, and vascular risk monitoring versus control to prevent cognitive decline in at-risk elderly people (FINGER): a randomised controlled trial. Lancet 2015; 385: 2255–63 Published Online March 12, 2015 http://dx.doi.org/10.1016/ S0140-6736(15)60461-5

19 Lourida I, Hannon E, Littlejohns TJ, et al. Association of Lifestyle and Genetic Risk With Incidence of Dementia. JAMA. Published online July 14, 2019322(5):430–437. doi:10.1001/jama.2019.9879

20 Kirk-Sanchez NJ, McGough EL. Physical exercise and cognitive performance in the elderly: current perspectives. Clinical Interventions in Aging. 2014;9:51-62. doi:10.2147/CIA.S39506.

21 Ahlskog JE, Geda YE, Graff-Radford NR, Petersen RC. Physical exercise as a preventive or disease-modifying treatment of dementia and brain aging. Mayo Clin Proc. 2011;86(9):876-84. doi: 10.4065/mcp.2011.0252.

22 Reynolds G. Sitting May Be Bad for Your Brain. New York Times. August 21, 2018.

23 Carter SE, Draijer R, Holder SM, et al. Regular walking breaks prevent the decline in cerebral blood flow associated with prolonged sitting. Journal of Applied Physiology 2018;125(3):790-798. doi: 10.1152/japplphysiol.00310.2018.

24 Adlard PA, Perreau VM, Pop V, Cotman CW. Voluntary Exercise Decreases Amyloid Load in a Transgenic Model of Alzheimer Disease. Journal of Neuroscience. 2005;25(17):4217– 4221

25 Erickson, KI, Voss MW, Prakash RS, et al. Exercise training increases size of hippocampus and improves memory PNAS 2011;108 (7):3017-3022; published ahead of print January 31, 2011, doi:10.1073/pnas.1015950108

26 DeFina LF, Willis BL, Radford NB, Gao A, Leonard D, Haskell WL, Weiner MF, Berry JD. The Association Between Midlife Cardiorespiratory Fitness Levels and Later-Life Dementia. A Cohort Study. Ann Intern Med. 2013;158(3):162-168

27 Abbott RD, White LR, Ross G, Masaki KH, Curb J, Petrovitch H. Walking and Dementia in Physically Capable Elderly Men. JAMA. 2004;292(12):1447-1453. doi:10.1001/jama.292.12.1447.

28 Weuve J, Kang JH, Manson JE, Breteler MM, Ware JH, Grodstein F. Physical activity, including walking, and cognitive function in older women. JAMA. 2004;292(12):1454–1461.

29 Kramer AF, Hahn S, Cohen NJ, Banich MT, McAuley E, Harrison CR, Chason J, Vakil E, Bardell L, Boileau RA. Ageing, fitness and neurocognitive function. Nature. 1999;400(6743):418–419.

30 Colcombe SJ, Erickson KI, Scalf PE, Kim JS, Prakash R, McAuley E, Elavsky S, Marquez DX, Liang Hu L, Kramer AF. Aerobic Exercise Training Increases Brain Volume in Aging Humans. J Gerontol A Biol

Sci Med Sci. 2006;61(11):1166-1170.

31 Raji CA, Merrill DA, Eyre H, et al. Longitudinal Relationships between Caloric Expenditure and Gray Matter in the Cardiovascular Health Study. Journal of Alzheimer Disease. 2016;52(2):719-729. doi:10.3233/JAD-160057.

32 Tari AR, Nauman J, Zisko N, et al. Temporal changes in cardiorespiratory fitness and risk of dementia incidence and mortality: a population-based prospective cohort study. Lancet Public Health. 2019; 4: e565–74

33 Bolandzadeh N, Tam R, Handy TC, et al. Resistance Training and White Matter Lesion Progression in Older Women: Exploratory Analysis of a 12-Month Randomized Controlled Trial. J Am Geriatr Soc. 2015;63(10):2052-60. doi: 10.1111/jgs.13644. Epub 2015 Oct 12.

34 Colcombe S, Kramer AF. Fitness effects on the cognitive function of older adults: A meta-analytic study. Psychol Sci. 2003;14(2):125–130.

35 Suwabe K, Byun K, Hyodo K, et al. Rapid stimulation of human dentate gyrus function with acute mild exercise. Proceedings of the National Academy of Sciences. 2018; 201805668 DOI: 10.1073/pnas.1805668115

36 Won J, Alfini AJ, Weiss LR, et al. Semantic Memory Activation After Acute Exercise in Healthy Older Adults. Journal of the International Neuropsychological Society. 2019;1 DOI: 10.1017/S1355617719000171

37 Kovacevic A, Fenesi B, Paolucci E, Heisz JJ. The effects of aerobic exercise intensity on memory in older adults. Applied Physiology, Nutrition, and Metabolism, 30 October 2019. https://doi.org/10.1139/apnm-2019-0495

38 Sink KM, Espeland MA, Castro CM, Church T, Cohen R, Dodson JA, Guralnik J, Hendrie HC, Jennings J, Katula J, Lopez OL, McDermott MM, Pahor M, Reid KF, Rushing J, Verghese J, Rapp S Williamson JD, for the LIFE Study Investigators. Effect of a 24-Month Physical Activity Intervention vs Health Education on Cognitive Outcomes in Sedentary Older AdultsThe LIFE Randomized Trial. JAMA. 2015;314(8):781-790. doi:10.1001/jama.2015.9617

39 2018 Physical Activity Guidelines Advisory Committee. 2018 Physical Activity Guidelines Advisory Committee Scientific Report. Washington, DC: U.S. Department of Health and Human Services, 2018.

40 Muller J, Chan K, Myers JN. Association Between Exercise Capacity and Late Onset of Dementia, Alzheimer Disease, and Cognitive Impairment. Mayo Clinic Proceedings. 2017;92 (2):211-217.

41 Crane PK, Walker R, Hubbard RA, et al.,Glucose Levels and Risk of Dementia. N Engl J Med. 2013; 369:540-548August 8, 2013DOI: 10.1056/NEJMoa1215740.

42 Arvanitakis Z, Wilson RS, Bienias JL, Evans DA, Bennett DA. Diabetes mellitus and risk of Alzheimer disease and decline in cognitive function. Arch. Neurol. 2004;61(5):661–666.

43 Ravona-Springer R, Schnaider-Beeri M. The association of diabetes and dementia and possible implications for nondiabetic populations. Expert review of neurotherapeutics. 2011;11(11):1609-1617. doi:10.1586/ern.11.152.

44 Luchsinger JA. Adiposity, hyperinsulinemia, diabetes and Alzheimer disease: an epidemiological perspective. Eur. J. Pharmacol. 2008;585(1):119–129.

45 Beeri, M Schnaider; Goldbourt, U.; Silverman, JM., et al. Diabetes mellitus in midlife and the risk of dementia three decades later. Neurology. 2004;63(10):1902–1907.

46 Yoon S, Cho H, Kim J, et al. Brain changes in overweight/obese and normal-weight adults with type 2 diabetes mellitus. Diabetologia. 2017;60(7):1207–1217.

47 Kril JJ and Halliday GM: Brain shrinkage in alcoholics: a decade on and what have we learned? Prog Neurobiol. 1999;58:381-387.

48 Meyer JS, Terayama Y, Konno S, Akiyama H, Margishvili GM, Mortel KF: Risk factors for cerebral degenerative changes and dementia. Eur Neurol. 1998;39(Suppl 1):7-16.

49 Hoang TD, Byers AL, Barnes DE, Yaffe K. Alcohol consumption patterns and cognitive impairment in older women. Am J Geriatr Psychiatry. 2014;22(12):1663-1667. doi:10.1016/j.jagp.2014.04.006.

50 Anstey KJ, Mack HA, Cherbuin N. Alcohol consumption as a risk factor for dementia and cognitive decline: meta-analysis of prospective studies. Am J Geriatr Psychiatry. 2009;17(7):542-55. doi: 10.1097/JGP.0b013e3181a2fd07.

51 Huang W-J, Zhang X, Chen W-W. Association between alcohol and Alzheimer disease. Experimental and Therapeutic Medicine. 2016;12(3):1247-1250. doi:10.3892/etm.2016.3455.

52 Topiwala A, Allan C, Valkanova V, et al. Moderate alcohol consumption as a risk factor for adverse brain outcomes and cognitive decline: longitudinal cohort study. BMJ. 2017;357:j2353.

53 Welch Killian A. Alcohol consumption and brain health BMJ. 2017;357:j2645

54 Topiwala A, Allan C, Valkanova V, et al. Moderate alcohol consumption as risk factor for adverse brain outcomes and cognitive decline: longitudinal cohort study. BMJ. 2017;357:j2353.

55 Reed BR, Marchant NL, Jagust WJ, DeCarli CC, Mack W, Chui HC. Coronary risk correlates with cerebral amyloid deposition. Neurobiol Aging. 2012;33(9):1979-1987.

56 Gottesman RF, Schneider ALC, Zhou Y, Coresh J, Green E, Gupta N, Knopman DS, Mintz A, Rahmim A, Sharrett AR, Wagenknecht LE, Wong DF, Mosley TH. Association Between Midlife Vascular Risk Factors and Estimated Brain Amyloid Deposition. JAMA. 2017;317(14):1443-1450. doi:10.1001/jama.2017.3090

57 Roeder A. Light in the Shadows. Harvard Public Health. Fall 2017.

58 Samieri C, Perier M, Gaye B, et al. Association of Cardiovascular Health Level in Older Age With Cognitive Decline and Incident Dementia. JAMA. 2018;320(7):657–664. doi:10.1001/jama.2018.11499

59 Saver JL, Cushman M. Striving for Ideal Cardiovascular and Brain Health It Is Never Too Early or Too Late. JAMA. 2018;320(7):645–647. doi:10.1001/jama.2018.11002

60 Williamson W, Lewandowski AJ, Forkert ND, et al. Association of cardiovascular risk factors with MRI indices of cerebrovascular structure and function and white matter hyperintensities in young adults. JAMA. 2018;320(7):665–673. doi:10.1001/jama.2018.11498

61 Healthy heart, healthy brain. University of California, Berkeley Wellness Letter. December 2018.

62 Williamson W, Lewandowski AJ, Forkert ND, et al. Association of Cardiovascular Risk Factors With MRI Indices of Cerebrovascular Structure and Function and White Matter Hyperintensities in Young Adults. JAMA. 2018;320(7):665–673. doi:10.1001/jama.2018.11498

63 Nam GE, Kim SM, Han K, Kim NH, Chung HS, et al. Metabolic syndrome and risk of Parkinson disease: A nationwide cohort study. PLOS Medicine. 2018;15(8):e1002640. https://doi.org/10.1371/journal.pmed.1002640

64 Sano M, Bell KL, Galasko D, et al. A randomized, double-blind, placebo-controlled trial of simvastatin to treat Alzheimer disease. Neurology. 2011;77(6):556-563.

65 Trompet S, van Vliet P, de Craen AJ, et al. Pravastatin and cognitive function in the elderly: results of the PROSPER study. J Neurol. 2010;257(1):85-90

66 Reed B, Villeneuve S, Mack W, DeCarli C, Chui HC, Jagust W. Associations Between Serum Cholesterol Levels and Cerebral Amyloidosis. JAMA Neurol. 2014;71(2):195-200. doi:10.1001/jamaneurol.2013.5390

67 Iadecola C, Yaffe K, Biller J, et al. On behalf of the American Heart Association Council on Hypertension; Council on Clinical Cardiology; Council on Cardiovascular Disease in the Young; Council

on Cardiovascular and Stroke Nursing; Council on Quality of Care and Outcomes Research; and Stroke Council. Impact of Hypertension on Cognitive Function: A Scientific Statement From the American Heart Association. Hypertension. 2016;HYP.0000000000000053, originally published October 10, 2016 https://doi.org/10.1161/HYP.0000000000000053

68 Launer LJ, Masaki K, Petrovitch H, Foley D, Havlik RJ. The association between midlife blood pressure levels and late-life cognitive function: the Honolulu-Asia Aging Study. JAMA. 1995;274(23):1846-1851.

69 Freitag MH, Peila R, Masaki K, et al. Midlife pulse pressure and incidence of dementia: the Honolulu-Asia Aging Study. Stroke. 2006;37(1):33-37.

70 Alonso A, Mosley TH, Gottesman RF, Catellier D, Sharrett AR, Coresh J. Risk of dementia hospitalisation associated with cardiovascular risk factors in midlife and older age: the Atherosclerosis Risk in Communities (ARIC) study. J Neurol Neurosurg Psychiatry. 2009;80(11):1194-1201.

71 Maillard P, Seshadri S, Beiser A, et al. Effects of systolic blood pressure on white-matter integrity in young adults in the Framingham Heart Study: a cross-sectional study. Lancet neurology. 2012;11(12):1039-1047. doi:10.1016/S1474-4422(12)70241-7.

72 Hughes D, Judge C, Murphy R, et al. Association of Blood Pressure Lowering With Incident Dementia or Cognitive Impairment: A Systematic Review and Meta-analysis. JAMA. 2020;323(19):1934–1944. doi:10.1001/jama.2020.4249

73 Walker KA, Sharrett AR, Wu A, et al. Association of Midlife to Late-Life Blood Pressure Patterns With Incident Dementia. JAMA. 2019;322(6):535–545. doi:10.1001/jama.2019.10575

74 The SPRINT MIND Investigators for the SPRINT Research Group. Effect of Intensive vs. Standard Blood Pressure Control on Probable Dementia: A Randomized Clinical Trial. JAMA. Published online January 28, 2019;321(6):553–561. doi:10.1001/jama.2018.21442

75 The SPRINT MIND Investigators for the SPRINT Research Group. Association of Intensive vs. Standard Blood Pressure Control With Cerebral White Matter Lesions. JAMA. 2019;322(6):524–534. doi:10.1001/jama.2019.10551

76 Prabhakaran S. Blood Pressure, Brain Volume and White Matter Hyperintensities, and Dementia Risk. JAMA. 2019;322(6):512–513. doi:10.1001/jama.2019.10849

77 Chuang YF, An Y, Bilgel M, Wong DF, Troncoso JC, O'Brien RJ, et al. Midlife adiposity predicts earlier onset of Alzheimer dementia, neuropathology and presymptomatic cerebral amyloid accumulation. Mol Psychiatry. 2016 Jul;21(7):910-915. doi: 10.1038/mp.2015.129. Epub 2015 Sep 1.

78 Whitmer RA, et al. "Central Obesity and Increased Risk of Dementia More Than Three Decades Later," Neurology (March 26, 2008): Electronic publication.

79 Barnes JL, Tian M, Edens NK, Morris MC. Consideration of nutrient levels in studies of cognitive decline: a review. Nutr Rev. 2014; 72:707–719.

80 Morris MC, Evans DA, Tangney CC, Bienias JL, Wilson RS. Associations of vegetable and fruit consumption with age-related cognitive change. Neurology. 2006;67:1370–1376.

81 Kang JH, Ascherio A, Grodstein F. Fruit and vegetable consumption and cognitive decline in aging women. Ann Neurol. 2005;57:713–720.

82 Morris MC, Evans DA, Bienias JL, Tangney CC, Bennett DA, Aggarwal N, Schneider J, Wilson RS. Dietary Fats and the Risk of Incident Alzheimer Disease. Arch Neurol. 2003;60(2):194-200. doi:10.1001/archneur.60.2.194

83 Grant WB. Using Multicountry Ecological and Observational Studies to Determine Dietary Risk Factors for Alzheimer Disease. J Am Coll Nutr. 2016;35(5):476-89. doi: 10.1080/07315724.2016.1161566.

84 van de Rest O, Wang Y, Barnes LL, Tangney C, Bennett DA, Morris MC. APOE ε4 and the associations

of seafood and long-chain omega-3 fatty acids with cognitive decline. Neurology. 2016;86(22):2063-70. doi: 10.1212/WNL.0000000000002719. Epub 2016 May 4.

85 Chew EY, Clemons TE, Agrón E, Launer LJ, Grodstein F, Bernstein PS, for the Age-Related Eye Disease Study 2 (AREDS2) Research Group. Effect of Omega-3 Fatty Acids, Lutein/Zeaxanthin, or Other Nutrient Supplementation on Cognitive FunctionThe AREDS2 Randomized Clinical Trial. JAMA. 2015;314(8):791-801. doi:10.1001/jama.2015.9677

86 Dangour AD, Allen E, Elbourne D, et al. Effect of 2-y n-3 long-chain polyunsaturated fatty acid supplementation on cognitive function in older people: a randomized, double-blind, controlled trial. Am J Clin Nutr. 2010;91(6):1725-1732.

87 Manson JE, Cook NR, Lee I-M, et al. Marine n−3 fatty acids and prevention of cardiovascular disease and cancer. N Engl J Med. DOI: 10.1056/NEJMoa1811403.

88 Hellmuth J, Rabinovici GD, Miller BL. The Rise of Pseudomedicine for Dementia and Brain Health. JAMA. Published online January 25, 2019321(6):543–544. doi:10.1001/jama.2018.21560

89 Lourida I, Soni M, Thompson-Coon J, et al. Mediterranean diet, cognitive function, and dementia: a systematic review. Epidemiology. 2013;24(4):479-489.

90 Sofi F, Abbate R, Gensini GF, Casini A. Accruing evidence on benefits of adherence to the Mediterranean diet on health: an updated systematic review and meta-analysis. Am J Clin Nutr. 2010;92:1189–1196

91 Scarmeas N, Luchsinger JA, Schupf N, et al. Physical activity, diet, and risk of Alzheimer disease. JAMA. 2009;302:627–637

92 Scarmeas N, Stern Y, Mayeux R, Manly JJ, Schupf N, Luchsinger JA. Mediterranean diet and mild cognitive impairment. Arch Neurol. 2009;66:216–225.

93 Luciano M, Corley J, Cox SR, et al. Mediterranean-type diet and brain structural change from 73 to 76 years in a Scottish cohort. Neurology. 2017; 88:1-10

94 Morris MC, Tangney CC, Wang Y, Sacks FM, Bennett DA, Neelum T, Aggarwal NT. MIND diet associated with reduced incidence of Alzheimer disease. Alzheimer & Dementia: The Journal of the Alzheimer Association. 2015;11(9), 1007 – 1014.

95 Morris MC, Tangney CC. Dietary fat composition and dementia risk. Neurobiol Aging. 2014;35(Suppl 2):S59–64.

96 Morris MC. Nutritional determinants of cognitive aging and dementia. Proc Nutr Soc. 2012;71:1–13.

97 Roberts RO, Geda YE, Cerhan JR, Knopman DS, Cha RH, Christianson TJ, et al. Vegetables, unsaturated fats, moderate alcohol intake, and mild cognitive impairment. Dement Geriatr Cogn Disord. 2010;29:413–23.

98 Nooyens AC, Bueno-de-Mesquita HB, van Boxtel MP, van Gelder BM, Verhagen H, Verschuren WM. Fruit and vegetable intake and cognitive decline in middle-aged men and women: the Doetinchem Cohort Study. Br J Nutr 2011;106:752–61.

99 Chen X, Huang Y, Cheng HG. Lower intake of vegetables and legumes associated with cognitive decline among illiterate elderly Chinese: a 3-year cohort study. J Nutr Health Aging 2012;16:549–52.

100 Devore EE, Kang JH, Breteler MM, Grodstein F. Dietary intakes of berries and flavonoids in relation to cognitive decline. Ann Neurol 2012;72:135–43.

101 Morris MC, Tangney CC, Wang Y, Sacks FM, Bennett DA, Neelum T, Aggarwal NT. MIND diet associated with reduced incidence of Alzheimer disease. Alzheimer & Dementia: The Journal of the Alzheimer Association. 2015;11(9):1007-1014

102 Morris MC, Tangney CC, Wang Y, Sacks F, Barnes LL, Bennett DA, et al. MIND diet score more predictive than DASH or Mediterranean diet scores. Alzheimer & Dementia 2014;10:P166.

103 Morris MC, Tangney CC, Wang Y, Sacks FM, Bennett DA, Neelum T, Aggarwal NT. MIND diet associated with reduced incidence of Alzheimer disease. Alzheimer & Dementia: The Journal of the Alzheimer Association, 2015;11(9):1007-1014.

104 H Gehlich, Kerstin & Beller, Johannes & Lange-Asschenfeldt, Bernhard & K€ Ocher D, Wolfgang & C Meinke, Martina & Lademann, Urgen. Consumption of fruits and vegetables: improved physical health, mental health, physical functioning and cognitive health in older adults from 11 European countries. Aging and Mental Health. Published online February 7, 2019. 10.1080/13607863.2019.1571011.

105 Shishtar E, Rogers GT, Blumberg JB, Au R, Jacques PF. Long-term dietary flavonoid intake and risk of Alzheimer disease and related dementias in the Framingham Offspring Cohort. Am J Clin Nutr. 2020 Aug 1;112(2):343-353. doi: 10.1093/ajcn/nqaa079. PMID: 32320019; PMCID: PMC7398772.

106 Akbaraly TN, Singh-Manoux A, Dugravot A, Brunner EJ, Kivimäki M, Sabia S. Association of Midlife Diet With Subsequent Risk for Dementia. JAMA. 2019;321(10):957–968. doi:10.1001/jama.2019.1432

107 Pase MP, Himali JJ, Jacques PF, et al. Sugary beverage intake and preclinical Alzheimer disease in the community. Alzheimer & Dementia. 2017;0(0):1-10. DOI: http://dx.doi.org/10.1016/j.jalz.2017.01.024.

108 Bernstein AM, de Koning L, Flint AJ, Rexrode KM, Willett WC. Soda consumption and the risk of stroke in men and women. Am J Clin Nutrition. 2012;95(5):1190-1199. https://doi.org/10.3945/ajcn.111.030205

109 Pase MP, Himali JJ, Beiser AS, et al. Sugar- and Artificially Sweetened Beverages and the Risks of Incident Stroke and Dementia Stroke. 2017;STROKE AHA.116.016027, originally published April 20, 2017 https://doi.org/10.1161/STROKEAHA.116.016027

110 Smith AD, Refsum H, Miller JW. Dietary Supplements for Brain Health. JAMA. 2019;321(24):2467. doi:10.1001/jama.2019.4963

111 Morris MC, Schneider JA, Tangney CC. Thoughts on B-vitamins and dementia. Journal of Alzheimer disease : JAD. 2006;9(4):429-433.

112 Hellmuth J, Rabinovici GD, Miller BL. Dietary Supplements for Brain Health—Reply. JAMA. 2019;321(24):2467–2468. doi:10.1001/jama.2019.4967

113 Morris MC, Schneider JA, Tangney CC. Thoughts on B-vitamins and dementia. Journal of Alzheimer disease : JAD. 2006;9(4):429-433.

114 Cobalamin CR. the stomach, and aging. Am J Clin Nutr. 1997;66:750–759.

115 Brody JE, A Vitamin to Protect the Aging Brain. New York Times, September 6, 2016.

116 Nedergaard M, Goldman SA. The Brain's Waste-Disposal System May Be Enlisted to Treat Alzheimer and Other Brain Illnesses. Scientific American. March 2016.

117 Osorio RS, Gumb T, Pirraglia E. et al. Sleep-disordered breathing advances cognitive decline in the elderly Neurology-2015:84;1964-1971.

118 Rebecca P. Gelber RP, Susan Redline S, Ross GW et al. Associations of brain lesions at autopsy with polysomnography features before death. Neurology 2014 : WNL.0000000000001163v1-10.1212/WNL.0000000000001163.

119 Brody JE, Aging's Solutions Outpace Proof They Work. New York Times, May 12, 2015.

120 Melby-Lervåg M, Hulme C. Is working memory training effective? A meta-analytic review. Dev Psychol. 2013 Feb;49(2):270-91. doi: 10.1037/a0028228. Epub 2012 May 21.

121 Parker-Pope T. Do Brain Workouts Work? Science Isn't Sure. New York Times, March 11, 2014.

122 Lampit A, Hallock H, Valenzuela M. Computerized Cognitive Training in Cognitively Healthy Older Adults: A Systematic Review and Meta-Analysis of Effect Modifiers. PLOS: November 18, 2014. http://dx.doi.org/10.1371/journal.pmed.1001756.

123 Rebok GW, Ball K, Guey LT, et al. Ten-Year Effects of the ACTIVE Cognitive Training Trial on Cognition and Everyday Functioning in Older Adults. Journal of the American Geriatrics Society. 2014;62(1):16-24. doi:10.1111/jgs.12607.

124 Anguera JL, Boccanfuso J, Rintoul JL, et al., Video game training enhances cognitive control in older adults. Nature 501, 97–101 (05 September 2013) doi:10.1038/nature12486

125 Thompson C. Keen Screen. New York Times Magazine. October 26, 2014, p. MM58

126 A Consensus on the Brain Training Industry from the Scientific Community," Max Planck Institute for Human Development and Stanford Center on Longevity, accessed (June 6, 2017), http://longevity3.stanford.edu/blog/2014/10/15/the-consensus-on-the-brain-training-industry-from-the-scientific-community/

127 A Consensus on the Brain Training Industry from the Scientific Community," Max Planck Institute for Human Development and Stanford Center on Longevity, accessed (June 6, 2017), http://longevity3.stanford.edu/blog/2014/10/15/the-consensus-on-the-brain-training-industry-from-the-scientific-community/

128 Rogalski EJ, Gefen T, Shi J, et al. Youthful memory capacity in old brains. J Cogn Neurosci. 2013;25(1):29-36.

129 Harrison TM, Weintraub S, Mesulam MM, Rogalski E. Superior memory and higher cortical volumes in unusually successful cognitive aging. J Int Neuropsychol Soc. 2012;18(6):1081-1085.

130 Cook AH, Sridhar J, Ohm D, Rademaker A, Mesulam M, Weintraub S, Rogalski E. Rates of Cortical Atrophy in Adults 80 Years and Older With Superior vs Average Episodic Memory. JAMA. 2017;317(13):1373-1375. doi:10.1001/jama.2017.0627

131 Barrett LF. How to Become a "Superager." New York Times. January 1, 2017; p SR10.

132 Komaroff AL. Can Infections Cause Alzheimer Disease? JAMA. 2020;324(3):239–240. doi:10.1001/jama.2020.4085

133 Lyon J. Alzheimer Outlook Far From Bleak. JAMA. 2017;317(9):896-898. doi:10.1001/jama.2017.0276

134 Bredesen DE, The End of Alzheimer. New York: Avery, Penguin Random House 2017.

135 Livingston G, Huntley J, Sommerlad A, et al. Dementia prevention, intervention, and care: 2020 report of the Lancet Commission. Lancet. 2020; 396: 413–46 Published Online July 30, 2020 https://doi.org/10.1016/ S0140-6736(20)30367-6

136 Sabayan B, Sorond F. Reducing Risk of Dementia in Older Age. JAMA. 2017;317(19):2028. doi:10.1001/jama.2017.2247

137 Winblad B, et al. Defeating Alzheimer disease and other dementias: a priority for European science and society. Lancet Neurology. 2016;15:455–532.

138 Bredesen DE, The End of Alzheimer. New York: Avery, Penguin Random House 2017.

Chapter 9 – Benefits of Physical Activity

1 Pontzer H, Evolved to exercise. Scientific American. January 2019.

2 Casperson CJ, Powell KE, Christenson GM. Physical activity, exercise, and physical fitness: definitions and distinctions for health-related research. Public Health Reports. 1985;100:126-131.

3 U.S. Department of Health and Human Services. Centers for Disease Control and Prevention. Physical Activity Guidelines Advisory Committee Report, 2008. http://www.health.gov/PAGuidelines/.

4 US Department of Health and Human Services. Centers for Disease Control and Prevention. 2008 Physical Activity Guidelines for Americans. http://www.health.gov/PAGuidelines/

5 2018 Physical Activity Guidelines Advisory Committee. 2018 Physical Activity Guidelines Advisory

Committee Scientific Report. Washington, DC: US Department of Health and Human Services, 2018.

6 US Department of Health and Human Services. Physical Activity Guidelines for Americans. 2nd ed. Washington, DC: US Dept of Health and Human Services; 2018.

7 Reynolds G. Guidelines That Need a Workout. New York Times. April 3, 2018.

8 Office of Disease Prevention and Health Promotion, US Department of Health and Human Services. Healthy People 2020: Data Search—Physical Activity. HealthyPeople.gov website. https://www.healthypeople.gov/2020/data-search/search-the-data#topic-area=3504. Updated September 13, 2018.

9 Piercy KL, Troiano RP, Ballard RM, et al. The Physical Activity Guidelines for Americans. JAMA.2018;320(19):2020–2028. doi:10.1001/jama.2018.14854

10 Ussery EN, Fulton JE, Galuska DA, Katzmarzyk PT, Carlson SA. Joint Prevalence of Sitting Time and Leisure-Time Physical Activity Among US Adults, 2015-2016. JAMA. 2018;320(19):2036–2038. doi:10.1001/jama.2018.17797

11 Yang L, Cao C, Kantor ED, et al. Trends in Sedentary Behavior Among the US Population, 2001- 2016. JAMA. 2019;321(16):1587–1597. doi:10.1001/jama.2019.3636

12 2018 Physical Activity Guidelines Advisory Committee. 2018 Physical Activity Guidelines Advisory Committee Scientific Report. Washington, DC: US Department of Health and Human Services, 2018.

13 Katzmarzyk PT (2010) Physical activity, sedentary behavior, and health: paradigm paralysis or paradigm shift? Diabetes. 59:2717–2725.

14 Katzmarzyk PT, Church TS, Craig CL, Bouchard C. Sitting time and mortality from all causes, cardiovascular disease, and cancer. Med Sci Sports Exerc. 2009;41: 998–1005.

15 Dunstan DW, Barr EL, Healy GN, Salmon J, Shaw JE, et al. Television viewing time and mortality: The Australian Diabetes, Obesity and Lifestyle Study (AusDiab). Circulation. 2010;121:384–391.

16 de Rezende LF, Rodrigues Lopes M, Rey-Lopez JP, Matsudo VK, Luiz Odo C. Sedentary behavior and health outcomes: an overview of systematic reviews. PLoS One. 2014;9(8):e105620.

17 Werner CM, Hecksteden A, Morsch A, Zundler J, et al. Differential effects of endurance, interval, and resistance training on telomerase activity and telomere length in a randomized, controlled study. European Heart Journal. 2019;40(1):34–46. https://doi.org/10.1093/eurheartj/ehy585

18 Gries KJ, Raue U, Perkins RK, Lavin KM, et al. Cardiovascular and skeletal muscle health with lifelong exercise. J Appl Physiol. 2018;125:1636–1645.

19 Reynolds G. Long after exercise, benefits persist. New York Times. April 23, 2019.

20 Du M. Do our cells pay a price when we sit too much? AJPH. 2017;107(9):1360-1361.

21 Hong-mei Xue, Qian-qian Liu, Guo Tian, Li-ming Quan, Yong Zhao, Guo Cheng, "Television Watching and Telomere Length Among Adults in Southwest China." American Journal of Public Health. 2017;107(9):1425-1432. DOI: 10.2105/AJPH.2017.303879

22 Du M, Prescott J, Kraft P, et al. Physical activity, sedentary behavior, and leukocyte telomere length in women. Am J Epidemiol. 2012;175(5):414–422.

23 Prevalence of Self-Reported Physical Inactivity Among US Adults by State and Territory, BRFSS, 2015–2018 https://www.cdc.gov/physicalactivity/data/inactivity-prevalence-maps/index.html#white

24 Lieberman DE. Is Exercise Really Medicine? An Evolutionary Perspective. Curr Sports Med Rep. 2015;14(4):313-9. doi: 10.1249/JSR.0000000000000168.

25 Shaw J. Born to Rest. Harvard Magazine. September-October 2016

26 Shaw J. Born to Rest. Harvard Magazine. September-October 2016

27 Lieberman DE. Is Exercise Really Medicine? An Evolutionary Perspective. Curr Sports Med Rep.

2015;14(4):313-9. doi: 10.1249/JSR.0000000000000168.

28 Shaw J. The Deadliest Sin. Harvard Magazine. March-April 2004.

29 Hagberg JM. Exercise, fitness, and hypertension. In: Bouchard C, Shephard RJ, Stephens T, Sutton JR, McPherson BD, eds. Exercise, Fitness, and Health. Champaign, Ill: Human Kinetics Publishers; 1990:455-566.

30 Haskell WL. The influence of exercise training on plasma lipids and lipoproteins in health and disease. Acta Med Scand. 1986;711 (suppl): 25-37.

31 Powell KE, Thompson PD, Caspersen CJ, Ford ES. Physical activity and the incidence of coronary heart disease. Annu Rev Public Health. 1987;8:253-287.

32 Leon AS, Connett J, Jacobs DR Jr, Rauramaa R. Leisure-time physical activity levels and risk of coronary heart disease and death: the Multiple Risk Factor Intervention trial. JAMA. 1987;258:2388-2395.

33 Cummings SR, Kelsey JL, Nevitt MD, O'Dowd KJ. Epidemiology of osteoporosis and osteoporotic fractures. Epidemiol Rev. 1985;7:178-208

34 Snow-Harter C, Marcus R. Exercise, bone mineral density, and osteoporosis. Exerc Sport Sci Rev. 1991;19:351-388.

35 Dalsky GP, Stoke KS, Ehsani AA, Slatopolsky E, Lee WC, Birge SJ. Weight-bearing exercise training and lumbar bone mineral content in postmenopausal women. Ann Intern Med. 1988;108:824-828.

36 Lee I, Paffenbarger RS, Hsieh C. Physical activity and risk of developing colorectal cancer among college alumni. J Natl Cancer Inst. 1991;83:1324-1329.

37 Moore SC, Lee I-M, Weiderpass E, et al. Association of leisure-time physical activity with risk of 26 types of cancer in 1.44 million adults [published online May 16, 2016]. JAMA Intern Med. doi:10.1001/jamainternmed.2016.1548.

38 King AC, Taylor CB, Haskell WL, DeBusk RF. Influence of regular aerobic exercise on psychological health. Health Psychol. 1989;8:305-324.

39 Taylor CB, Sallis JF, Needle R. The relationship of physical activity and exercise to mental health. Public Health Rep. 1985;100:195-201.

40 Manson JE, Nathan DM, Krolewski AS, Stampfer MJ, Willett WC, Hennekens CH. A prospective study of exercise and incidence of diabetes among US male physicians. JAMA.1992;268:63-67

41 2018 Physical Activity Guidelines Advisory Committee. 2018 Physical Activity Guidelines Advisory Committee Scientific Report. Washington, DC: US Department of Health and Human Services, 2018.

42 Reynolds G. The Super-Short Workout and Other Fitness Trends. The Well Blog. December 31, 2014. http://well.blogs.nytimes.com/2014/12/31/the-super-short-workout-and-other-fitness-trends/

43 Paffenbarger RS, Hyde RT, Wing AL, Hsieh C-C. Physical activity, all-cause mortality, and longevity of college alumni. N Engl J Med. 1986;314:605-613.

44 Paffenbarger RS, Hyde RT, Wing AL, Lee I, Jung DL, Kampert JB. The association of changes in physical-activity level and other lifestyle characteristics with mortality among men. N Engl J Med. 1993;328:538-545.

45 Blair SN, Kohl HW, Paffenbarger RS, Clark DG, Cooper KH, Gibbons LW. Physical fitness and all-cause mortality. JAMA. 1989;262:2395-2401.

46 Sandvik L, Erikssen J, Thaulow E, Erikssen G, Mundal R, Rodhal K. Physical fitness as a predictor of mortality among healthy, middle-aged Norweigan men. N Engl J Med. 1993;328:533-537.

47 Bassuk SS, Church TS, Manson JE. We all know we should exercise. Scientific American, August 2013.

48 Khan KM, et al. Sport and exercise as contributors to the health of nations. Lancet. 380;9836:59-64.

49 Centers for Disease Control and Prevention. Physical Activity and Health. http://www.cdc.gov/physicalactivity/basics/pa-health/

50 Hahn RA, Teutsch SM, Rothenberg RB, Marks JS. Excess deaths from nine chronic diseases in the United States. JAMA. 1986;264:2654-2659.

51 McGinnis JM, Foege WH. Actual causes of death in the United States. JAMA. 1993;270:2207-2212.

52 Mandsager K, Harb S, Cremer P, Phelan D, Nissen SE, Jaber W. Association of Cardiorespiratory Fitness With Long-term Mortality Among Adults Undergoing Exercise Treadmill Testing. JAMA Network Open.2018;1(6):e183605. doi:10.1001/jamanetworkopen.2018.3605

53 Rockhill B, Willett WC, Manson JE, et al. Physical activity and mortality: a prospective study among women. American Journal of Public Health. 2001;91(4):578-583.

54 Holme I, Anderssen SA. Increases in physical activity is as important as smoking cessation for reduction in total mortality in elderly men: 12 years of follow-up of the Oslo II study. Br J Sports Med. 2015;49:743-748. originally published online May 14, 2015. doi: 10.1136/bjsports-2014-094522.

55 Slomski A. Physical Ability at Midlife May Predict Mortality. JAMA. 2014;311(24):2472. doi:10.1001/jama.2014.7449.

56 Cooper R, Strand BH, Hardy R, et al. Physical capability in mid-life and survival over 13 years of follow-up: British birth cohort study. BMJ. 2014;348:g2219 doi: 10.1136/bmj.g2219 (Published 29 April 2014).

57 Lee D, Pate RR, Lavie CJ, Sui X, Church TS, Blair SN. Leisure-Time Running Reduces All-Cause and Cardiovascular Mortality Risk. Journal of the American College of Cardiology. 2014;64(5):472-481. doi:10.1016/j.jacc.2014.04.058.

58 Lee DC, Brellenthin AG, Thompson PD, Sui X, Lee IM, Lavie CJ. Running as a Key Lifestyle Medicine for Longevity. Prog Cardiovasc Dis. 2017;60(1):45-55. doi: 10.1016/j.pcad.2017.03.005. Epub 2017 Mar 30.

59 Sabia S, Dugravot A, Kivimaki M, Brunner E, Shipley MJ, Singh-Manoux A. Effect of intensity and type of physical activity on mortality: results from the Whitehall II cohort study. Am J Public Health. 2012;102(4):698-704. doi: 10.2105/AJPH.2011.300257. Epub 2011 Nov 28.

60 Kujala UM, Kaprio J, Sarna S, Koskenvuo M. Relationship of Leisure-Time Physical Activity and Mortality: The Finnish Twin Cohort. JAMA. 1998;279(6):440-444. doi:10.1001/jama.279.6.440.

61 Wen CP, Wai JP, Tsai MK, et al., Minimum amount of physical activity for reduced mortality and extended life expectancy: A prospective cohort study. Lancet. 2011;378(9798):1244-1253.

62 Patterson R, McNamara E, Tainio M, et al. Sedentary behaviour and risk of all-cause, cardiovascular and cancer mortality, and incident type 2 diabetes: a systematic review and dose response meta-analysis. Eur J Epidemiol. 2018;33:811-829.

63 Ekelund U, Tarp J, Steene-Johannessen J, et al. Dose-response associations between accelerometry measured physical activity and sedentary time and all cause mortality: systematic review and harmonised meta-analysis. BMJ. 2019 Aug 21;366:l4570. doi: 10.1136/bmj.l4570.

64 LaCroix AZ, Bellettiere J, Rillamas-Sun E, et al. Association of Light Physical Activity Measured by Accelerometry and Incidence of Coronary Heart Disease and Cardiovascular Disease in Older Women. JAMA Netw Open. Published online March 15, 20192(3):e190419. doi:10.1001/jamanetworkopen.2019.0419

65 Lee IM, Shiroma EJ, Kamada M, Bassett DR, Matthews CE, Buring JE. Association of Step Volume and Intensity With All-Cause Mortality in Older Women. JAMA Intern Med. Published online May 29, 2019. 179(8):1105–1112. doi:10.1001/jamainternmed.2019.0899

66 Tudor-Locke C, Bassett DR Jr. How many steps/day are enough? Preliminary pedometer indices for

public health. Sports Med. 2004;34(1):1-8. doi:10.2165/00007256-200434010-00001

67 Saint-Maurice PF, Troiano RP, Bassett DR, et al. Association of Daily Step Count and Step Intensity With Mortality Among US Adults. JAMA. 2020;323(12):1151–1160. doi:10.1001/jama.2020.1382

68 Jeff K. Vallance JK, Paul A. Gardiner PA, Brigid M. Lynch BM, et al. Evaluating the Evidence on Sitting, Smoking, and Health: Is Sitting Really the New Smoking? Am J Pub Hlth. 2018;108:1478-1482. https://doi.org/10.2105/AJPH.2018.304649

69 Gebel K, Ding D, Chey T, Stamatakis E, Brown WJ, Bauman AE. Effect of Moderate to Vigorous Physical Activity on All-Cause Mortality in Middle-aged and Older Australians. JAMA Intern Med. 2015;175(6):970-977. doi:10.1001/jamainternmed.2015.0541

70 Lee IM, Paffenbarger RS. Associations of light, moderate, and vigorous intensity physical activity with longevity: the Harvard Alumni Health Study. Am J Epidemiol. 2000;151(3):293-299.

71 Saint-Maurice PF, Troiano RP, Matthews CE, Kraus WE. Moderate-to-igorous Physical Activity and All-Cause Mortality: Do Bouts Matter? Journal of the American Heart Association. 2018;7:e007678

72 Saint-Maurice PF, Coughlan D, Kelly SP, et al. Association of Leisure-Time Physical Activity Across the Adult Life Course With All-Cause and Cause-Specific Mortality. JAMA Netw Open. Published online March 08, 20192(3):e190355. doi:10.1001/jamanetworkopen.2019.0355

73 Arem H, Moore SC, Patel A, Hartge P, Berrington de Gonzalez A, Visvanathan K, Campbell PT, Freedman M, Weiderpass E, Adami HO, Linet MS, Lee IM, Matthews CE. Leisure Time Physical Activity and Mortality A Detailed Pooled Analysis of the Dose-Response Relationship. JAMA Intern Med. 2015;175(6):959-967. doi:10.1001/jamainternmed.2015.0533

74 Reynolds G. Internally Fit, How exercising keeps your cells young. New York Times Magazine January 31, 2010 p.17.

75 American Heart Association. Long-term physical activity has an anti-aging effect at the cellular level. ScienceDaily, 2 December 2009. <www.sciencedaily.com/releases/2009/11/091130161806.htm>.

76 Reynolds G. Make Some More Effort. New York Times. January 2, 2018.

77 Gries KJ, Raue U, Perkins RK, et al. Cardiovascular and skeletal muscle health with lifelong exercise. Journal of applied Physiology. 2018;125(5) 1636-1645. https://doi.org/10.1152/japplphysiol.00174.2018

78 Reynolds G. Pumping Iron. New York Times Magazine. December 9, 2018.

79 June 2014 June in Medicine & Science in Sports & Exercise,

80 Nes BM, Vatten LJ, Nauman J, Janszky I, Wisløff U. A simple nonexercise model of cardiorespiratory fitness predicts long-term mortality. Med Sci Sports Exerc. 2014;46(6):1159-65. doi: 10.1249/MSS.0000000000000219.

81 Reynolds G. A Gold Standard of Health. New York Times, July 7, 2015.

82 Stamatakis E, Hamer M, O'Donovan G, Batty GD, Kivimaki M. A non-exercise testing method for estimating cardiorespiratory fitness: associations with all-cause and cardiovascular mortality in a pooled analysis of eight population-based cohorts. Eur Heart J. 2013;34(10):750-8. Epub 2012 May 3.

83 Pollock RD, Carter S, Velloso CP, Duggal NA, Lord JM, Lazarus NR, Harridge SDR. An investigation into the relationship between age and physiological function in highly active older adults. The Journal of Physiology. 2015;593:657–680. doi: 10.1113/jphysiol.2014.282863

84 Pollock RD, O'Brien KA, Daniels LJ, et al., Properties of the vastus lateralis muscle in relation to age and physiological function in master cyclists aged 55-79 years. Aging Cell, 2018; e12735 DOI: 10.1111/acel.12735

85 Duggal NA, Pollock RD, Lazarus NR, Harridge S, Lord JM. Major features of Immunesenescence, including Thymic atrophy, are ameliorated by high levels of physical activity in adulthood. Aging Cell. 2018

Apr;17(2). doi: 10.1111/acel.12750. Epub 2018 Mar 8.

86 Denham J, Nelson CP, O'Brien BJ, Nankervis SA, Denniff M, et al. (2013) Longer Leukocyte Telomeres Are Associated with Ultra-Endurance Exercise Independent of Cardiovascular Risk Factors. PLoS ONE. 2013;8(7): e69377. doi:10.1371/journal.pone.0069377

87 Reynolds G. Powerhouse Renovation. New York Times Magazine, March 26, 2017.

88 Song J, Lindquist LA, Chang RW, et al. Sedentary Behavior as a Risk Factor for Physical Frailty Independent of moderate activity: results from the osteoarthritis initiative. AJPH 2015;105(7):1439-1444.

89 Cassel CK. Use it or lose it, activity may be the best treatment for aging. JAMA. 2013;288:2333-2335.

90 Dalsky GP, Stoke KS, Ehsani AA, Slatopolsky E, Lee WC, Birge SJ. Weight-bearing exercise training and lumbar bone mineral content in postmenopausal women. Ann Intern Med. 1988;108:824-828.

91 Ekelund LG, Haskell WL, Johnson JL, Wholey FS, Criqui MH, Sheps DS. Physical fitness as a prevention of cardiovascular mortality in asymptomatic North American men. N Engl J Med. 1988; 319:1379-1384.

92 Centers for Disease Control and Prevention. Public health focus: physical activity and the prevention of coronary heart disease. MMWR Morb Mortal Wkly Rep. 1993;42:669-672.

93 Bassuk SS, Church TS, Manson JE. We all know we should exercise. Scientific American, August 2013, 76-79.

94 Lee IM, Paffenbarger RS, Hennekens CH. Physical activity, physical fitness and longevity. Aging (Milano). 1997;9:2–11.

95 Blair SN, Jackson AS. Physical fitness and activity as separate heart disease risk factors: a meta-analysis. Med Sci Sports Exerc. 2001;33:762–764.

96 Thompson PD, Buchner D., Piña, IL, Balady G J, Williams MA, Marcus, BH, Wenger, NK. Exercise and physical activity in the prevention and treatment of atherosclerotic cardiovascular disease: A statement from the Council on Clinical Cardiology (Subcommittee on Exercise, Rehabilitation, and Prevention) and the Council on Nutrition, Physical Activity, and Metabolism (Subcommittee on Physical Activity). Circulation. 2003;107(24):3106-3116. DOI: 10.1161/01.CIR.0000075572.40158.77

97 Gebel K, Ding D, Chey T, Stamatakis E, Brown WJ, Bauman AE. Effect of Moderate to Vigorous Physical Activity on All-Cause Mortality in Middle-aged and Older Australians. JAMA Intern Med. 2015;175(6):970-977. doi:10.1001/jamainternmed.2015.0541

98 Rankin AJ, Rankin AC, MacIntyre P, Hillis WS. Walk or run? Is high-intensity exercise more effective than moderate-intensity exercise at reducing cardiovascular risk? Scott Med J. 2012;57 (2):99-102.

99 Sabia S, Dugravot A, Kivimaki M, Brunner E, Shipley MJ, Singh-Manoux A. Effect of intensity and type of physical activity on mortality: results from the Whitehall II cohort study. Am J Public Health. 2012;102(4):698-704.

100 Wen CP, Wai JP, Tsai MK, Chen CH. Minimal amount of exercise to prolong life: to walk, to run, or just mix it up? J Am Coll Cardiol. 2014;64(5):482-484.

101 Kodama S, Saito K, Tanaka S, Maki M, Yachi Y, Asumi M, Sugawara A, Totsuka K, Shimano H, Ohashi Y, et al. Cardiorespiratory fitness as a quantitative predictor of all-cause mortality and cardiovascular events in healthy men and women: a meta-analysis. JAMA. 2009 May 20; 301(19):2024-35.

102 Brown WJ, Pavey T, Bauman AE. Comparing population attributable risks for heart disease across the adult lifespan in women Br J Sports Med doi:10.1136/bjsports-2013-093090

103 O'Keefe JH. et al. Potential Adverse Cardiovascular Effects From Excessive Endurance Exercise. Mayo Clinic Proceedings. 2012;87(6):587 - 595

104 Maron BJ. The Paradox of Exercise. N Engl J Med. 2000;343:1409-1411November 9, 2000DOI:

10.1056/NEJM200011093431911.

105 Eijsvogels TMH, Fernandez AB, Thompson PD. Are There Deleterious Cardiac Effects of Acute and Chronic Endurance Exercise? Physiol Rev. 2016;96:99–125. https://doi.org/10.1152/physrev.00029.2014

106 Hoffman MD, Krishnan E. Health and Exercise-Related Medical Issues among 1,212 Ultramarathon Runners: Baseline Findings from the Ultrarunners Longitudinal Tracking (ULTRA) Study. PLoS ONE. 2014;9(1): e83867. doi:10.1371/journal.pone.0083867

107 Sanchis-Gomar F, Fiuza-Luces C, Lucia A. Exercise Intensity, Dose, and Cardiovascular Disease. JAMA. 2016;315(15):1658-1659. doi:10.1001/jama.2016.0306.

108 Eijsvogels TM, Thompson PD. Exercise is medicine: at any dose? JAMA. 2015;314(18):1915-1916.

109 Eijsvogels TMH, Thompson PD. Exercise Intensity, Dose, and Cardiovascular Disease—Reply. JAMA. 2016;315(15):1659. doi:10.1001/jama.2016.0312.

110 Garatachea N, Santos-Lozano A, Sanchis-Gomar F, et al. Elite athletes live longer than the general population: a meta-analysis. Mayo Clin Proc. 2014;89(9):1195-1200.

111 Sanchis-Gomar F, Lucia A, Levine BD. Relationship between strenuous exercise and cardiac "morbimortality": benefits outweigh the potential risks [published online August 5, 2015]. Trends Cardiovasc Med. doi:10.1016/j.tcm.2015.07.008.PubMed

112 Reynolds G. A New Target: 15,000 Steps. New York Times. March 28, 2017.

113 Reynolds G. A New Target: 15,000 Steps. New York Times. March 28,2017.

114 Tigbe WW, Granat MH, Sattar N, Lean MEJ. Time spent in sedentary posture is associated with waist circumference and cardiovascular risk. Int J Obes (Lond). 2017;41(5):689-696. doi: 10.1038/ijo.2017.30. Epub 2017 Jan 31.

115 Stefanick ML, Mackey S, Sheehan M, et al. Effects of diet and exercise in men and postmenopausal women with low levels of HDL cholesterol and high levels of LDL cholesterol. N Engl J Med. 1998;339:12-20.

116 Kokkinos PF, Faselis C, Myers J, Panagiotakos D, Doumas M. Interactive effects of fitness and statin treatment on mortality risk in veterans with dyslipidaemia: a cohort study. www.thelancet.com Published online November 28, 2012 http://dx.doi.org/10.1016/S0140-6736(12)61426-3

117 Liu Y, Lee D, Li Y, Zhu W, et al. Associations of Resistance Exercise with Cardiovascular Disease Morbidity and Mortality. Medicine & Science in Sports & Exercise, 2019;51(3):499-508. 1 DOI: 10.1249/MSS.0000000000001822

118 Moore SC, Lee I-M, Weiderpass E, et al. Association of leisure-time physical activity with risk of 26 types of cancer in 1.44 million adults [published online May 16, 2016]. JAMA Intern Med. doi:10.1001/amainternmed.2016.1548.

119 Kirk-Sanchez NJ, McGough EL. Physical exercise and cognitive performance in the elderly: current perspectives. Clinical Interventions in Aging. 2014;9:51-62. doi:10.2147/CIA.S39506.

120 Ahlskog JE, Geda YE, Graff-Radford NR, Petersen RC. Physical exercise as a preventive or disease- modifying treatment of dementia and brain aging. Mayo Clin Proc. 2011;86(9):876-84. doi: 10.4065/mcp.2011.0252.

121 Raji CA, Merrill DA, Eyre H, et al. Longitudinal Relationships between Caloric Expenditure and Gray Matter in the Cardiovascular Health Study. Journal of Alzheimer's Disease. 2016;52(2):719-729. doi:10.3233/JAD-160057.

122 Bolandzadeh N, Tam R, Handy TC, Nagamatsu LS, Hsu CL, Davis JC1, Dao E1, Beattie BL, Liu-Ambrose T. Resistance Training and White Matter Lesion Progression in Older Women: Exploratory Analysis of a 12-Month Randomized Controlled Trial. J Am Geriatr Soc. 2015;63(10):2052-60. doi: 10.1111/

jgs.13644. Epub 2015 Oct 12.

123 Colcombe S, Kramer AF. Fitness effects on the cognitive function of older adults: A meta-analytic study. Psychol Sci. 2003;14(2):125–130.

124 Muller J, Chan K, Myers JN. Association Between Exercise Capacity and Late Onset of Dementia, Alzheimer Disease, and Cognitive Impairment. Mayo Clinic Proceedings, 2017;92 (2):211-217.

125 Taylor CB, Sallis JF, Needle R. The relationship of physical activity and exercise to mental health. Public Health Rep. 1985;100:195-201.

126 Sanchis-Gomar F, Fiuza-Luces C, Lucia A. Exercise Intensity, Dose, and Cardiovascular Disease. JAMA. 2016;315(15):1658-1659. doi:10.1001/jama.2016.0306

127 Sharma A, Madaan V, Petty FD. Exercise for mental health. Prim Care Companion J Clin Psychiatry. 2006;8(2):106.

128 Pinto Pereira SM, Geoffroy M, Power C. Depressive Symptoms and Physical Activity During 3 Decades in Adult LifeBidirectional Associations in a Prospective Cohort Study. JAMA Psychiatry. 2014;71(12):1373-1380. doi:10.1001/jamapsychiatry.2014.1240

129 Cooney G, Dwan K, Mead G. Exercise for Depression. JAMA. 2014;311(23):2432-2433. doi:10.1001/jama.2014.4930.

130 Bailey C. Fit or Fat. Boston: Houghton Mifflin, 1977.

131 Pavlou K, Krey S, Steffee WP. Exercise as an adjunct to weight loss and maintenance in moderately obese subjects. Am J Clin Nutr. 1989;49: 1115-1123.

132 Bouchard C, Depres JP, Tremblay A. Exercise and obesity. Obesity Res. 1993;1:133-147.

133 Bassuk SS, Church TS, Manson JE. We all know we should exercise. Scientific American, August 2013, 76-79.

134 Beavers KM, Ambrosius WT, Rejeski WJ, et al. Effect of Exercise Type During Intentional Weight Loss on Body Composition in Older Adults with Obesity. Obesity. 2017;25(7):1823-1829. https://doi.org/10.1002/oby.21977

135 Liao CD, Tsauo JY, Wu YT, et al. Effects of protein supplementation combined with resistance exercise on body composition and physical function in older adhttp://www.health.harvard.edu/diet-and-weight- loss/calories-burned-in-30-minutes-of-leisure-and-routine-activities.ults: a systematic review and meta-analysis, The American Journal of Clinical Nutrition. 2017;106(4):1078–1091, https://doi.org/10.3945/ajcn.116.143594

136 Morton RW, Murphy KT, McKellar SR. A systematic review, meta-analysis and meta-regression of the effect of protein supplementation on resistance training-induced gains in muscle mass and strength in healthy adults. Br J Sports Med 2018;52:376–384. doi:10.1136/bjsports-2017-097608

137 Williams PT. Greater weight loss from running than walking during a 6.2-yr prospective follow-up. Medicine & Science in Sports & Exercise. 2013 Apr;45(4):706-13. doi: 10.1249/MSS.0b013e31827b0d0a.

138 Larson-Meyer DE, Palm S, Bansal A, Austin KJ, Hart A, Alexander BM. Influence of Running and Walking on Hormonal Regulators of Appetite in Women. Journal of obesity 04/2012; 2012(5):730409. DOI: 10.1155/2012/730409

139 Edinburgh RM, Bradley HE, Abdullah N-F, et al. Lipid metabolism links nutrient-exercise timing to insulin sensitivity in men classified as overweight or obese, The Journal of Clinical Endocrinology & Metabolism. October 19, 2019. dgz104, https://doi.org/10.1210/clinem/dgz104

140 US Department of Health and Human Services. Centers for Disease Control and Prevention. Physical Activity Guidelines Advisory Committee Report, 2008. http://www.health.gov/PAGuidelines/.

141 2018 Physical Activity Guidelines Advisory Committee. 2018 Physical Activity Guidelines Advisory

Committee Scientific Report. Washington, DC: US Department of Health and Human Services, 2018.

142 Saint-Maurice PF, Troiano RP, Berrigan D, et al. Volume of Light Versus Moderate-to-Vigorous Physical Activity: Similar Benefits for All-Cause Mortality? J Am Heart Assoc. 2018;7:e008815. DOI: 10.1161/JAHA.118.008815

143 Schmidt D, Ricci D, Baumeister SE, Leitzmann MF. Replacing Sedentary Time with Physical Activity in Relation to Mortality. Medicine & Science in Sports & Exercise. 2016;48(7):1312-1319. doi: 10.1249/MSS.0000000000000913

144 O'Donovan G, Lee I, Hamer M, Stamatakis E. Association of "Weekend Warrior" and Other Leisure Time Physical Activity Patterns With Risks for All-Cause, Cardiovascular Disease, and Cancer Mortality. JAMA Intern Med. 2017;177(3):335-342. doi:10.1001/jamainternmed.2016.8014.

145 Reynolds G. Weekend Warriors' Live Longer. New York Times January 17, 2017.

146 Fyfe JJ, Broatch JR, Trewin AJ, et al. Cold water immersion attenuates anabolic signaling and skeletal muscle fiber hypertrophy, but not strength gain, following whole-body resistance training. Journal of Applied Physiology. 2019;127(5):1403-1418. https://doi.org/10.1152/japplphysiol.00127.2019

147 Cooper K. The New Aerobics. New York: Bantam Books, 1970.

148 Galloway J. Galloway's Book on Running. Bolinas, California: Shelter Publications, 1984.

149 Burgomaster KA, Hughes SC, Heigenhauser GJ, Bradwell SN, Gibala MJ. Six sessions of sprint interval training increases muscle oxidative potential and cycle endurance capacity in humans. J. Appl. Physiol. 2005;98:1985–1990.

150 Jakeman J, Adamson S, Babraj JA. Extremely short duration high-intensity training substantially improves endurance performance in triathletes. Appl. Physiol. Nutr. Metab. 2012;37:976–981.

151 Adamson SB, Lorimer R, Cobley JN, Babraj JA. Extremely Short–Duration High-Intensity Training Substantially Improves the Physical Function and Self-Reported Health Status of Elderly Adults. Journal of the American Geriatrics Society. 2014;62(7):1380–1381, July 2014 Article first published online: 12 JUL 2014.DOI: 10.1111/jgs.12916

152 2018 Physical Activity Guidelines Advisory Committee. 2018 Physical Activity Guidelines Advisory Committee Scientific Report. Washington, DC: US Department of Health and Human Services, 2018.

153 Reynolds G. Making every minute count. New York Times June 25, 2013.

154 Adamson SB, Lorimer R, Cobley JN, Lloyd R, Babraj JA. High Intensity Training Improves Health and Physical Function in Middle Aged Adults. Biology. 2014;3(2):333-344. doi:10.3390/biology3020333.

155 Reynolds G. An Interval Regimen to Keep. New York Times August 4, 2015.

156 T. P. Gunnarsson, J. Bangsbo. The 10-20-30 training concept improves performance and health profile in moderately trained runners. Journal of Applied Physiology. 2012;113(1):16-24. DOI: 10.1152/japplphysiol.00334.2012

157 Reynolds G. The Shortest Workout Possible. New York Times, February 7, 2017.

158 High Intensity Training. University of California, Berkeley Wellness Letter. 32(6), February 2013.

159 Klika B, Jordan C. "High-Intensity Circuit Training Using Body Weight: Maximum Results With Minimal Investment. ACSM's Health & Fitness Journal. 17(3):8–13, May/June 2013. doi:10.1249/FIT.0b013e31828cb1c8

Chapter 10 – Stress and Mental Health

1 World Health Organization. Strengthening Mental Health Promotion. Geneva: World Health Organiztion (Fact sheet no. 220); 2001.

2 Ryff CD, Keyes CLM. The structure of psychological well–being revisited. J Pers Soc Psychol 1995;69:719–727.

3 Ryff CD. Happiness is everything, or is it? Explorations on the meaning of psychological well–being. J Pers Soc Psychol 1989;57:1069–1081.

4 Keyes CLM. Social well–being. Soc Psychol Quart 1998;61:121–140. http://www.cdc.gov/mentalhealth/basics.htm

5 U.S. Department of Health and Human Services. Mental Health: A Report of the Surgeon General. Rockville, MD: U.S. Department of Health and Human Services; Substance Abuse and Mental Health Services Administration, Center for Mental Health Services, National Institutes of Health, National Institute of Mental Health, 1999.

6 U.S. Department of Health and Human Services. Mental Health: A Report of the Surgeon General. Rockville, MD: U.S. Department of Health and Human Services; Substance Abuse and Mental Health Services Administration, Center for Mental Health Services, National Institutes of Health, National Institute of Mental Health, 1999.

7 Parikh SG, Depression and Anxiety, Scientific American White Paper; 2015.

8 Center for Disease Control and Prevention, Mental Health Basics. http://www.cdc.gov/mentalhealth/basics.htm

9 Stein MB, Craske MG. Treating Anxiety in 2017 Optimizing Care to Improve Outcomes. JAMA. 2017;318(3):235–236. doi:10.1001/jama.2017.6996

10 Kessler RC, Berglund P, Demler O, Jin R, Merikangas KR, Walters EE. Lifetime prevalence and age-of-onset distributions of DSM-IV disorders in the National Comorbidity Survey Replication. Arch Gen Psychiatry. 2005;62:593-602.

11 Kamal R, Cox C, Rousseau D, for the Kaiser Family Foundation. Costs and Outcomes of Mental Health and Substance Use Disorders in the US. JAMA. 2017;318(5):415. doi:10.1001/jama.2017.8558

12 Kamal R, Cox C, Rousseau D, for the Kaiser Family Foundation. Costs and Outcomes of Mental Health and Substance Use Disorders in the US. JAMA. 2017;318(5):415. doi:10.1001/jama.2017.8558

13 Peterson-Kaiser Health System Tracker. https://www.healthsystemtracker.org/chart-collection/current-costs-outcomes-related-mental-health-substance-abuse-disorders/#item-mental-health-leading-cause-disease-burden-females-third-leading-cause-males.

14 U.S. Department of Health and Human Services. Mental Health: A Report of the Surgeon General. Rockville, MD: U.S. Department of Health and Human Services; Substance Abuse and Mental Health Services Administration, Center for Mental Health Services, National Institutes of Health, National Institute of Mental Health, 1999.

15 Center for Disease Control and Prevention, Mental Health Basics. http://www.cdc.gov/mentalhealth/basics.htm

16 Rampell C. The Half-Trillion-Dollar Depression. New York Times Magazine, July 7, 2013, p.MM14

17 Heikkilä K, Fransson EI, Nyberg ST, et al. Job Strain and Health-Related Lifestyle: Findings From an Individual-Participant Meta-Analysis of 118 000 Working Adults. Am J. Public Health. 2013;103(11):2090-2105.

18 Cohen S, Janicki-Deverts D, Miller GE. Psychological Stress and Disease. JAMA. 2007;298(14):1685-1687. doi:10.1001/jama.298.14.1685.

19 Lee BK, Glass TA, McAtee MJ, et al. Associations of Salivary Cortisol With Cognitive Function in the Baltimore Memory Study. Arch Gen Psychiatry. 2007;64(7):810-818. doi:10.1001/archpsyc.64.7.810.

20 Friedman RA. Born to Be Happy, Through a Twist of Human Hard Wire. New York Times. December 31, 2002.

21 Parikh SG. Depression and Anxiety, University of California, Berkeley White Paper. 2020.

22 Zimmerman M. Using the 9-Item Patient Health Questionnaire to Screen for and Monitor Depression. JAMA. 2019;322(21):2125–2126. doi:https://doi.org/10.1001/jama.2019.15883

23 Parikh SG, Depression and Anxiety, Scientific American White Paper, 2015. p.5

24 Kessler RC, Chiu WT, Demler O, Walters EE. Prevalence, severity, and comorbidity of 12-month DSM-IV disorders in the National Comorbidity Survey Replication. Arch Gen Psychiatry. 2005;62:617–627

25 Pratt LA, Brody DJ. Depression in the United States household population, 2005–2006. NCHS Data Brief. 2008(7):1–8.

26 Bipolar Disorder. The Mayo Clinic. https://www.mayoclinic.org/diseases-conditions/bipolar-disorder/symptoms-causes/syc-20355955

27 Carvalho AF, Firth J, Vieta E. Bipolar Disorder. N Engl J Med. 2020;383(1):58-66. doi: 10.1056/NEJMra1906193. PMID: 32609982

28 Rabins PV. How to Protect Your Memory & Brain Health, 8 Key Strategies. Johns Hopkins Medicine. Remedy Health Media 2011; p. 70

29 Parikh SG. Depression and Anxiety, University of California, Berkeley White Paper. 2020.

30 Russek LG, Schwartz GE. Feelings of parental caring predict health status in midlife: a 35-year follow-up of the Harvard Mastery of Stress Study. J Behav Med. 1997;20(1):1-13.

31 Lassale C, Batty GD, Baghdadli A, Jacka F, et al. Healthy dietary indices and risk of depressive outcomes: a systematic review and meta-analysis of observational studies. Molecular Psychiatry. 2019;24:965–986 https://doi.org/10.1038/s41380-018-0237-8

32 Berk M, Jacka FN. Diet and Depression—From Confirmation to Implementation. JAMA. 2019;321(9):842–843. doi:10.1001/jama.2019.0273

33 Sarris J, Byrne GJ, Stough C, et al. Nutraceuticals for major depressive disorder—more is not merrier. J Affect Disord. 2019;245:1007-1015. doi:10.1016/j.jad.2018.11.092

34 Bot M, Brouwer IA, Roca M, et al. Effect of Multinutrient Supplementation and Food-Related Behavioral Activation Therapy on Prevention of Major Depressive Disorder Among Overweight or Obese Adults With Subsyndromal Depressive Symptoms: The MooDFOOD Randomized Clinical Trial. JAMA. 2019;321(9):858–868. doi:10.1001/jama.2019.0556

35 Exercising to relax. Harvard Health Publications, Harvard Medical School, Harvard Men's Health Watch. February 2011. http://www.health.harvard.edu/newsletters/Harvard_Mens_Health_Watch/2011/February/ exercising-to-relax

36 Choi KW, Chen C, Stein MB, et al. Assessment of Bidirectional Relationships Between Physical Activity and Depression Among Adults: A 2-Sample Mendelian Randomization Study. JAMA Psychiatry. Published online January 23, 2019;76(4):399–408. doi:10.1001/jamapsychiatry.2018.4175

37 Gordon BR, McDowell CP, Hallgren M, Meyer JD, Lyons M, Herring MP. Association of Efficacy of Resistance Exercise Training With Depressive Symptoms Meta-analysis and Meta-regression Analysis of Randomized Clinical Trials. JAMA Psychiatry. 2018;75(6):566–576. doi:10.1001/jamapsychiatry.2018.0572

38 2018 Physical Activity Guidelines Advisory Committee. 2018 Physical Activity Guidelines Advisory Committee Scientific Report. Washington, DC: U.S. Department of Health and Human Services, 2018.

39 Pinto Pereira SM, Geoffroy M, Power C. Depressive Symptoms and Physical Activity During 3 Decades in Adult Life Bidirectional Associations in a Prospective Cohort Study. JAMA Psychiatry. 2014;71(12):1373-1380. doi:10.1001/jamapsychiatry.2014.1240

40 Cooney GM, Dwan K, Greig CA, Lawlor DA, Rimer J, Waugh FR, McMurdo M, Mead GE, Exercise for Depression, Cochrane Review 12 September 2013

41 Benson H, Klipper MZ, The Relaxation Response. New York: Harper Collins; 1975.

42 Ornish D, The Spectrum. New York: Ballantine Books; 2007.

43 Russek LG, Schwartz GE. Feelings of parental caring predict health status in midlife: a 35-year follow-up of the Harvard Mastery of Stress Study. J Behav Med. 1997;20(1):1-13.

44 Vaillant, GE. Aging Well, Boston: Little, Brown, and Company; 2002.

45 Vaillant, GE. Triumphs of Experience. Cambridge: Harvard University Press; 2012.

46 Shenk JW. What Makes Us Happy, The Atlantic. June 2009. http://www.theatlantic.com/magazine/toc/2009/06/

47 Parikh SG, Depression and Anxiety, Scientific American White Paper, 2015. p. 15-16

48 Carvalho AF, Firth J, Vieta E. Bipolar Disorder. N Engl J Med. 2020;383(1):58-66. doi: 10.1056/NEJMra1906193. PMID: 32609982

49 Bohnert ASB, Ilgen MA. Understanding Links among Opioid Use, Overdose, and Suicide. N Engl J Med. 2019; 380:71-79. DOI: 10.1056/NEJMra1802148

50 Fazel S, Runeson B. Suicide. N Engl J Med. 2020;382(3):266-274.

51 Miron O, Yu K, Wilf-Miron R, Kohane IS. Suicide Rates Among Adolescents and Young Adults in the United States, 2000-2017. JAMA. 2019;321(23):2362–2364. doi:10.1001/jama.2019.5054

52 Fazel S, Runeson B. Suicide. N Engl J Med. 2020;382(3):266-274.

53 Swanson JW, Bonnie RJ, Appelbaum PS. Getting Serious About Reducing Suicide: More "How" and Less "Why." JAMA. 2015;314(21):2229–2230. doi:10.1001/jama.2015.15566

54 Studdert DM, Zhang Y, Swanson SA, et al. Handgun ownership and suicide in California. N Engl J Med 2020;382:2220-2229

55 Brown GK, Ten Have T, Henriques GR, Xie SX, Hollander JE, Beck AT. Cognitive therapy for the pr vention of suicide attempts: a randomized controlled trial. JAMA. 2005;294:563-570

56 Bohnert ASB, Ilgen MA. Understanding Links among Opioid Use, Overdose, and Suicide. N Engl J Med. 2019; 380:71-79. DOI: 10.1056/NEJMra1802148

57 Fazel S, Runeson B. Suicide. N Engl J Med. 2020; 382(3):266-274.

58 Cuijpers P. The Challenges of Improving Treatments for Depression. JAMA. 2018;320(24):2529–2530. doi:10.1001/jama.2018.17824

59 Parikh SG, Depression and Anxiety, Scientific American White Paper, 2015. p. 1

60 Chapman DP, Perry GS, Strine TW.The vital link between chronic disease and depressive disorders. Prev Chronic Dis. 2005;2(1):A14.

61 Parikh SG. Depression and Anxiety, University of California, Berkeley White Paper. 2020.

62 Shining a light on depression. University of California, Berkeley Wellness Letter. Spring 2018.

63 Brunoni AR, Moffa AH, Sampaio-Junior B, et al. Trial of electrical direct-current therapy versus esci alopram for depression. N Engl J Med. 2017;376:2523-33.

64 Lisanby SH. Noninvasive Brain Stimulation for Depression — The Devil Is in the Dosing. N Engl J Med. 2017; 376:2593-2594. DOI: 10.1056/NEJMe1702492

65 Sanacora G, Frye MA, McDonald W, Mathew SJ, Turner MS, Schatzberg AF, Summergrad P, Nemeroff CB, for the American Psychiatric Association (APA) Council of Research Task Force on Novel Biomarkers and Treatments. A Consensus Statement on the Use of Ketamine in the Treatment of Mood Disorders. JAMA Psychiatry. 2017;74(4):399–405. doi:10.1001/jamapsychiatry.2017.0080

66 Golzari SEJ, Mahmoodpoor A. Ketamine for the Treatment of Depression. JAMA Psychiatry.

2017;74(9):971. doi:10.1001/jamapsychiatry.2017.1779

67 Kim J, Farchione T, Potter A, Chen Q, Temple R. Esketamine for Treatment-Resistant Depression — First FDA-Approved Antidepressant in a New Class. N Engl J Med. 2019; 381:1-4 DOI: 10.1056/NEJMp1903305

68 Parikh SG. Depression and Anxiety, University of California, Berkeley White Paper. 2020.

69 http://www.nimh.nih.gov/health/topics/panic-disorder/index.shtml

70 Parikh SG, Depression and Anxiety, University of California, Berkeley White Paper; 2020.

71 Hirschtritt ME, Bloch MH, Mathews CA. Obsessive-Compulsive Disorder Advances in Diagnosis and Treatment. JAMA. 2017;317(13):1358-1367. doi:10.1001/jama.2017.2200

72 Parikh SG. Depression and Anxiety, University of California, Berkeley White Paper. 2020.

73 http://www.nimh.nih.gov/health/topics/attention-deficit-hyperactivity-disorder-adhd/index.shtml

74 http://www.nimh.nih.gov/about/director/2010/attention-on-adhd-awareness-week.shtml

75 Cortese S. Pharmacologic Treatment of Attention Deficit–Hyperactivity Disorder. N Engl J Med. 2020;383:1050-1056. DOI: 10.1056/NEJMra1917069

76 http://www.nimh.nih.gov/health/topics/attention-deficit-hyperactivity-disorder-adhd/index.shtml

77 A Parent's Guide to Autism Spectrum Disorder, available at: http://www.nimh.nih.gov/health/publications/a-parents-guide-to-autism-spectrum-disorder/index.shtml

78 https://www.nami.org/Learn-More/Mental-Health-Conditions/Related-Conditions/Psychosis

79 Lieberman JA, First MB. Psychotic disorders. N Engl J Med. 2018;379(3):270–80

80 https://www.nami.org/Learn-More/Mental-Health-Conditions/Related-Conditions/Psychosis

81 Marder SR, Cannon TD. Schizophrenia. N Engl J Med. 2019;381(18):1753-1761.

82 http://www.nimh.nih.gov/health/topics/schizophrenia/index.shtml

83 http://www.nimh.nih.gov/health/topics/schizophrenia/index.shtml

84 http://www.nimh.nih.gov/health/topics/schizophrenia/index.shtml

85 Insel T. Directors Blog: Can We Prevent Psychosis? November 20, 2014. http://www.nimh.nih.gov/about/director/2014/can-we-prevent-psychosis.shtml

86 Stafford MR et al. Early interventions to prevent psychosis: systematic review and meta-analysis. BMJ. 2013;18;346:f185.

87 McFarlane WR et al. Clinical and Functional Outcomes After 2 Years in the Early Detection and Intervention for the Prevention of Psychosis Multisite Effectiveness Trial. Schizophr Bull. 2014 Jul 26. pii: sbu108. [Epub ahead of print]

88 Substance Abuse Center for Behavioral Health Statistics and Quality. Results from the 2015 National Survey on Drug Use and Health: Detailed Tables. SAMHSA. https://www.samhsa.gov/data/sites/default/files/NSDUH-DetTabs-2015/NSDUH-DetTabs-2015/NSDUH-DetTabs-2015.pdf. Published September 8, 2016. Accessed January 18, 2017.

89 Johnston, L. D., Miech, R. A., O'Malley, P. M., Bachman, J. G., Schulenberg, J. E., & Patrick, M. E. Monitoring the Future national survey results on drug use 1975-2018: Overview, key findings on adolescent drug use. Ann Arbor: Institute for Social Research, University of Michigan. 2019.

90 Marijuana. Drug Facts. National Institute of Drug Abuse. December 2019. https://www.drugabuse. gov/publications/drugfacts/marijuana

91 National Academies of Sciences, Engineering, and Medicine. The Health Effects of Cannabis and Cannabinoids: The Current State of Evidence and Recommendations for Research. Washington, DC: National

Academies Press; 2017. doi:10.17226/24625

92 Whiting PF, Wolff RF, Deshpande S, et al. Cannabinoids for medical use. JAMA. 2015;313(24):2456-2473. doi:10.1001/jama.2015.6358

93 D'Souza DC, Ranganathan M. Medical Marijuana: Is the Cart Before the Horse? JAMA. 2015;313(24):2431–2432. doi:10.1001/jama.2015.6407

94 Scott JC, Slomiak ST, Jones JD, Rosen AFG, Moore TM, Gur RC. Association of cannabis with cognitive functioning in adolescents and young adults: a systematic review and meta-analysis. JAMA Ps chiatry. 2018;75(6):585-595. doi:10.1001/jamapsychiatry.2018.0335

95 Hill KP. Medical Use of Cannabis in 2019. JAMA. Published online, August 09, 2019. 322(10):974–975. doi:10.1001/jama.2019.11868

96 Volkow ND, Baler RD, Compton WM, Weiss SRB. Adverse Health Effects of Marijuana Use. N Engl J Med. 2014; 370:2219-2227. DOI: 10.1056/NEJMra1402309.

97 Parikh SG, Depression and Anxiety, University of California, Berkeley White Paper; 2020.

98 Rubin R. Cannabidiol Products Are Everywhere, but Should People Be Using Them? JAMA. 2019;322(22):2156–2158. doi:https://doi.org/10.1001/jama.2019.17361

99 Bonn-Miller MO, Loflin MJE, Thomas BF, Marcu JP, Hyke T, Vandrey R. Labeling Accuracy of Cannabidiol Extracts Sold Online. JAMA. 2017;318(17):1708–1709. doi:10.1001/jama.2017.11909

100 NCHS, National Vital Statistics System. Estimates for 2018 and 2019 are based on provisional data. Estimates for 2015-2017 are based on final data (available from https://www.cdc.gov/nchs/nvss/mortality_public_use_data.htm).

101 Katz J U.S. Drug Deaths Climbing Faster Than Ever. New York Times. June 6, 2017.

102 Babu KM, Brent J, Juurlink DN. Prevention of Opioid Overdose. N Engl J Med. 2019; 380:2246-2255. DOI: 10.1056/NEJMra1807054

103 Chou R, Turner JA, Devine EB, et al. The effectiveness and risks of long-term opioid therapy for chronic pain: a systematic review for a National Institutes of Health Pathways to Prevention Workshop. Ann Intern Med. 2015;162:276-286.

104 Dowell D, Haegerich TM, Chou R. CDC guideline for prescribing opioids for chronic pain — United States, 2016. MMWR Recomm Rep. 2016;65:1-49.

105 Wakeman SE, Larochelle MR, Ameli O, et al. Comparative Effectiveness of Different Treatment Pathways for Opioid Use Disorder. JAMA Netw Open. 2020;3(2):e1920622. doi:10.1001/jamanetworkopen.2019.20622

Chapter 11 - Preventing Infectious Disease

1 Infectious diseases. World Health Organization. www.who.int/topics/infectious_diseases/en/

2 Johns Hopkins Coronavirus Resource Center. https://coronavirus.jhu.edu/

3 Janeway CA, Travers P, Walport M, et al. Infectious agents and how they cause disease. Immunobiology: The Immune System in Health and Disease. 5th edition. New York: Garland Science; 2001. http://www.ncbi.nlm.nih.gov/books/NBK27114/

4 Moyer MW. The Looming Threat of Factory-Farm Superbugs. Scientific American, December 2016. pp71-79.

5 Antibiotic Resistance Threats in the United States. Centers for Disease Control and Prevention.; 2019. https://www.cdc.gov/drugresistance/pdf/threats-report/2019-ar-threats-report-508.pdf

6 Bradley SF. What Is Known About Candida auris. JAMA. 2019;322(15):1510–1511. doi:https://doi.

org/10.1001/jama.2019.13843

7 Peter Sands P, Mundaca-Shah C, Dzau VJ. The Neglected Dimension of Global Security — A Framework for Countering Infectious-Disease Crises. N Engl J Med. 2016; 374:1281-1287. DOI: 10.1056/NEJMsr1600236

8 Disease Outbreaks. World Health Organization, http://www.who.int/csr/disease/en/

9 Pandemic and Epidemic Diseases. 2014. World Health Organization. http://www.who.int/csr/disease/WHO_PED_flyer_2014.PDF?ua=1

10 Guan W, Ni Z, Hu Y, et al. Clinical characteristics of coronavirus disease 2019 in China. N Engl J Med. February 28, 2020. DOI: 10.1056/NEJMoa2002032.

11 Disease Burden of Influenza. Centers for Disease Control and Prevention. https://www.cdc.gov/flu/about/burden/index.html

12 Key Facts About Influenza (Flu). Centers for Disease Control and Prevention. http://www.cdc.gov/flu/keyfacts.htm

13 Skin Infections. Medline Plus. http://www.nlm.nih.gov/medlineplus/skininfections.html#summary

14 Magill SS, O'Leary E, Janelle SJ, et al. Changes in prevalence of health care-associated infections in U.S. hospitals. N Engl J Med. 2018;379:1732-1744.

15 Magill SS, Edwards JR, Bamberg W, et al. Multistate Point-Prevalence Survey of Health Care–Associated Infections. N Engl J Med 2014;370:1198-208.

16 Whitney CG, Zhou F, Singleton J, et al. Benefits from Immunization During the Vaccines for Children Program Era — United States, 1994–2013. Morbidity and Mortality Weekly Report (MMWR). 2014; 63(16):352-355.

17 Vaccines & Immunizations. Centers for Disease Control and Prevention. http://www.cdc.gov/vaccines/default.htm

18 Travelers Health. Centers for Disease Control and Prevention. http://wwwnc.cdc.gov/travel/destinations/ list

19 Vaccine Side Effects. Vaccines.gov. U.S. Department of Health & Human Services.http://www.vaccines. gov/basics/safety/side_effects/index.html

20 Offit PA, The Anti-Vaccination Epidemic. Wall St. Journal September 25, 2014.

21 Who Should NOT Get Vaccinated with these Vaccines? Centers for Disease Control and Prevention. http://www.cdc.gov/vaccines/vpd-vac/should-not-vacc.htm

22 Immunization Schedules. Centers for Disease Control and Prevention. http://www.cdc.gov/vaccines/default.html

23 Adults. Vaccines.gov. U.S. Department of Health & Human Services. https://www.vaccines.gov/ who_and_when/adults

24 Adults age 65 and older. Vaccines.gov. U.S. Department of Health & Human Services. https://www.vaccines.gov/who_and_when/adults/seniors

Chapter 12- Preventing Osteoporosis

1 Facts and Statistics. International Osteoporosis Foundation http://www.iofbonehealth.org/facts-statistics#category-14

2 NIH Osteoporosis and Related Bone Diseases National Resource Center http://www.niams.nih.gov/Health_Info/Bone/Osteoporosis/overview.asp#Prevention

3 National Osteoporosis Foundation: Facts. http://nof.org/

4 Nutrition for Everyone: Basics: Calcium and Bone Health, Center for Disease Control and Prevention, http://www.cdc.gov/nutrition/everyone/basics/vitamins/calcium.html

5 U.S. Department of Health and Human Services. Bone Health and Osteoporosis: A Report of the Surgeon General. Rockville, MD: U.S. Department of Health and Human Services, Office of the Surgeon General, 2004. http://www.ncbi.nlm.nih.gov/books/NBK45513/pdf/TOC.pdf

6 Facts and Statistics. International Osteoporosis Foundation http://www.iofbonehealth.org/facts-statistics#category-14

7 Bone loss: what to do about it. U.C. Berkeley Wellness Letter. Summer 2017.

8 Facts and Statistics. International Osteoporosis Foundation http://www.iofbonehealth.org/facts-statistics#category-14

9 Bone loss: what to do about it. U.C. Berkeley Wellness Letter. Summer 2017.

10 Licata AA, bone density, bone quality, and FRAX: changing concepts in osteoporosis management. Am J Ob Gyn. 2013:92-95.

11 NIH Osteoporosis and Related Bone Diseases National Resource Center http://www.niams.nih.gov/Health_Info/Bone/Osteoporosis/overview.asp#Prevention

12 Nutrition for Everyone: Basics: Calcium and Bone Health, Center for Disease Control and Prevention, http://www.cdc.gov/nutrition/everyone/basics/vitamins/calcium.html

13 NIH Osteoporosis and Related Bone Diseases National Resource Center http://www.niams.nih.gov/Health_Info/Bone/Osteoporosis/overview.asp#Prevention

14 Nutrition for Everyone: Basics: Calcium and Bone Health, Center for Disease Control and Prevention, http://www.cdc.gov/nutrition/everyone/basics/vitamins/calcium.html

15 Bone loss: what to do about it. U.C. Berkeley Wellness Letter. Summer 2017.

16 Warren MP Health issues for women athletes: exercise-induced amenorrhea. J Clin Endocrinol Metab. 1999;84:1892.

17 Preisinger E, Alacamlioglu Y, Pils K, et al. Therapeutic exercise in the prevention of bone loss. A controlled trial with women after menopause. Am J Phys Med Rehabil. 1995;74:120.

18 Hartard M, Haber P, Ilieva D, et al. Systematic strength training as a model of therapeutic intervention. A controlled trial in postmenopausal women with osteopenia. Am J Phys Med Rehabil. 1995;75:21.

19 Kemmler W, Lauber D, Weineck J, et al. Benefits of 2 years of intense exercise on bone density, physical fitness, and blood lipids in early postmenopausal osteopenic women: results of the Erlangen Fitness Osteoporosis Prevention Study (EFOPS). Arch Intern Med. 2004;164:1084.

20 Kanis JA, Johnell O, Oden A, et al. Smoking and fracture risk: a meta-analysis. Osteoporos Int 2005;16:155.

21 NIH Osteoporosis and Related Bone Diseases National Resource Center http://www.niams.nih.gov/Health_Info/Bone/Osteoporosis/overview.asp#Prevention

22 Nutrition for Everyone: Basics: Calcium and Bone Health, Center for Disease Control and Prevention, http://www.cdc.gov/nutrition/everyone/basics/vitamins/calcium.html

23 Kanis JA, Johansson H, Johnell O, et al. Alcohol intake as a risk factor for fracture. Osteoporos Int. 2005;16:737.

24 Felson DT, Kiel DP, Anderson JJ, Kannel WB. Alcohol consumption and hip fractures: the Framingham Study. Am J Epidemiol. 1988;128:1102

25 Melhus H, Michaelsson K, Kindmark A. et al. Excessive dietary intake of vitamin A is associated with reduced bone mineral density and increased risk for hip fracture. Ann Intern Med.1998;129:770-778.

26 Feskanich D, Singh V, Willett WC, Colditz GA. Vitamin A Intake and Hip Fractures Among Postmenopausal Women. JAMA. 2002;287(1):47–54. doi:10.1001/jama.287.1.47

27 Soyka LA, Misra M, Frenchman A, et al. Abnormal bone mineral accrual in adolescent girls with anorexia nervosa. J Clin Endocrinol Metab. 2002;7:4177.

28 Legroux-Gerot I, Vignau J, Collier F, Cortet B (2005) Bone loss associated with anorexia nervosa. Joint Bone Spine 72:489.

29 Ellis FR, Holesh S, Ellis JW. Incidence of osteoporosis in vegetarians and omnivores. Am J Clin Nutr. 1972;25(6):555-558.

30 New SA (2004) Do vegetarians have a normal bone mass? Osteoporos Int. 2004;15:679.

31 Tucker KL, Hannan MT, Chen H, et al. Potassium, magnesium, and fruit and vegetable intakes are associated with greater bone mineral density in elderly men and women. Am J Clin Nutr. 1999;69:727.

32 Hannan MT, Tucker KL, Dawson-Hughes B, et al. Effect of dietary protein on bone loss in elderly men and women: the Framingham Osteoporosis Study. J Bone Miner Res. 2000;15:2504.

33 Fuhrman J. Eat to live. Little Brown & Co.. New York 2011 pp.104-111

34 Feskanich D, Willett WC, Stampfer MJ, Colditz GA. Protein consumption and bone fractures in women. Am J Epidemiol. 1996;143:472–479

35 Beasley JM, Ichikawa LE, Ange BA et al. Is protein intake associated with bone mineral density in young women? Am J Clin Nutr. 2010;91:1311-1316

36 Darling AL, Millward DJ, Torgerson DJ, Hewitt CE, Lanham-New SA. Dietary protein and bone health: a systematic review and meta-analysis. Am J Clin Nutr. 2009;90:1674–92

37 Shams-White MM, Chung M, Du M, Fu Z, Insogna KL, Karlsen MC, LeBoff MS, Shapses SA, Sackey J, Wallace TC, Weaver CM. Dietary protein and bone health: a systematic review and meta-analysis from the National Osteoporosis Foundation. Am J Clin Nutr. 2017;105(6):1528-1543. doi: 10.3945/ajcn.116.145110. Epub 2017 April 12.

38 National Osteoporosis Foundation: Facts. http://nof.org/

39 Nutrition for Everyone: Basics: Calcium and Bone Health, Center for Disease Control and Prevention, http://www.cdc.gov/nutrition/everyone/basics/vitamins/calcium.html

40 McDougall JA, McDougall MA. The McDougall Plan. Clinton NJ: New Win Publishing; 1983, pp. 95-109

41 Campbell CT, Campbell TM. The China Study, Dallas TX: Benbella Books; 2006, pp. 204-211

42 Michaëlsson K, Wolk A, Langenskiöld S, Basu S, Warensjö Lemming E, Melhus H et al. Milk intake and risk of mortality and fractures in women and men: cohort studies BMJ. 2014; 349:g6015

43 Facts and Statistics. International Osteoporosis Foundation http://www.iofbonehealth.org/facts-statistics#category-14

44 Chapuy MC, Arlot ME, Duboeuf F, et al. Vitamin D3 and calcium to prevent hip fractures in the elderly women. N Engl J Med. 1992;327:1637.

45 Dawson-Hughes B, Harris SS, Krall EA, Dallal GE (1997) Effect of calcium and vitamin D supplementation on bone density in men and women 65 years of age or older. N Engl J Med. 337:670.

46 Feskanich D, Willett WC, Colditz GA. Calcium, vitamin D, milk consumption, and hip fractures: a prospective study among postmenopausal women. Am J Clin Nutr. 2003;77:504–511.

47 Moyer VA. U.S. Preventive Services Task Force. Vitamin D and calcium supplementation to prevent fractures in adults: U.S. Preventive Services Task Force recommendation statement. Ann Intern Med. 2013;158:691–6.

48 Bischoff-Ferrari HA, Willett WC, Wong JB, Giovannucci E, Dietrich T, Dawson-Hughes B. Fracture Prevention With Vitamin D Supplementation: A Meta-analysis of Randomized Controlled Trials. JAMA.2005;293(18):2257–2264. doi:10.1001/jama.293.18.2257

49 Burt LA, Billington EO, Rose MS, Raymond DA, Hanley DA, Boyd SK. Effect of High-Dose Vitamin D Supplementation on Volumetric Bone Density and Bone Strength: A Randomized Clinical Trial. JAMA.2019;322(8):736–745. doi:10.1001/jama.2019.11889

50 Moyer VA. U.S. Preventive Services Task Force. Vitamin D and calcium supplementation to prevent fractures in adults: U.S. Preventive Services Task Force recommendation statement. Ann Intern Med. 2013;158:691–6.

51 Jia-Guo Zhao, Xian-Tie Zeng, Jia Wang, Lin Liu. Association Between Calcium or Vitamin D Supplementation and Fracture Incidence in Community-Dwelling Older Adults A Systematic Review and Meta-analysis. JAMA.2017;318(24):2466–2482. doi:10.1001/jama.2017.19344

52 Bolland MJ, Grey A, Avenell A. Effects of vitamin D supplementation on musculoskeletal health: a systematic review, meta-analysis, and trial sequential analysis. Lancet Diabetes & Endocrinology. Published Online October 4, 2018 http://dx.doi.org/10.1016/ S2213-8587(18)30265-1

53 Yao P, Bennett D, Mafham M, et al. Vitamin D and Calcium for the Prevention of Fracture: A Systematic Review and Meta-analysis. JAMA Netw Open. 2019;2(12):e1917789. doi:https://doi.org/10.1001/jamanetworkopen.2019.17789

54 Bischoff-Ferrari, HA, et al. Dietary calcium and serum 25-hydroxyvitamin D status in relation to BMD among U.S. adults. J of Bone Miner Res. 2009;24(5):935-942.

55 Bischoff-Ferrari, HA, et al. 2007. Calcium intake and hip fracture risk in men and women: A meta-analysis of prospective cohort studies and randomized controlled trials. Am J Clin Nutr, 86:17980-90.

56 Hegsted DM. Calcium and Osteoporosis. The Journal of Nutrition. 1986;116(11):2316–2319. https://doi.org/10.1093/jn/116.11.2316

57 NIH Osteoporosis and Related Bone Diseases National Resource Center http://www.niams.nih.gov/Health_Info/Bone/Osteoporosis/overview.asp#Prevention

58 Nutrition for Everyone: Basics: Calcium and Bone Health, Center for Disease Control and Prevention, http://www.cdc.gov/nutrition/everyone/basics/vitamins/calcium.html

59 Bone loss: what to do about it. U.C. Berkeley Wellness Letter. Summer 2017.

60 Cauley JA. Screening for Osteoporosis. JAMA. 2018;319(24):2483–2485. doi:10.1001/jama.2018.5722

61 US Preventive Services Task Force. Screening for osteoporosis to prevent fractures: US Preventive Services Task Force Recommendation Statement. JAMA. 2018;319(24):2521-2531. doi:10.1001/jama.2018.7498

62 Bone loss: what to do about it. U.C. Berkeley Wellness Letter. Summer 2017.

63 Bone loss: what to do about it. U.C. Berkeley Wellness Letter. Summer 2017.

64 Licata AA, bone density, bone quality, and FRAX: changing concepts in osteoporosis management. Am J Ob Gyn. 2013:92-95.

65 Crandall CJ, Ensrud KE. Osteoporosis Screening in Younger Postmenopausal Women. JAMA. 2020;323(4):367–368. doi:10.1001/jama.2019.18343

66 Reid IR, Horne AM, Mihov B, et al. Fracture prevention with zoledronate in older women with osteopenia. N Engl J Med 2018;379:2407-2416.

67 Berry SD, Kiel DP, Colón-Emeric C. Hip Fractures in Older Adults in 2019. JAMA. Published online May 10, 2019;321(22):2231–2232. doi:10.1001/jama.2019.5453

68 Drugs for Postmenopausal Osteoporosis. JAMA. 2019;321(22):2233–2234. doi:10.1001/jama.2019.6077

69 Rosen CJ, Ingelfinger JR. Building Better Bones with Biologics - A New Approach to Osteoporosis? N Engl J Med. 2016;375(16):1583-1584. Epub 2016 Sep 18.

70 NIH Osteoporosis and Related Bone Diseases National Resource Center http://www.niams.nih.gov/Health_Info/Bone/Osteoporosis/overview.asp#Prevention

71 National Osteoporosis Foundation: Facts. http://nof.org/

72 Nutrition for Everyone: Basics: Calcium and Bone Health, Center for Disease Control and Prevention, http://www.cdc.gov/nutrition/everyone/basics/vitamins/calcium.html

73 Black DM, Rosen CJ. Postmenopausal Osteoporosis. N Engl J Med 2016;374:254-62. DOI: 10.1056/NEJMcp1513724

74 Bellows L, Moore R, Gross A. Dietary Supplements: Vitamins and Minerals. Colorado State University Extension Publication no. 9.338 (9/13) http://www.ext.colostate.edu/pubs/foodnut/09338.html

Chapter 13- Sexual and Reproductive Health

1 SIECUS (the Sexuality Information and Education Council of the United States) http://www.siecus.org

2 SIECUS (the Sexuality Information and Education Council of the United States) http://www.siecus.org

3 Guttmacher In Brief. Facts on American Teens' Sexual and Reproductive Health. http://www.guttmacher.org/pubs/FB-ATSRH.html

4 Tsui AO, McDonald-Mosley R, Burke AE. Family planning and the burden of unintended pregnancies. Epidemiol Rev. 32(1):152-74; 2010.

5 Finer LB and Zolna MR, Declines in unintended pregnancy in the United States, 2008–2011, New England Journal of Medicine, 2016, 374(9):843–852, http://nejm.org/doi/full/10.1056/NEJMsa1506575.

6 Mosher WD, Jones J, Abma, JC. Intended and unintended births in the United States: 1982-2010. National Center for Health Statistics. 2012; Vital Health Stat (55). from http://www.cdc.gov/nchs/data/nhsr/nhsr055.pdf.

7 Maternal mortality, World Health Organization Fact sheet N°348 Updated May 2014

8 Frost JJ, Darroch JE, Remez L. Improving contraceptive use in the United States. In Brief. New York, NY: Guttmacher Institute, 2008, No. 1.

9 Hoffman, S.D. By the Numbers: The Public Costs of Adolescent Childbearing. The National Campaign to Prevent Teen Pregnancy, 2006, Washington, DC.

10 Frost JJ, Darroch JE, Remez L. Improving contraceptive use in the United States. In Brief. New York, NY: Guttmacher Institute, 2008, No. 1.

11 Finer LB and Zolna MR, Unintended pregnancy in the United States: incidence and disparities, 2006, Contraception. 2011, doi: 10.1016/j.contraception.2011.07.013

12 Frost JJ, Singh S and Finer LB, U.S. women's one-year contraceptive use patterns, 2004, Perspectives on Sexual and Reproductive Health, 2007, 39(1):48–55, http://onlinelibrary.wiley.com/doi/10.1363/3904807/pdf

13 Trussell J. Contraceptive Failure in the United States. Contraception. 2011; 83:397-404.

14 Raine TR, Foster-Rosales A, Upadhyay UD, Boyer CB, Brown BA, Sokoloff A, Harper CC. Oneyear contraceptive continuation and pregnancy in adolescent girls and women initiating hormonal contraceptives. Obstet Gynecol. 2011;117:363-371.

15 Frost JJ, Singh S and Finer LB, U.S. women's one-year contraceptive use patterns, 2004, Per-

spectives on Sexual and Reproductive Health, 2007, 39(1):48–55, http://onlinelibrary.wiley.com/doi/10.1363/3904807/pdf

16 Hatcher RA, Trussell J, Nelson AL, Cates W, Kowal D, Policar MS. Contraceptive Technology, Twentieth Revised Edition: Ardent Media, Inc.; 2011.

17 Hatcher RA, Trussell J, Nelson AL, Cates W, Kowal D, Policar MS. Contraceptive Technology, Twentieth Revised Edition: Ardent Media, Inc.; 2011.

18 Speidel JJ, Rocca CH, Thompson MJK, Harper CC, Pregnancy: not a disease but still a health risk. Contraception. 2013; 88(4):481-4.

19 Trussell J, Jordan B, Reproductive health risks in perspective. Contraception. 2006; 73: 437-439.

20 Speidel JJ. Barriers to Contraceptives Development. Testimony presented to 102nd Congress Committee on Small Business Subcommittee on Regulation, Business Opportunities, and Energy, Camden, NJ. 1992.

21 Darroch JE, Sedgh G and Ball H, Contraceptive Technologies: Responding to Women's Needs, New York: Guttmacher Institute, 2011.

22 Nelson A L, Rezvzn A. A pilot study of women's knowledge of pregnancy health risks: implications for contraception. Contraception. 2012;85:78-82.

23 Hatcher RA, Trussell J, Nelson AL, Cates W, Kowal D, Policar MS. Contraceptive Technology, Twentieth Revised Edition: Ardent Media, Inc.; 2011.

24 Hatcher RA, Trussell J, Nelson AL, Cates W, Kowal D, Policar MS. Contraceptive Technology, Twentieth Revised Edition: Ardent Media, Inc.; 2011: 438-462.

25 Fraser IS. Non-contraceptive health benefits of intrauterine hormonal systems. Contraception. 2010; 82(5): 396-403.

26 Hubacher D, Grimes DA. Noncontraceptive health benefits of intrauterine devices: a systematic review. Obstet Gynecol Surv. 2002;57:120–8.

27 Hatcher RA, Trussell J, Nelson AL, Cates W, Kowal D, Policar MS. Contraceptive Technology, Twent eth Revised Edition: Ardent Media, Inc.; 2011.

28 Centers for Disease Control and Prevention. U.S. Medical Eligibility Criteria for Contraceptive Use, 2010 . MMWR 2010;59,RR-4 :1-86.

29 Wu JP, Moniz MH, Ursu AN. Long-acting Reversible Contraception—Highly Efficacious, Safe, and Underutilized. JAMA. 2018;320(4):397–398. doi:10.1001/jama.2018.8877

30 Farley TM, Rosenberg MJ, Rowe PJ, Chen JH, Meirik O. Intrauterine devices and pelvic inflammatory disease: an international perspective. Lancet. 1992;339:785–8.

31 Hatcher RA, Trussell J, Nelson AL, Cates W, Kowal D, Policar MS. Contraceptive Technology, Twentieth Revised Edition: Ardent Media, Inc.; 2011

32 Evidence for Contraceptive Options and HIV Outcomes (ECHO) Trial ConsortiumHIV incidence among women using intramuscular depot medroxyprogesterone acetate, a copper intrauterine device, or a levonorgestrel implant for contraception: a randomised, multicentre, open-label trial. Lancet. 2019; 394: 303–13 published online June 13. http://dx.doi.org/10.1016/S0140-6736(19)31288-7

33 Hatcher RA, Trussell J, Nelson AL, Cates W, Kowal D, Policar MS. Contraceptive Technology, Twentieth Revised Edition: Ardent Media, Inc.; 2011

34 Burkman R, Bell C, Serfaty D. The evolution of combined oral contraception: improving the risk-to-benefit ratio. Contraception. 2011;84:19-34.

35 Maguire K, Westhoff C. The state of hormonal contraception today: established and emerging noncontraceptive health benefits. Am J Obstet Gynecol. 2011;205:S4-S8.

36 Robert L Reid, Carolyn Westhoff, Diana Mansour, et al., Oral contraceptives and Venous Thromboembolism: Consensus Opinion from an International Workshop held in Berlin, Germany in December 2009. J Fam Plann Reprod Health Care. 2010;36:117-122. doi: 10.1783/147118910791749425

37 Heinemann K, Heinemann L A J. Comparative risks of venous thromboembolism among users of oral contraceptives containing drospirenone and levonorgesterel. J Fam Plann Reprod Health Care. 2011;37:132-135 originally published online June 9, 2011. doi: 10.1136/jfprhc-2011-14524

38 Hatcher RA, Trussell J, Nelson AL, Cates W, Kowal D, Policar MS. Contraceptive Technology, Twentieth Revised Edition: Ardent Media, Inc.; 2011, p.219

39 Iversen L, Sivasubramaniam S, Lee AJFielding S, Hannaford PC. Lifetime cancer risk and combined oral contraceptives: the Royal College of General Practitioners' Oral Contraception Study. Am J Obstet and Gynecol, 2017;216(6):580.e1-580.e9.

40 Westhoff CL, Pike MC. Hormonal contraception and breast cancer. Am J Obstet Gynecol. 2018 Aug;219(2):169.e1-169.e4. doi: 10.1016/j.ajog.2018.03.032. Epub 2018 May 17.

41 Schwarz EB, Foster DG, Grossman D. Contemporary Hormonal Contraception and the Risk of Breast Cancer. N Engl J Med. 2017;378(13):1263-4.

42 Bassuk SS, Manson JE. Oral contraceptives and menopausal hormone therapy: relative and attributable risks of cardiovascular disease, cancer, and other health outcomes. Ann Epidemiol. 2015;25:193-200.

43 Iversen L, Sivasubramaniam S, Lee AJ, Fielding S, Hannaford PC. Lifetime cancer risk and combined oral contraceptives: the Royal College of General Practitioners' Oral Contraception Study. Am J Obstet and Gynecol. 2017;216(6):580.e1-580.e9.

44 Raymond EG, Grimes DA. The comparative safety of legal induced abortion and childbirth in the United States. Obstet Gynecol. 2012;119:215-9.

45 Schwingl PJ, Ory HW, Visness CM. Estimates of the risk of cardiovascular death attributable to lowdose oral contraceptives in the United States. Am J Obstet Gynecol. 1999;180:241-9.

46 Hatcher RA, Trussell J, Nelson AL, Cates W, Kowal D, Policar MS. Contraceptive Technology, Twentieth Revised Edition: Ardent Media, Inc.; 2011.

47 Induced Abortion in the United States, Guttmacher Fact Sheet, July 2014, www.guttmacher.org/pubs/fb_induced_abortion.html

48 Jones RK and Jerman J, Abortion incidence and service availability in the United States, 2011, Perspectives on Sexual and Reproductive Health. 2014;46(1):3-14

49 Grimes DA, Brandon LG. Every Third Woman In America: How Legal Abortion Transformed Our Nation

50 Ahman E, Shah IH. New estimates and trends regarding unsafe abortion mortality. International Journal of Gynaecology and Obstetrics. 2011;115(2):121-126.

51 Pazol K, Creanga AA, Kim D. Burley KD, Jamieson DJ. Abortion Surveillance — United States, 2011. MMWR Surveillance Summaries November 28, 2014 / 63(SS11);1-41

52 Trussell J, Jordan B, Reproductive health risks in perspective. Contraception. 2006;73:437-439.

53 Bartlett LA1, Berg CJ, Shulman HB, Zane SB, Green CA, Whitehead S, Atrash HK. Risk factors for legal induced abortion-related mortality in the United States. Obstet Gynecol. 2004;103(4):729-37.

54 Rossouw JE, Anderson GL, Prentice RL, et al.; Writing Group for the Women's Health Initiative Investigators. Risks and benefits of estrogen plus progestin in healthy postmenopausal women: principal results from the Women's Health Initiative randomized controlled trial. JAMA. 2002;288(3):321-333.

55 Manson JE, Aragaki AK, Rossouw JE, et al. Menopausal Hormone Therapy and Long-term All-Cause and Cause-Specific MortalityThe Women's Health Initiative Randomized Trials. JAMA. 2017;318(10):927–

938. doi:10.1001/jama.2017.11217

56 McNeil M. Menopausal Hormone TherapyUnderstanding Long-term Risks and Benefits. JAMA.2017;318(10):911–913. doi:10.1001/jama.2017.11462

57 Is hormone therapy okay, again? University of California, Berkeley Wellness Letter. December 2017.

58 Grady D. Evidence for Postmenopausal Hormone Therapy to Prevent Chronic ConditionsSuccess, Failure, and Lessons Learned. JAMA Intern Med. 2018;178(2):185–186. doi:10.1001/jamainternmed.

2017.7861

59 Pinkerton JV, Hormone therapy for postmenopausal women. N Engl J Med. 2020;382(5):446-455.

60 Hormone therapy: new findings. University of California, Berkeley Wellness Letter. May 2019.

61 The 2017 hormone therapy position statement of The North American Menopause Society. Menopause. 2017;24(7):0000000000000921.

62 Pinkerton JV, Hormone therapy for postmenopausal women. N Engl J Med. 2020;382(5):446-455.

63 US Preventive Services Task Force. Hormone Therapy for the Primary Prevention of Chronic Conditions in Postmenopausal Women. US Preventive Services Task Force Recommendation Statement. JAMA.2017;318(22):2224–2233. doi:10.1001/jama.2017.18261

64 Garnick MB. Testosterone Replacement Therapy Faces FDA Scrutiny. JAMA. 2015;313(6):563-564. doi:10.1001/jama.2014.17334

65 Layton JB, Kim Y, Alexander GC, Emery SL. Association Between Direct-to-Consumer Advertising and Testosterone Testing and Initiation in the United States, 2009-2013. JAMA. 2017;317(11):1159-1166. doi:10.1001/jama.2016.21041

66 Sugerman DT. Low Testosterone. JAMA. 2013;310(17):1872. doi:10.1001/jama.2013.280724

67 The lowdown on "low T" University of California, Berkeley Wellness Letter Vol 27, Issue 8, May 2011.

68 Snyder PJ, Bhasin S, Cunningham GR, et al. Effects of testosterone treatment in older men. N Engl J Med. 2016;374:611-24.

69 Orwoll ES. Establishing a Framework — Does Testosterone Supplementation Help Older Men? N Engl J Med. 2016;374:682-683February 18, 2016DOI: 10.1056/NEJMe1600196

70 Vigen R, O'Donnell CI, Barón AE, Grunwald GK, Maddox TM, Bradley SM, Barqawi A, Woning G, Wierman ME, Plomondon ME, Rumsfeld JS, Ho PM. Association of Testosterone Therapy With Mortality, Myocardial Infarction, and Stroke in Men With Low Testosterone Levels. JAMA. 2013;310(17):1829-1836. doi:10.1001/jama.2013.280386

71 Basaria S, Coviello AD, Travison TG, et al. Adverse events associated with testosterone administration. N Engl J Med. 2010;363(2):109-122.

72 Finkle WD, Greenland S, Ridgeway GK, et al. Increased Risk of Non-Fatal Myocardial Infarction Following Testosterone Therapy Prescription in Men. PLOS ONE. 2014;9(1): e85805. https://doi.org/10.1371/journal.pone.0085805

73 Walker RF, Zakai NA, MacLehose RF, et al. Association of Testosterone Therapy With Risk of Venous Thromboembolism Among Men With and Without Hypogonadism. JAMA Intern Med. 2020;180(2):190–197. doi:10.1001/jamainternmed.2019.5135

74 Safety of Testosterone Replacement Therapy. JAMA. 2016;315(14):1512-1513. doi:10.1001/jama.2016.3450

75 Sharma R, Oni OA, Gupta K, et al. Normalization of testosterone level is associated with reduced incidence of myocardial infarction and mortality in men. Eur Heart J. 2015;36(40):2706-2715

76 Snyder PJ, Bhasin S, Cunningham GR, et al. Effects of testosterone treatment in older men. N Engl J

Med. 2016;374:611-24.

77 Orwoll ES. Establishing a Framework — Does Testosterone Supplementation Help Older Men? N Engl J Med. 2016;374:682-683February 18, 2016DOI: 10.1056/NEJMe1600196

78 WHO, Sexually transmitted infections (STIs) Fact sheet N°110 Updated November 2013 www.who.int/mediacentre/factsheets/.../en/

79 Hook EW. A Recommendation Against Serologic Screening for Genital Herpes Infection—What Now?. JAMA.2016;316(23):2493-2494. doi:10.1001/jama.2016.17139.

80 CDC Fact Sheet, Incidence, Prevalence and Cost of Sexually Transmitted Infections in the United States, http://www.cdc.gov/std/stats/sti-estimates-fact-sheet-feb-2013.pdf

81 Satterwhite CL, et al. Sexually transmitted infections among U.S. women and men: Prevalence and incidence estimates, 2008. Sex Transm Dis. 2013; 40(3): pp. 187-193.

82 http://www.cdc.gov/nchhstp/newsroom/docs/std-trends-508.pdf

83 Hook EW. A Recommendation Against Serologic Screening for Genital Herpes Infection—What Now?. JAMA.2016;316(23):2493-2494. doi:10.1001/jama.2016.17139.

84 Sexually Transmitted Disease Surveillance, 2013. www.cdc.gov/std/stats.

85 Owusu-Edusei K, et al. The estimated direct medical cost of selected sexually transmitted infections in the United States, 2008. Sex Transm Dis. 2013;40(3):197-201.

86 Centers for Disease Control and Prevention. Sexually Transmitted Disease Surveillance 2017. Atlanta: U.S. Department of Health and Human Services; 2018.

87 Centers for Disease Control and Prevention. Sexually Transmitted Disease Surveillance 2017. Atlanta: U.S. Department of Health and Human Services; 2018

88 Centers for Disease Control and Prevention. HIV/AIDS Basic Statistics. 2018. https://www.cdc.gov/hiv/basics/statistics.html.

89 Centers for Disease Control and Prevention. Sexually Transmitted Disease Surveillance 2017. Atlanta: U.S. Department of Health and Human Services; 2018.

90 CDC. Disease Burden from Viral Hepatitis A, B, and C in the United States. Atlanta: U.S. Department of Health and Human Services; 2016. https://www.cdc.gov/hepatitis/statistics/index.htm

91 CDC. Disease Burden from Viral Hepatitis A, B, and C in the United States. Atlanta: U.S. Department of Health and Human Services; 2016. https://www.cdc.gov/hepatitis/statistics/index.htm.

92 CDC. Genital HPV Infection. Atlanta: U.S. Department of Health and Human Services; 2018. https://www.cdc.gov/std/hpv/stdfact-hpv.htm

93 Sexually transmitted infections More than 1 million sexually transmitted infections occur every day. Evidence brief. World Health Organization. 2019. https://apps.who.int/iris/bitstream/handle/10665/329888/WHO-RHR-19.22-eng.pdf?ua=1

94 Tanksley A, Cifu AS. Screening for Gonorrhea, Chlamydia, and Hepatitis B. JAMA. 2016;315(12):1278-1279. doi:10.1001/jama.2016.0223.

95 Centers for Disease Control and Prevention. HIV/AIDS Basic Statistics. 2018. https://www.cdc.gov/hiv/basics/statistics.html.

96 Centers for Disease Control and Prevention. Estimated HIV incidence and prevalence in the United States, 2010–2015. HIV Surveillance Supplemental Report 2018;23(No. 1). http://www.cdc.gov/hiv/library/reports/hiv-surveillance.html. Published March 2018.

97 Centers for Disease Control and Prevention. HIV/AIDS Basic Statistics. 2018. https://www.cdc.gov/hiv/basics/statistics.html

98 Frieden TR, Foti KE, Mermin J. Applying Public Health Principles to the HIV Epidemic — How Are We Doing?. N Engl J Med. 2015; 373:2281-2287December 3, 2015DOI: 10.1056/NEJMms1513641

99 Kuehn B. HIV Underdiagnosed. JAMA. 2019;321(18):1760. doi:10.1001/jama.2019.4922

100 Eisinger RW, Dieffenbach CW, Fauci AS. HIV Viral Load and Transmissibility of HIV Infection: Undetectable Equals Untransmittable. JAMA. Published online January 10, 2019;321(5):451–452. doi:10.1001/jama.2018.21167

101 Katz I, Jha AK. HIV in the United States: Getting to Zero Transmissions by 2030. JAMA. Published online March 08, 2019;321(12):1153–1154. doi:10.1001/jama.2019.1817

102 Kazi DS, Katz IT, Jha AK. PrEParing to End the HIV Epidemic — California's Route as a Road Map or the United States. N Engl J Med. 2019;381:2489-2491. DOI: 10.1056/NEJMp1912293

103 Centers for Disease Control and Prevention. HIV/AIDS Basic Statistics. 2018. https://www.cdc.gov/hiv/basics/statistics.html

104 US Preventive Services Task Force. Screening for HIV Infection: US Preventive Services Task Force Recommendation Statement. JAMA. Published online June 11, 2019;321(23):2326–2336. doi:10.1001/jama.2019.6587

105 Nelson AL, Rezvan A. A pilot study of women's knowledge of pregnancy health risks: implications for contraception. Contraception. 2012;85:78-90.

106 Raymond EG, Grimes DA. The comparative safety of legal induced abortion and childbirth in the United States. Obstet Gynecol. 2012;119:215-9.

107 Berg CJ, Callaghan WM, Syverson C, Henderson Z. Pregnancy-related mortality in the United States, 1998 to 2005. Obstet Gynecol. 2010;116:1302-9.

108 Slomski A. Why Do Hundreds of US Women Die Annually in Childbirth? JAMA. 2019:321(13):1239–1241. doi:10.1001/jama.2019.0714

109 Trussell J, Jordan B, Reproductive health risks in perspective. Contraception. 2006;73: 437-439.

110 Callaghan WM, Creanga AA, Kuklina EV. Severe maternal morbidity among delivery and postpartum hospitalizations in the United States. Obstet Gynecol. 2012;120:1029-36.

111 WHO, Adolescent pregnancy, Fact sheet N°364. Updated September 2014 www.who.int/mediacentre/factsheets/.../en/

112 Hayes DK, Fan AZ, Smith RA, Bombard JM. Trends in selected chronic conditions and behavioral risk factors among women of reproductive age, Behavioral Risk Factor Surveillance System, 2001–2009. Prev Chronic Dis. 201;8(6):A120.Epub 2011 Oct 17.

113 Martin JA, Hamilton BE, Ventura SJ, Osterman MJK, Wilson EC, Mathews T. Births: final data for 2010. Natl Vital Stat Rep 2012:61.

114 Berg CJ, MacKay AR, Qin C, Callaghan WM. Overview of maternal morbidity during hospitalization for labor and delivery in the United States 1993–1997 and 2001–2005. Obstet Gynecol. 2009;113:1075-81.

115 Earls MF; Committee on Psychosocial Aspects of Child and Family Health. American Academy of Pediatrics. Incorporating recognition and management of perinatal and postpartum depression into pediatric practice. Pediatrics 2010;126(5):1032-9.

116 Brody J. When Bathroom Runs Rule the Day (and Night). New York Times, December 13, 2016, on Page D5.

117 Lifestyle changes. Overactive bladder. The Urology Care Foundation. http://urologyhealth.org/urologic-conditions/overactive-bladder-(oab)/treatment/lifestyle-changes.

118 Brody J. When Bathroom Runs Rule the Day (and Night). New York Times, December 13, 2016, on Page D5.

Chapter 14 – Environmental Pollutants and Toxins

1 Samoli E, Peng R, Ramsay T, et al. Acute effects of ambient particulate matter on mortality in Europe and North America: results from the APHENA study. Environ Health Perspect. 2008;116:1480-1486.

2 Atkinson RW, Kang S, Anderson HR, Mills IC, Walton HA. Epidemiological time series studies of PM2.5 and daily mortality and hospital admissions: a systematic review and meta-analysis. Thorax. 2014;69:660-665.

3 Payne-Sturges DC, Marty MA, Perera F, et al. Healthy Air, Healthy Brains: Advancing Air Pollution Policy to Protect Children's Health. American Journal of Public Health. 2019;109, 550_554. https://doi.org/10.2105/AJPH.2018.304902

4 International Agency for Research on Cancer. PDQ® - IARC's Comprehensive Cancer Database. Outdoor air pollution a leading environmental cause of cancer deaths. World Health Organization. 2013. https://www.iarc.fr/en/ media-centre/iarcnews/pdf/pr221_E.pdf

5 Gharibvand et al. The association between ambient fine particulate matter and incident adenocarcinoma subtype of lung cancer. Environmental Health. 2017;16:71 DOI 10.1186/s12940-017-0268-7

6 Air Pollution, National Institute of Environmental Health Sciences. https://www.niehs.nih.gov/health/topics/agents/air-pollution/index.cfm.

7 Levin D. Change in the Air. Harvard Public Health. Fall 2017:15-23.

8 Mannino DM, Sanderson WT. Using Big Data to Reveal Chronic Respiratory Disease Mortality Patterns and Identify Potential Public Health Interventions. JAMA. 2017;318(12):1112–1114. doi:10.1001/jama.2017.11746

9 Dwyer-Lindgren L, Bertozzi-Villa A, Stubbs RW, Morozoff C, Shirude S, Naghavi M, Mokdad AH, Murray CJL. Trends and Patterns of Differences in Chronic Respiratory Disease Mortality Among US Counties, 1980-2014. JAMA. 2017;318(12):1136–1149. doi:10.1001/jama.2017.11747

10 Gauderman WJ, Urman R, Avol E, Berhane K, McConnell R, Rappaport E, et al. Association of improved air quality with lung development in children. N Engl J Med. 2015;372(10):905–13.

11 Dockery DW, Pope CA, Xu X, et al. An association between air pollution and mortality in six US cities. N Engl J Med. 1993;329:1753–9.

12 Di Q, Wang Y, Zanobetti A, et al. Air Pollution and Mortality in the Medicare Population. N Engl J Med. 2017;376(26):2513-2522.

13 Di Q, Dai L, Wang Y, et al. Association of Short-term Exposure to Air Pollution With Mortality in Older Adults. JAMA. 2017;318(24):2446–2456. doi:10.1001/jama.2017.17923

14 Liu C, Chen R, Sera F, et al. Ambient particulate air pollution and daily mortality in 652 cities. N Engl J Med. 2019;381:705-715.

15 Environmental Protection Agency. the Federal Insecticide, Fungicide, and Rodenticide Act (FIFRA). https://www.epa.gov/laws-regulations/summary-federal-insecticide-fungicide-and-rodenticide-act

16 American Chemical Council. https://www.americanchemistry.com/Policy/Chemical-Safety/TSCA/.

17 Orzech D. Chemical Kids — Environmental Toxins and Child Development. Social Work Today. 2007;7(2):37. http://www.socialworktoday.com/archive/marapr2007p37.shtml.

18 Center for Disease Control and Prevention. Fourth National Report on Human Exposure to Environmental Chemicals, 2009. https://www.cdc.gov/exposurereport/pdf/fourthreport.pdf

19 Center for Disease Control and Prevention. Updated Tables, February 2015. http://www.cdc.gov/biomonitoring/ pdf/FourthReport_UpdatedTables_Feb2015.pdf

20 Brody J. A Book Links Parkinson's to Toxic Chemicals. New York Times. July, 21, 2020.

21 World Health Organization. http://www.who.int/ceh/capacity/Children_are_not_little_adults.pdf

22 National Research Council (US); Institute of Medicine (US). Children's Health, The Nation's Wealth: Assessing and Improving Child Health. Washington (DC): National Academies Press (US); 2004. 3, Influences on Children's Health. Available from: http://www.ncbi.nlm.nih.gov/books/NBK92200/

23 Grigg J. Environmental toxins; their impact on children's health. Arch Dis Child. 2004;89:244-250 doi:10.1136/adc.2002.022202 http://adc.bmj.com/content/89/3/244.full.pdf

24 PFOA, PFOS and Other PFASs. Basic Information on PFAS | Per- and Polyfluoroalkyl Substances (PFAS). United States Environmental Protection Agency.

25 Felton R. "Your Guide to Safer Drinking Water." Consumer Reports. November 2020. p.26-33.

26 Janesick AS, Blumberg B, Obesogens: an emerging threat to public health. American J. Obstetrics & Gynecology. 2016:559-565.

27 Groopman J. The Plastic Panic. The New Yorker. May 31, 2010 http://jeromegroopman.com/ny-articles/PlasticPanic-053110.pdf.

28 FDA Regulations No Longer Authorize the Use of BPA in Infant Formula Packaging Based on Abandonment; Decision Not Based on Safety. FDA 2013. https://www.fda.gov/food/newsevents/constituentupdates/ ucm360147.htm

29 Abbasi J. Scientists Call FDA Statement on Bisphenol A Safety Premature. JAMA. 2018;319(16):1644–1646. doi:10.1001/jama.2018.328

30 University of California, Berkeley Wellness Newsletter. July, 2019.

31 Superfund: National Priorities List (NPL). Environmental Protection Agency. https://www.epa.gov/superfund/superfund-national-priorities-list-npl

32 CDC Agency for Toxic Substances and Disease Registry http://www.atsdr.cdc.gov/spl/index.html

33 Get Toxic Chemicals Out of Cosmetics. Scientific American. November 2017:10.

34 Eat the peach, not the pesticide. Consumer Reports. May 2015, 29-32.

35 Roberts C. Stop Eating Pesticides. Consumer Reports. October 2020. p.24-33.

Chapter 15 - More Advice about Healthy Living

1 Martin WH, Sobel J, Griest SE, Howarth L, Yong-bing SID. Noise induced hearing loss in children: Preventing the silent epidemic. Journal of Otology 2006 Vol 1 No 1

2 Goman AM, Lin FR. Prevalence of Hearing Loss by Severity in the United States. American J. of Public Health, 2016;106(10): 1820-1822.

3 Fink DJ. What is a Safe Noise Level for the Public? American J. of Public Health, 2017;107(1): 44-45.

4 Visual impairment and blindness. World Health Organization. Fact Sheet N°282 Updated August 2014. http://www.who.int/mediacentre/factsheets/fs282/en/

5 Brody JE. The Worst That Could Happen? Going Blind. New York Times, February 21, 2017.

6 Reynolds G. Let There Be Light. New York Times Magazine, January 22, 2017.

7 Rabin RC. Lasik's Risks, in Focus. New York Times. June 12, 2018.

8 McKay B. Routine Eye Surgery Can Take a Heavy Toll. Wall St. Journal. July 2, 2019.

9 Kates MM, Tuli S. What Is LASIK Eye Surgery? JAMA. 2020;324(8):815. doi:10.1001/jama.2020.1286

10 Chakravarthy U, Peto T. Current Perspective on Age-Related Macular Degeneration. JAMA. 2020;324(8):794–795. doi:10.1001/jama.2020.5576

11 Simple tips for healthy eyes. National Eye Institute. https://nei.nih.gov/healthyeyes/eyehealthtips

12 Age-Related Eye Disease Study Research Group. The relationship of dietary carotenoid with vitamin

A, E, and C intake with age-related macular degeneration in a case-control study. Archives of Ophthalmology; 2007; 125(9):1225-1232.

13 Pieramici DJ. Sports-Related Eye Injuries. JAMA. 2017;318(24):2483–2484. doi:10.1001/jama.2017.17560

14 Age-Related Eye Disease Study Research Group. Risk factors associated with age-related nuclear and cortical cataract. Ophthalmology; 2001;108(8):1400-1408.

15 U.S. Department of Health and Human Services, Office of the Surgeon General. The Health Consequences of Smoking: A Report of the Surgeon General. Washington, D.C., 2004.

16 Reynolds G. Let There Be Light. New York Times Magazine, January 22, 2017.

17 Oral Health Basics. CDC https://www.cdc.gov/oralhealth/basics/index.html

18 Dye BA, Xianfen L, Beltrán-Aguilar ED. Selected Oral Health Indicators in the United States 2005–2008. NCHS Data Brief, no. 96. Hyattsville, MD: National Center for Health Statistics, Centers for Disease Control and Prevention; 2012.

19 U.S. Department of Health and Human Services. Oral Health in America: A Report of the Surgeon General. National Institute of Dental and Craniofacial Research, National Institutes of Health. Rockville, MD: National Institute of Dental and Crainiofacial Research. 2000.

20 Dye BA, Thornton-Evans G, Xianfen L, Iafolla TJ. Dental Caries and Tooth Loss in Adults in the United States, 2011-2012. NCHS Data Brief, no 197. Hyattsville, MD: National Center for Health Statistics; 2015.

21 Dye BA, Thornton-Evans G, Li X, Iafolla TJ. Dental caries and tooth loss in adults in the United States, 2011–2012. NCHS data brief, no 197. Hyattsville, MD: National Center for Health Statistics. 2015.

22 Eke PI, Dye, BA, Wei L, et. al. Update on prevalence of periodontitis in adults in the United States: NHANES 2009 to 2012. J of Periodontology. 2015;86(5):611-622.

23 Dye BA, Tan S, Smith V, et al. Trends in oral health status, United States, 1988–1994 and 1999–2004. Vital Health Stat. 2007;11(248).

24 National Cancer Institute. Surveillance, Epidemiology, and End Results (SEER) Program. (N.D.) SEER Stat Fact Sheets: Oral Cavity and Pharynx Cancer website. http://seer.cancer.gov/statfacts/html/oralcav.html. Accessed July 5, 2016.

25 Five Year Survival, All Sites. National Program of Cancer Registries. https://nccd.cdc.gov/uscs/Survival/ Relative_Survival_Tables.pdf

26 US Department of Health and Human Services. Oral Health in America: A Report of the Surgeon General. Rockville, MD: US Department of Health and Human Services, National Institute of Dental and Craniofacial Research, National Institutes of Health; 2000.

27 US Department of Health and Human Services. Oral Health in America: A Report of the Surgeon General. Rockville, MD: US Department of Health and Human Services, National Institute of Dental and Craniofacial Research, National Institutes of Health; 2000.

28 A Dental Checkup. University of California, Berkeley Wellness Letter. 32(5), Winter 2015.

29 Carroll AE. Questionable Wisdom on How to Care for Teeth. New York Times. August 30, 2016.

30 US Department of Health and Human Services. Oral Health in America: A Report of the Surgeon General. Rockville, MD: US Department of Health and Human Services, National Institute of Dental and Craniofacial Research, National Institutes of Health; 2000.

31 http://www.ada.org/en/publications/ada-news/2016-archive/august/association-responds-to-news-story-challenging-benefits-of-dental-floss-use?nav=news.

32 Huang GJ, Cunha-Cruz J, Rothen M, Spiekerman C, Drangsholt M, Anderson L, Roset GA. A prospective study of clinical outcomes related to third molar removal or retention. Am J Public Health. 2014;104(4):728-34. doi: 10.2105/AJPH.2013.301649.

33 Friedman JW. The prophylactic extraction of third molars: a public health hazard. Am J Public Health. 2007;97(9):1554-1559.

34 Osborn TP, Frederickson G Jr, Small IA, Torgerson TS. A prospective study of complications related to mandibular third molar surgery. J Oral Maxillofac Surg. 1985;43(10):767-769.

35 Healthy Sleep. Division of Sleep Medicine. Harvard Medical School. http://healthysleep.med.harvard.edu/healthy/.

36 The ABCs of sleep. University of California, Berkeley Wellness Letter. 30(2), Fall 2013.

37 Healthy Sleep. Division of Sleep Medicine. Harvard Medical School. http://healthysleep.med.harvard.edu/healthy/

38 Sigurdson K, Ayas N. The public health and safety consequences of sleep disorders. Canadian J Physiol Pharmacol. 2007; 85:179-183.

39 Liu Y, Wheaton AG, Chapman DP, Cunningham TJ, Lu H, Croft JB. Prevalence of Healthy Sleep Duration among Adults — United States, 2014. MMWR Morb Mortal Wkly Rep 2016;65:137–141. DOI: http://dx.doi.org/10.15585/mmwr.mm6506a1.

40 Czeisler CA, Wickwire EM, Barger LK, et al. Sleep Health: Journal of the National Sleep Foundation. 2016; 2(2): 94–99.

41 Nedergaard M, Goldman SA. The Brain's Waste-Disposal System May Be Enlisted to Treat Alzheimer's and Other Brain Illnesses. Scientific American. March 2016.

42 Osorio RS, Gumb T, Pirraglia E. et al. Sleep-disordered breathing advances cognitive decline in the elderly Neurology-2015:84;1964-71.

43 Rebecca P. Gelber RP, Susan Redline S, Ross GW et al. Associations of brain lesions at autopsy with polysomnography features before death. Neurology 2014 : WNL.0000000000001163v1-10.1212/WNL.0000000000001163.

44 Healthy Sleep. Division of Sleep Medicine. Harvard Medical School. http://healthysleep.med.harvard.edu/healthy/

45 Sigurdson K, Ayas N. The public health and safety consequences of sleep disorders. Canadian J Physiol Pharmacol. 2007; 85:179-183.

46 Hublin C, Partinen M, Koskenvuo M, Kaprio J. Sleep and mortality: a population-based 22-year follow- up study. Sleep. 2007; 30(10):1245-53.

47 Patel SR, Ayas NT, Malhotra MR, White DP, Schernhammer ES, Speizer FE, Stampfer MJ, Hu FB. A prospective study of sleep duration and mortality risk in women. Sleep. 2004; 27(3):440-4.

48 Gallicchio L, Kalesan B. Sleep duration and mortality: a systematic review and meta-analysis. J Sleep Res 2009;18:148–58.

49 Healthy Sleep. Division of Sleep Medicine. Harvard Medical School. http://healthysleep.med.harvard.edu/healthy/.

50 Healthy Sleep. Division of Sleep Medicine. Harvard Medical School. http://healthysleep.med.harvard.edu/healthy/

51 Peppard PE, Young T, Barnet JH, Palta M, Hagen EW, Hla KM. Increased prevalence of sleep-disordered breathing in adults. Am J Epidemiol. 2013;177(9):1006-1014.

52 Redline S. Screening for Obstructive Sleep Apnea Implications for the Sleep Health of the Population. JAMA.2017;317(4):368-370. doi:10.1001/jama.2016.18630.

53 Veasey SC, Rosen IM. Obstructive Sleep Apnea in Adults. N Engl J Med. 2019;380:1442-1449 DOI: 10.1056/NEJMcp1816152

54 Medalie L, Cifu AS. Management of Chronic Insomnia Disorder in Adults. JAMA. 2017;317(7):762-763. doi:10.1001/jama.2016.19004

55 National Sleep Foundation. https://www.thensf.org/

56 Watson NF, Badr MS, Belenky G, et al. ; Consensus Conference Panel. Joint consensus statement of the American Academy of Sleep Medicine and Sleep Research Society on the recommended amount of sleep for a healthy adult: methodology and discussion. Sleep 2015;38:1161–83.

57 Healthy Sleep. Division of Sleep Medicine. Harvard Medical School. http://healthysleep.med.harvard.edu/healthy/

58 Rubin R. Sleeping In Doesn't Mitigate Metabolic Changes Linked to Sleep Deficit. JAMA. Published online May 15, 2019;321(21):2062–2063. doi:10.1001/jama.2019.4701

59 Pahor M. Falls in Older Adults: Prevention, Mortality, and Costs. JAMA. 2019;321(21):2080–2081. doi:10.1001/jama.2019.6569

60 Hartholt KA, Lee R, Burns ER, van Beeck EF. Mortality From Falls Among US Adults Aged 75 Years or Older, 2000-2016. JAMA. 2019;321(21):2131–2133. doi:10.1001/jama.2019.4185

61 https://www.cdc.gov/safechild/poisoning/index.htm

62 Jones CM, Einstein EB, Compton WM. Changes in Synthetic Opioid Involvement in Drug Overdose Deaths in the United States, 2010-2016. JAMA. 2018;319(17):1819–1821. doi:10.1001/jama.2018.2844

63 National Center for Health Statistics. CDC. https://www.cdc.gov/nchs/fastats/accidental-injury.htm

64 Ganz DA, Latham NK. Prevention of falls in community-dwelling older adults. N Engl J Med. 2020; 38(8):734-743.

65 Pahor M. Falls in Older Adults: Prevention, Mortality, and Costs. JAMA. 2019;321(21):2080–2081. doi:10.1001/jama.2019.6569

66 Liu-Ambrose T, Davis JC, Best JR, et al. Effect of a Home-Based Exercise Program on Subsequent Falls Among Community-Dwelling High-Risk Older Adults After a Fall: A Randomized Clinical Trial. JAMA. 2019;321(21):2092–2100. doi:10.1001/jama.2019.5795

67 Shumway-Cook A, Silver IF, LeMier M, York S, Cummings P, Koepsell TD. Effectiveness of a community-based multifactorial intervention on falls and fall risk factors in community-living older adults: a randomized, controlled trial. J Gerontol A Biol Sci Med Sci. 2007;62(12):1420-1427.

68 Sherrington C, Fairhall NJ, Wallbank GK, Tiedemann A, Michaleff ZA, Howard K, Clemson L, Hopewell S, Lamb SE. Exercise for preventing falls in older people living in the community. Cochrane Database of Systematic Reviews. 2019, Issue 1. Art. No.: CD012424. DOI: 10.1002/14651858.CD012424.pub2

69 Torpy, JM, Lynm, C, Glass, RM. Burn Injuries. JAMA. 2009;302(16):1828

70 https://www.cdc.gov/safechild/burns/index.html

71 Statista. 2019. https://www.statista.com/statistics/376703/us-civilian-fire-deaths/

72 Drowning prevention. CDC. https://www.cdc.gov/safechild/drowning/index.html

73 https://www.cdc.gov/safechild/Sports_Injuries/index.html

74 https://www.cdc.gov/motorvehiclesafety/distracted_driving/

75 National Highway Traffic Safety Administration. https://crashstats.nhtsa.dot.gov/Api/Public/ViewPublication/ 812747

76 Boudette NE. Traffic Deaths in Estimate, Pass 40,000 for First Time Since '07. New York Times, Feb-

ruary

16, 2017.

77 Traffic Safety Facts, 2012 Data: Speeding. National Highway Traffic Safety Administration. https://crashstats.nhtsa.dot.gov/Api/Public/Publication/812021

78 Distracted Driving. National Highway Traffic Safety Administration. https://www.nhtsa.gov/ risky-driving/distracted-driving

79 Compton RP, Berning A. National Highway Traffic Safety Administration. Traffic Safety Facts Research Note: drugs and alcohol crash risk. U.S. Department of Transportation, Washington, DC; 2015 Available at: http://www.nhtsa.gov/staticfiles/nti/pdf/812117-Drug_and_Alcohol_Crash_Risk.pdf.

80 Asbridge M, Hayden JA, Cartwright JL. Acute cannabis consumption and motor vehicle collision risk: systematic review of observational studies. BMJ. 2012;344:e536 doi: 10.1136/bmj.e536

81 Hartman RL, Huestis MA. Cannabis effects on driving skills. Clin Chem. 2013;59(3):478-492.

82 Ramaekers JG. Driving Under the Influence of CannabisAn Increasing Public Health Concern. JAMA.2018;319(14):1433–1434. doi:10.1001/jama.2018.1334

83 Calvert S. Drug Use Is Up in Fatal Crash Study. Wall St. Journal. June 18, 2018.

84 Santaella-Tenorio J, Mauro CM, Wall MM, et al. US Traffic Fatalities, 1985–2014, and Their Relationship to Medical Marijuana Laws, American Journal of Public Health. 2017;107(2):336-342. DOI: 10.2105/AJPH.2016.303577.

85 Aydelotte JD, Brown LH, Luftman KM, et al. Crash Fatality Rates After Recreational Marijuana Legalization in Washington and Colorado. American Journal of Public Health. 2017; 107(8):1329-1331. DOI: 10.2105/AJPH.2017.30848.

86 Monte AA, Zane RD, Heard KJ. The Implications of Marijuana Legalization in Colorado. JAMA.2015;313(3):241–242. doi:10.1001/jama.2014.17057.

87 Blincoe LJ, Miller TR, Zaloshnja E, Lawrence BA. National Highway Traffic Safety Administration. The economic and societal impact of motor vehicle crashes, 2010. (Revised). U.S. Department of Transportation, Washington, DC; 2015. Available at: http://www-nrd.nhtsa.dot.gov/pubs/812013.pdf

88 Wonder database. Centers for Disease Control and Prevention. https://wonder.cdc.gov/controller/ saved/D76/D48F344

89 Kalesan B, Adhikarla C, Pressley JC, et al. The hidden epidemic of firearm injury: increasing firearm injury rates during 2001–2013. Am J Epidemiol. 2017;185(7):546–553.

90 Cook PJ, Rivera-Aguirre AE, Cerdá M, et al. Constant lethality of gunshot injuries from firearm assault: United States, 2003–2012. Am J Public Health. 2017;107(8):1324–1328.

91 Mervosh S. Nearly 40,000 deaths from firearms in 2017. New York Times. December 19, 2018.

92 Doucette ML, Crifasi CK, Frattaroli S. Right-to-carry laws and firearm workplace homicides: a longitudinal analysis (1992-2017). AJPH. 2019;109(12):1747-1753.

93 Miller M, Azrael D, Hemenway D. State-Level Homicide Victimization Rates In The U.S. In Relation To Survey Measures Of Household Firearm Ownership, 2001-2003. Social Science And Medicine. 2007; 64:656-64.

94 Miller M, Hemenway D, Azrael D. State-level homicide victimization rates in the US in relation to survey measures of household firearm ownership, 2001-2003. Soc Sci Med. 2007 Feb;64(3):656-64. Epub 2006 Oct 27. https://doi.org/10.1016/j.socscimed.2006.09.024

95 Butkus R, Doherty R, Daniel H; Health and Public Policy Committee of the American College of Physicians. Reducing firearm-related injuries and deaths in the United States: executive summary of a policy position paper from the American College of Physicians. Ann Intern Med. 2014;160(12):858-860.

doi:10.7326/M14-0216

96 Weinberger SE, Hoyt DB, Lawrence HC III, et al. Firearm-related injury and death in the United States: a call to action from 8 health professional organizations and the American Bar Association. Ann Intern Med. 2015;162(7):513-516. doi:10.7326/M15-0337

97 Bauchner H, Rivara FP, Bonow RO, et al. Death by Gun Violence—A Public Health Crisis. JAMA. 2017;318(18):1763–1764. doi:10.1001/jama.2017.16446

Chapter 16 - Understanding Scientific Data

1 Frieden TR. Evidence for Health Decision Making — Beyond Randomized, Controlled Trials. N Engl J Med 2017; 377:465-475. DOI: 10.1056/NEJMra1614394

2 Research Study Types. Harvard T. H. Chan School of PublicHealth. https://www.hsph.harvard.edu/nutri-tionsource/ research-study-types/

3 Berlin JA, Golub RM. Meta-analysis as EvidenceBuilding a Better Pyramid. JAMA. 2014;312(6):603–606. doi:10.1001/jama.2014.8167

4 Greco T, Zangrillo A, Biondi-Zoccai G, Landoni G. Meta-analysis: pitfalls and hints. Heart Lung Vessel. 2013; 5(4): 219–225.

5 van den Brandt PA. The impact of a Mediterranean diet and healthy lifestyle on premature mortality in men and women Am J Clin Nutr doi: 10.3945/ajcn.110. 008250.

6 Vance E. Mind over Matter. National Geographic December 2016. p 30-55.

Index

D

N

U

V

X

Y

Z

Made in the USA
Middletown, DE
09 January 2021

31226236R00336